Ocular Differential Diagnosis

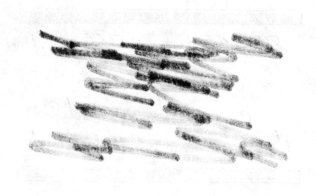

SIXTH EDITION

Ocular Differential Diagnosis

Frederick Hampton Roy, M.D., F.A.C.S.

Department of Ophthalmology University of Arkansas Medical Center Little Rock, Arkansas

Baptist Medical Center St. Vincent Infirmary Arkansas Children's Hospital Little Rock Surgery Center

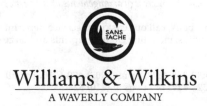

Williams & Wilkins

A WAVERLY COMPANY

BALTIMORE • PHILADELPHIA • LONDON • PARIS • BANGKOK
BUENOS AIRES • HONG KONG • MUNICH • SYDNEY • TOKYO • WROCLAW

Editor: Darlene Barela Cooke
Managing Editor: Frances M. Klass
Production Coordinator: Peter J. Carley
Project Editor: Robert Magee
Designer: Cathy Cotter
Cover Designer: Cathy Cotter
Typesetter: Peirce Graphic Services
Printer: Port City Press, Inc.
Binder: Port City Press, Inc.

Copyright © 1997 Williams & Wilkins

351 West Camden Street
Baltimore, Maryland 21201-2436 USA

Rose Tree Corporate Center
1400 North Providence Road
Building II, Suite 5025
Media, Pennsylvania 19063-2043 USA

Printed in the United States of America

First Edition, 1972
Second Edition, 1975
    Reprinted, 1978, 1980
Third Edition, 1984
Fourth Edition, 1989
Fifth Edition, 1993
Sixth Edition, 1997

Library of Congress Cataloging-in-Publication Data

Roy, Frederick Hampton.
    Ocular differential diagnosis / Frederick Hampton Roy. — 6th ed.
        p.   cm
    Includes bibliographical references and index.
    ISBN 0-683-07415-6
    1. Eye—Diseases—Diagnosis.   2. Diagnosis, Differential.
I. Title
    [DNLM: 1. Eye Diseases—diagnosis—outlines.   2. Diagnosis,
Differential—outlines.   WW 18.2 R888o 1996]
RE76.R68   1996
617.7'15—dc20
DNLM/DLC
for Library of Congress   96-13229
                                                                                CIP

The publishers have made every effort to trace the copyright holders for borrowed material. If they have inadvertently overlooked any, they will be pleased to make the necessary arrangements at the first opportunity.

To purchase additional copies of this book, call our customer service department at **(800) 638-0672** or fax orders to **(800) 447-8438.** For other book services, including chapter reprints and large quantity sales, ask for the Special Sales department.

Canadian customers should call **(800) 268-4178,** or fax **(905) 470-6780.** For all other calls originating outside of the United States, please call **(410) 528-4223** or fax us at **(410) 528-8550.**

Visit Williams & Wilkins on the Internet: **http://www.wwilkins.com** or contact our customer service department at **custserv@wwilkins.com.** Williams & Wilkins customer service representatives are available from 8:30 am to 6:00 pm, EST, Monday through Friday, for telephone access.

97 98 99
2 3 4 5 6 7 8 9 10

To Mary Michelle
To my children:
Nichola, Robert, Kimberly, Frederick, Jr., and Charles

To Dr. Arlington Krause, molder and questioner
in my early formative academic life

To Dr. Philip Lewis and Dr. Roger Hiatt
for guidance and direction

PREFACE

The 6th edition of Ocular Differential Diagnosis is a milestone.

The 1st edition of Ocular Differential Diagnosis was published in 1972 and various editions have been translated in Spanish, Turkish, Chinese, Portuguese, and Italian.

All previous editions have been my work. Dr. Gonzolo Murillo of La Paz, Bolivia helped in edition 4 and 5 with the diagnostic decision tables. These have been retained. In this new edition I have selected highly qualified doctors to be section editors for each chapter. These section editors have done an excellent job of updating each chapter in terms of entries, references and terminology.

I feel this is the best edition of Ocular Differential Diagnosis thus far.

This text would not have been possible without the superb efforts of both Renee Tindall and Loyette Davis.

I hope the ophthalmologist and optometrist using this book will bring any errors in this edition to my attention.

Little Rock, Arkansas

Frederick Hampton Roy, M.D.

SECTION EDITORS

Richard Ward Allinson, M.D.
Clinical Assistant Professor
Department of Ophthalmology
University of Arizona
Staff Surgeon, Ophthalmology Section
Carl T. Hayden Veterans Affairs Medical
  Center
Phoenix, Arizona

Richard Anderson, M.D.
Professor of Ophthalmology
Chief, Division of Ophthalmic Plastic Surgery
Salt Lake City, Utah

Edward G. Buckley, M.D.
Professor of Ophthalmology
Associate Professor of Pediatrics
Pediatric Ophthalmology and Strabismus
Duke Eye Center
Durham, North Carolina

G. A. Cioffi, M.D.
Devers Glaucoma Service
Devers Eye Institute
Portland, Oregon

Mandi D. Conway, M.D.
Assistant Professor LSU Eye Center
Vitreoretinal Surgery
Director Medical Retina & Uveitus Service
New Orleans, Louisiana

David E. Cowen, M.D.
Assistant Professor
Director, Opthalmic Plastic and
Reconstructive Surgery Service
Director, Lacrimal and Orbital Disorders Clinic
University of Kentucky
Department of Ophthalmology
Lexington, Kentucky

Vinay N. Desai, M.D.
Department of Ophthalmology
Washington University School of Medicine
St. Louis, Missouri

Kenneth M. Goins, M.D.
Assistant Professor of Ophthalmology
Corneal and Refractive Diseases
University of Chicago
Chicago, Illinois

Tamas Halda, PhD.
Senior Research Associate
Helen Keller Eye Research Foundation
Birmingham, Alabama

Leonard S. Kirsch, M.D., F.R.C.S.(C)
Attending Vitreoretinal Surgeon
Largo Medical Center
Morton Plant Hospital
Doctors Hospital of Sarasota
Sarasota Memorial Hospital
Largo, Florida

Ferenc Kuhn, M.D.
Assistant Professor of Clinical Ophthalmology
Department of Ophthalmology
University of Alabama at Birmingham/Eye
  Foundation Hospital
Director of Research, United States Eye Injury
  Registry
Associate Director of Clinical Research
Helen Keller Eye Research Foundation
Birmingham, Alabama

Nick Mamalis, M.D.
Professor of Ophthalmology
Director of Ophthalmic Pathology
Moran Eye Center
University of Utah
Salt Lake City, Utah

Fernando Murillo-Lopez, M.D.
Hampton Roy Eye Center
Little Rock, Arkansas
Miami, Florida

Bhupendra C.K. Patel, M.D., F.R.C.S.,
    F.R.C.Ophth.
Assistant Professor
Division of Opthalmic Plastic, Reconstructive,
Orbital & Lacrimal Surgery
Department of Ophthalmology
Moran Eye Center
University of Utah
Salt Lake City, Utah

Christopher J. Rapuano, M.D.
Associate Surgeon, Cornea Service
Wills Eye Hospital
Associate Professor of Ophthalmology
Jefferson Medical College
Thomas Jefferson University
Philadelphia, Pennsylvania

James A. Savage, M.D.
Associate Clinical Professor
University of Texas-Southwestern Medical
    Center
Dallas, Texas

Kristin Tarbet, M.D.
University of Utah School of Medicine
Ophthalmology Residency - Washington
    University
Barnes Hospital
St. Louis, Missouri

David T. Tse, M.D., F.A.C.S.
Professor, Department of Ophthalmology
Ophthalmic Plastic, Orbital Surgery and
    Oncology
Bascom Palmer Eye Institute
University of Miami School of Medicine
Miami, Florida

Douglas Witherspoon, M.D.
Assistant Professor of Clinical Ophthalmology
University of Alabama at Birmingham
Birmingham, Alabama

CONTENTS

CONTENTS

HOW TO USE THIS BOOK

This book can be used easily and quickly by following the directions presented below.

1. If the sign or symptom relates to a particular region of the eye, turn to the table of contents preceding this page to find the number of the page on which listings of the signs and symptoms pertaining to the specific region begins. This latter page (or those immediately following) will refer the user to that (or those) on which the various causes of the condition are listed. For example, let us assume that the patient has *pigmentation of the cornea*. The table of contents on page ix shows that the *cornea* section begins on page 276. Turning to page 276 the user finds references to page 284 on which the causes of corneal pigmentation are listed according to type. In the index, this topic is listed as Cornea, pigmentation of, 284–287.

2. If the symptom, such as *binocular diplopia* or *night blindness* does not relate to a particular region of the eye, look for it either in the Index at the back of the book or under General Signs and Symptoms beginning on page 683.

   Various features of a disease may be crosschecked. For instance, a "pulsating exophthalmos with orbital bruit and conjunctival edema" may be sought under *orbit*, page 3, where the user of the book is referred to *exophthalmos*, page 5, and *orbital bruit*, page 35, and under *conjunctiva*, page 210, where the user is referred to *conjunctival edema*, page 233. The terms "exophthalmos," "orbital bruit" (under *orbit, bruit of*) and "conjunctival edema" (under *conjunctiva, edema of*) may also be found in the Index. Terms such as "secondary glaucoma" are indexed under the noun, e.g., *glaucoma, secondary*.

3. Following some of the differential diagnosis lists are diagnostic decision tables. These tables list the history, physical signs, and laboratory tests that differentiate each of the possible diagnosis. These can be identified in the Index because they are in italics.

Regional Signs
and Symptoms

Orbit

DAVID E. COWEN MD

Contents

Pseudoproptosis (Appearance of Exophthalmos)

*1. Asymmetry of bony orbits

2. Congenital cystic eyeball

*3. Contralateral enophthalmos (see p. 18)

4. Facial asymmetry as progressive facial hemiatrophy (Parry-Romberg syndrome)

5. Harlequin orbit (shallow orbit with arched superior and lateral wall) as with hypophosphatasia

6. Hypoplastic supraorbital ridges as in trisomy (Edwards syndrome)

7. Retraction of upper lid as with thyroid disease

8. Slight blepharoptosis as with Horner syndrome of contralateral eye

9. Shallow orbit as in Crouzon disease (craniofacial dysostosis)

10. Unilateral congenital glaucoma

11. Unilateral high-axial myopia

12. Unilateral secondary glaucoma resulting from ocular trauma during childhood

Newell, F.W.: Ophthalmology, Principles and Concepts. 7th ed. St. Louis, C.V. Mosby, 1992.
Rootman, J.: Diseases of the Orbit. Philadelphia. J.B. Lippincott, 1988.

Exophthalmos

1. Drugs, including:

adrenal cortex injection
aldosterone
betamethasone
carbimazole
cocaine
cortisone
desoxycorticosterone
dexamethasone
dextrothyroxine
fludrocortisone
fludprednisolone
hydrocortisone
iodide and iodine solution and compounds
levothyroxine
liothyronine
liotrix
lithium carbonate

meprednisone
methimazole
methylprednisolone
methylthiouracil
oral contraceptives
paramethasone
poliovirus vaccine
prednisolone
prednisone
propranolol
propylthiouracil
radioactiveiodides
thyroglobulin
thyroid
triamcinolone
vitamin A

2. Inflammation
   A. Acute—orbital cellulitis
   B. Acute suppurative—mucormycosis (diabetic or debility)
   C. Benign lymphoepithelial lesion (Mikulicz disease)
   *D. Chronic (nongranulomatous—pseudotumor)
   E. Chronic (granulomatous—tuberculosis, sarcoid (Schaumann syndrome), syphilis (lues), parasites, aspergillosis)
   F. Relapsing polychondritis

3. Injuries
   A. Foreign body
   B. Orbital hemorrhage
   C. Orbital roof fracture
   D. Secondary carotid cavernous sinus fistula
   E. Thermal burns

4. Systemic disease
   A. Acute intracranial hypertension
   B. Amyloidosis (Lubarsch-Pick syndrome)
   C. Chloroma
   D. Cretinism (hypothyroidism)
   E. Hypervitaminosis A
   F. Hypophosphatasia (phosphoethanolaminuria)
   *G. Thyroid disorder

* = most important

H. Myasthenia gravis (Erb-Goldflam syndrome)

I. Obesity

5. Tumors

A. Cartilaginous tumors
   (1) Cartilaginous hamartoma
   (2) Chondroma
   (3) Chondrosarcoma
   (4) Mesenchymal chondrosarcoma

B. Cystic lesions
   (1) Colobomatous cyst
   (2) Dermoid cyst
   (3) Hematocele
   (4) Hydatid cyst
   (5) Meningocele and meningoencephalocele
   (6) Mucocele
   (7) Optic nerve sheath cyst
   (8) Simple epithelial cyst
   (9) Teratoma

C. Fibrocytic tumors
   (1) Fibroma
   (2) Fibrosarcoma
   (3) Fibrous histiocytoma
   (4) Juvenile fibromatosis
   (5) Nodular fasciitis

D. Histiocytic lesions
   (1) Others
      a. Juvenile xanthogranuloma (JXG, nevoxanthoendothelioma)
      b. Sinus histiocytosis with massive lymphadenopathy
   (2) Systemic histiocytoses (histiocytosis X) (Hand-Schüller-Christian disease)

E. Inflammatory pseudotumor of orbit
   (1) Ectopic cerebellar tissue in orbit
   (2) Local, such as fungus or foreign body
   (3) Systemic such as sarcoidosis syndrome (Schaumann syndrome) or collagen disease
   (4) Unknown cause

F. Lacrimal gland (fossa) lesions
   (1) Epithelial tumors
      a. Adenoid cystic carcinoma
      b. Mucoepidermoid carcinoma
      c. Pleomorphic adenocarcinoma (malignant mixed tumor)
      d. Pleomorphic adenoma (benign mixed tumor)

    (2) Nonepithelial lesions
       a. infectious
       b. inflammatory
       c. lymphoid and leukemia
       d. systemic (sarcoid)

G. Lipocytic and myxoid tumors
    (1) Lipoma
    (2) Liposarcoma
    (3) Myxoid liposarcoma
    (4) Myxoma

H. Lymphoid tumors and leukemias (excluding lacrimal gland lesions)
    (1) Benign reactive lymphoid hyperplasia
    (2) Burkitt lymphoma
    (3) Lymphoblastic leukemia
    (4) Myelogenous leukemia (granulocytic sarcoma)
    (5) Non-Hodgkin lymphoma

I. Metastatic tumors of the orbit
    (1) Malignant melanoma of skin
    (2) Neuroblastoma (child)
    (3) Other sites such as Ewing sarcoma
    (4) Primary in breast (adult female)
    (5) Primary in lung (adult male)
    (6) Primary in prostate (adult male)

J. Nonepithelial lesions
    (1) Benign reactive lymphoid hyperplasia
    (2) Inflammatory pseudotumors (dacryoadenitis)
    (3) Lymphoma
    (4) Plasmacytoma

K. Optic nerve and meningeal tumors
    (1) Juvenile pilocytic astrocytoma (optic nerve glioma)
    (2) Meningioma
       a. Primary optic nerve sheath
       b. Secondary
    (3) Malignant optic nerve glioma

L. Osseous and fibro-osseous tumors
    (1) Aneurysmal bone cyst
    (2) Benign osteoblastoma
    (3) Brown tumor of hyperparathyroidism
    (4) Fibrous dysplasia (Albright syndrome)
    (5) Giant-cell granuloma

(6) Giant-cell tumor (osteoclastoma)

(7) Infantile cortical hyperostosis

(8) Ossifying fibroma

(9) Osteoma

(10) Osteosarcoma

M. Peripheral nerve tumors

(1) Alveolar soft-part sarcoma

(2) Amputation neuroma

(3) Granular cell myoblastoma

(4) Neurilemoma

   a. Benign

   b. Malignant

(5) Neurofibroma

   a. Plexiform

   b. Solitary

(6) Paraganglioma (chemodectoma)

N. Primary melanocytic tumors

(1) Blue nevus

(2) Melanocytic hamartoma

(3) Melanotic progonoma (retinal tumor)

(4) Primary orbital melanoma

O. Rhabdomyoma and rhabdomyosarcoma

(1) Rhabdomyoma

(2) Rhabdomyosarcoma

P. Secondary orbital tumors from adjacent structures

(1) Conjunctival origin

   a. Melanoma

   b. Mucoepidermoid carcinoma

   c. Squamous-cell carcinoma

(2) Eyelid origin

   a. Basal-cell carcinoma

   b. Melanoma

   c. Sebaceous carcinoma

   d. Squamous-cell carcinoma

(3) Intracranial origin

   a. Astrocytoma

   b. Meningioma

(4) Intraocular origin

   a. Medulloepithelioma

   b. Neurilemoma

   c. Retinoblastoma

   d. Uveal melanoma

  (5) Nasopharyngeal origin

   a. Angiofibroma

   b. Carcinoma

   c. Melanoma

  (6) Paranasal sinus origin

   a. Ethmoid sinus carcinoma

   b. Inverting papilloma

   c. Maxillary sinus carcinoma

   d. Rhabdomyosarcoma

 Q. Vasculogenic lesions

  (1) Capillary hemangioma

  (2) Cavernous hemangioma

  (3) Hemangiopericytoma

  (4) Hemangiosarcoma

  (5) Kaposi sarcoma

  (6) Lymphangioma

  (7) Varices

  (8) Vascular leiomyoma

  (9) Vascular leiomyosarcoma

6. Vascular disorders

 A. Allergic vasculitis

 B. Angioedema (Quincke disease)

 C. Arteriovenous aneurysm or varices

 D. Arteriovenous fistula (varicose aneurysm)

 E. Collagen disease—lupus erythematosus (Kaposi Libman-Sacks syndrome), periarteritis nodosa (Kussmaul disease), or dermatomucomyositis (Wagner-Unverricht syndrome)

 F. Cranial arteritis

 G. Thrombophlebitis

Alper, M.G.: Computed tomography in planning and evaluating orbital surgery. Ophthalmology, 87:419, 1980.

Archer, K.F. et al.: Orbital Nonchromaffin Paraganglioma. Ophthalmology, 96:1659–1666, 1989.

Bullock, J.D., and Yanes, B.: Metastatic tumors of the orbit. Ann. Ophthalmol., 12:1392, 1980.

Carlson, R.E.: Transient exophthalmos. Ann. Ophthalmol., 14:724–729, 1982.

Carriere, V.M., et al.: A case of prostate carcinoma with bilateral orbital metastases and the review of the literature. Ophthalmology, 89:402, 1982.

Grove, A.S.: Orbital trauma and computed tomography. Ophthalmology, 87:403, 1980.

Fraunfelder, F.T.: Drug-Induced Ocular Side Effects and Drug Interactions. 4th Ed. Philadelphia, Williams & Wilkins, 1996.

Howard, G.M., et al.: Pulsating metastatic tumor of the orbit. Am. J. Ophthalmol., 85:767, 1978.

Luxenberg, M.N.: Chloroma. Arch. Ophthalmol., 109:734–736, 1991. Lyon, D.B. et. al.: Epithelioid Hemangioendothelioma of the Orbital Bones. Ophthalmology 99:1773–1778, 1993.

Morales, A.G., et al.: Hydatid Cysts of the Orbit. Ophthalmol., 95:1027–1032, 1988.

Newman, N.J., et al.: Ectopic brain in the orbit. Ophthalmology, 93:268–272, 1986.

Newis-Levin, L., et al.: Plasma cell myeloma of the orbit. Ann. Ophthalmol., 18:477, 1981.

Rawlings, E.F., et al.: Polypoid sinusitis mimicking orbital malignancy. Am. J. Ophthalmol., 87:694–697, 1979.

Shields, J.A., et al.: Classification and incidence of space-occupying lesions of the orbit. Arch Ophthalmol., 102:1606–1611, 1984.

Skalka, H.W., and Callahan, M.A.: Congenital hematic cyst of the orbit. Ann. Ophthalmol., 11:1103, 1979.

Syndromes and Diseases Associated with Exophthalmos

1. Actinomycosis
2. Albright syndrome (fibrous dysplasia)
3. Amyloidosis (Lubarsch-Pick syndrome)
4. Apert syndrome (sphenoacrocraniosyndactyly)
5. Arteriovenous fistula (varicose aneurysm)
6. Aspergillosis
7. Bacillus cereus
8. Bloch-Sulzberger disease (incontinentia pigment I)
9. Bonnet-Dechaume-Blanc syndrome (neuroretinoangiomatosis syndrome)
10. Bourneville syndrome (tuberous sclerosis)
11. Caffey syndrome (infantile cortical hyperostosis)
12. Carotid artery-cavernous sinus fistula
13. Clostridium perfringens
14. Coenurosis
15. Craniostenosis
16. Cretinism (hypothyroidism)
17. Crouzon disease (craniofacial dysostosis)
18. Cryptococcosis
19. Cushing syndrome (adrenocortical syndrome)
20. Dejean sign (orbital floor fracture)
21. de Lange syndrome (congenital muscular hypertrophy-cerebral syndrome)
22. Dermatomucomyositis (polymyositis dermatomyositis)
23. Dermoid
24. Diencephalic epilepsy syndrome (autonomic epilepsy syndrome)
25. Dirofilariasis
26. Dracontiasis (Guinea worm infection)
27. Engelmann syndrome (diaphyseal dysplasia)
28. Ewing sarcoma
29. Feer disease (infantile acrodynia)

30. Fibrosarcoma
31. Fibrous dysplasia (Albright syndrome)
32. Foix syndrome (cavernous sinus thrombosis)
33. Gardner syndrome
34. Grönblad-Strandberg syndrome (pseudoxanthoma elasticum)
35. Hallermann-Streiff-François syndrome (oculomandibulofacial dyscephaly)
36. Hand-Schüller-Christian disease (histiocytosis X)
37. Heerfordt syndrome (uveoparotid fever)
38. Hemangiomas
39. Herpes zoster
40. Hodgkin disease
41. Hollenhorst syndrome (chorioretinal infarction syndrome)
42. Horner syndrome (cervical sympathetic paralysis syndrome)
43. Hunter syndrome (MPS II)
44. Hurler (MPS I-H) syndrome
45. Hutchinson disease (adrenal cortex neuroblastoma with orbital metastasis)
46. Hydatid cyst
47. Hydrocephalus chondrodystrophicus congenita (extreme hydrocephalus syndrome)
48. Hypertension
49. Hyperthyroidism (Basedow syndrome)
50. Hypervitaminosis A
51. Hypophosphatasia (phosphoethanolaminuria)
52. Jansen disease (metaphyseal dysostosis)
53. Juvenile xanthogranuloma (JXG, nevoxanthoendothelioma)
54. Kleeblattschädel syndrome (cloverleaf skull)
55. Leiomyoma
56. Leopard syndrome (multiple lentigines syndrome)
57. Leprechaunism
58. Leukemia
59. Linear nevus sebaceous of Jadassohn
60. Lupus erythematosus (Kaposi-Libman-Sacks syndrome)
61. Lymphoid hyperplasia
62. Lymphangioma
63. Lymphosarcoma
64. Melnick-Needles syndrome (osteodysplasty)
65. Meningioma
66. Mikulicz syndrome (dacryosialoadenopathy)
67. Mobius' disease (congenital paralysis of 6th and 7th nerves)
68. Mucocele
69. Mucormycosis

70. Multiple myeloma
71. Mumps
72. Myasthenia gravis (Erb-Goldflam syndrome)
73. Neurilemoma
74. Noonan syndrome (male Turner syndrome)
75. Osteopetrosis (Albers-Schönberg syndrome)
76. Paget syndrome (osteitis deformans)
77. Periarteritis nodosa (Kussmaul syndrome)
78. Periocular and ocular metastatic tumors
79. Pierre-Robin syndrome (micrognathia-glossoptosis syndrome)
80. Progeria (Hutchinson-Gilford syndrome)
81. Pyknodysostosis
82. Quincke disease (angioedema)
83. Relapsing polychondritis
84. Retinoblastoma
85. Rhabdomyosarcoma
86. Rochon-Duvigneaud syndrome (superior orbital fissure syndrome)
87. Rollet syndrome (orbital apex-sphenoidal syndrome)
88. Sarcoidosis syndrome (Schaumann syndrome)
89. Scaphocephaly syndrome
90. Scheie syndrome (MPS I-S)
91. Scurvy (avitaminosis C)
92. Sebaceous gland carcinoma
93. Seckel syndrome (bird-headed dwarf syndrome)
94. Sezary syndrome (mycosis fungoides syndrome)
95. Shy-Gonatas syndrome (orthostatic hypotension syndrome)
96. Siegrist sign (pigmented choroidal vessels)
97. Silverman syndrome (battered baby syndrome)
98. Sphenocavernous syndrome
99. Streptococcus
100. Sturge-Weber syndrome (encephalofacial angiomatosis)
101. Syphilis (lues)
102. Thermal burns
103. Trichinellosis
104. Trisomy syndrome (Edward syndrome)
105. Tuberculosis
106. Turner syndrome (gonadal dysgenesis)
107. von Hippel-Lindau syndrome (retinocerebral angiomatosis)
108. von Recklinghausen disease (neurofibromatosis)
109. Wegener syndrome (Wegener granulomatosis)

Geeraets, W.J.: Ocular Syndromes. 3rd Ed. Philadelphia, Lea & Febiger, 1976.

Goodman, R.M., and Gorlin, R.J.: The Face in Genetic Disorders. St. Louis, C.V. Mosby, 1970.

Roy, F.H.: Ocular Syndromes and Systemic Diseases. 2nd Ed. Philadelphia, W.B. Saunders, 1989.

Specific Exophthalmos

1. Age

   A. Newborn—most common

   *(1) Orbital sepsis

   (2) Orbital neoplasm

   B. Neonatal—osteomyelitis of the maxilla

   C. Early childhood (up to year of age—most common

   *(1) Dermoid

   *(2) Hemangioma

   (3) Dermolipoma

   (4) Histiocytosis X including Hand-Schüller-Christian disease

   *(5) Orbital extension of retinoblastoma

   D. One to five years—most common

   *(1) Dermoid

   (2) Metastatic neuroblastoma

   (3) Rhabdomyosarcoma

   (4) Epithelial cyst, such as sebaceous cyst and epithelial inclusion cyst

   (5) Glioma of optic nerve

   (6) Sphenoid wing meningioma

   *(7) Orbital extension of retinoblastoma

   (8) Fibrous dysplasia (Albright syndrome)

   (9) Metastatic embryonal sarcoma

   *(10) Hemangioma

   E. Five to ten years—most common

   (1) Pseudotumor

   (2) Orbital extension of retinoblastoma

   (3) Malignant lymphomas and leukemias

   *(4) Dermoid

   *(5) Hemangioma

   (6) Meningioma

   (7) Fibrous dysplasia (Albright syndrome)

   (8) Rhabdomyosarcoma

   (9) Orbital hematoma

   (10) Glioma of optic nerve

   F. Ten to thirty years—most common

   *(1) Pseudotumor

* = most important

    (2) Mucocele

    (3) Meningioma

  *(4) Endocrine ophthalmopathy (thyroid related ophthduropathy)

    (5) Lacrimal gland tumor

    (6) Malignant lymphomas and leukemias

    (7) Dermoid

    (8) Hemangioma

    (9) Peripheral nerve tumors

  (10) Undifferentiated sarcomas

  (11) Osteoma

  (12) Fibrous dysplasia (Albright syndrome)

  (13) Rhabdomyosarcoma

  (14) Glioma of optic nerve

G. Thirty to fifty years—most common

  *(1) Pseudotumor

    (2) Mucocele

    (3) Malignant lymphomas and leukemias

  *(4) Hemangioma

  *(5) Endocrine ophthalmopathy (thyroid related ophthduropathy)

    (6) Lacrimal gland tumors

    (7) Rhinogenic carcinoma

    (8) Malignant melanoma

    (9) Osteosarcoma

  (10) Fibrosarcoma

  (11) Metastatic carcinoma

  (12) Meningioma

  (13) Dermoid

H. Fifty to seventy years—most common

  *(1) Pseudotumor

  *(2) Mucocele

  *(3) Malignant lymphomas and leukemias

    (4) Dermoid

    (5) Carcinoma of palpebral or epibulbar origin

  *(6) Meningioma

  *(7) Endocrine ophthalmopathy (thyroid related abitopathy)

    (8) Lacrimal gland tumor

    (9) Osteosarcoma

  (10) Fibrosarcoma

  (11) Undifferentiated sarcoma

  (12) Metastatic carcinoma

  (13) Osteoma

(14) Fibrous dysplasia (Albright syndrome)

(15) Neurofibroma

(16) Hemangioma

I. More than seventy years—most common

(1) Melanoma

(2) Pseudotumor

*(3) Lymphoma

*(4) Metastatic tumor

(5) Basal cell carcinoma

(6) Mucocele

2. Unilateral exophthalmos—most common

A. Anatomical conditions

(1) Unilateral myopia of high degree

(2) Defects in the vault of the orbit: meningocele, encephalocele, hydroencephalocele

(3) Exophthalmos associated with arterial hypertension

(4) Recurrent exophthalmos from retrobulbar hemorrhage, lymphangioma

(5) Intermittent exophthalmos associated with venous anomalies within the cranium

(6) Disease of the pituitary gland; meningiomas involving sphenoid ridge

*(7) Unilateral exophthalmos associated with endocrine or thyroid-related ophthalmopathy

B. Traumatic conditions

(1) Contralateral floor fracture with enophthalmos

(2) Fracture of the orbit with retrobulbar hemorrhage

(3) Laceration and rupture of the tissues of the orbit and the extraocular muscles

(4) Intracranial trauma sustained at birth; aneurysm in orbit

(5) Pulsating exophthalmos from carotid-cavernous aneurysm

(6) Spontaneous retrobulbar hemorrhage as seen in whooping cough

(7) Chronic subdural hematoma bulging into orbit

(8) Posterior exophthalmos (orbital apex lesion)

    a. Pseudotumor

    b. Malignant tumor

    c. Benign tumor

    d. Vascular disease

    e. Infection

C. Inflammatory conditions

(1) Retrobulbar abscess and cellulitis

(2) Thrombophlebitis of the orbital veins

(3) Cavernous sinus thrombosis

(4) Erysipelas (St. Anthony fire)

(5) Tenonitis

(6) Periostitis (syphilitic or tuberculous)

* = most important

(7) Orbital mucocele, pyocele; cholesteatoma

(8) Orbital exostosis

(9) Paget disease with hyperostosis

(10) Actinomycosis, trichinosis, mycotic pseudotumor

D. Disease of blood, lymph, and hematopoietic system

(1) Rickets (avitaminosis D)

(2) Scurvy (avitaminosis C)

(3) Hemophilia (factor VIII deficiency)

(4) Lymphosarcoma

(5) Chloroma

(6) Hodgkin disease

E. Space-taking lesions

(1) Vascular anomalies

a. Congenital orbital varix (young patient with systemic abnormalities)

b. Cavernous hemangioma (middle age)

c. Capillary hemangioma (young children) Kasabach-Merrit syndrome

(2) Orbital tumors: pseudotumors; orbital cysts; meningocele; lymphangioma; orbital meningioma; lacrimal gland tumor; sarcoma; metastatic carcinoma; metastatic adrenal tumors; osteomas arising in the accessory nasal sinuses; tumors of the nasopharynx, benign and malignant

(3) Intracranial tumor with orbital extension including chordoma and meningioma

F. Unilateral exophthalmos in children

(1) Inflammation

(2) Vascular disorders

(3) Neoplasms

(4) Metabolic diseases

(5) Developmental anomalies

(6) Others

*(7) Orbital cellulitis

3. Bilateral exophthalmos—most common

*A. Thyroid or endocrine ophthalmopathy

B. Orbital myositis (owing to causes other than thyroid dysfunction)

C. Cavernous sinus thrombosis (Foix syndrome)

D. Metastatic neuroblastoma

E. Hand-Schüller-Christian disease (histiocytosis X)

F. Crouzon disease (dysostosis craniofacialis)

G. Paget disease (osteitis deformans)

4. Type proptosis—most common

A. Straight forward—glioma of optic nerve, intraconal cavernous hemangioma

B. Down and temporal—mucocele of frontal sinus

     C. Down and nasal—lacrimal gland lesion

     D. Downward—tumor of roof of orbit

     E. Upward—tumor of floor of orbit

5. Transient exophthalmos

    *A. Orbital varices

     B. Orbital varices with intracranial extension

     C. Arteriovenous malformations

     D. Cavernous hemangioma

6. Pulsating exophthalmos—most common

    *A. Carotid-cavernous fistula

     B. von Recklinghausen disease associated with bony defect of skull

     C. Large frontal mucocele

     D. Meningoencephalocele

     E. Blow-in fracture of roof of orbit

     F. Neurofibromatosis

     G. Fistula

     H. Malignancies

      I. Mucoceles

      J. Orbital varix

     K. Dermoid cysts

     L. Aneurysm

7. Recurrent exophthalmos

     A. Recurrent orbital inflammation (pseudotumor) or hemorrhage

     B. Orbital cysts that rupture

     C. Lymphangioma (children)

     D. Syndrome of intermittent exophthalmos-congenital venous malformations of the orbit: venous angioma and orbital varix

     E. Temporal lobe tumor with orbital extension

     F. Neurofibromatosis

     G. Vascular neoplasm

8. Intermittent exophthalmos

     A. Orbital varices

     B. Recurrent hemorrhage

     C. Vascular neoplasm

     D. Lymphangioma

9. Exophthalmos associated with conjunctival chemosis, restricted movement of eyes because of pain—pseudotumor

10. Exophthalmos in an acutely ill patient—cavernous sinus thrombosis

11. Exophthalmos associated with engorged conjunctival episcleral vessels

* = most important

    A. Nonpulsating-cerebral arteriovenous angioma, ophthalmic vein thrombosis, or cavernous sinus thrombosis

    B. Pulsating exophthalmos-carotid-cavernous sinus fistula

12. Exophthalmos associated with a palpable mass in region of the lacrimal gland

    A. Primary inflammatory exophthalmos

    B. Neoplasm

    C. Sarcoidosis syndrome (Schaumann syndrome)

    D. Hodgkin disease

13. Exophthalmos in patient with uncontrolled diabetes, usually with acidosis, who develops unilateral lid edema, ptosis, internal and external ophthalmoplegia, proptosis, and severe vision loss—orbital mucormycosis

14. Exophthalmos in an infant with ecchymosis of the eyelids

    A. Metastatic neuroblastoma

    B. Orbital leukemia infiltration

15. Bilateral exophthalmos from bilateral orbital pseudotumor

    A. Eosinophilic granuloma

    B. Retroperitoneal fibrosis

    C. Myasthenia gravis (Erb-Goldflam syndrome)

Bullock, J.D., and Bartley, G.B.: Dynamic proptosis. Am. J. Ophthalmol., 102:104–110, 1986.

Ferry, A.P., et al.: Orbital invasion by an intracranial chordoma. Am. J. Ophthalmol., 92:7–12, 1981.

Henderson, J.W.: Orbital Tumors. New York, Thieme-Stratton, 1980.

Hoopes, P.C., et al.: Giant cell granuloma of the orbit. Ophthalmology, 88:1361, 1981.

Jones, I.S., and Jakobiec, F.A.: Diseases of the Orbit. Philadelphia, Harper and Row, 1979.

Krohel, G.B., et al.: Orbital Disease: A Practical Approach. Stewart, William B. and Chavis, Richard M., eds. (Illus). New York, Grune & Stratton, 1981.

Macy, J.I., et al.: Orbital cellulitis. Ophthalmology, 87:1309, 1980.

Musarella, M.A., et al.: Ocular involvement in neuroblastoma: Prognostic implications. Ophthalmology, 91:936–940, 1984.

Nicholson, D.H., and Green, W.R. (ed.): Pediatric Ocular Tumors. New York, Masson, 1981.

Richards, A.B., et al.: Pseudotumor of the orbit and retroperitoneal fibrosis. Arch. Ophthamol., 98:1617–1620, 1980.

Walsh, F.B., and Hoyt, W.F.: Clinical Neuro-ophthalmology. 4th Ed. Baltimore, Williams & Wilkins, 1985.

Enophthalmos

1. Senility (common)

2. Wasting diseases—loss of orbital fat

*3. Injury—blow-out fracture of floor of orbit (most common)

4. Orbital varices—transient exophthalmos with fat atrophy

5. Chronic or severe liver or gallbladder disease (usually in right eye owing to increased tone of orbicularis muscle and extraocular muscles)

6. Superior sulcus deformity

    A. Traumatic bony loss

    B. Atrophy of the orbital tissues

    C. Levator detachment with ptosis

Exophthalmos (Up to One Year)

	Dermoid	Hemangioma	Histiocytosis X on Hand-Schüller-Christian Disease	Retinoblastoma (Orbital Extension)
History				
1. Bilateral				S
2. Congenital	S	U		S
3. Familial				U
4. More in females		U		
5. More in males			U	
6. Present at birth		S		
Physical Findings				
1. Astigmatism	S	S		
2. Bluish lid/conjunctiva		U		U
3. Bullous keratopathy			S	
4. Cataract			S	
5. Corneal opacity				S
6. Glaucoma		R		U
7. Hypopyon	U			S
8. Keratitis	S	S		
9. Lid ecchymosis	S			R
10. Microphthalmos	S			
11. Papilledema			S	R
12. Phthisis bulbi				S
13. Ptosis	S	S		
14. Retinal detachment			S	
15. Retinal hemorrhage			U	
16. Uveitis			U	
17. Vitreous hemorrhage				S
Laboratory Data				
1. Biopsy	U	U	S	U
2. Computed tomographic scan				
A. Calcific densities	U			U
B. Tumor	S	U	S	S
3. Orbital roentigenogram				
A. Cystic defects	U			
B. Diffusely enlarged orbit		U		
C. Enlarged optic canal				U
D. Expansion of orbital margin	U	U		
E. Fossa formation of orbit	U			
F. Orbital bone destruction			U	U
G. Orbital mass				U
4. Thrombocytopenia		U		
5. Ultrasonography				
A. Cystic tumor	U			
B. Orbital mass		U		

R = rarely; S = sometimes; and U = usually.

Exophthalmos (One to Five Years)

	Dermoid*	Metastatic Neuroblastoma	Rhabdomyosarcoma	Sebaceous Carcinoma	Glioma of Optic Nerve	Sphenoid Wing Meningioma	Retinoblastoma (Orbital Extension)*	Fibrous Dysplasia	Metastatic Embryomal Sarcoma	Hemangioma*
History										
1. Bilateral		U			S	S	S			
2. Congenital		S					S			U
3. Familial			U				U			
4. More in females				U	U	S				U
5. More in males		U							S	
6. Painful		S					S			
7. Painless					U	S		U		
Physical Findings										
1. Anosmia						S		S		
2. Associated with neurofibromatosis					S	S		S		
3. Astigmatism	S									S
4. Bluish lid/conjunctiva							U			U
5. Corneal opacity							S			
6. Choroidal folds			S		S					
7. Edema lids/conjunctiva	S	S					S			
8. Extraocular muscle paralysis	S		S	S	S					
9. Glaucoma		R	S		S		U			S
10. Hearing defects, nasal obstruction, and epiphora			S					S		
11. Heterochromia of iris		S								
12. Horner syndrome		S								
13. Hypermetropia					S	S				
14. Hypopyon	U						S			
15. Keratitis	S		S	S					S	S
16. Lid ecchymosis	S	U	S				R		U	
17. Located in superior nasal quadrant		U								
18. Located in superior temporal quadrant	U									
19. Marcus Gunn pupil sign					S	U				
20. Microphthalmos	S									
21. Nystagmus					S					
22. Optic nerve atrophy		S			S	S		U		
23. Optic neuritis		S								
24. Papilledema		S	S		U		R	S		
25. Palsy of third cranial nerve						U				
26. Palsy of sixth and seventh cranial nerves		S								
27. Phthisis bulbi							S			
28. Ptosis	S	S	U							S
29. Retinal hemorrhage		U								
30. Strabismus		S	S	S	S	S	S	S		
31. Vitreous hemorrhage							S		U	

Exophthalmos (One to Five Years) *Continued*

	Dermoid*	Metastatic Neuroblastoma	Rhabdosarcoma	Sebaceous Carcinoma	Glioma of Optic Nerve	Sphenoid Wing Meningioma	Retinoblastoma (Orbital Extension)*	Fibrous Dysplasia	Metastatic Embryomal Sarcoma	Hemangioma*
Laboratory Data										
1. Biopsy	S	U	S	U	R	U	U	S	U	S
2. Computed tomographic scan										
A. Enlargement optic nerve/sheath					U					
B. Orbital mass	U	S			U			S	S	U
C. Tumor between optic nerve and lateral rectus										U
D. Tumor with bony erosion			U							
3. In urine										
A. Catecholamines		U								
B. Vanillylmandelic acid		U								
4. Orbital roentgenogram										
A. Calcific densities	S	U					U			
B. Cystic defect	S									
C. Diffusely enlarged orbit						U		U	U	U
D. Enlargement of superior orbital fissure								U		
E. Expansion of optic canal					U	U				
F. Expansion of orbital margin	U					U				U
G. Fossa formation of orbit	U									
H. Hyperostosis						U	U			
I. Narrowing of superior orbital fissure								U		
J. Orbital mass that involves sphenoid bone								U		
K. Osteolysis	U									
5. Ultrasonography										
A. Cystic tumor	U						U			U
B. Orbital mass		S	U					S	U	S
C. Enlarged optic nerve shadow					U	U				

* R = rarely; S = sometimes; and U = usually.

Exophthalmos (Five to Ten Years)

	Pseudotumor	Retinoblastoma*	Leukemia and Lymphomas	Dermoid*	Hemangioma*	Meningioma	Fibrous Dysplasia	Rhabdomyosarcoma	Orbital Hematoma	Glioma of Optic Nerve
History										
1. Bilateral	S	S	S				S			S
2. Familial		U								
3. Following blunt trauma								S	U	
4. More in females					U	U				U
5. More in males			U					U		
6. Painful	U					S		S	S	
7. Painless		U	U	U	U	U	U	U		S
8. Rapid onset	S								U	S
Physical Findings										
1. Anosmia						S				
2. Associated with neurofibromatosis						S	S			S
3. Astigmatism				S	S					
4. Bluish lid/conjunctiva		U			U				S	
5. Central retinal artery thrombosis	S									
6. Corneal opacity		S								
7. Choroidal folds						S		S		S
8. Edema of lids/conjunctiva	U	S		S		S		S	S	
9. Epibulbar lesions			U							
10. Extraocular muscle paralysis: Limitation/Restriction	S		S	S		S		S		S
11. Glaucoma	S	U	U		S			S		S
12. Globe displacement (down)	S									
13. Hypermetropia	S				S	U				S
14. Hypopyon		S	S							
15. Involvement of trigeminal nerve	U									
16. Intraorbital bleeding		S								
17. Keratitis				S	S	S	S	S		
18. Lid ecchymosis	S	R	R	S				S	S	
19. Located in superior nasal quadrant								U		
20. Marcus Gunn pupil sign						S				S
21. Microphthalmos				S						
22. Nystagmus										S
23. Ophthalmoplegia	S									
24. Optic nerve atrophy	S		S			U	U			S
25. Optic neuritis	S		S							
26. Optociliary venous shunts on disc						S				S
27. Orbital myositis	S									
28. Papilledema	S	R	S			S	S	S		S
29. Phthisis bulbi		S	S							
30. Ptosis	S			S	S	R	S	U	S	
31. Retinal detachment		S								
32. Soft retinal exudate			U							
33. Strabismus		S				S	S			S
34. Uveitis		S	U							
35. Vitreous hemorrhage		S							S	

Exophthalmos (Five to Ten Years) *Continued*

	Pseudotumor	Retinoblastoma*	Leukemia and Lymphomas	Dermoid*	Hemangioma*	Meningioma	Fibrous Dysplasia	Rhabdomyosarcoma	Orbital Hematoma	Glioma of Optic Nerve
Laboratory Data										
1. Biopsy	U	S	U	U	U	S	S	S	S	R
2. Computed tomographic scan										
A. Calcific densities		U			U			U		
B. Diffuse radiodensity blends with normal structure	U									
C. Enlargement optic nerve/sheath						U				U
D. Extraocular muscle enlargement	U							S		
E. Orbital mass		S	S	U	U		S		S	S
F. Tumor with bony erosion							S	U		
3. Orbital roentgenogram										
A. Calcific densities		U			U			U		
B. Diffusely enlarged orbit		S				S		R		
C. Enlarged optic canal						S				S
D. Expansion of orbital margin					U					
E. Fossa formation of orbit					U					
F. Hyperostosis		S				S	S			S
G. Hyperostosis sphenoid bone						S	U			
H. Narrowing of superior orbital fissure							U			
I. Osteolysis			S	S						
J. Periosteal reaction										
4. Thrombocytopenia					S					
5. Ultrasonography										
A. Cystic tumor					U	U				
B. Enlarged optic nerve							U			U
C. Orbital mass		S	U	S	S		U	U		
D. Uniform dense diffuse mass	U		U				U			

R = rarely; S = sometimes; and U = usually.

Exophthalmos (Ten to Thirty Years)

	Pseudotumor*	Mucocele	Meningioma	Thyroid Ophthalmopathy*	Lacrimal Gland Tumor	Malignant Lymphomas and Leukemias	Dermoid	Hemangioma	Peripheral Nerve Tumors	Undifferentiated Sarcomas	Osteoma	Fibrous Dysplasia	Rhabdomyosarcoma	Glioma of Optic Nerve
History														
1. Bilateral	S			S		S								R
2. Common in females			U	S				U						S
3. Common in males						U			U		S		U	
4. Familial													U	
5. Painful	U		S		S								S	
6. Painless		U	U				U	U	U	U	U	U	U	R
7. Slow onset									U					
Physical Findings														
1. Anosmia			S									S		
2. Associated with neurofibromatosis									U			S		S
3. Astigmatism					R		S	S						
4. Bluish lids/conjunctiva								U						
5. Central retinal artery occlusion	S													
6. Corneal opacity												R		
7. Choroidal folds		S	S					S					R	S
8. Edema lids/conjunctiva	U		S	S			R					S	S	
9. Epibulbar lesion						U			S					
10. Extraocular muscle restriction	S	S	S	U	R	S	S	S	R				S	
11. Glaucoma	S		S			S		R				R	S	R
12. Globe displacement (down)	S	S			U		S		R		S	S		
13. Hemangioma of conjunctiva, iris, or disc								U						
14. Hyperopia	S		U					S						
15. Hypopyon						S								
16. Infrequent blinking				U										
17. Intraorbital bleeding						S			R	S				
18. Involvement of trigeminal nerve	U				S									
19. Keratitis			S	U		S	S	S						
20. Lacrimation	S	S		S	S									
21. Lid ecchymosis	S						R	S					S	
22. Lid lag				U										
23. Lid retraction				U										
24. Marcus Gunn pupil sign			S											S
25. Microphthalmos							S							
26. Nystagmus														S
27. Neurocutaneous melanosis										U				
28. Optic nerve atrophy	S	R	U			S		S			S	S		S
29. Optic neuritis	S					S								
30. Optociliary venous shunts on disc			S											
31. Orbital myositis	S				S									
32. Panophthalmitis														

Exophthalmos (Ten to Thirty Years) *Continued*

	Pseudotumor*	Mucocele	Meningioma	Thyroid Ophthalmopathy*	Lacrimal Gland Tumor	Malignant Lymphomas and Leukemias	Dermoid	Hemangioma	Peripheral Nerve Tumors	Undifferentiated Sarcomas	Osteoma	Fibrous Dysplasia	Rhabdomyosarcoma	Glioma of Optic Nerve
Physical Findings														
33. Papilledema	S	R	S	R		S		S			S	S	S	
34. Poor fixation on lateral gaze	S			U										
35. Ptosis			S	S			S	S					S	
36. Retinal detachment						S					S			
37. Soft retinal exudate						U								
38. Strabismus	S		S	S										S
39. Tremor of closed lids				U										
40. Uveitis	R					U								

R = rarely; S = sometimes; and U = usually.

Exophthalmos (Thirty to Fifty Years)

	Pseudotumor*	Mucocele	Malignant Lymphomas and Leukemias	Hemangioma	Thyroid Ophthalmopathy*	Lacrimal Gland Tumor	Rhinogenic Carcinoma	Malignant Melanoma	Osteosarcoma	Fibrosarcoma	Metastatic Carcinoma	Meningioma	Dermoid
History													
1. Bilateral	S		S		S						S		
2. Chinese extraction							U						
3. Common in females				S	S							U	
4. Common in males			U				U						
5. Familial					S				S	S	S		
6. More in whites					S				U				
7. Painful	U					S	S			U	S		
Physical Findings													
1. Astigmatism					S	S					S		S
2. Bluish lids/conjunctiva					U								
3. Central retinal artery occlusion	S												
4. Choroidal folds		S			S						S	S	

* = most important

Exophthalmos (Thirty to Fifty Years) *Continued*

Physical Findings

	Pseudotumor*	Mucocele	Malignant Lymphomas and Leukemias	Hemangioma	Thyroid Ophthalmopathy*	Lacrimal Gland Tumor	Rhinogenic Carcinoma	Malignant Melanoma	Osteosarcoma	Fibrosarcoma	Metastatic Carcinoma	Meningioma	Dermoid
5. Choroidal nevus								S					
6. Conjunctivitis	S				S								
7. Cranial nerve palsies							S				R		
8. Degenerative changes in retinal pigment epithelium								S			S		
9. Edema of lids/conjunctiva	S				S				S	S		S	R
10. Epibulbar subconjunctival lesion			S								R		
11. Fibrosarcoma of lids, lacrimal sac, or sclera										U			
12. Glaucoma	S		S	S				R	S		R		
13. Globe displacement (down)	S	S	R	R	S	U				S	S		R
14. Hemangioma of conjunctiva, iris, or disc				S									
15. Horner syndrome							S						
16. Hypermetropia	S											U	
17. Hypopyon			S										U
18. Increased pigmentation of lids				S	S			S					
19. Infrequent blinking					U								
20. Intraorbital bleeding			S						R		R		
21. Involvement of trigeminal nerve	U					S			S				
22. Keratitis				S	U				S			R	R
23. Lacrimation	S				S	S							
24. Lid ecchymosis	S		R										S
25. Lid lag					U								
26. Marcus Gunn pupil sign					S							S	
27. Microphthalmos													S
28. Nasolacrimal obstruction						U			S	S	R		
29. Orbital myositis	S				S				S	S			
30. Ophthalmoplegia	S	R			S	R	U		S	S	S		
31. Optic nerve atrophy	R	R	S	R	S				S	S		U	
32. Optic neuritis	S		S								R		
33. Optociliary venous shunts on the disc												S	
34. Panophthalmitis									S		S		
35. Papilledema	S		S	R						S		U	
36. Phthisis bulbi			S										
37. Pigmented or amelanotic choroidal mass								U					
38. Poor fixation on lateral gaze		S			U								

R = rarely; S = sometimes; and U = usually.

Exophthalmos (Fifty to Seventy Years)

	Pseudotumor*	Mucocele	Malignant Lymphomas and Leukemias	Dermoid	Carcinoma of Palpebral and Epibulbar Origin	Meningioma	Thyroid Ophthalmopathy	Lacrimal Gland Tumor	Osteosarcoma	Fibrosarcoma	Undifferentiated Sarcoma	Metastatic Carcinoma	Osteoma	Fibrous Dysplasia	Neurofibroma	Hemangioma
History																
1. Bilateral	S		S				S					S				
2. Common in females						U	S									U
3. Common in males			U										S			
4. Familial							S									
5. Painful	S		S		S	R	S	U				S	S		S	
Physical Findings																
1. Associated with neurofibromatosis														S	U	
2. Bluish lids/conjunctiva																U
3. Central retinal artery occlusion	S		R									R				
4. Chalazions					S											
5. Choroidal folds		S				S						S			S	S
6. Chronic blepharitis					S											
7. Conjunctivitis	S				S											
8. Disc pallor	R					S										
9. Ectropion					S										S	
10. Edema of lids/conjunctiva	S		S			S	S		S					S	S	
11. Entropion					S										S	
12. Epibulbar subconjunctival vessels			U		U											
13. Extraocular muscle paralysis	S	R	S				S			S					S	
14. Fibrosarcoma of lids, lacrimal sac, and sclera											U					
15. Glaucoma	S		U						S			R			S	S
16. Globe displacement (down and temporal)	S	S										S	S		S	
17. Globe displacement (down and nasal)								U				S			S	
18. Hemangioma of conjunctiva, iris, or disc																S
19. Hypermetropia	S					U										S
20. Hypopyon			S		S							S				
21. Involvment of trigeminal nerve	U							S	S						S	
22. Increased pigmentation of lids							S									
23. Intraorbital bleeding			S						S			S				
24. Infrequent blinking							U									
25. Keratitis				S	S	S	U		U	S		S		S	S	S
26. Lacrimation	S						S	S								
27. Lid ecchymosis	S		R	S	S										S	
28. Lid lag							U									
29. Lid notching					S											
30. Lid retraction					S		U									
31. Loss of vision	S	S				U	S		S		S	S		U	S	
32. Madarosis					U											
33. Marcus Gunn pupil sign						S	S									
34. Microphthalmos			S													
35. Nasolacrimal obstruction									S			R			S	

* = most important

Exophthalmos (Fifty to Seventy Years) *Continued*

	Pseudotumor*	Mucocele	Malignant Lymphomas and Leukemias	Dermoid	Carcinoma of Palpebral and Epibulbar Origin	Meningioma	Thyroid Ophthalmopathy	Lacrimal Gland Tumor	Osteosarcoma	Fibrosarcoma	Undifferentiated Sarcoma	Metastatic Carcinoma	Osteoma	Fibrous Dysplasia	Neurofibroma	Hemangioma
Physical Findings																
36. Nodular or nodular ulcerative lid lesion					U											
37. Nystagmus														S		
38. Ophthalmoplegia	S						S	R	S							
39. Optic nerve atrophy	S	R	S			U			S			S	S	U	S	
40. Optic neuritis	S		S									R				
41. Optociliary venous shunts on the disc						S										
42. Orbital myositis	S							S		S						
43. Panophthalmitis						S						S				
44. Papilledema	S	R	S						S				S	S	S	
45. Phthisis bulbi			S													
46. Poor fixation on lateral gaze	S						U									
47. Ptosis				S			S	S							S	S
48. Retinal detachment	R		S									S				
49. Soft retinal exudates			U									S				
50. Tremor of closed lids							U									
51. Uveitis	S		U						S			S			S	
52. Vitreous hemorrhage												S				U
Laboratory Data																
1. Biopsy	U	U	U	U	U	S		U	S	S	S	U	U	S	U	U
2. Computed tomographic scan																
A. Calcific densities		S			S				S			R				
B. Diffuse radiodensity blends with normal structure	U															
C. Enlargement optic nerve sheath						U										
D. Extraocular muscle enlargement	U						U					S				
E. Orbital mass		U	U	U	U			U	U	U	U		U	S	U	U
F. Tumor between optic nerve and lateral rectus																U
G. Tumor superior lateral orbit				R				U				S				
3. In blood																
A. 32 Phosphorus uptake elevated												U				
B. T3–T4 level increased, thyrotropin-releasing hormone test positive							S									
4. Orbital roentgenogram																
A. Calcific densities		S		S									U	S		
B. Cystic defects				S												
C. Diffusely enlarged orbit	S													S		
D. Expansion of optic canal						U									U	
E. Expansion of orbital margins						S		U							U	U
F. Fossa formation of orbit				S				S								
G. Frontal sinus bone dense/destruction		U												S		

Exophthalmos (Fifty to Seventy Years) *Continued*

	Pseudotumor*	Mucocele	Malignant Lymphomas and Leukemias	Dermoid	Carcinoma of Palpebral and Epibulbar Origin	Meningioma	Thyroid Ophthalmopathy	Lacrimal Gland Tumor	Osteosarcoma	Fibrosarcoma	Undifferentiated Sarcoma	Metastatic Carcinoma	Osteoma	Fibrous Dysplasia	Neurofibroma	Hemangioma
Laboratory Data																
H. Hyperostosis							S						U			
I. Narrowing of superior orbital fissure						U		U					U	U		
J. Orbital mass											S	S		S		
K. Osteolysis		U	S	U	S											
L. Periosteal reaction	S															
5. Ultrasonography																
A. Cystic tumor		U		U												U
B. Enlarged extraocular muscle	S															
C. Orbital mass			U							U	U	U	U	U		
D. Uniform diffuse dense mass	U		U		U								U			

R = rarely; S = sometimes; and U = usually.

Exophthalmos (More Than Seventy Years)

	Malignant Melanoma	Pseudotumor	Malignant Lymphoma and Leukemia*	Metastatic Carcinoma*	Basal Cell Carcinoma	Mucocele
History						
1. Bilateral		S		S		
2. Common in females				S		S
3. Common in males			S		S	
4. More in whites	U				U	
5. Ocular pain		U	S	S	S	
Physical Findings						
1. Central retinal artery occlusion				S	R	
2. Choroidal folds				S	S	
3. Choroidal nevus	S					
4. Degenerative changes in retinal pigment epithelium	S					
5. Ectropion					S	S
6. Edema of lids/conjunctiva			S	U	S	
7. Entropion					S	S

* = most important

Exophthalmos (More Than Seventy Years) *Continued*

	Malignant Melanoma	Pseudotumor	Malignant Lymphoma and Leukemia*	Metastatic Carcinoma*	Basal Cell Carcinoma	Mucocele
Physical Findings						
8. Extraocular muscle limatation	S	S	S	S		S
9. Glaucoma	S	S		S		
10. Globe displacement (down and temporally)		S				S
11. Hypermetropia	U	S				
12. Increased lid pigmentation	S					
13. Intraorbital bleeding				S		
14. Involvement of trigeminal nerve		U		S		S
15. Lacrimation					S	U
16. Lid ecchymosis		S		S	S	
17. Nodular/ulcerative lid lesion					U	
18. Optic nerve atrophy	S	R		S		S
19. Optic neuritis		S				
20. Orbital myositis		S		S		
21. Papilledema	S	S	S	S		S
22. Pigmented or amelanotic choroidal mass	S					
23. Retinal detachment	S	S				
24. Retinal hemorrhages			S	S		
25. Uveitis		S	U	S		
26. Vitreous hemorrhage	U					
Laboratory Data						
1. Biopsy	U	U	U	U	U	U
2. Computed tomographic scan						
A. Diffuse radiodensity blends with normal structures		S				
B. Extraocular muscle enlargement		U		U		U
C. Orbital mass	U		U	U		U
3. Orbital roentgenogram						
A. Calcific densities						U
B. Diffusely enlarged orbit	U	U	U	U	U	
C. Enlargement of superior orbital fissure				U		
D. Erosion of optic canal	U					U
E. Frontal sinus bone dense/destruction						U
F. Osteolysis	U		U	U		
G. Periosteal reaction		U				
4. Ultrasonography						
A. Orbital mass			S	U	S	
B. Uniform dense diffuse mass		U		U		

R = rarely; S = sometimes; and U = usually.

Pulsating Exophthalmos (Most Common)

	Carotid-cavernous Aneurysm	Von-Recklinhausen Disease with Bony Defect of Skull	Large Frontal Mucocele	Meningoencephalocele	Blow-out Fracture of Orbital Root
History					
1. Activated at puberty, pregnancy, and menopause		S			
2. Congenital				U	
3. Diplopia			U		U
4. Hereditary		U			
5. Ocular pain	S				U
6. Slow progression	U				
7. Trauma					U
8. Unilateral	U	R	U		S
Physical Findings					
1. Cataracts		S			
2. Displacement of the globe		U	U	U	U
3. Elephantiasis of lids		U			
4. Hamartoma of retina		S			
5. Hydrophthalmos		S			
6. Hypertelorism				U	
7. Intraorbital hemorrhage					U
8. Lacrimation, excessive			U		
9. Lid ecchymosis/edema					U
10. Loss of facial sensation	U				
11. Mass fluctuant to palpation in the orbid				U	
12. Nodular swelling of corneal nerves		U			
13. Ophthalmoplegia	U				U
14. Optic atrophy		S			S
15. Optic nerve edema	S				
16. Orbital edema					U
17. Orbital emphysema					U
18. Ptosis		U			S
Laboratory Data					
1. Carotid angiography	U			S	
2. Cerebral arteriography	U				
3. Computed tomographic orbit scan	U	U	U	U	U
4. Pneumoencephalography	U			S	
5. Roentgenogram, orbit	U	U	U	U	U
6. Ultrasonography (ocular)			U		
7. Venography	S				

R = rarely; S = sometimes; and U = usually.

* = most important

Recurrent Exophthalmos

	Recurrent Ocular Inflammation or Hemorrhage	Orbital Cysts That Rupture	Lymphangioma	Syndrome of Intermittent Exophthalmos—Congenital Malformation of Orbit, Venous Angioma, Orbital Varix	Temporal Lobe Tumor with Orbital Extension	Neurofibromatosis	Vascular Neoplasms
History							
1. Alterations in visual field					U		
2. Apparently healthy individuals	U				U		
3. Associated with upper respiratory infection		S					
4. Congenital				S			
5. Diplopia	S		S	S			S
6. Hematologic history	U	R					
7. Hereditary						U	
8. More in males	S	S					U
9. Most in children					U		
10. Traumatic history		U	S				R
11. Unilateral	U	S	U		R		
12. Visual hallucinations					U		
Physical Findings							
1. Blood cysts of orbit	S	U	U				
2. Bluish color lids/conjunctiva							U
3. Conjunctival ecchymosis	U	R					
4. Ectropion uvea						U	
5. Glaucoma				S		S	S
6. Hemangioma conjunctiva/disc							U
7. Keratitis						S	S
8. Lid ecchymosis	U	R					
9. Narrowing of the palpebral fissure				U			
10. Neurofibroma of eyelids						U	
11. Nystagmus					S		S
12. Optic nerve atrophy			S	S	S	S	S
13. Prominent corneal nerves						S	
14. Ptosis		R			R	U	S
15. Pupil dilated				U			
16. Retrobulbar hemorrhage	S	R		R	R		S
17. Venous malformation in lids, fornix, and canthal areas				U			
18. Vitreous hemorrhage							S
Laboratory Data							
1. Carotid angiography					U		R
2. Complete blood count	U						
3. Computed tomographic scan	U	U	U		U	S	U
4. Histopathology			S	U	U	U	S
5. Ultrasonography	U	U	U		S	U	U
6. Venous angiography				U			
7. Roentgenogram (orbit and skull)		R		U	S	S	S

R = rarely; S = sometimes; and U = usually.

C. Migration of muscle cone implant

D. Herniated orbital fat secondary to an orbital fracture

7. Associated syndromes

    A. Arthrogryposis (amyoplasia congenita)

    B. Babinski-Nageotte syndrome (medullary tegmental paralysis)

    C. Cestan-Chenais syndrome (lesion in the lateral portion of medulla oblongata)

    D. Cockayne syndrome (dwarfism with retinal atrophy and deafness)

    E. Craniocervical syndrome (whiplash injury)

    F. Cretinism (hypothyroidism)

    G. Cryptophthalmia syndrome

    H. Dejean syndrome (orbital floor syndrome)

    I. Dejerine-Klumpke syndrome (thalamic hyperesthetic anesthesia)

    J. Freeman-Sheldon syndrome (craniocarpotarsal dysplasia)

    K. General fibrosis syndrome

    L. Greig syndrome (ocular hypertelorism syndrome)

    M. Hemifacial microsomia syndrome (François-Haustrate syndrome)

    N. Horner syndrome (cervical sympathetic paralysis syndrome)

    O. Klippel-Trenaunay-Weber syndrome (angio-osteohypertrophy syndrome)

    P. Krause syndrome (encephalo-ophthalmic syndrome)

    Q. Maple syrup urine disease (branched chain ketoaciduria)

    R. Morquio syndrome (MPS IV)

    S. Naffziger syndrome (scalenus anticus syndrome)

    T. Pancoast syndrome (superior pulmonary sulcus syndrome)

    U. Parry-Romberg syndrome (progressive facial hemiatrophy)

    V. Passow syndrome (Bremer status dysraphicus)

    W. Raeder syndrome (paratrigeminal paralysis)

    X. Retroparotid space syndrome

    Y. Vernet syndrome (jugular foramen syndrome)

    Z. von Herrenschwand syndrome (sympathetic heterochromia)

    AA. Wallenberg syndrome (dorsolateral medullary syndrome)

8. Apparent enophthalmos with horizontal conjugate gaze

9. Metastatic adenocarcinoma of orbit (cicatricial)

10. Neurofibromatosis: pulsating enophthalmos

11. Typhoid fever (abdominal typhus)

Albert, D.M. and Jakobiec, F.A.: Principles and Practice of Ophthalmology. Philadelphia. W.B. Saunders Co. 1881–2095, 1994.

Baylis, H.I., and Call, N.B.: Severe enophthalmos following irradiation of the anophthalmic socket: surgical approaches. Ophthalmology, 86:1647, 1982.

Bello, V.M., and Levine, M.R.: Superior sulcus deformity. Arch. Ophthalmol., 98:2215, 1980.

Cline, R.A.,and Rootman, J.: Enophthalmos: A clinical review. Ophthalmology, 91:229–237, 1984.

Roy, F.H.: Ocular Syndromes and Systemic Diseases. 2nd Ed. Philadelphia, W.B. Saunders, 1989.

Stasior, O.G., and Roen, J.L.: Traumatic enophthalmos. Ophthalmology, 89:1267, 1982.

Wilkins, R.B., and Kulwin, D.R.: Spontaneous enophthalmos associated with chronic maxillary sinusitis. Ophthalmology, 88:981, 1981.

Intraorbital Calcifications

1. Calcification of more irregular configuration and texture
   - A. Cysticercosis
   - B. Orbital hematoma
   - C. Plexiform neurofibroma
   - D. Toxoplasmosis
   - E. Tuberculosis
2. Calcification of orbital vessels
   - A. Atheromatous plaque
   - B. Monkeberg sclerosis
   - C. Secondary to metabolic-endocrine disturbances such as hyperparathyroidism or hypervitaminosis
   - D. Band-shaped keratopathy
3. Chronic inflammatory and parasitic disease of the orbit
4. Hemangiopericytoma
5. Intraocular calcifications following
   - A. Congenital deformity
   - B. Malignant lacrimal gland tumor
   - C. Recurrent iritis and keratitis
   - D. Retinal detachment
   - E. Trauma (perforating, nonperforating, or surgical)
6. Intraocular sarcoma
7. Mucocele
8. Myositis ossificans
9. Orbital phleboliths: helical form in veins—smooth, round, or oval
10. Organized hematomas of the orbit
*11. Retinoblastoma
12. Retrolental fibroplasia
13. Sites of intraocular calcification
    - A. Cyclitic membrane
    - B. Lens
    - C. Peripapillary choroid
    - D. Posterior pole to ora serrata in region of choroid and pigment epithelium
    - E. Retina
    - F. Vitreous

Albert, D.M. and Jakobiec, F.A.: Principles and Practice of Ophthalmology. Philadelphia. W.B. Saunders Co. 1881–2095, 1994.

Basta, L.L., et al.: Focal choroidal calcification. Ann. Ophthalmol., 13:447–450, 1981.

Garrity, J.A., and Kennerdell, J.S.: Orbital calcification associated with hemangiopericytoma. Am. J. Ophthalmol., 102:126, 1986.

Zizmor J., and Lombardi, G.: Atlas of Orbital Radiology. Birmingham, Aesculapius, 1973.

Orbital Bruit (Noise Heard over Orbit with Stethoscope)

1. Bilateral

    A. Hyperthyroidism

    B. Severe anemias

2. Unilateral

    *A. Abnormal communication in the cavernous sinus, i.e. bilateral carotid-cavernous sinus

    B. Aneurysmal angioma of orbit or fundus such as in Wyburn-Mason syndrome (Bonnet-Dechaume-Blanc syndrome)

    C. Arteriovenous aneurysm (arteriovenous fistula)

    D. Intermittent or pulsating exophthalmos

    E. Stenosis of carotid artery including thrombosis, sclerosis, or external pressure such as that due to an outer-ridge sphenoidmeningioma

Albert, D.M. and Jakobiec, F.A.: Principles and Practice of Ophthalmology. Philadelphia. W.B. Saunders Co. 1881–2095, 1994.

Grobb, W.E., et al.: Facial Hamantomas in Children: Neurofibroma, lymphangioma and hemangiomia. Plast. Reconstr. Surg. 66: 509, 1980.

Kushner, F.H.: Carotid-cavernous fistula as a complication of carotid endarterectomy. Ann. Ophthalmol., 13:979, 1981.

Lloyd, G.A: Vascular anomalies in the Orbit: C T and Angiographic diagnosis. Orbit 1: 45, 1982.

Malzone, W.F., and Gonyea, E.F.: Exophthalmos with intracranial arteriovenous malformations. Neurology, 28:531–538, 1973.

Murali, R., et al.: Intraorbital arteriovenous malformation with spontaneous thrombosis. Ann. Ophthalmol., 13:457, 1981.

Orbital Bruit (Noise Heard over Orbit with Stethoscope)

	Hyperthyroidism	Severe Anemias	Arteriovenous Aneurysm	Stenosis of Carotid Artery	Aneurysmal Angiomas of Orbit or Fundus	Abnormal Communication in Cavernous Sinus	Intermittent or Pulsating Exophthalmos
History							
1. Amaurosis fugax				U			
2. Bilateral	U	S					S
3. Congenital						S	S
4. Diplopia	S						
5. Familial	U						
6. Middle age	U				U		
7. Older patients				U			
8. Traumatic						U	S
Physical Findings							
1. Arteriovenous malformations of retina					U	S	S
2. Central or branch retinal artery occlusion				U			
3. Chemosis of conjunctiva	S					U	S
4. Conjunctival vessels dilated						U	S
5. Cotton-wool spots		U			U		
6. Enlargement periorbital veins of lids, forehead, temple						S	U
7. Exposure keratopathy	S						
8. Hollenhorst plaques				U			
9. Increased intraocular pressure						U	S
10. Increased lid pigmentation	U						
11. Infrequent blinking	U						
12. Lid edema	S						
13. Lid lag	U						
14. Neurofibromas in lids, conjunctiva, and cornea							S
15. Nodules in iris							S
16. Ophthalmoplegia	S						
17. Restriction of extraocular myaels	U						
18. Papilledema		U					
19. Retinal hemorrhage		S	U	S			
20. Retraction of upper lid	U						
21. Tremor of closed lids	U						
Laboratory Data							
1. Carotid arteriography					S		
2. Cerebral angiography					U	U	
3. Computed tomographic scan	U						
4. Orbital ultrasonogram	U						
5. Orbital venography							U
6. Orbital roentgenogram							S
7. Platelet levels and hemoglobin low counts		U					
8. T3–T4	U						

R = rarely; S = sometimes; and U = usually.

Orbital Emphysema (Air Found in Orbital Tissues and Adnexa Usually Demonstrable by Palpation)

*1. Due to fracture of ethmoid sinuses or orbital floor

2. Following forceful blowing of nose

3. Injury from compressed air

4. Orbital cellulitis and abscess with gas formation by infecting organism

5. Osteomyelitis and infected sinus with fistulous communication with gas formation by infecting organism

6. Resulting from use of high-speed dental drill and air-water spray during oral operation

7. Subconjunctival emphysema seen with mechanical ventilation

Buckley, M.J., et al.: Orbital emphysema causing vision loss after a dental extraction. J. Amer. Dental Assoc. 120: 421–422, 1990.

Hunts, J.H., et al.: Orbital emphysema. Staging and acute management. Ophthal.101: 960–966, 1994.

Zimmer-Galler, I.E., and Bartley, G.B.: Orbital Emphysema: case reports and review of the literature. Mayo Clinic Proceedings. 69: 115–121, 1994.

Orbital Pain

1. Acute dacryoadenitis

2. Amputation neuroma of the orbit

3. Associated syndromes

    A. Cavernous sinus thrombosis syndrome

    B. Charlin syndrome (nasal nerves syndrome)

    C. Erysipelas

    D. Ophthalmoplegic migraine syndrome

    E. Raeder syndrome (paratrigeminal paralysis)

    F. Tolosa-Hunt syndrome (painful ophthalmoplegia)

4. Break-bone fever (dengue fever)

5. Clostridium perfringens

6. Eye strain from uncorrected errors of refraction

7. Myositis

    A. Collagen diseases

    B. Infectious myositis

    C. Trichinosis

8. Orbital cellulitis or abscess

9. Orbital periostitis because of injury, tuberculosis, syphilis, extension of sinus disease, or other conditions

*10. Pseudotumor or tumor of the orbit—pain infrequently present

11. Retrobulbar neuritis

12. Trauma

13. Tumors of cerebellopontine angle, frequent lesion of seventh nerve

* = most important

Albert, D.M. and Jakobiec, F.A.: Principles and Practice of Ophthalmology. Philadelphia. W.B. Saunders Co. 1881–2095, 1994.

Bullen, C.L., and Younge, B.R.: Chronic orbital myositis. Ophthalmology, 89:1749, 1982.

Kline, L.B.: The Tolosa-Hunt syndrome. Surv. Ophthalmol., 27:79, 1982.

Lanzino, G., et al.: Orbital pain and unruptured carotid-posterior communicating artery aneurysms: the role of sensory fibers of the third cranial nerve. Acta Neurochirurgica. 120: 7–11, 1993.

Roy, F.H.: Ocular Syndromes and Systemic Diseases. 2nd Ed. Philadelphia, W.B. Saunders, 1989.

Shallow Orbits or Diminished Orbital Volume (Illusion of Proptosis or Glaucoma)

1. Aminopterin-induced syndrome
2. Apert syndrome (acrocephalosyndactyly)
3. Carpenter syndrome
4. Cerebrohepatorenal syndrome (Smith-Lemli-Opitz syndrome)
5. Craniostenosis
6. Crouzon disease (dysostosis craniofacialis)
7. Diseases of nasal passages and sinuses
    A. Dentigenous cysts
    B. Fibrous dysplasia (Albright syndrome)
    C. Hypoplasia of maxilla associated with chronic maxillary sinusitis
    D. Rhinoscleroma
8. Dubowitz syndrome
9. Early enucleation of eye
*10. Familial hypoplasia of orbital margin
11. Frontometaphyseal dysplasia (FMD)
12. Hyperostosis (hypertrophy of orbital bones)
13. Hypophosphatasia—harlequin orbit (shallow orbit with arched superior and lateral wall)
14. Kleeblattschädel syndrome
15. Lateral displacement of medial orbital wall by hypertrophic polypoid nasal sinus disease
16. Marshall-Smith syndrome
17. Oculoauriculovertebral dysplasia (Goldenhar syndrome)
18. Osteogenesis imperfecta (van der Hoeve syndrome)
19. Radiation injury of bone
20. Robert syndrome (pseudothalidomide syndrome)
21. Saethre-Chotzen syndrome
22. Secondary to fracture
23. Stanesco dysostosis syndrome
24. Trisomy 13-(trisomy D) (Patau syndrome)
25. Trisomy (Edward syndrome)
26. Zellweger syndrome

27. 6q- D syndrome
28. 9p- syndrome

Roy, F.H.: Ocular Syndromes and Systemic Diseases. 2nd Ed. Philadelphia, W.B. Saunders, 1989.

Smith, D.W.: Recognizable Patterns of Human Malformation. 4th Ed. Philadelphia, W.B. Saunders, 1988.

Pseudohypertelorism (Illusion of Increased Distance between Bony Orbits and Increased Interpupillary Distance)

1. Blepharophimosis
*2. Epicanthal skin folds
3. Exotropia
*4. Flat nasal bridge of nose
5. Increased distance between the inner canthi (telecanthus)
6. Widely spaced eyebrows

DeMyer, W.: The median cleft face syndrome. Neurology, 17:961, 1967.

Hypertelorism (Increased Distance between Bony Orbits and Increased Interpupillary Distance)

1. Aarskog syndrome (facial-digital-genital syndrome)
2. Acrocollosal syndrome
3. Acrodysostosis syndrome
4. Albers-Schonberg disease (osteopetrosis)
5. Aminopterin-induced syndrome
*6. Apert syndrome (acrodysplasia)
*7. Association of hypertelorism, microtia, and facial clefting
*8. Baraitser-Winter syndrome
9. BBB syndrome (hypertelorism-hypospadias syndrome)
10. Blatt syndrome (cranio-orbito-ocular dysraphia)
11. Blepharonosofacial syndrome
12. Camptomelic dysplasia syndrome
13. Carpenter syndrome (acrocephalopolysyndactyly II)
14. Cat-eye syndrome (Schachenmann syndrome)
15. Cerebral gigantism (Sotos syndrome)
16. Cerebrohepatorenal syndrome (Zellweger)
17. Cherubism
18. Chromosome partial long-arm deletion syndrome (de Grouchy syndrome)
19. Chromosome partial short-arm deletion syndrome (monosomy partial [short-arm] syndrome)
20. Chromosome short-arm deletion
21. Chondrodystrophia calcificans congenita (Conradi syndrome)
22. Cleft lip and palate sequence

* = most important

23. Clefting, ectropion, and conical teeth syndrome
24. Cleidocranial dysostosis syndrome
25. Coffin Lowry syndrome
26. Congenital hemihypertrophy
27. Craniocarpotarsal syndrome (Freeman-Sheldon syndrome)
28. Craniocleidodysostosis syndrome (Marie-Sainton syndrome)
29. Craniosynostosis-radial aplasia (Baller-Gerold syndrome)
30. Cretinism (hypothyroidism)
31. Cri du chat syndrome (Cry of the cat syndrome)
32. Crouzon disease (dysostosis craniofacialis)
33. Cryptophthalmos syndrome
34. Curtius syndrome (ectodermal dysplasia with ocular malformations)
35. DiGeorge sequence
36. Down syndrome (mongolism)
37. Dubowitz syndrome (dwarfism-eczema-peculiar facies)
38. Ehlers-Danlos syndrome (fibrodysplasia elastica generalisata)
39. Engelmann syndrome (diaphyseal dysplasia)
40. Facio-oculoacousticorenal syndrome
41. Familial characteristic
42. Familial metaphyseal dysplasia (Pyle disease)
43. Fetal alcohol syndrome
44. Fetal aminopterin effects
45. Fetal hydantoin effects
46. Fish odor syndrome
47. Frontonasal dysplasia syndrome (median cleft face syndrome)
48. Frontal encephaloceles
49. Gorlin syndrome (orodigitofacial dysostosis)
50. Greig syndrome (hypertelorism)
51. Haney-Falls syndrome (congenital keratoconus posticus circumscriptus)
52. Holt-Oram syndrome
53. Hurler syndrome (MPS I-H)
54. Hydrocephalus
55. Hypomelanosis of Ito syndrome (systematized achromic nevus)
56. Ichthyosis (collodion baby)
57. Infantile gigantism
58. Infantile hypercalcemia with supravalvular aortic stenosis (Williams-Beuren syndrome)
59. Iris dysplasia-hypertelorism-psychomotor retardation syndrome
60. Jacobs' syndrome (triple X syndrome)
61. KBG syndrome (initials of family studied)

62. Kleeblattschädel syndrome (extreme hydrocephalus syndrome)

63. Klein syndrome

64. Klinefelter XXY syndrome (gynecomastia-aspermatogenesis syndrome)

65. Klippel-Feil syndrome (synostosis cervical vertebrae)

66. Larsen syndrome

67. Leprechaunism

68. Lissencephalia (Miller-Dieker syndrome)

69. Little syndrome (nail-patella syndrome)

70. Mandibulofacial dysostosis (Franceschetti syndrome)

71. Maple syrup urine disease (branched chain ketoaciduria)

72. Marfan syndrome (arachnodactyly-dystrophia-mesodermalis congenita)

73. Meckel-Gruber syndrome

74. Melnick-Needles syndrome (osteodysplasty)

75. Metaphyseal dysostosis (Jansen disease)

76. McFarland syndrome

77. Morquio-Ullrich syndrome (MPS IV)

78. Multiple basal cell nevi (Gorlin-Goltz syndrome)

79. Multiple lentigenes syndrome (Leopard syndrome)

80. Myelomeningocele-Chiari malformations

81. Noonan syndrome (male Turner syndrome)

82. Oculodentodigital syndrome

83. Oculomandibulofacial dyscephaly (Hallermann-Streiff syndrome)

84. Optic nerve hypoplasia

85. Orofaciodigital (OFD) type I and type II (Mohr syndrome)

86. Osteogenesis imperfecta (van der Hoeves syndrome)

87. Otopalatodigital syndrome (OPD syndrome)

88. Pena-shokeir type I syndrome

89. Pfeiffer syndrome

90. Potter syndrome (renofacial syndrome)

91. Ring B chromosome

92. Ring chromosome

93. Rieger syndrome (dysgenesis mesostromalis)

94. Robert syndrome (pseudothalidomide syndrome)

95. Robinow syndrome (fetal face syndrome)

96. Saethre-Chotzen syndrome (acrocephalosyndactyly type III)

97. Sjögren-Larson syndrome (oligophrenia-ichthyosis-spastic diplegia syndrome)

98. Sprengel syndrome

99. Traumatic naso-orbital fracture

100. Triploidy syndrome

101. Trisomy syndrome

102. Trisomy 9q syndrome

103. Trisomy 13-(Patau's syndrome)

104. Trisomy syndrome

105. Turner-Bonnevie-Ullrich-Nielsen syndrome

106. Turner syndrome (gonadal dysgenesis)

107. Waardenburg syndrome (embryonic fixation syndrome)

108. Weaver syndrome

109. Williams syndrome

110. XXXX syndrome

111. XXXXX syndrome

112. XXXXY syndrome

113. 4p- syndrome (Wolf syndrome)

114. 4p- D syndrome

115. 6p- D syndrome

116. 9p- syndrome

117. 10q- syndrome

118. 13q- syndrome

119. 18q- syndrome

Chrousos, G.A., et al.: Ocular findings in Turner syndrome. Ophthalmology, 91:926–928, 1984.

DeJong, P., et al.: Medullated nerve fibers: A sign of multiple basal cell nevi (Gorlin's) syndrome. Arch. Ophthalmol., 103:1833–1836, 1985.

Isenberg, S.J.: The Eye in Infancy. Chicago, Year Book Medical Publishers, 1989.

McKusick, V.A.: Mendelian Inheritance in Man. 9th Ed. Baltimore, Johns Hopkins University Press, 1994.

Pallotta, R.: Iris coloboma ptosis, hypertelorism, and mental retardation: a new syndrome posibly localized on chromosome 2. Journal of Medical Genetics. 28: 342–344.1991.

Roy, F.H.: Ocular Syndromes and Systemic Diseases. 2nd Ed. Philadelphia, W.B. Saunders, 1989.

Seaver, L.H. and Cassidy S.B.: New Syndrome: mother and son with hypertelorism, downslanting palpebral fissures, malar hypoplasia, and apparently low-set ears associated with joint and scrotal anomalies. American Journal Medical Genetics. 41: 405–409, 1991.

Verloes, A.: Iris coloboma, ptosis, hypertelorism, and mental retardation: Baraitser-Winter syndrome or Noonan syndrome. Journal of Medical Genetics. 30: 425–426, 1993.

Hypotelorism (Decreased Distance between Bony Orbits and Decreased Interpupillary Distance)

1. Arrhinencephaly (holoprosencephaly)

2. Cebocephalia

3. Cockayne syndrome (dwarfism with retinal atrophy and deafness)

4. Coffin-Siris syndrome

5. Ethmocephalus

*6. Familial

7. François diencephalic syndrome (Hallerman-Streiff syndrome)

8. Goldenhar syndrome (oculoauriculovertebral dysplasia)

9. Maternal phenylketonuria fetal effects

10. Meckel-Gruber syndrome

11. Median cleft lip (frontonasal dysplasia syndrome)

12. Median philtrum-premaxilla anlage

13. Ocular-dental-digital dysplasia (Meyer-Schivickerath and Weyers syndrome)

14. Ring syndrome

15. Trigonocephaly (C syndrome, Opitz trigonocephaly syndrome)

16. Trisomy 13-(Patau syndrome, trisomy D syndrome)

17. Trisomy 20p syndrome

18. Trisomy (Down syndrome, mongolism)

19. Turner syndrome (gonadal dysgenesis)

20. Williams syndrome

21. Wolf syndrome (monosomy partial syndrome)

22. 5p- D syndrome

23. 18p- syndrome

Evans, D.G.: Dominantly inherited microcephaly, hypotelorism and normal intelligence. Clinical Genetics. 39: 178–180, 1991.

Isenberg, S.J.: The Eye in Infancy. Chicago, Year Book Medical Publishers, 1989. Judisch, G.F., et al.: Orbital hypotelorism. Arch. Ophthalmol., 102:995–997, 1984.

Richieri-Costa, A., et al.: Mental retardation, microbrachycephaly, hypotelorism, palpebral ptosis, thin/long face, cleft lip, and lumbosacral/pelvic anomalies. American Journal of Medical Genetics. 43: 565–568, 1992.

Roy, F.H.: Ocular Syndromes and Systemic Diseases. 2nd Ed. Philadelphia, W.B. Saunders, 1989.

Deep-set Eyes

1. Cockayne syndrome (dwarfism with retinal atrophy and deafness)

2. Craniocarpotarsal syndrome (Freeman-Sheldon syndrome) *

3. Familial

4. Marfan syndrome (dolichostenomelia-arachnodactylyhyperchon-droplasia-dystrophia mesodermalis congenita)

5. Mesodermal dysmorphodystrophy (Weill-Marchesani syndrome)

6. Oculocerebrorenal syndrome (Lowe syndrome)

7. Pycnodysostosis

8. Syndrome of blepharophimosis with myopathy

Aita, J.A.: Congenital Facial Anomalies with Neurologic Defects. Springfield, Ill., Charles C. Thomas, 1969.

Prominent Supraorbital Ridges

1. Apert syndrome (acrocephalosyndactylism syndrome)

2. Basal cell nevus syndrome (Gorlin-Goltz syndrome)

3. Cleidocranial dysostosis (Marie Sainton syndrome)

4. Congenital lipodystrophy

* = most important

5. Congenital syphilis (congenital lues)

6. Ectodermal dysplasia (Curtius syndrome)

*7. Frontometaphyseal dysplasia

8. Hurler syndrome (MPS I-H)

9. Marfan syndrome (arachnodactyly-dystrophia mesodermalis congenita)

10. Otopalatodigital syndrome (Taybi syndrome)

11. Pyle metaphyseal dysplasia syndrome

Albert, D.M. and Jakobiec, F.A.: Principles and Practice of Ophthalmology. Philadelphia. W.B. Saunders Co. 1881–2095, 1994.

Roy, F.H.: Ocular Syndromes and Systemic Diseases. 2nd Ed. Philadelphia, W.B. Saunders, 1989.

Stern, S.D., et al.: The ocular and cosmetic problems in frontometaphyseal dysplasia. J. Pediatr. Ophthalmol., 9:151–161, 1972.

Wilson, F.M., et al.: Corneal changes in ectodermal dysplasia: Case report, histopathology, and differential diagnosis. Am. J. Ophthalmol., 75:17–27, 1973.

Osteolysis of Bony Orbit

1. Autoimmune diseases, such as Wegener granulomatosis

2. Congenital

3. Hyperparathyroidism

4. Injury, such as blow-out fracture of orbital floor

5. Meningocele and encephalocele of orbit

6. Metastasis from remote primary neoplasms

7. Primary orbital disease

   A. Infectious, including tuberculosis and syphilis

   B. Neoplastic, including neurofibroma and lacrimal gland tumor

   C. Cystic, including dermoid and epidermoid cyst

8. Reticuloendotheliosis as histiocytosis X (Hand-Schüller-Christian disease)

9. Secondary extension of infectious or neoplastic disease from adjacent sinuses, brain, skin, bone, and nasopharynx

10. Sinus disease including mucoceles

Albert, D.M. and Jakobiec, F.A.: Principles and Practice of Ophthalmology. Philadelphia. W.B. Saunders Co. 1881–2095, 1994.

Jacobs, L., et al.: Computerized Tomography of the Orbit and Sella. Turcica, New York. Raven, 1980.

Margo, C.E., et al.: Psammomatoid ossifying fibroma. Arch. Ophthalmol., 107:1347–1351, 1986.

Fossa Formation of Orbit (Local Expansion of Bony Orbital Wall Caused by Persistent Pressure; Bony Cortex is Intact)

1. Encapsulated benign lacrimal gland tumor

2. Encapsulated malignant lacrimal gland tumor

3. Orbital dermoid

Albert, D.M. and Jakobiec, F.A.: Principles and Practice of Ophthalmology. Philadelphia. W.B. Saunders Co. 1881–2095, 1994.

Jacobs, L., et al.: Computerized Tomography of the Orbit and Sella Turcica. New York, Raven Press, 1980.

Zizmor, J.: Orbital Radiology in Unilateral Exophthalmos. In Turtz, A.I. Proceedings of the Centennial Symposium; Manhattan Eye, Ear, and Throat Hospital. Vol. I. St. Louis, C.V. Mosby, 1969.

Expansion of Orbital Margins (Usually Associated with Benign Tumors of the Orbit)

1. Dermoid
2. Hemangioma
3. Lacrimal gland tumors
4. Meningioma
5. Neurofibroma

Albert, D.M. and Jakobiec, F.A.: Principles and Practice of Ophthalmology. Philadelphia. W.B. Saunders Co. 1881–2095, 1994.

Coleman, D.J., et al.: Ultrasonography of the Eye and Orbit. Philadelphia, Lea & Febiger, 1977.

Zizmor, J.: Orbital Radiology in Unilateral Exophthalmos. In Turtz, A. I. (ed.): Proceedings of the Centennial Symposium: Manhattan Eye, Ear, and Throat Hospital. Vol. I. St. Louis, C.V. Mosby, 1969.

Hypertrophy of Orbital Bones (Hyperostosis and/or Sclerosis)

1. Acromegaly
2. Anemias of childhood (severe: Cooley, sickle cell, spherocytosis, iron deficiency)
3. Cerebral atrophy (childhood)
4. Craniostenosis
5. Engelmann disease (hereditary diaphyseal dysplasia)
6. Hyperostosis frontalis interna
7. Idiopathic
8. Infantile cortical hyperostosis (Caffey disease)
9. Microcephaly
10. Myotonia atrophica (myotonic dystrophy, Curschmann-Steinert syndrome)
11. Osteopetrosis (Albers-Schönberg disease)
12. Paget disease (osteitis deformans)
13. Tumors of orbit, including osteoma, fibrous dysplasia (Albright syndrome), meningioma, metastatic neuroblastoma, mixed tumors of lacrimal gland, transitional cell carcinomas of the nasopharynx

Albert, D.M. and Jakobiec, F.A.: Principles and Practice of Ophthalmology. Philadelphia. W.B. Saunders Co. 1881–2095, 1994.

Jacobs, L. et al.: Computerized Tomography of the Orbit and Sella Turcica. New York, Raven, 1980.

Minton, L.R., and Elliot, J.H.: Ocular manifestations of infantile cortical hyperostosis. Am. J. Ophthalmol., 64:902, 1967.

Morse, P.H., et al.: Ocular findings in hereditary diaphyseal dysplasia (Engelmann's disease. Am. J. Ophthalmol., 68:100–104,1969.

Teplick, J.G., and Hoskin, M.E.: Roentgenologic Diagnosis. 3rd Ed. Philadelphia, W.B. Saunders, 1976.

* = most important

Expansion of Optic Canal

1. Increased intracranial pressure
2. Inflammatory lesions
   A. Chiasmatic arachnoiditis
   B. Nonspecific granuloma
   C. Sarcoid granuloma
   D. Tuberculoma
3. Tumors
   A. Meningioma
   B. Metastatic sarcoma to choroid
   C. Neurofibromatosis (von Recklinghausen syndrome)
   D. Optic nerve glioma
   E. Retinoblastoma
4. Vascular lesions
   A. Arteriovenous malformation
   B. Ophthalmic artery aneurysm

Levin, L.A. and Rubin, P.D: Advances in Orbital Imaging. Int. Ophthal. Clin. 32: 1–25, 1992.

Potter, G.D., and Trakel, S.L.: Optic canal. In Newton, T.H., and Potts, D.G. (eds.): Radiology of the Skull and Brain. Vol. 1. Book 2. St. Louis, C.V. Mosby, 1971.

Zizmor, J.: Orbital radiology in unilateral exophthalmos. In Turtz, A.I. (ed.): Proceedings of the Centennial Symposium: Manhattan Eye, Ear, and Throat Hospital. Vol. I. St. Louis, C.V. Mosby, 1969.

Small Optic Canals

1. Developmental abnormalities
   A. Anophthalmos or microphthalmos
   B. Enucleation
   C. Craniosynostosis (CSO)
2. Dysostoses
   A. Osteopetrosis (Albers-Schönberg syndrome)
   B. Fibrous dysplasia (Albright syndrome)
   C. Pyle disease (craniometaphyseal dysplasia syndrome)
   D. Paget disease (osteitis deformans)
3. Inflammatory lesions—osteitis
4. Tumor—meningioma

Albert, D.M. and Jakobiec, F.A.: Principles and Practice of Ophthalmology. Philadelphia. W.B. Saunders Co. 1881–2095, 1994.

Potter, G.D., and Trakel, S.L.: Optic canal. In Newton, T.H., and Potts, D.G. (eds.): Radiology of the Skull and Brain. Vol. 1. Book 2. St. Louis, C.V. Mosby, 1971.

Erosion of Optic Canal

1. Lateral wall

    A. Pituitary tumor

    B. Aneurysm of internal carotid artery

    C. Craniopharyngioma

    D. Tumor of orbital apex

2. Medial wall

    A. Carcinoma of sphenoid sinus

    B. Mucocele of sphenoid sinus

    C. Granuloma of sphenoid sinus

3. Roof

    A. Tumor of anterior cranial fossa

    B. Surgical unroofing

4. Decrease in length

    A. Tumor of orbital apex

5. Complete destruction

    A. Malignant tumor

    B. Eosinophilic granuloma

Albert, D.M. and Jakobiec, F.A.: Principles and Practice of Ophthalmology. Philadelphia. W.B. Saunders Co. 1881–2095, 1994.

Potter, G.D., and Trakel, S.L.: Optic canal. In Newton, T.H., and Potts, D.G. (eds.): Radiology of the Skull and Brain. Vol. 1. Book 2. St. Louis, C.V. Mosby, 1971.

Zizmor, J.: Orbital radiology in unilateral exophthalmos. In Turtz, A.I. (ed.): Proceedings of the Centennial Symposium: Manhattan Eye, Ear, and Throat Hospital. Vol. I. St. Louis, C.V. Mosby, 1969.

Enlargement of Superior Orbital Fissure

1. Carotid cavernous fistula

2. Chronic increased intracranial pressure

3. Extension of infraorbital mass into fissure

4. Intracavernous carotid aneurysm

5. Intracranial chordoma

6. Masses within middle fossa

7. Metastatic carcinoma to sphenoid wings

8. Nasopharyngeal carcinoma—rare

9. Neurofibromatosis including optic nerve glioma

10. Orbital dysplasia

11. Orbital varix

12. Pituitary neoplasm—changes in sella and clinoid process

13. Posterior orbital encephalocele

14. Sarcomas, neurilemoma, or other orbital malignancies

Albert, D.M. and Jakobiec, F.A.: Principles and Practice of Ophthalmology. Philadelphia. W.B. Saunders Co. 1881–2095, 1994.

Ferry, A.P., et al.: Orbital invasion by an intracranial chordoma. Am. J. Ophthalmol., 92:7–12, 1981.

Grimson, B.S., and Perry, D.D.: Enlargement of the optic disk in childhood optic nerve tumors. Am. J. Ophthalmol., 97:627–631, 1984.

Shields, J.A., et al.: Orbital neurilemoma with extension through the superior orbital fissure. Arch. Ophthalmol., 104:871–873, 1986.

Narrowing of the Superior Orbital Fissure

1. Chronic hemolytic anemias of childhood
2. Fibrous dysplasia (Albright syndrome)
3. Meningioma
4. Osteitis
5. Osteoblastoma
6. Osteoma
7. Osteopetrosis (Albers-Schönberg syndrome)
8. Paget disease (osteitis deformans)

Albert, D.M. and Jakobiec, F.A.: Principles and Practice of Ophthalmology. Philadelphia. W.B. Saunders Co. 1881–2095, 1994.

Jacobs, L., et al.: Computerized Tomography of the Orbit and Sella Turcica. New York, Raven Press, 1980.

Kieffer, S.A.: Superior orbital fissure. In Newton, T.H., and Potts, D.G. (eds.): Radiology of the Skull and Brain. Vol. 1. Book 2. St. Louis, C.V. Mosby, 1971.

Small Orbit

1. Anophthalmos
2. Enucleation
3. Microphthalmos
4. Mucocele

Kieffer, S.A.: Orbit. In Newton, T.H., and Potts, D.G. (eds.): Radiology of the Skull and Brain. Vol.1. Book 2. St. Louis, C.V. Mosby, 1971.

Sarnat, B.G.: Eye and orbital size in the young and adult. Ophthalmologica, 185:74–89, 1982.

Large Orbit

1. Congenital
    A. Dysplasia
    B. Glaucoma
    C. Serous cysts
2. Pseudotumor
3. Tumors within muscle cone
    A. Hemangiomas
    B. Neurofibroma
    C. Optic glioma
    D. Orbital varix
    E. Retinoblastoma

Albert, D.M. and Jakobiec, F.A.: Principles and Practice of Ophthalmology. Philadelphia. W.B. Saunders Co. 1881–2095, 1994.

Kieffer, S.A.: Orbit. In Newton, T.H., and Potts D.G. (eds.): Radiology of the Skull and Brain. Vol. 1. Book 2. St. Louis, C.V. Mosby, 1971.

Hematic Orbital Cysts (Blood Cyst of Orbit)

1. Blood dyscrasia
2. Cavernous hemangioma
3. Childbirth
4. Lymphangioma
5. Orbital blunt trauma
6. Spontaneous hemorrhage
7. Vascular disease

Albert, D.M. and Jakobiec, F.A.: Principles and Practice of Ophthalmology. Philadelphia. W.B. Saunders Co. 1881–2095, 1994.

Jacobson, D.M., et al.: Maternal orbital hematoma associated with labor. Am. J. Ophthalmol. 105:547–553, 1988.

Shapiro, A., et al.: A clinicopathologic study of hematic cysts of the orbit. Am. J. Ophthalmol., 102:237–241, 1986.

Lids

BHUPENDRA PATEL MD

Contents

Mongoloid Palpebral Fissure (Temporal Canthus Is Higher Than Nasal Canthus)

1. A esotropia syndrome
2. A exotropia syndrome
3. Amniogenic band syndrome (Streeter dysplasia)
4. Anhidrotic ectodermal dysplasia
5. Cebocephalia (fetalis hypoplastica)
6. Chondrodystrophia (Conradi syndrome)
7. Chromosome short-arm deletion

8. Congenital spherocytic anemia

9. Crouzon syndrome (hereditary craniofacial dysostosis)

10. Femoral-facial syndrome

11. Fetal hydantoin syndrome

12. Hereditary ectodermal dysplasia syndrome (Siemen syndrome)

13. Jacobs syndrome (triple X syndrome)

14. Jarcho-Levin syndrome

15. Klinefelter XXY syndrome (gynecomastia-aspermatogenesis syndrome)

16. Laurence-Moon-Biedl syndrome *(retinitis pigmentosa-polydactyl-adiposogenital syndrome)

17. Meckel syndrome (dysencephalia-splanchnocystic syndrome)

18. Miller-Dieker syndrome

*19. Mongoloid (trisomy or Down syndrome)

*20. Orientals

21. Peters' trisomy 5p (Peters' anomaly)

22. Oto-palatao-digital syndrome

23. Pfeiffer syndrome

24. Pleonosteosis syndrome (Leri syndrome, carpal tunnel syndrome)

25. Prader-Willi syndrome

26. Rhizomelic chondrodysplasia punctata syndrome

27. Trisomy mosaic and 9p- syndromes

28. Trisomy syndrome

29. Trisomy and 18q syndrome

30. Trisomy 20p syndrome

31. XXXXX syndrome

32. XXXXY syndrome

33. 4p- syndrome

34. 5p- syndrome

Isenberg, S.J. The Eye in Infancy. Chicago, Year Book Medical Publishers, 1989.

Roy, F.H.: Ocular Syndromes and Systemic Diseases. 2nd Ed. Philadelphia, W.B. Saunders, 1989.

Antimongoloid Palpebral Fissure (Downward Displacement of Temporal Canthus)

1. Aarskog syndrome (facial-digital-genital syndrome)

2. Acrocephalosyndactylia (Apert syndrome)

3. A esotropia and A exotropia

4. Bird-headed dwarf syndrome (Seckel syndrome)

5. Cardio-facio cutaneous syndrome

6. Cerebral gigantism (Sotos syndrome)

7. Cleft-palate

8. Chromosome short-arm deletion

9. Cloverleaf cranium

10. Coffin-Lowry syndrome

11. Cohen syndrome

12. Congenital facial hemiatrophy (Mobius syndrome)

13. Craniocarpotarsal dysplasia (Freeman-Sheldon syndrome; whistling face syndrome)

14. Craniofacial dysostosis (Crouzon syndrome)

15. Cri du chat syndrome (cat cry syndrome)

16. De Lange syndrome (congenital muscular hypertrophy-cerebral syndrome)

17. Di George syndrome

18. Epidermal nevus syndrome (ichthyosis hystrix)

19. Lethal multiple pterygium syndrome (LMPS)

20. Linear nevus sebaceous of Jadassohn (Jadassohn-type anetoderma)

21. Mandibulofacial dysostosis (Franceschetti syndrome and Treacher-Collins syndrome)

22. Marchesani syndrome (dystrophia mesodermalis congenita hyperplastica)

23. Maxillofacial dysostosis

24. Nager syndrome

25. Noonan syndrome (male Turner syndrome)

26. Oculoauriculovertebral dysplasia (Goldenhar syndrome)

27. Oculomandibulofacial dyscephaly (Hallermann-Streiff syndrome)

28. Otopalatodigital syndrome (OPD)

29. Pyknodysostosis

30. Partial trisomy of long arm of chromosome 630. Pseudo-Ullrich-Turner syndrome

31. Ring D chromosome

32. Rubinstein-Taybi syndrome (broad thumbs syndrome)

33. Ruvalcaba syndrome

34. Saethre-Chotzen syndrome

*35. Trauma

36. Trisomy 9p syndrome

37. Trisomy syndrome

38. Trisomy 17p syndrome

39. Trisomy syndrome (E syndrome)

40. Turner syndrome (gonadal dysgenesis)

41. Wolf syndrome (chromosome partial deletion syndrome)

42. 4q- syndrome

43. 21q syndrome

Isenberg, S.J.: The Eye in Infancy. Chicago, Year Book Medical Publishers, 1989.

Roy, F.H.: Ocular Syndromes and Systemic Diseases. 2nd Ed. Philadelphia, W.B. Saunders, 1989.

* = most important

Pseudoptosis (Conditions Simulating Ptosis, but Lid Droop Is Not the Result of Levator Malfunction, and Ptosis Is Usually Corrected When the Causative Factors Are Cleared Up or Removed)

1. Due to globe displacement
    A. Anophthalmia including poorly fitting prosthesis
    *B. Enophthalmos such as that resulting from blow-out fracture of the floor of the orbit or atrophy of orbital fat
    *C. Microphthalmia
    *D. Phthisis bulbi
    E. Hypotony and inward collapse of eye
    F. Cornea plana
    G. Hypotropia of that eye or hypertropia of the other eye

2. Due to mechanical displacement of the lid
    A. Inflammation
        (1) Trachoma—thick, heavy lid
        *(2) Chalazion or hordeolum
        (3) Elephantiasis
        (4) Chronic conjunctivitis—conjunctival thickening
        (5) Traumatic or infectious edema involving the lid
        *(6) Blepharitis
        (7) Corneal foreign body
        (8) Contact lens
        (9) Sinusitis, cellulitis
    B. Tumors, especially fibromas, lipomas, or hemangiomas
    C. Scar tissue due to burns, physical trauma, and lacerations may bind the lid down
    D. Tumors of lacrimal gland—S-shaped lid

*3. Dermatochalasis (ptosis adiposa, baggy lids, "puffs"—senile atrophy of the lid skin)

4. Blepharochalasis—rare condition occurring in young individuals, characterized by recurrent bouts of inflammatory lid edema with subsequent stretching of the skin

5. The oriental lid—the palpebral fissure is narrower than normal and the upper lid rarely has a furrow; hence, the fold usually hangs down to or over the lid margin

6. Dissociated vertical deviation (DVD)

7. Duane syndrome (retraction syndrome)

8. Blepharospasm—eyebrow lower than normal, hemifacial spasm

9. Contralateral widening of the lid fissure as pseudoproptosis (see p. 4), exophthalmos, or lid retraction (p. 71)

10. Vertical strabismus

Beard, C.: Ptosis. St. Louis, C.V. Mosby, 1969.

Beyer, C. K., et. al.: Naso-orbital Fractures, Complications, and Treatment. Ophthalmology, 89:456, 1982.

Crawford, J.S.: Ptosis: Is it correctable and how? Ann. Ophthalmol., 3:452–456, 1971.

Hawkins, W.R.: Inward collapse of an eye. Arch. Ophthalmol., 84:385–386, 1970.

Huber, A.: Eye Symptoms in Brain Tumors. 2nd Ed. St. Louis, C.V. Mosby, 1971.

Blepharoptosis (Ptosis, Droopy Upper Lid) (Weak Levator Palpebrae Superioris Muscle)

1. Congenital ptosis
   *A. Simple (most congenital ptosis)—may be the result of autosomal dominant inheritance
   B. Complicated ptosis
      (1) Ptosis with ophthalmoplegia (most congenital ptosis)—the most commonly involved muscle is the superior rectus
      (2) Ptosis with other lid deformities such as epicanthus, blepharophimosis, microphthalmia, and lid coloboma—may be hereditary
      (3) Synkinetic (paradoxical) ptosis-aberrant nervous connections from the other extrinsic muscles of the eye and jaw to the levator muscle
         a. Marcus Gunn phenomenon (jaw winking reflex)—motor root of the fifth cranial nerve to the muscle of mastication also is misdirected through the third nerve to the levator muscle
         b. Phenomenon of Marin Amat (reverse jaw winking reflex)
         c. Misdirected third nerve syndrome—bizarre eyelid movements that may accompany various eye movements; the ptotic eyelid may rise as the medial rectus, the inferior rectus, or the superior rectus muscle contracts
   C. Involutional ptosis
2. Acquired ptosis
   A. Traumatic ptosis
      (1) Eyelid laceration
      (2) Postsurgical ptosis
         a. Enucleation
         b. Orbital operation
         c. Cataract operation
         d. Radial keratotomy
      (3) Foreign bodies lying in the roof of the orbit
      (4) Fracture of orbital roof, also following contusion with resulting hematoma but without fracture
      (5) Air blast injury
      (6) Botulinum toxin treatment of strabismus and blepharospasm
      (7) Prolonged hard contact lens wear
   B. Neurogenic ptosis
      (1) Peripheral involvement of the third nerve
      (2) Basilar, cortical, and nuclear lesions
      (3) Cerebral hemorrhages, tumors, or abscesses

* = most important

    (4) Multiple neuritis, nerve syphilis, or multiple sclerosis

    (5) Horner syndrome—lower lid higher than other lower lid

    (6) Familial dysautonomia (Riley-Day syndrome)

    (7) Misdirected third nerve syndrome—following third nerve palsy the fibers do not regrow into their respective muscles

    (8) Aseptic meningitis, transient

    (9) Pituitary tumor

C. Myogenic ptosis

    (1) Primary muscular atrophy (late familial ptosis), in which ptosis is usually the only symptom

    (2) Dystrophia myotonia, in which there is dystrophia not only of the extraocular muscles but also of the face, neck, and extremities

    (3) Myasthenia gravis, non-familial acquired ptosis

    (4) The congenital fibrosis syndrome characterized by bilateral ptosis and gradual fibrosis of all the extraocular muscles

    (5) Oculopharyngeal muscular dystrophy characterized by dysphagia and progressive bilateral ptosis

    (6) Progressive familial myopathic ptosis and involvement of one, some, or all extraocular (and no other) muscles of one or both eyes

    (7) Late spontaneous unilateral ptosis

    (8) Amyloid degeneration with involvement of the levator muscle

  *(9) Senility—loss of general muscle tone and atrophy of orbital fat

  (10) Ptosis and normal pregnancy

  (11) Hyperthyroidism and ptosis—following active stages

  (12) Drugs, including:

adenine arabinoside

adrenal cortex injection

alcohol

aldosterone

allobarbital

amobarbital

amodiaquine

aprobarbital

aurothioglucose

aurothioglycanide

barbital

betamethasone

butabarbital

butalbital

butallylonal

butethal

carbon dioxide

carbromal

chloral hydrate

chloroquine

cocaine(?)

cortisone

cyclobarbital

cyclopentyl allylbarbituric acid

cyclopentobarbital

desoxycorticosterone

dexamethasone

dextrothyroxine

digitalis

dimethyl tubocurarine

diphtheria and tetanus toxoids and pertussis (DPT)

disulfiram(?)

fludrocortisone

fluorometholone

flu-prednisolone

F3T

gold Au-198

gold sodium thiomalate

heptabarbital

hexethal

hexobarbital

hydrocortisone

hydroxychloroquine

idoxuridine

isocarboxazid

isosorbide dinitrate(?)

loxapine

measles virus vaccine (live)

medrysone

mephenesin

mephobarbital

metharbital

methitural

methohexital

methyl alcohol

methylpentynol

metocurine iodide

methylprednisolone

nalidixic acid(?)

nialamide

opium

oral contraceptives

paramethasone

pentobarbital

phencyclidine

phenelzine

phenobarbital

phenoxybenzamine

prednisolone

prednisone

primidone

probarbital

secobarbital

succinylcholine

sulthiame

talbutal

tetraethylammonium

thiamylal

thiopental

tolazoline

tranylcypromine

triamcinolone

trichloroethylene

trifluorothymidine

tubocurarine

vidarabine

vinbarbital

vinblastine

vincristine

*(13) Corticosteroid ptosis—prolonged use of topical corticosteroid therapy

(14) Mascara ptosis—due to subconjunctival deposits of mascara

(15) Ptosis associated with chronic conjunctivitis and uveitis

(16) Use of botulinum toxin

D. Protective ptosis-following injury to the eye

E. Mechanical ptosis

(1) Tumor

a. Benign tumor—such as neurofibroma or hemangioma

b. Malignant tumor—such as basal cell carcinoma, squamous cell carcinoma, malignant melanoma, or rhabdomyosarcoma

c. Metastatic lesion—such as from breast or lung

d. Sinus extension—such as mucocele of frontal sinus

(2) Blepharochalasis—hereditary with recurrent attacks of severe edema and residual damage to the tissues

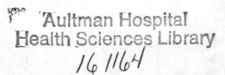

* = most important

   (3) Cicatricial ptosis—such as that secondary to cicatricial conjunctivitis (see p. 224) or surgical trauma to the superior fornix

   (4) Contact lens migration

   (5) Palpebral form of vernal conjunctivitis

   (6) Intracranial extension—such as chordoma

Bodker, F.S, et al.: Acquired blepharoptosis secondary to essential blepharospasm. Ophthalmic Surgery, 24: 546–550, 1993.

Burns, C. L., et al.: Ptosis associated with botulinum toxin treatment of strabismus and blepharospasm. Ophthalmology, 93:1621–1627, 1986.

Carroll, R.P., and Lindstrom, R.L.: Blepharoptosis after radial keratotomy. Am. J. Ophthalmol., 102:800, 1986.

Fraunfelder, F.T.: Drug-Induced Ocular Side Effects and Drug Interactions. 4th Ed. Philadelphia, Williams & Wilkins, 1996.

Frueh, B.R.: The mechanistic classification of ptosis. Ophthalmology, 87:1019, 1980.

Hertle, R.W., et al.: Congenital unilateral fibrosis, blepharoptosis, and enophthalmos syndrome. Ophthalmology, 99:347–355, 1992.

Perman, K.I., et al.: The use of botulinum toxin in the medical management of benign essential blepharospasm. Ophthalmology, 93:1–3, 1986.

Roy, F.H.: Ocular Syndromes and Systemic Diseases. 2nd Ed. Philadelphia, W.B. Saunders, 1989.

Smith, K.W., and Buckley, E.G.: Recurrent blepharoptosis secondary to a pituitary tumor. Am. J. Ophthalmol. 106:760–761, 1988.

van den Bosch, W., and Lemij, H.G.: Blepharoptosis Induced by Prolonged Hard Contact Lens Wear. Ophthalmology, 99:1759–1765, 1993.

Vaughn, G.L., et al.: Variable diplopia and blepharoptosis after orbital floor fracture repair. American Journal of Ophthalmology, 117:407–409, 1994.

Syndromes and Diseases Associated with Ptosis

1. Aarskog syndrome (faciogenital dysplasia)—x-linked
2. Acquired immunodeficiency syndrome
3. Addison disease (idiopathic hypoparathyroidism)
4. Alacrima congenital with distichiasis, conjunctivitis, keratitis-autosomal dominant
5. Albers-Schonberg syndrome (marble bone disease)
6. Albright syndrome (osteitis fibrosa disseminata)
7. Amyloidosis (Lubarsch-Pick syndrome)
8. Apert syndrome (acrocephalosyndactylia syndrome)
9. Arteriovenous fistula
10. Axenfeld-Schurenberg syndrome (cyclic oculomotor paralysis)
11. Babinski-Nageotte syndrome (medullary tegmental paralysis)
12. Basal cell carcinoma
13. Bassen-Kornzweig syndrome (abetalipoproteinemia)
14. Bell palsy (idiopathic facial paralysis)
15. Bing-Neel syndrome (Bing disease)
16. Blepharophimosis syndrome
17. Bonnet-Dechaume-Blanc syndrome (neuroretinoangiomatosis)

18. Bonnevie-Ullrich syndrome (pterygolymphangiectasia)
19. Botulism
20. Brown syndrome (superior oblique tendon sheath syndrome)
21. Carpenter syndrome (acrocephalopolysyndactyly II)
22. Cavernous sinus syndrome (Foix syndrome)
23. Cerebral palsy
24. Cestan-Chenais syndrome (Cestan syndrome)
25. Chromosome long arm deletion syndrome
26. Chromosome partial deletion (long arm) syndrome (de Grouchy syndrome)
27. Chromosome short arm deletion syndrome
28. Congenital fibrosis syndrome (all extraocular muscles)
29. Congenital fibrosis of the inferior rectus with ptosis-autosomal dominant
*30. Congenital ptosis
    A. Simple, failure of peripheral differentiation of muscles—dominant
    B. Ptosis with blepharophimosis—dominant
    C. Ptosis due to ophthalmoplegia—autosomal dominant
31. Craniocarpotarsal dysplasia (Freeman-Sheldon syndrome)
32. Craniocervical syndrome (whiplash injury)
33. Cretinism (juvenile hypothyroidism)
34. Creutzfeldt-Jakob syndrome (spastic pseudosclerosis)
35. Cri du chat syndrome (crying cat syndrome)
36. Crouzon syndrome (dysostosis craniofacialis)
37. Cushing syndrome(2) (cerebellopontine angle syndrome)
38. Dandy-Walker syndrome (atresia of foramen Magendie)
39. Dawson disease (subacute sclerosing panencephalitis)
40. Dejerine-Klumpke syndrome (lower radicular syndrome)
41. de Lange syndrome (congenital muscular hypertrophy—cerebral syndrome)
42. Devic syndrome (ophthalmoencephalomyelopathy)
43. Diphtheria
44. Dubowitz syndrome (dwarfism-eczema-peculiar facies)
45. Duck-bill lips, low-set ears—autosomal dominant
46. Eaton-Lambert syndrome (myasthenic syndrome)
47. Eclampsia and pre-eclampsia
48. Ehlers-Danlos syndrome (fibrodysplasia elastic generalisata)
49. Engelmann syndrome (osteopathia hyperostotica scleroticans multiplex infantalis)
50. Epidermal nevus syndrome (ichthyosis hystrix)
51. Erb-Goldflam syndrome (myasthenia gravis)
52. Erysipelas (St. Anthony fire)
53. Fabry syndrome
54. Facio-renal-acromesometic syndrome

* = most important

55. Fisher syndrome (ophthalmoplegia-ataxia-areflexia syndrome)
56. Fetal alcohol syndrome
57. Fetal trimethadione
58. Foramen lacerum syndrome (aneurysm of internal carotid artery syndrome)
59. Freeman-Sheldon syndrome
60. Garcin syndrome (half base syndrome)
61. Gerlier disease (paralytic vertigo)
62. Gillum-Anderson syndrome (dominant blepharoptosis, high myopia)
63. Guillain-Barré syndrome (acute infectious neuritis)
64. Hairy elbow syndrome
65. Hemangiomas
66. Herpes zoster
67. Hodgkin disease
68. Horner syndrome (cervical sympathetic paralysis)
69. Hunter syndrome (mucopolysaccharidosis II)
70. Hurler disease (mucopolysaccharides type I [MPS I])
71. Hyperammonemia
72. Hyperparathyroidism
73. Hyperthyroidism (Basedow syndrome)
74. Hypocalcemia
*75. Hypoparathyroidism
76. Hysteria
77. Infectious mononucleosis
78. Influenza
79. Jugular foramen syndrome (Vernet syndrome)
80. Kearns Jayne syndrome
81. Kiloh-Nevin syndrome (muscular dystrophy of external ocular muscles)
82. Kohn-Romano syndrome (blepharoptosis, blepharophimosis, epicanthus inversus, telecanthus)
83. Komoto syndrome (congenital eyelid tetrad)
84. Krause syndrome (congenital encephalo-ophthalmic dysplasia)
85. Kugelberg-Welander syndrome (progressive proximal muscle atrophy)
86. Kussmaul disease (necrotizing angiitis)
87. Laurence-Moon-Bardet-Biedl syndrome (retinitis pigmentosa-polydactyly-adiposogenital syndrome)
88. Leigh disease (subacute necrotizing encephalomyelopathy)
89. Little syndrome (nail-patella syndrome)
90. Lymphangioma
91. Lymphedema
92. Malaria

93. Malignant hyperthermia syndrome

94. Maple syrup urine disease (branched chain ketoaciduria)

95. Marcus Gunn syndrome (jaw winking syndrome)

96. Marin Amat syndrome (inverted Marcus Gunn syndrome)

97. Misdirected third nerve syndrome

98. Mobius syndrome (congenital paralysis of the sixth and seventh nerves)

99. Morquio syndrome (keratosulfaturia)

100. Mucormycosis

101. Multiple sclerosis (disseminated sclerosis)

102. Myopathy, centronuclear with external ophthalmoplegia—autosomal dominant

103. Myotonic dystrophy syndrome (Curschmann-Steinert syndrome)

104. Myotubular myopathy—autosomal recessive or x-linked

105. Naffiziger syndrome (scalenus anticus syndrome)

106. Neurilemoma

107. Neuroblastoma

108. Neurofibromatosis

109. Nonne-Milroy-Meige disease (congenital trophedema)

110. Noonan syndrome (male Turner syndrome)

111. Oculopharyngeal muscular dystrophy

112. Ophthalmoplegic migraine syndrome

113. Ophthalmoplegic—retinal degeneration (Kearns-Sayre syndrome)

114. Orodigital-facial syndrome (Papillon-Leage and Psaume syndrome)

115. Pachydermoperiostosis (Touraine-Solente-Gole syndrome)

116. Pancoast syndrome (superior pulmonary sulcus syndrome)

117. Parinaud syndrome (paralysis of vertical movements)

118. Parkinson syndrome (paralysis agitans)

119. Parry-Romberg syndrome (progressive facial hemiatrophy)

120. Periocular and ocular metastatic tumors

121. Pierre-Robin syndrome (micrognathia-glossoptosis syndrome)

122. Poliomyelitis

123. Progressive intracranial arterial occlusion syndrome

124. Purpura and ptosis—combined inheritance with male to male transmission

125. Raeder syndrome (paratrigeminal paralysis)

126. Retraction syndrome (Duane syndrome)—autosomal dominant

127. Retroparotid space syndrome

128. Riley-Day syndrome (congenital familial dysautonomia)

129. Ring D chromosome

130. Rollet syndrome (orbital apex-sphenoidal syndrome)

131. Rubinstein-Taybi syndrome (broad thumbs syndrome)

132. Scleroderma (progressive systemic sclerosis)

* = most important

133. Scurvy (vitamin C deficiency)

134. Shy-Gonatas syndrome (similar to Hunter and Refsum syndrome)

135. Smith-Lemli-Opitz syndrome (cerebrohepatorenal syndrome)

136. Smith syndrome (facioskeletogenital dysplasia)

137. Sparganosis

138. Spider bites

139. Strabismus and ectopic pupils-autosomal dominant

140. Subclavian steal syndrome

141. Syphilis (acquired lues)

142. Syringomyelia (Passow syndrome)

143. Temporal arteritis syndrome (Hutchinson-Horton-Magath-Brown syndrome)

144. Thirteen Q syndrome (microcephaly, high nasal bridge, thumb hypoplasia)

145. Tolosa-Hunt syndrome (painful ophthalmoplegia)

146. 3p syndrome

147. Trachoma

148. Treft syndrome (optic atrophy and hearing loss)

149. Triploidy (chromosomes instead of 46)

150. Trisomy (E syndrome)

151. Tuberculosis

152. Tunbridge-Paley disease (juvenile diabetes, optic atrophy and hearing loss)

153. Turner syndrome (gonadal dysgenesis)

154. van Bogaert-Hozay syndrome

155. Vertebral fusion, posterior lumbosacral with ptosis—autosomal dominant

156. von Herrenschwand syndrome (sympathetic heterochromia)

157. von Recklinghausen syndrome (neurofibromatosis)

158. Waardenburg syndrome (embryonic fixation syndrome)

159. Wallenberg syndrome (dorsolateral medullary syndrome)

160. Weber syndrome (cerebellar peduncle syndrome)

161. Wernicke syndrome (hemorrhagic polioencephalitis superior syndrome)

Larned, D.C., et al.: The association of congenital ptosis and congenital heart disease. Ophthalmology, 93:492–494, 1986.

McKusick, V.A.: Mendelian Inheritance in Man. 9th Ed. Baltimore, Johns Hopkins University Press, 1994.

Roy, F.H.: Ocular Syndromes and Systemic Diseases. 2nd Ed. Philadelphia, W.B. Saunders, 1989.

Ptosis

	Congenital Ptosis	Traumatic Ptosis	Neurogenic Ptosis as Horner Syndrome	Myogenic Ptosis as Myasthenia Gravis	Drugs as Steroid Ptosis	Mechanical Ptosis as Neurofibroma	Cicatricial Ptosis as Following Conjunctivitis
History							
1. Bilateral	S			U	S		U
2. Birth injury		U					
3. Familial	S			S		S	
4. Trauma/surgery		U					
5. More in females				U			S
6. Photophobia							U
7. Prolonged use of topical corticosteroids					U		
8. Transient diplopia				U		S	
9. Visual loss		S					
10. Weakness/fatigability	S	S		U		S	
Physical Findings							
1. Accomodative insufficiency					R		
2. Amblyopia	S						
3. Astigmatism	S					S	S
4. Blepharophimosis-ptosis syndrome	S						
5. Conjunctival discharge							U
6. Disc hypoplasia	R						
7. Enophthalmos	S		U				
8. Epiphora							U
9. Extraocular muscle fibrosis	S						
10. Heterochromia of iris			S				
11. Involved lid higher in downgaze	U						
12. Lagophthalmos	S						
13. Levator disinsertion		U				S	S
14. Lid crease absent	U	S	U				
15. Lid crease present		U			U	U	U
16. Lid lag in downgaze	U	S					
17. Lower lid somewhat elevated			U				
18. Miotic pupil			U				
19. Moderate/marked ptosis with fair/poor levator function	S						
20. Myopia	S						
21. Nystagmus	S				S		
22. Orbicularis oculi weakness				U			
23. Paradoxical lid retraction				U			
24. Ptosis decreases downgaze	U						
25. Ptosis increases upgaze	U					U	U
26. Ptosis same in upgaze and downgaze		U					
27. Slight ptosis with good levator function	U		U		U	U	U
28. S-shaped lid margin						U	

Ptosis

	Congenital Ptosis	Traumatic Ptosis	Neurogenic Ptosis as Horner Syndrome	Myogenic Ptosis as Myasthenia Gravis	Drugs as Steroid Ptosis	Mechanical Ptosis as Neurofibroma	Cicatricial Ptosis as Following Conjunctivitis
Physical Findings							
29. Strabismus	S						
30. Transient hyperemic, anhidrotic, warm ipsilateral face			U				
31. Transient increased accommodation			S				
32. Upper salcus deeper uninvolved side		U					
Laboratory Data							
1. Hydroxyamphetamine or cocaine 4% drops pharmacologic test			U				
2. Positive tensilon test				U			

R = rarely; S = sometimes; and U = usually.

Specific Blepharoptosis

1. Unilateral ptosis with dilated pupil—tumor or abscess of temporal lobe and third nerve palsy
2. Unilateral ptosis with miosis-midbrain lesion near the posterior commissure and Horner syndrome
3. Ptosis with disturbance of integrated ocular movement—lesion near superior colliculus
4. Bilateral ptosis with small immobile pupils and loss of upward rotation of eyeballs—lesion near posterior commissure
5. Ptosis with loss of voluntary elevation but normal involuntary elevation of the lid when the eye looks up—supranuclear lesion
6. Ptosis in repose and normal elevation with active motion—hereditary cerebellar ataxia of Pierre-Marie
7. Ptosis onset in adolescent—familial chronic external ophthalmoplegia
8. Ptosis may be early and only sign of nuclear paralysis in:
    A. Botulism
    B. Multiple sclerosis (disseminated sclerosis)
    C. Hemorrhagic superior poliomyelitis of Wernicke
    D. Tabes
    E. Vasospasm of ophthalmoplegic migraine
9. Ptosis with cranial nerve dysfunction suggests a basal lesion such as:
    A. Aneurysm
    B. Epidemic paralyzed vertigo (Gerlier disease)
    *C. Herpes zoster
    D. Meningitis
    E. Polyneuritis of cranial nerves
    *F. Trauma
10. Transient ptosis
    A. Acute exanthema
    B. Acute infection such as erysipelas
    *C. Botulinum toxin injection
    D. Eclampsia
    E. Exogenous poisons such as those due to alcohol, lead, carbon monoxide, arsenic, snake venom
    F. Hematoma
    G. Influenza
    H. Scurvy (vitamin C deficiency)
11. Ptosis with orbicularis weakness—muscle disease
12. S-shaped ptosis
    A. Chronic chalazion
    B. Cyst on lateral border of tarsus
    C. Dermoid

* = most important

D. Floppy eyelid syndrome

E. Lacrimal gland enlargement or prolapse

F. Lateral levator palpebrae superioris muscle dehiscence

G. Neurofibromatosis

H. Trachoma

Dunn, W.J., et al. Botulinum toxin for the treatment of dysthyroid ocular myopathy. Ophthalmology, 93:4770–4775, 1986.

Gerner, E.W., and Hughes, S.M.: Floppy eyelid with hyperglycinemia. Am. J. Ophthalmol., 98:614–615, 1984.

Haessler, F.H.: Eye Signs in General Disease. Springfield, IL, Charles C. Thomas, 1960.

Horner Syndrome (Paralysis of Sympathetic Nerve Supply with Lid Ptosis, Miosis, Apparent Enophthalmos; Frequently Dilatation of the Vessels, with Absence of Sweating [Anhidrosis] on Homolateral Side; Pupil Demonstrates a Decreased Sensitivity to Cocaine and Hypersensitivity to Adrenalin; Patient May Have Heterochromia with Congenital Horner Syndrome)

1. Region of first neuron—lesions of hypothalamus and diencephalic region also suggest diabetes insipidus, disturbed temperature regulation, adiposogenital syndrome, and autonomic epidemic epilepsy of Penfield

    A. Arnold-Chiari malformation

    B. Basal meningitis, such as in syphilis

    C. Base of skull tumors e.g., melanoma

    D. Multiple sclerosis

    E. Pituitary tumor

    F. Tumor of third ventricle

    G. Midbrain, such as in syphilis

    H. Pons, such as in intrapontine hemorrhage

    I. Medulla, such as in Wallenberg syndrome (lateral medullary syndrome)—thrombosis of posterior inferior cerebellar artery

    J. Cervical region

        (1) Syringomyelia

        (2) Tumor

        (3) Injury

        (4) Syphilis (acquired lues)

        (5) Poliomyelitis

        (6) Meningitis

        (7) Amyotrophic lateral sclerosis

        (8) Related to scleroderma and facial hemiatrophy

        (9) Vascular malformation

2. Region of second neuron

    A. Spinal birth injury-Klumpke paralysis with injured lower brachial plexus

    B. Cervical rib

    C. Charcoast-Tobias syndrome

D. Thoracic lesions

    (1) Pancoast tumor—in apex of lung, such as carcinoma or tuberculosis

    (2) Aneurysm of aorta, subclavian or carotid artery

    (3) Central venous catheterization

    (4) Mediastinal tumors

    (5) Lymphadenopathy of Hodgkin disease, leukemia, lymphosarcoma, or tuberculosis

    (6) Stellate ganglion block

    (7) Tube thoracostomy

E. Neck

    *(1) Enlarged lymph gland, tumors, aneurysm, and thyroid gland

    (2) Carcinoma of esophagus

    (3) Retropharyngeal tumors

    (4) Neuroma of sympathetic chain

    (5) Intraoral trauma with damage to internal carotid plexus

    (6) Thin intervertebral foramina of spinal cord, such as in pachymeningitis, hypertrophic spinal arthritis, ruptured intervertebral disc, and meningeal tumors

    (7) Traction of sternocleidomastoid muscle such as from positioning on operating table

    (8) Complications of tonsillectomy

    (9) Mandibular tooth abscess

    *(10) Lesions of middle ear, such as in acute purulent otitis media and petromastoid operation

    (11) Carotid artery dissection

    (12) Internal carotid artery occlusion

3. Region of third neuron

    A. Aneurysm of internal carotid and its branches

    B. Paratrigeminal syndrome (Raeder syndrome)

    C. Cavernous sinus syndrome (Foix syndrome)

    D. Tumors of cysts of orbit

    E. Drugs can affect any region and include:

acetophenazine	lidocaine	propiomazine
alseroxylon	mepivacaine	propoxycaine
bupivacaine	mesoridazine	rauwolfia serpentina
butaperazine	methdilazine	rescinnamine
carphenazine	methotrimeprazine	reserpine
chlorpromazine	oral contraceptives	syrosingopine
deserpidine	perazine	thiethylperazine
diacetyl-morphine	pericyazine	thiopropazate
diethazine	perphenazine	thioproperazine
ethopropazine	piperacetazine	thioridazine
etidocaine	prilocaine	trifluoperazine
fluphenazine	procaine	triflupromazine
guanethidine	prochlorperazine	trimeprazine
influenza virus vaccine	promazine	
levodopa	promethazine	

* = most important

F. Cluster headaches (migrainous neuralgia)

G. Herpes zoster

H. Migraine

I. Fetal varicella syndrome

Fraunfelder, F.T.: Drug-Induced Ocular Side Effects and Drug Interactions. 4th Ed. Philadelphia, Williams & Wilkins, 1996.

Gibbs, J., et al.: Congenital Horner syndrome associated with non-cervical neuroblastoma. Developmental Medicine & Child Neurology, 34: 642–644, 1992.

Kline, L.B., et. al.: Painful Horner's syndrome due to spontaneous carotid artery dissection. Ophthalmology, 94:226–230, 1987.

Roy, F.H.: Ocular Syndromes and Systemic Diseases, 2nd Ed. Philadelphia, W.B. Saunders, 1989.

Smith, E.F., et al.: Herpes zoster ophthalmicus as a cause of Horner syndrome. Journal of Clinical Neuro-Ophthalmology, 13: 250–253, 1993.

Horner Syndrome

	Region of First Neuron as Pituitary Tumor	Region of Second Neuron as Pancoast Tumor	Region of Third Neuron as Cluster Headaches
History			
1. Begins during second to third decades			U
2. Cervical trauma/surgery		U	
3. Common during fourth to seventh decades	U		
4. Common—bronchogenic carcinoma		S	
5. Common in males		U	U
6. Common—meningioma and internal carotid aneurysm			U
7. Common—single intracranial neoplasm (adenoma)	U		
8. Family			U
9. Head trauma			S
10. Visual loss in one or both eyes	S		
Physical Findings			
1. Anhidrosis homolateral side	U	U	S
2. Apparent enophthalmos	U	U	S
3. Bitemporal hemianopia	U		
4. Extraocular muscle palsies	U		S
5. Failure of pupil dilation with hydroxyamphetamine 1%			U
6. Heterochromia of iris	R	R	
7. Increased accommodation	U	U	
8. Ipsilateral lacrimation			U
9. Miosis	U	U	U
10. Narrowing of palpebral fissure		U	
11. Ocular hypotony	U	U	S
12. Optic disc pallor	S		
13. Papilledema	R		
14. Proptosis	S		
15. Ptosis	U	U	U
16. Pupil dilates little with cocaine 4%	U	U	U
17. Recurrent ocular pain			U
18. Third nerve palsy			U
19. Transient dilated vessels conjunctiva/face	U	U	U
20. Trigeminal anesthesia	S		U
Laboratory Data			
1. Carotid arteriography			U
2. Computed tomographic scan of head	U	U	U
3. Cervical planigrams		U	
4. Pituitary panel—serum prolactin, growth hormone, adrenocorticotropic hormone, follicle-stimulating hormone, luteinizing hormone, thyroid-stimulating hromone	S		
5. Pneumoencephalography	S		S
6. Visual field test	U		
7. Roentgenogram of chest		U	
8. Roentgenogram of skull	U		S

R = rarely; S = sometimes; and U = usually

Ptosis of Lower Lid (Uncommon-Drooping of Lower Lid So that Lid Margin Is Adjacent to Globe but Below Limbus)

1. Blepharophimosis syndrome
*2. Cicatricial with mechanical displacement by scar, tumor, or skin disease; may be associated with ectropion
*3. Paralytic due to lower lid lagophthalmos
4. Pseudoptosis such as in exophthalmos and higher degrees of myopia
5. Idiopathic

Fox, S.A.: Idiopathic blepharoptosis of lower eyelid. Am. J. Ophthalmol., 74:330–331, 1972.
Leatherbarron, B., and Collin, J.R.: Eyelid surgery in facial palsy. Eye, 5: 585–590, 1991.

Lagophthalmos (Inability to Voluntarily Close Eyelids)

*1. Physiologic—many people sleep with their eyes open, especially orientals
2. Orbital—extreme proptosis
3. Mechanical—scarring of the lids or retractor muscles
4. Paralytic
   A. VII nerve palsy (see p. 75)
   B. Leprosy
   C. Lesions of cerebral cortex and its projections, including bilateral frontal lesions
5. Psychological
   A. Failure to comprehend the command
   *B. Unwillingness to comply with the command

Harvey, J.T., and Anderson, R.L.: Lid lag and lagophthalmos. Ophthalmol. Surg., 12:338, 1981.
Lessell, S.: Supranuclear paralysis of voluntary lid closure. Arch. Ophthalmol., 88:241–244, 1972.

Pseudo-lid Retraction

*1. Exophthalmos
2. Unilateral high axial myopia
3. Unilateral congenital glaucoma
4. Congenital cystic eyeball
5. Abnormalities of orbit
   A. Asymmetry
   B. Shallow such as in Crouzon disease (dysostosis craniofacialis)
   C. Harlequin (shallow orbit with arched superior and lateral wall), such as in hypophosphatasia
6. Ptosis of other eyelid

Fox, S.A.: The palpebral fissure. Am. J. Ophthalmol., 62:73–78, 1966.
Walsh, F.B., and Hoyt, W.F.: Clinical Neuro-ophthalmology. 4th Ed. Baltimore, Williams & Wilkins, 1985.

Lid Retraction (Normally More Than 85% of Vertical Palpebral Fissures 10 mm or Less with the Eyelids Just Concealing the Corneoscleral Limbus at the 12 and 6 o'clock Meridians)

1. Lid retraction with upward movement of eye

    A. Congestive dysthyroid disease

    B. Deficiency in upward gaze—following rectus operation or weakness of superior rectus

    C. Excessive stimulation of levator muscles in Bell phenomenon with seventh nerve palsy

    D. Levator muscles receive excessive stimuli from nerve fiber of superior rectus

    E. Pretectal or peri-aqueductal lesion in midbrain

2. Lid retraction with downward movement of eye

    A. Aberrant regeneration of third nerve of inferior rectus to levator (pseudo-Graefe phenomenon)—elevation of lid in downward gaze

    B. Brown syndrome (superior oblique tendon sheath syndrome)

    C. Extrapyramidal syndrome of postencephalic parkinsonism and progressive supranuclear palsy

    D. Failure of levator to relax on downward movement of eye

    (1) Secondary neuromuscular

    *(2) Mechanical, such as from a scar

    E. Non-congestive type of dysthyroid exophthalmos (Graefe sign)—lid lag in downward gaze

3. Lid retraction with horizontal gaze

    A. Duane syndrome (retraction syndrome)

    B. Underaction of lateral rectus muscle and spillover to levator causing widening

4. Lid retraction because of supranuclear lesions—usually bilateral when due to lesion in or about posterior commissure (Collier sign, tucked lids, posterior fossa stare)

    A. Bulbar poliomyelitis

    B. Chorea (Huntington hereditary chorea)

    C. Closed head injury associated with defective adduction of eyes, coarse nystagmus, nuclear palsy, pyramidal signs

    D. Coma due to disease of ventral midbrain and pons

    E. Craniostenosis

    F. Epidemic encephalitis

    G. Hydrocephalic infants

    H. Hydrophobia

    I. Hysteria

    J. Malingering

    K. Meningitis

    L. Multiple sclerosis (disseminated sclerosis)

    M. Parinaud syndrome (divergence paralysis)

* = most important

N. Parkinson disease (paralysis agitans)

O. Russell syndrome

P. Sylvian aqueduct syndrome (Koerber-Solus-Elschnig syndrome)

Q. Syphilis (tabes)

R. Tumors of midbrain; meningiomas of sphenoid wing; sellar, parasellar, and suprasellar tumors; and frontal or temporal lobe tumors

S. von Economo syndrome (encephalitis lethargica)

5. Lid retraction because of neuromuscular disease—commonly asymmetric or unilateral

    A. Drugs

        (1) Phenylephrine and other sympathomimetics

        (2) Prostigmin and tensilon, especially with myasthenic levator involvement

        (3) Succinylcholine, subparalytic doses

        (4) Thyroid extract

    B. Fuch phenomenon—healing of injured third nerve, previously ptotic lid has involuntarily spastic raising with movements of eyes

    C. Infant lid retraction—transient because of maternal hyperthyroidism

    D. Irritation of cervical sympathetic nerve (Horner syndrome)

  *E. Mechanical suspension of lid such as that due to scar, tumor, surgical attachment to frontalis muscle, or shortening of levator muscle, or following glaucoma filtering procedures

    F. Peripheral seventh nerve paresis with loss of orbicularis oculi muscle tone

6. Lid retraction with myopathic disease

    A. Associated with hepatic cirrhosis

    B. Thyroid myopathy (Graves disease, Basedow syndrome)

        (1) Dalyrumple sign—widening of palpebral fissure

        (2) Stellwag sign—retraction of upper lid associated with infrequent or incomplete blinking

7. Lid retraction following operations on vertical muscles, such as recession of superior rectus muscle or simultaneous recession and restriction of the levator by common fascial check ligament between the two muscles

8. Paradoxical lid retraction because of paradoxical levator innervation

    A. Defective ocular abduction with abducens palsy

    B. Lid retraction associated with ptosis of the opposite eyelid (levator denervation supersensitivity)

    C. Misdirection of third nerve axons (following acquired or congenital lesions)—occurs on attempt to adduct, elevate, or depress eye

    D. Movement of lower jaw

        (1) Contraction of external pterygoid muscle by opening mouth (Marcus Gunn)

        (2) Contraction of internal pterygoid muscle by closing mouth

9. Physiologic

    A. Act of surprise

B. Slow onset of blindness, such as that secondary to glaucoma and optic atrophy

C. Time of attention

Collins, J.R., et al.: Congenital eyelid retraction. Brit. J. Ophthal., 74: 542–544, 1990.

Dixon, R.: The surgical management of thyroid-related upper eyelid retraction. Ophthalmology, 89:52, 1982.

Roy, F.H.: Ocular Syndromes and Systemic Diseases. 2nd Ed. Philadelphia, W.B. Saunders, 1989.

Walsh, F.B., and Hoyt, W.F.: Clinical Neuro-ophthalmology. 4th Ed. Baltimore, Williams & Wilkins, 1985.

Lid Lag (When Patient Looks Down, the Eyelids Lag Behind Briefly)

1. Congenital—usually in association with congenital ptosis

2. Hepatic failure

3. Iatrogenic—following ptosis surgery

4. Mechanical—scars of the upper lid

5. Myopathic disease

　　*A. Graefe sign—thyroid myopathy—the upper lid pauses and then follows the eye downward (Basedow syndrome)

　　B. Myotonic dystrophia

　　C. Periodic myotonic lid lag—familial (hyperkalemic) myotonic periodic paralysis

6. Neuromuscular disease

　　A. Excessive intake of thyroid extract

　　B. Physiologic lagophthalmos—short upper tarsus in Asians and some Caucasians with incomplete descent of the lid during sleep

7. Supranuclear origin—extrapyramidal syndromes have defective inhibition of lids in downward gaze

　　A. Congenital supranuclear lid lag

　　B. Guillain-Barre syndrome

　　C. Postencephalitic parkinsonism, Parkinson syndrome (shaking palsy)

　　D. Progressive supranuclear palsy

Kirkali, P., and Kansu, T.: Lid lag in hyperkalemic periodic paralysis. Annals of Ophthal., 23:422–423, 1991.

Roy, F.H.: Ocular Syndromes and Systemic Diseases. 2nd Ed. Philadelphia, W.B. Saunders, 1989.

Tan, E., et al.: Lid lag and the Guillain-Barre syndrome. J. of Clinical Neuro-Ophthal., 10:121–123, 1990.

Blepharospasm (Spasmodic Eyelid Closure)

Most common and important: Psychogenic-onset commonly in children and young adults.

1. Addison disease (adrenal cortical insufficiency)

2. Associated with syphilis, tetanus, and tetany

3. Basal ganglion dysfunction—onset usually after middle age; including Parkinson disease (shaking palsy)

* = most important

4. Cerebral palsy

5. Cogan syndrome (non-syphilitic interstitial keratitis) with vestibulo-auditory symptoms

6. Drugs, including:

acetophenazine
amitriptyline
amodiaquine
amoxapine(?)
amphetamine
antazoline
brompheniramine
butaperazine
carbinoxamine
carphenazine
chloroquine
chlorpheniramine
chlorpromazine
clemastine
clomipramine
desipramine
dexbrompheniramine
dexchlorpheniramine
dextroamphetamine
dextrothyroxine
diethazine
dimercaprol
dimethindene
diphenhydramine
diphenylpyraline
doxepin

doxylamine
dronabinol
droperidol
emetine
ethopropazine
fluphenazine
haloperidol
hashish
hydroxychloroquine
imipramine
levodopa
levothyroxine
liothyronine
liotrix
lorazepam
marihuana
mesoridazine
methamphetamine
methdilazine
methotrimeprazine
nortriptyline
pentylenetetrazol
perazine
pericyazine
perphenazine
pheniramine

phenmetrazine
phenylephrine
piperacetazine
prochlorperazine
promazine
promethazine
propiomazine
protriptyline
pyrilamine
tetrahydrocannabinol
thiethylperazine
thiopropazate
thioproperazine
thioridazine
thyroglobulin
thyroid
trifluoperazine
trifluperidol
triflupromazine
trimeprazine
trimipramine
tripelennamine
triprolidine
vidarabine
vinblastine

7. Electrical injury

8. Encephalitis

9. Epidemic keratoconjunctivitis

10. Hallervorden-Spatz

11. Hereditary reflex blepharospasm

12. Idiopathic (essential)

13. Leprosy (Hansen disease)

14. Meige's syndrome

15. Obsessive-compulsive disorder

*16. Pain or light sensitivity following injury, inflammation, or foreign bodies of lids, conjunctiva, cornea, or iris

17. Photosensitivity and sunburn

18. Poison ivy dermatitis

19. Postencephalitic blepharospasm

20. Psychogenic-obsessive-compulsive disorder-onset commonly in children and young adults

21. Psychologic reflex blepharospasm—seen in premature infants with tactile stimulation of lids

22. Sparganosis

23. Systemic scleroderma (progressive systemic sclerosis)

24. Thomsen syndrome (congenital myotonia syndrome)

25. Tourette syndrome (coprolalia, generalized tic)

Bihari, K., et al.: Blepharospasm and obsessive-compulsive disorder. J Nervous and Mental Disease., 180:130–132, 1992.

Coppeto, J.R., and Lessell, S.: A familial syndrome of dystonia blepharospasm and pigmentary retinopathy. Neurology, 40:1359–1363, 1990.

Defazio, G., et al.: Genetic contribution to idiopathic adult-onset blepharospasm and cranial-cervical dystonia. European Neurology, 33:345–350, 1993.

Johnston, J.S.: A New Variant of Blepharospasm., Amer. J. Ophthal. 114:524, 1992.

Fraunfelder, F.T.: Drug-Induced Ocular Side Effects and Drug Interactions. Philadelphia, Williams & Wilkins, 1996.

Gray, A.R., and Barker, G.R.: Idiopathic blepharospasm-oromandibular dystonia syndrome (Meige's syndrome) presenting as chronic temporomandibular joint dislocation. Brit. J. Oral & Maxillofacial Surgery, 29:97–99, 1991.

Larumbe, R., et al.: Reflex blepharospasm associated with bilateral basal ganglia lesion. Movement Disorders, 8:198–200, 1993.

Patel, B.C., and Anderson, R.L.: Blepharospasm. Ophthalmic Practice, 11: 293–302, 1993.

Persing, J.A., et al.: Blepharospasm-oromandibular dystonia associated with a left cerebellopontine angle meningioma. J Emergency Medicine, 8: 571–574, 1990.

Roy, F.H.: Ocular Syndromes and Systemic Diseases. 2nd Ed. Philadelphia, W.B. Saunders, 1989.

Facial Palsy (Paralysis of Facial Muscles Supplied by Seventh Nerve; Orbicularis Oculi Paralysis May Result in Epiphora and Ectropion)

1. Congenital

2. Birth injury with nerve crushed at exit of stylomastoid foramen

3. Myogenic paralysis

   A. Myotonic atrophia

   B. Facioscapulohumeral type of muscular dystrophy

   C. Myasthenia gravis (Erb-Goldflam syndrome)

   D. Hypokalemia, periodic

   E. Curare poisoning

   F. Botulism

   G. Congenital facial diplegia (Mobius syndrome)

   H. Infants, from maternal ingestion of thalidomide

   I. Kugelberg-Welander syndrome

* = most important

4. Neurologic paralysis

   A. Supranuclear paralysis—upper face including orbicularis relatively unaffected with affected lower face

     (1) Voluntary movement—pyramidal fibers involved, such as in Weber syndrome, with contralateral hemiplegia of face and limbs and ipsilateral oculomotor paralysis

     (2) Weakness or abolition of the emotional movements of the face with retention of full voluntary activity, such as with lesion of anterior part of frontal lobe or near optic thalamus

   B. Peripheral paralysis—involvement of upper and lower face

     (1) Pontine lesion—associated structures involved include sixth nerve, conjugate ocular deviation to the same side, ipsilateral paralysis of jaw muscles, and pyramidal tract in paralysis of limb of opposite side

       a. Acute nuclear lesions, such as with anterior poliomyelitis, Landry paralysis, or degenerative conditions

       b. Foville syndrome—ipsilateral sixth nerve with loss of conjugate deviation to same side and hemiplegia of the opposite limbs

       c. Millard-Gubler syndrome—ipsilateral sixth nerve paralysis and hemiplegia of the opposite limbs.

       d. Parotid gland surgery

       e. Progressive muscular atrophy

       f. Syringobulbia

       g. Tumors

       h. Vascular lesions

     (2) Posterior fossa—associated with nerve deafness, loss of taste on anterior two thirds of tongue, and occasionally diminution of tears

       a. Acoustic neuroma

       b. CHARGE association

       c. Facial neuritis due to polyneuritis cranialis, beriberi, encephalitis, diabetes or intrathecal anesthesia

       d. Fracture of the skull

       e. Meningitis, including syphilitic and tuberculous

       f. Preauricular cyst associated with congenital cholesteatoma

       g. Tumors of facial nerve

     (3) Petrous temporal bone—associated with decreased lacrimation and salivary secretion, loss of taste on anterior two thirds of tongue, and intensified sensation of loud noises

       *a. Arteriosclerosis

       *b. Bell palsy—inflammation of facial nerve of unknown etiology

       c. Cephalic tetanus

       d. Diabetes mellitus (Willis disease)

       e. Fractures

       f. Herpes zoster, spread from geniculate ganglion

      g. Hypertension

      h. Nerve leprosy (Hansen disease)

     *i. Otitis media

      j. Secondary syphilis

   (4) Facial lesions at or beyond the stylomastoid foramen

      a. Fracture of the ramus of the mandible

      b. Melkersson-Rosenthal syndrome (Melkersson idiopathic fibroedema)

      c. Neoplasia or inflammatory swelling of parotid, such as in uveoparotid fever (Heerfordt disease) and Mikulicz disease

      d. Supporting lymph nodes behind the angle of the jaw

Eggenberger, E.R.: Facial palsy in Lyme disease. New England J. of Medicine, 328:1571, 1993.

George, M.K., and Pahor, A.L.: Sarcoidosis: a cause for bilateral facial palsy. Ear, Nose & Throat Journal, 70:492–493, 1991.

Lacombe, D.: Facial palsy and cranial nerve abnormalities in CHARGE association. American J. of Medical Genet., 15: 351–353, 1993.

Landers, S.A.: Preauricular cyst associated with congenital cholesteatoma: an unusual cause of facial palsy. Amer. J of Otology, 15:273–275, 1994.

Roy, F.H.: Ocular Syndromes and Systemic Diseases. 2nd Ed. Philadelphia, W.B. Saunders, 1989.

Infrequent Blinking

  *1. Contact lens usage

   2. Encephalitis, acute

   3. Encephalitis or mild postencephalitic states

  *4. Ethanol intake

   5. Infants in first few months of life

   6. Parkinson syndrome including mycostatic paresis of parkinsonism

   7. Psychotic states

   8. Progressive supranuclear palsy

   9. Thyrotoxicosis including exophthalmic ophthalmoplegia (Stellwag sign)

Roy, F.H.: Ocular Syndromes and Systemic Diseases. 2nd Ed. Philadelphia, W.B. Saunders, 1989.

Walsh, F.B., and Hoyt, W.F.: Clinical Neuro-ophthalmology. 4th Ed. Baltimore, Williams & Wilkins, 1985.

Frequent Blinking

  *1. Reflex—strong lights, sudden approach of objects toward eyes, loud noises, and touching the cornea; reflex blinking common in albinos and light intolerance

   2. Spontaneous—mental state and environment

     A. Children with habit spasm and facial tic

     B. Blepharospasm

    *C. Older persons with inadequate lacrimation and local irritation of the eyes

   3. Disorders of central nervous system disease such as parkinsonism or various forms of pseudobulbar palsy

* = most important

4. Drugs including:

acetylcholine
allobarbital
ambenonium
amobarbital
amodiaquine
aprobarbital
barbital bupivacaine
butabarbital
butalbital
butallylonal
butethal
carbachol
carbamazepine
chloroprocaine
chloroquine
clofibrate
cyclobarbital
cyclopentobarbital
demecarium

dibucaine
echothiophate
edrophonium
etidocaine
heptabarbital
hexethal
hexobarbital
hydroxychloroquine
isoflurophate
levodopa
lidocaine
mephobarbital
mepivacaine
methacholine
metharbital
methitural
methohexital
methylphenidate
neostigmine

pentobarbital
phenobarbital
physostigmine
pilocarpine
piperocaine
prilocaine
primidone
probarbital
procaine
propoxycaine
pyridostigmine
secobarbital
talbutal
tetracaine
thiamylal
thiopental
vinbarbital

Fraunfelder, F.T.: Drug-Induced Ocular Side Effects and Drug Interactions. 4th Ed. Philadelphia, Williams & Wilkins, 1996.

Moses, R.A.: Adler's Physiology of the Eye. 8th Ed. St. Louis, C.V. Mosby, 1986.

Walsh, F.B., and Hoyt, W.F.: Clinical Neuro-ophthalmology. 4th Ed. Baltimore, Williams & Wilkins, 1985.

Lid Edema (Puffiness or Bagginess of Lids)

*1. Noninflammatory or minimally inflammatory swelling

  A. Acosta syndrome (Mountain climbers syndrome)

  B. Allergic gastroenteropathy with protein loss

  C. Arteriovenous fistula

  D. Cardiac and renal disease

    (1) Nephrosis and acute glomerulonephritis—early morning edema

    (2) Starvation and cachexia

  E. Dermatochalasis

  F. Elephantiasis

    (1) Chronic eczema or infection (erysipelas)

    (2) Hemolymphangioma

    (3) Leprosy (Hansen disease)

    (4) Lues (syphilis)

    (5) Melkersson-Rosenthal syndrome (Melkersson idiopathic fibroedema)

(6) Nonne-Milroy-Meige disease (idiopathic hereditary lymphedema)

(7) von Recklinghausen disease (neurofibromatosis)

(8) Traumatic disruption of the lymph drainage system

(9) Tuberculosis

G. Endocrine exophthalmos (hyperthyroidism)

H. Foix syndrome (Cavernous sinus syndrome)

I. Granulomatous ileocolitis

J. Hutchinson syndrome (adrenal cortex neuroblastoma with orbital metastasis)

K. Infectious generalized diseases

    (1) Diphtheria

    (2) Infectious mononucleosis

    (3) Malaria

    (4) Meningococcal meningitis

    (5) Pertussis (whooping cough)

    (6) Rheumatic fever

    (7) Scarlet fever

    (8) Trypanosomiasis

    (9) Tuberculosis

  (10) Yellow fever

L. Nasal nerve syndrome (Charlin syndrome)

M. Parasitic infestations

    (1) Anthrax

    (2) Ascariasis

    (3) Chlamydia

    (4) Dermatophytosis

    (5) Myiasis

    (6) Onchocerciasis syndrome (river blindness)

    (7) Tapeworms

    (8) Toxocariasis

    (9) Trichinosis

N. Protrusion of fat through orbital fascia

O. Retinoblastoma

P. Stasis, including premenstrual edema

Q. Superior vena cava syndrome

R. Systemic scleroderma (progressive systemic scleroderma)

*S. Tumors and pseudotumors

    (1) Benign and malignant ectodermal and mesodermal tumors

    (2) Brill-Symmer disease (lymphosarcoma)

    (3) Hemangiomas

    (4) Hodgkin disease

* = most important

(5) Leukemic deposit

(6) Liposarcoma

(7) Meningiomas of sphenoid ridge with impediment of venous circulation of ophthalmic veins or cavernous sinus

(8) Neurofibromatosis

(9) Pseudotumors

    a. Amyloid degeneration

    b. Eosinophilic or basophilic granulomas

T. Trauma

(1) Basilar skull fractures

(2) Injury

*(3) Surgery

U. Angioneurotic edema caused by drugs, including:

acenocoumarol

acetaminophen

acetanilid

acetophenazine

acetyldigitoxin

acyclovir

adrenal cortex injection

albuterol

aldosterone

allobarbital

alprazolam

aluminum nicotinate

aminosalicylate(?)

aminosalicylic acid(?)

amiodarone

amitriptyline

amobarbital

amoxapine

amoxicillin

ampicillin

anisindione

antazoline

antimony lithium thiomalate

antimony potassium tartrate

antimony sodium tartrate

antimony sodium thioglycolate

antipyrine

aprobarbital

aspirin

auranofin

aurothioglucose

aurothioglycanide

azatadine

bacitracin

barbital

bendroflumethiazide

benzathine penicillin G

benzphetamine

benzthiazide

betamethasone

betaxolol

bleomycin

brompheniramine

bupivacaine

busulfan

butabarbital

butalbital

butallylonal

butaperazine

butethal

capreomycin

captopril

carbamazepine

carbenicillin

carbimazole

carbinoxamine

carisoprodol

carphenazine

cefaclor

cefadroxil

cefamandole

cefazolin

cefonicid

cefoperazone

ceforanide

cefotaxime

cefotetan

cefoxitin

cefsulodin

ceftazidime

ceftizoxime

ceftriaxone

cefuroxime

cephalexin

cephaloglycin

cephaloridine

cephalothin

cephapirin

cephradine

chlorambucil

chloramphenicol

chlordiazepoxide

chloroprocaine

chlorothiazide

chlorpheniramine

chlorphentermine

chlorprothixene

chlortetracycline

chlorthalidone

clindamycin

clonazepam

clonidine

clorazepate

cloxacillin

cobalt

codeine

cortisone

cyclobarbital

cyclopentobarbital

cyclophosphamide

cyclosporine

cyclothiazide

cyproheptadine

cytarabine

dacarbazine

dactinomycin

danazol

dantrolene

dapsone

daunorubicin

deferoxamine

demeclocycline

desipramine

deslanoside

desoxycorticosterone

dexamethasone

dexbrompheniramine

dexchlorpheniramine

dextran

diacetylmorphine

diatrizoate meglumine and sodium

diazepam

dichlorphenamide

dicloxacillin

dicumarol

diethylcarbamazine

diethylpropion

diethazine

digitalis

digitoxin

digoxin

diltiazem

dimethindene

dimethyl sulfoxide

diphenadione

diphenhydramine

diphenylpyraline

diphtheria and tetanus toxoids (adsorbed)

diphtheria and tetanus toxoids and pertussis vaccine (adsorbed)

disulfiram

doxepin

doxorubicin

doxycycline

* = most important

doxylamine

measles and rubella virus vaccine (live)

droperidol

measles, mumps, and rubella virus vaccine (live)

emetine

enalapril

measles virus vaccine (live)

erythromycin

melphalan

ethionamide

mephenytoin

ethopropazine

mephobarbital

ethosuximide

meprednisone

ethotoin

meprobamate

ethyl biscoumacetate

mesoridazine

etidocaine

methacycline

etretinate

metharbital

fenfluramine

methdilazine

flecainide

methicillin

fludrocortisone

methitural

fluorescein

methohexital

fluphenazine

methotrimeprazine

fluprednisone

methsuximide

flurazepam

methylprednisolone

gitalin

metoclopramide

gold Au 198

metrizamide

gold sodium thiomalate

metronidazole

gold sodium thiosulfate

mexiletine

griseofulvin

mianserin

halazepam

midazolam

haloperidol

minocycline

heparin

moxalactam

heptabarbital

mumps virus vaccine (live)

hetacillin

nafcillin

hexethal

nalidixic acid

hexobarbital

niacinamide

hydrabamine penicillin V

nicotinic acid

hydrocortisone

nicotinyl alcohol

ibuprofen

nifedipine

indomethacin

nitrazepam

insulin

nitrofurantoin

iodide and iodine solution and compounds

oral contraceptives

iron dextran

ouabain

isoniazid

oxacillin

lanatoside C

oxytetracycline

lincomycin

paramethadione

lorazepam

paramethasone

maprotiline

pentobarbital

perazine

pericyazine

perphenazine

phenacetin

phenobarbital

phenoxymethyl penicillin

phensuximide

piperacetazine

piroxicam

poliovirus vaccine

potassium penicillin G

potassium penicillin V

potassium phenethicillin

potassium phenoxymethyl
penicillin

prazepam

prednisolone

prednisone

primidone

probarbital procaine penicillin G

prochlorperazine

promazine

promethazine

propiomazine

quinidine

quinine

rabies immune globulin

rabies vaccine

radioactive iodides

ranitidine

rifampin

rubella and mumps virus vaccine (live)

rubella virus vaccine (live)

secobarbital

sodium salicylate

streptomycin

sulindac

talbutal

temazepam

tetanus immune globulin

tetanus toxoid

tetracycline

thiabendazole

thiamylal

thiethylperazine

thiopental

thiopropazate

thioproperazine

thioridazine

thiotepa

thiothixene

tocainide

triamcinolone

triazolam

trifluoperazine

trifluperidol

triflupromazine

trimeprazine

trimethadione

vancomycin

verapamil

vinbarbital

2. Inflammatory edema

   A. Acute hemorrhagic conjunctivitis

   B. Allergic eczema (contact dermatitis)

     (1) Anesthetics

    *(2) Atropine (topical)

     (3) Eczematous keratoconjunctivitis

     (4) Iodine

     (5) Mercury

     (6) Neurodermatitis

     (7) Penicillin

* = most important

~~(8) Photodermatitis~~

(9) Quincke edema

(10) Tuberculosis (scrofula)

C. Anthrax

D. Bee sting of the cornea

E. Dacryoadenitis

    (1) Acute dacryoadenitis

    (2) Chronic dacryoadenitis

F. Epidemic keratoconjunctivitis

G. Erysipelas

H. Herpes simplex

I. Hollenhorst syndrome (Chorioretinal infarction syndrome)

J. Hordeolum, chalazion

K. Lymphogranuloma venereum

L. Mycoses

M. Ophthalmic zoster

N. Other causes of lid edema

    (1) Conjunctival inflammations

        a. Diphtheria

        b. Newcastle disease (fowlpox)

        c. Ophthalmia neonatorum

        d. Parinaud syndrome (conjunctiva-adenitis syndrome)

    (2) Keratitis

    (3) Orbital inflammation

    (4) Periostitis

    (5) Scleritis (see p. 272)

        a. Posterior scleritis

        b. Scleromalacia perforans

    (6) Thermal, chemical, mechanical, or radiation injury

        a. Hypothermal injury

        b. Polychlorinated biphenyl (PCB)

O. Scalded skin syndrome (Ritter disease)

P. Serum sickness—systemic reaction to foreign serum, serum products, vaccines, penicillin, and sulfa drugs

Q. Silverman syndrome (battered-baby syndrome)

R. Spider bites

S. Urticaria due to drugs including:

acenocoumarin	acetazolamide
acetaminophen	acyclovir
acetanilid	albuterol

allobarbital

allopurinol

alprazolam

aluminum nicotinate

amiodarone

amitriptyline

amobarbital

amoxapine

amoxicillin

ampicillin

anisindione

antazoline

antimony lithium thiomalate

antimony potassium tartrate

antimony sodium tartrate

antimony sodium thioglycollate

antipyrine

aprobarbital

aspirin

auranofin

aurothioglucose

aurothioglycanide

azatadine

bacitracin

barbital

BCG vaccine

bendroflumethiazide

benzathine penicillin G

benzphetamine

benzthiazide

betamethasone

betaxolol

bleomycin

brompheniramine

bupivacaine

busulfan

butabarbital

butalbital

butallylonal

cactinomycin

capreomycin

captopril

carbamazepine

carbenicillin

carbimazole

carbinoxamine

carisoprodol

cefaclor

cefadroxil

cefamandole

cefazolin

cefonicid

cefoperazone

ceforanide

cefotaxime

cefotetan

cefoxitin

cefsulodin

ceftazidime

ceftizoxime

ceftriaxone

cefuroxime

cephalexin

cephaloglycin

cephaloridine

cephalothin

cephapirin

cephradine

chlorambucil

chloramphenicol

chlordiazepoxide

chloroprocaine

chlorothiazide

chlorpheniramine

chlorphentermine

chlorporthixen

chlortetracycline

chlorthalidone

cimetidine

cisplatin

clemastine

clindamycin

clofibrate

clomiphene

clomipramine

clonazepam

clonidine

clorazepate

cloxacillin

cobalt

codeine

cyclobarbital

cyclopentobartibal

cyclophosphamide

cyclosporine

cyclothiazide

cyproheptadine

cytarabine

dacarbazine

dactinomycin

danazol

dantrolene

dapsone

daunorubicin

deferoxamine

demeclocycline

desipramine

dexamethasone

dexbrompheniramine

dexchlorpheniramine

dextran

diacetylmorphine

diatrizoate meglumine and sodium

diazepam

DIC

dichlorphenamide

dicloxacillin

dicumarol

diethylcarbamazine

diethylpropion

digitalis

diltiazem

dimethindene

dimethyl sulfoxide

diphenadione

diphenhydramine

diphenylpyraline

diphtheria and tetanus toxoids (adsorbed)

diphtheria and tetanus toxoids and pertussis
(DPT) vaccine (adsorbed)

diphtheria toxoids (adsorbed)

disulfiram

DMSo

DPT vaccine

doxepin

doxorubicin

doxycycline

doxylamine

emetine

enalapril

erythromycin

ethionamide

ethotoin

ethoxzolamide

ethyl biscoumacetate

etidocaine

etretinate

fenfluramine

fenoprofen

flecainide

fluorescein

fluorouracil

flurazepam

flurbiprofen

framycetin

furosemide

gentamicin

glutethimide

gold Au 198

gold sodium thiomalate

gold sodium thiosulfate

griseofulvin

halazepam

heparin

heptabarbital

hetacillin

hexethal

hexobarbital

hydrabamine penicillin V

hydralazine

hydrochlorothiazide

hydrocortisone

hydroflumethiazide

hydromorphone

ibuprofen

imipramine

indapamide

indomethacin

influenza virus vaccine

insulin

interferon

iodide and iodine solutions and compounds

iodipamide meglumine

iophendylate

iothalamate meglumine and sodium

iothalamic acid

iron dextran

isoniazid

isosorbide

isotretinoin

ketoprofen

labetalol

levallorphan

levobunolol

lidocaine

lincomycin

lorazepam

loxapine

mannitol

maprotiline

measles and rubella virus vaccine (live)

measles, mumps, and rubella virus vaccine
  (live)

measles virus vaccine (live)

melphalan

meperidine

mephenytoin

mephobarbital

mepivacaine

meprobamate

mercuric oxide

methacycline

methadone

methaqualone

metharbital

methazolamide

methicillin

methimazole

methitural

methocarbamol

methohexital

methotrexate

methyclothiazide

methyldopa

methylphenidate

methylprednisolone

methylthiouracil

methyprylon

metoclopramide

metocurine iodide

metolazone

metoprolol

metrizamide

metronidazole

mianserin

midazolam

minocycline

mitomycin

morphine

moxalactam

mumps virus vaccine (live)

nafcillin

nalidixic acid

nalorphine

naloxone

naltrexone

naproxen

neomycin

neostigmine

niacin

niacinamide

nicotinyl alcohol

nifedipine

nitrazepam

nitrofurantoin

nitromersol

nortriptyline

opium

oral contraceptives

oxacillin

oxazepam

oxymorphone

oxyphenbutazone
oxytetracycline
penicillamine
pentazocine
pentobarbital
phenacetin
phendimetrazine
phenindione
pheniramine
phenobarbital
phenprocoumon
phentermine
phenylbutazone
phenylmercuric acetate
phenylmercuric nitrate
piperazine
piroxicam
poliovirus vaccine
polythiazide
potassium penicillin G
potassium penicillin V
potassium phenethicillin
practolol
prazepam
prazosin
prilocaine
primidone
probarbital
procaine
procaine penicillin G
procarbazine
propoxycaine
propranolol
propylthiouracil
protriptyline
pyrilamine
quinacrine
quinethazone
quinidine
quinine
rabies immune globulin
rabies vaccine
radioactive iodides

ranitidine
rifampin
rubella and mumps virus vaccine (live)
rubella virus vaccine (live)
secobarbital
smallpox vaccine
sodium antimonylgluconate
sodium salicylate
stibocaptate
stibogluconate
stibophen
streptomycin
succinylcholine
sulfacetamide
sulfachlorpyridazine
sulfacytine
sulfadiazine
sulfadimethoxine
sulfamerazine
sulfameter
sulfamethazine
sulfamethizole
sulfamethoxazole
sulfamethoxypyridazine
sulfanilamide
sulfaphenazole
sulfapyridine
sulfasalazine
sulfathiazole
sulfisoxazole
sulindac
suramin
talbutal
temazepam
tetanus immune globulin
tetanus toxoid
tetracycline
thiabendazole
thiamylal
thimerosal
thiopental
thiotepa
thiothixene

timolol
triamcinolone
triazolam
trichlormethiazide
trimethaphan
trimipramine
tripelennamine

triprolidine
tubocurarine
vancomycin
verapamil
vinbarbital
warfarin

   T. Wegener syndrome (Wegener granulomatosis)

   U. Vaccination

      (1) Ocular vaccina

      (2) Postvaccinial ocular syndrome

      (3) Variola

Flach, A.J., et al.: Photosensitivity to topically applied sulfisoxazole ointment. Arch. Ophthalmol., 100:1286–1287, 1982.

Fraunfelder, F.T.: Drug-Induced Ocular Side Effects and Drug Interactions. 4th Ed. Philadelphia, Williams & Wilkins, 1996.

Isenberg, S.J.: The Eye in Infancy. Chicago, Year Book Medical Publishers, 1989.

Newell, F.: Ophthalmology, Principles and Concepts. 7th Ed. St. Louis, C.V. Mosby, 1991.

Pau, H.: Differential Diagnosis of Eye Diseases. 2nd Ed. New York, Thieme Med. Pub., 1988.

Roy, F.H.: Ocular Syndromes and Systemic Diseases. 2nd Ed. Philadelphia, W.B. Saunders, 1989.

Yao-an, F.U.: Ocular manifestation of polychlorinated biphenyl (PCB) intoxication. Arch. Ophthalmol., 101:379–381, 1983.

Bleeding of the Eyelid

   1. Drugs including:

acetazolamide
acetohexamide
allopurinol
alprazolam
amantadine
amitriptyline
aspirin
auranofin
aurothioglucose
aurothioglycanide
BCG vaccine
bendroflumethiazide
benzthiazide
betamethasone
betaxolol
carbamazepine

chlordiazepoxide
chlorothiazide
chlorpropamide
chlorthalidone
cimetidine
clofibrate
clonazepam
clorazepate
cyclothiazide
cytarabine
danazol
dapsone
desipramine
dexamethasone
diazepam
dichlorphenamide

diltiazem

emetine

ethoxzolamide

flurazepam

furosemide

glutethimide

glyburide

gold Au 198

gold sodium thiomalate

gold sodium thiosulfate

halazepam

hydrochlorothiazide

hydrocortisone

hydroflumethiazide

ibuprofen

imipramine

indapamide

indomethacin

influenza virus vaccine

interferon

ketoprofen

levobunolol

lorazepam

measles and rubella virus vaccine (live)

measles, mumps, and rubella virus vaccine (live)

measles virus vaccine (live)

methaqualone

methazolamide

methyclothiazide

methylprednisolone

methyprylon

metolazone

metoprolol

midazolam

mumps virus vaccine (live)

naproxen

nifedipine

nitrazepam

nortriptyline

oxazepam

oxprenolol

phenytoin

piperazine

piroxicam

polythiazide

prazepam

procarbazine

propranolol

protriptyline

quinethazone

quinine

rifampin

rubella and mumps virus vaccine (live)

rubella virus vaccine (live)

smallpox vaccine

sodium salicylate

sulfacetamide

sulfachlorpyridazine

sulfacytine

sulfadiazine

sulfadimethoxine

sulfamerazine

sulfameter

sulfamethazine

sulfamethizole

sulfamethoxazole

sulfamethoxypyridazine

sulfanilamide

sulfaphenazole

sulfapyridine

sulfasalazine

sulfathiazole

sulfisoxazole

temazepam

tetanus immune globulin

tetanus toxoid

timolol

tolazamide

tolbutamide

triamcinolone

triazolam

trichlormethiazide

verapamil

2. Hutchinson syndrome (adrenal cortex neuroblastoma with orbital metastasis)

*3. Trauma

Fraunfelder, F.T.: Drug-Induced Ocular Side Effects and Drug Interactions. 4th Ed. Philadelphia, Williams & Wilkins, 1996.

Ectropion (Lid Margin Turned Outward from the Eyeball)

1. Congenital ectropion

    A. With distichiasis

    B. With tight septum; microblepharon

    C. With partial coloboma

    D. With mandibulofacial dysostosis (Franceschetti syndrome)

    E. With megaloblepharon (euryblepharon)

    F. With microphthalmos or buphthalmos

    G. Cerebro-oculo-facio-skeletal syndrome

    H. Down syndrome (mongolism)

    I. Hartnup syndrome (niacin deficiency)

    J. Lowe syndrome (oculocerebrorenal syndrome)

    K. Miller syndrome

    L. Milroy disease (oromandibular dystonia)

    M. Robinow syndrome

    N. Sjögren-Larrson syndrome

2. Acquired ectropion

    A. Spastic ectropion

      *(1) Acute spastic ectropion

      (2) Blepharophimosis syndrome

      *(3) Chronic spastic ectropion becoming cicatricial ectropion

      (4) Hypothermal injury

      (5) Myasthenia gravis—afternoon onset (Erb-Goldflam syndrome)

      (6) Siemen syndrome (hereditary ectodermal dysplasia syndrome)

    B. Atonic ectropion

      (1) Bell palsy (Idiopathic facial paralysis)

      (2) Guillain-Barré syndrome (acute infectious neuritis)

      (3) Paralytic ectropion—lagophthalmos, such as in seventh nerve palsy

      *(4) Senile ectropion—tissue relaxation

    C. Cicatricial ectropion, including scars and leprosy

      (1) Amendola syndrome

      (2) Blastomycosis

      (3) Collodion baby syndrome (congenital ichthyosis)

      (4) Etretinate therapy

      (5) Hydroa vacciniforme

* = most important

    (6) Kabuki makeup syndrome

    (7) Leprosy (Hansen disease)

    (8) Palmoplantar keratodermia

    (9) Postblepharoplasty ectropion

    (10) Psoriasis (psoriasis vulgaris)

    (11) Radiation

    (12) Sezary syndrome (malignant cutaneous reticulosis syndrome)

    (13) Systemic fluorouracil

    (14) Thermal burns

    (15) Transformation from chronic spastic ectropion

    (16) Zinsser-Engman-Cole syndrome (dyskeratosis congenita with pigmentation)

D. Allergic ectropion-anaphylactic, contact, and microbial (usually temporary)

    (1) Danbolt-Closs syndrome (acrodermatitis enteropathica)

    (2) Elschnig syndrome

E. Mechanical

    (1) Kaposi disease (multiple idiopathic hemorrhagic sarcoma)

    (2) Leiomyoma

    (3) Lumps (chalazion, cysts, neurofibroma)

Barr, C.C., and Gamel, J.W.: Blastomycosis of the eyelid. Arch. Opthalmol., 104:96–97, 1986.

Hurwitz, B.S.: Cicatricial ectropion: a complication of systemic fluorouracil. Arch Ophthal. 111:1608–1609, 1993.

Isenberg, S.J.: The eye in infancy. Chicago, Year Book Medical Publishers, 1989.

Roy, F.H.: Ocular Syndromes and Systemic Diseases. 2nd Ed. Philadelphia, W.B. Saunders, 1989.

Stratakis, C.A., et al.: A variant of the cerebro-oculo-facio-skeletal syndrome with congenital ectropion and a case of lamellar ichthyosis in the same family. Clinical Genetics, 45:162–163, 1994.

Entropion (Inversion of Lid Margin)

1. Congenital, including congenital epiblepharon—inferior oblique insufficiency; ectrodactyly, ectodermal dysplasia, cleft lip-palate syndrome, including with and without lower eyelid retractor insertion

    A. Inferior oblique insufficiency syndrome

    B. Dental-ocular-cutaneous syndrome

    C. Siemen syndrome (anhidrotic ectodermal dysplasia)

2. Acquired

    *A. Spastic entropion—acute, affecting lower lid, precipitated by acute inflammation or prolonged patching

    B. Mechanical entropion

        (1) Anophthalmos

        (2) Enophthalmos

        (3) Microphthalmos

        (4) Lymphedema

    *C. Senile entropion—relative enophthalmos secondary to fat atrophy

D. Cicatricial entropion—physical and chemical burns of conjunctiva and cicatrizing diseases, including trachoma and leprosy

  (1) Chronic cicatricial conjunctivitis

  (2) Leprosy (Hansen disease)

  (3) Radiation

  (4) Thermal burns

  (5) Trachoma

  (6) Following cryosurgery of the eyelid

  (7) Amendola syndrome

  (8) Variola

Bartley, G.B., et al.: Congenital entropion with intact lower eyelid retractor insertion. Am. J. Ophthalmol., 112:437–441, 1991.

Biglan, A.W., and Buerger, G.F.: Congenital horizontal tarsal kink. Am. J. Ophthalmol., 89:522–524, 1980.

Fraunfelder, F.T., et al.: Cryosurgery for malignancies of the eyelid. Ophthalmology, 87:461, 1982.

Roy, F.H.: Ocular Syndromes and Systemic Diseases. 2nd Ed. Philadelphia, W.B. Saunders, 1989.

Westfall, C.T., et al.: Operative Complications of the Transconjunctival inferior fornix approach. Ophthalmology, 98:1525–1528, 1991.

Epicanthus (Fold of Skin over Inner Canthus of Eye)

1. Types

    A. Epicanthus inversus—fold arises in the lower lid and extends upward to a point slightly above the inner canthus; it is accompanied by long medial canthal tendons, blepharophimosis, and ptosis—autosomal dominant

    *B. Epicanthus palpebralis (common type)—epicanthal fold arises from the upper lid above the tarsal region and extends to the lower margin of the orbit

    C. Epicanthus supraciliaris (unusual type)—epicanthal fold arises near brow and runs toward tear sac

    *D. Epicanthus tarsalis (Mongolian eye)—epicanthal fold arises from the tarsal (lid) fold and loses itself in the skin close to the inner canthus—autosomal dominant

2. Associated conditions

    A. Aminopterin-induced syndrome

    B. Basal cell nevus syndrome (Gorlin syndrome)

    C. Bassen-Kornzweig syndrome (familial hypolipoproteinemia)

    D. Bilateral renal agenesis

    E. Blepharophimosis, ptosis, epicanthus inversus syndrome

    F. Bonnevie-Ullrich syndrome (pterygolymphangiectasia)

    G. Carpenter syndrome (acrocephalopolysyndactyly II)

    H. Cat-eye syndrome (partial G-trisomy syndrome)

    I. Cerebro-facio-articular syndrome of van Maldergen

    J. Cerebrohepatorenal syndrome (Smith-Lemli-Opitz syndrome)

    K. Chondrodystrophia (Conradi syndrome)

    L. Chromosome long-arm deletion syndrome

* = most important

M. Chromosome deletion (deletion 18)

N. Chromosome partial short-arm deletion syndrome (Wolf syndrome)

O. Chromosome short-arm deletion syndrome

P. Chromosome 13q partial deletion syndrome

Q. Congenital facial paralysis (Mobius syndrome)

R. Craniocarpotarsal syndrome (whistling face syndrome)

S. Craniosynostosis-radial aplasia (Baller-Gerold syndrome)

T. Cri du chat syndrome (cry of the cat syndrome)

U. Dubowitz syndrome

V. Down syndrome (trisomy 21, mongolism)

W. Drummond syndrome (idiopathic hypercalcemia, blue diaper syndrome)

X. Ehlers-Danlos syndrome (fibrodysplasia elastica generalisata)

Y. 18q syndrome

Z. Familial blepharophimosis

AA. Fetal alcohol syndrome

BB. Freeman-Sheldon syndrome (whistling face syndrome)

CC. Gansslen syndrome (hematologic-metabolic bone disorder)

DD. Greig syndrome (ocular hypertelorism syndrome)

EE. Hurler syndrome (dysostosis multiplex)

FF. Infantile hypercalcemia

GG. Jacobs syndrome (triple X syndrome)

HH. Klinefelter XXY syndrome (gynecomastia-aspermatogenesis syndrome)

II. Kohn-Romano syndrome (ptosis, blepharophimosis, epicanthus inversus, and telecanthus)

JJ. Komoto syndrome (congenital eyelid tetrad)

KK. Laurence-Moon-Bardet-Biedl syndrome (retinitis pigmentosa-polydactyly-adiposogenital)

LL. Leopard syndrome (multiple lentigines syndrome)

MM. Leroy syndrome (mucopolysaccharide excretion)

NN. Little syndrome (nail patella syndrome)

OO. Michel's syndrome

PP. Mohr-Claussen syndrome (similar to orodigital-facial syndrome)

QQ. Noonan syndrome (Turner syndrome in males)

RR. Oculocerebrorenal syndrome (Lowe syndrome)

SS. Oculodentodigital dysplasia (microphthalmos syndrome)

TT. Potter syndrome (renofacial syndrome)

UU. Ring chromosome syndrome

VV. Ring chromosome syndrome

WW. Ring chromosome (microcephaly, hypertelorism, epicanthus)

XX. Ring chromosome in the D group (13–15)

YY. Robinow-Silverman-Smith syndrome

ZZ. Rubinstein-Taybi syndrome (broad thumbs syndrome)

AAA. Schonenberg syndrome (dwarf-cardiopathy syndrome)

BBB. Smith syndrome (facioskeletogenital dysplasia)

CCC. TAR syndrome

DDD. Thalassemia

EEE. Trisomy syndrome (Edward syndrome)

FFF. Turner syndrome (gonadal dysgenesis)

GGG. Waardenburg syndrome (embryonic fixation syndrome)

HHH. X-linked mental retardation syndrome

McKusick, V.A.: Mendelian Inheritance in Man, 9th Ed. Baltimore, Johns Hopkins University Press, 1994.

Roy, F.H.: Ocular Syndromes and Systemic Diseases. 2nd Ed. Philadelphia, W.B. Saunders, 1989.

Hypopigmentation (Depigmentation of Eyelids)

1. Drugs, including:

amodiaquine	fluorometholone	methotrexate
arsenic	gentamicin(?)	methylprednisolone
betamethasone	hydroquinone	methylthiouracil
carbimazole	hydrocortisone	neostigmine
chloramphenicol	hydroxychloroquine	physostigmine
chloroquine	isoflurophate	prednisolone
corticosteroids	medrysone	propylthiouracil
cortisone	mercaptoethylamine	thiotepa
dexamethasone	methimazole	triamcinolone

2. Genetic factors

   A. Albinism

   B. Chediak-Higashi syndrome (anomalous leukocytic inclusions with constitutional stigmata)

   C. Cross-McKusick-Breen syndrome

   D. Fanconi syndrome (amino diabetes)

   E. Hermansky-Pudlak syndrome (oculocutaneous albinism and hemorrhagic diathesis)

   F. Histidinemia

   G. Homocystinuria

   H. Incontinentia pigmenti achromians (hypomelanosis of Ito syndrome)

   I. Menkes syndrome (kinky hair syndrome)

   J. Nevus depigmentosuses

   K. Phenylketonuria (Folling syndrome)

   L. Tuberous sclerosis (Bourneville syndrome)

    M. Vitiligo

    N. Vogt-Koyanagi-Harada syndrome (uveitis-vitiligo-alopecia-poliosis syndrome)

    O. Waardenburg syndrome (embryonic fixation syndrome)

    P. Woolf syndrome (chromosome partial deletion syndrome)

    Q. Ziprkowski-Margolis syndrome

3. Following cryosurgery of the eyelid

4. Burns (thermal, ultraviolet, ionizing, radiation)

5. Trauma

6. Kwashiorkor—malnutrition in children

7. Chronic protein deficiency or loss and malabsorption of vitamin B_{12}

8. Endocrine factors

    A. Hypopituitarism (Simmond syndrome)

    B. Addison disease (adrenal cortical insufficiency)

    C. Hyperthyroidism (Grave disease)

9. Inflammation and infection

    A. Discoid lupus erythematosus

    B. Eczematous dermatitis

    C. Leprosy (Hansen disease)

    D. Onchocerciasis syndrome (river blindness)

    E. Pinta

    F. Pityriasis alba

    G. Post-inflammatory hypomelanoses

    H. Post-kala-azar

    I. Psoriasis

    J. Sarcoidosis syndrome (Schaumann syndrome)

    K. Syphilis (acquired lues)

    L. Tinea versicolor

    M. Vagabond leukoderma

    N. Vitiligo

    O. Yaws

10. Scleroderma (progressive systemic sclerosis)

Fraunfelder, F.T.: Drug-Induced Ocular Side Effects and Drug Interactions. 4th Ed. Philadelphia, Williams & Wilkins, 1996.

Fraunfelder, F.T., et al.: Cryosurgery for malignancies of the eyelid. Ophthalmology, 87:461, 1982.

Roy, F.H.: Ocular Syndromes and Systemic Diseases. 2nd Ed. Philadelphia, W.B. Saunders, 1989.

Hyperpigmentation (Discoloration of Lids)

1. Deposits of the eyelids as caused by drugs, including:

acetophenazine	butaperazine	colloidal silver
aurothioglucose	carphenazine	diethazine
aurothioglycanide	chlorpromazine	ethopropazine

ferrocholinate
ferrous sulfate
ferrous gluconate
ferrous succinate
ferrous sulfate
fluphenazine
gold Au 198
gold sodium thiomalate
iron dextran
iron sorbitex
mercuric oxide
mesoridazine

methdilazine
methotrimeprazine
mild silver protein
nitromersol
perazine
pericyazine
perphenazine
phenylmercuric acetate
phenylmercuric nitrate
piperacetazine
polysaccharide-iron complex
prochlorperazine

promazine
promethazine
propiomazine
silver nitrate
silver protein
thiethylperazine
thimerosal thiopropazate
thioproperazine
thioridazine
triflupromazine
trifluoperazine
trimeprazine

2. Hyperpigmentation as caused by drugs, including:

actinomycin C
aluminum nicotinate
aminopterin
bleomycin
busulfan
calcitriol
cyclophosphamide
cytarabine
dactinomycin
dromostanolone
epinephrine
ergocalciferol
ferrous fumarate

floxuridine
fluorouracil
fluoxymesterone
gold sodium thiosulfate
mercaptopurine
methotrexate
niacinamide
nicotinic acid
nicotinyl alcohol
pipobroman
practolol
procarbazine
quinacrine

sulfacetamide
sulfamethizole
sulfisoxazole
testolactone
testosterone
thimerosal
thioquanine
uracil mustard
vitamin A
vitamin D_2
vitamin D_3

3. Periorbital hyperpigmentation—dark circles around the eye

*A. Allergic rhinitis

*B. Familial (autosomal dominant)

C. Medium and dark complexioned Caucasians

4. Brown hyperpigmentation

A. Genetic factors

(1) Acanthosis nigricans

(2) Albright syndrome (fibrous dysplasia)

(3) Cafe-au-lait and freckle-like macules in neurofibromatosis

(4) Dyskeratosis congenita

(5) Fanconi syndrome (amino diabetes)

(6) Freckles

(7) Lentigines

(8) Melanocytic nevus

(9) Neurocutaneous melanosis

* = most important

(10) Seborrheic keratosis

(11) Xeroderma pigmentosum

B. Metabolic factors

(1) Gaucher syndrome (cerebroside lipidosis)

(2) Hemochromatosis

(3) Niemann-Pick disease (essential lipoid histiocytosis)

(4) Porphyria (cutanea tarda)

(5) Wilson disease (hepatolenticular degeneration)

C. Endocrine factors

(1) ACTH therapy

(2) Addison disease (adrenal cortical insufficiency)

(3) Estrogen therapy

(4) Melanoma

(5) Pituitary tumors

(6) Pregnancy

D. Nutritional factors

(1) Kwashiorkor (hypoproteinemia syndrome)

(2) Pellagra (avitaminosis B_2)

(3) Sprue

(4) Vitamin B_{12} deficiency (Addison pernicious anemia)

E. Chemical and pharmacologic agents

(1) Arsenic

(2) Berlock dermatosis

(3) Bleomycin

(4) Busulfan

(5) Nitrogen mustard, topical

(6) Photochemical agents

F. Physical agents

(1) Ionizing radiation

(2) Thermal radiation

*(3) Trauma

(4) Ultraviolet light

G. Inflammation and infection

(1) Atopic dermatitis

(2) Lichen planus

(3) Lichen simplex chronicus

(4) Lupus erythematosus discoid (Kaposi-Libman-Sacks syndrome)

(5) Psoriasis

(6) Tinea versicolor

H. Neoplasms

      (1) Acanthosis nigricans

      (2) Malignant melanoma

      (3) Mastocytosis

  I. Miscellaneous factors

      (1) Autosomal recessive ectodermal dysplasia

      (2) Catatonic schizophrenia

      (3) Chronic hepatic insufficiency

      (4) Cronkhite-Canada syndrome

      (5) Encephalitis

      (6) Erythema dyschromicum perstans

      (7) Liver spots

      (8) Systemic scleroderma (progressive systemic sclerosis)

      (9) Whipple syndrome (intestinal lipodystrophy)

5. Blue, gray or slate hyperpigmentation

  A. Genetic factors

      (1) Blue melanocytic nevus

      (2) Dermal melanocytosis (Mongolian spot)

      (3) Franceschetti-Jadassohn syndrome (reticular pigmented dermatosis)

      (4) Incontinentia pigmenti (Bloch-Sulzberger syndrome)

      (5) Oculodermal melanocytosis

  B. Metabolic factors

      (1) Amyloidosis, cutaneous macular (Lubarsch-Pick syndrome)

      (2) Hemochromatosis

  C. Nutritional factors

      (1) Chronic nutritional insufficiency

  D. Inflammation and infection

      (1) Erythema dyschromicum perstans

      (2) Pinta

      (3) Riehl melanosis

  E. Chemical and pharmacologic agents

      (1) Chlorpromazine

      (2) Gold

      (3) Phenothiazines

      (4) Sulfonamides

      (5) Tetracyclines

  F. Neoplasms

      (1) Slate-gray dermal pigmentation with metastatic melanoma and melanogenuria

  G. Other

      (1) Blue dye

      (2) Cyanosis

* = most important

Ellis, D.S.: Congenital neurocutaneous melanosis with metastatic orbital malignant melanoma. Ophthalmology, 93:1639–1642, 1986.

Fitzpatrick, T.B., et al.: Dermatology in general medicine. New York, McGraw-Hill Book Co., 1982.

Fraunfelder, F.T.: Drug Induced Ocular Side Effects and Drug Interactions. 4th ed. Philadelphia, Williams & Wilkins, 1996.

Haddock, N., and Wilkin, J.K.: Periorbital hyperpigmentation. J.A.M.A., 246:835, 1981.

Pau, H.: Differential diagnosis of eye diseases. 2nd ed. New York, Thieme Med. Pub., 1988.

Schwartz, M.P.: Blue Christmas. J.A.M.A., 257:3229–3230, 1987.

Tumors of Eyelids

1. Molluscum contagiosum—small, greasy-appearing elevation that is usually umbilicated, or any other granuloma
2. Neoplasm
   A. Basal cell epithelioma—very common; may be a red, circumscribed, lobulated growth involving the lid margin, or may have an umbilicated center (rodent ulcer)
   B. Squamous cell or Zeis cell epithelioma—hard pearly-appearing lesion, usually without increased vascularity
   C. Meibomian-gland carcinoma—resembles a chalazion
   D. Metastatic tumors of the lid—respiratory tract, breast, skin (melanoma), gastrointestinal tract, or kidney
   E. Keratoacanthoma—benign, hemispherical, elevated tumor with a central keratin-filled crater; develops within several months
   F. Hemangioma—rubor of vascular tumor, usually having a smooth surface with tufts of vessels near the surface
   G. Benign mixed tumor of the lacrimal (palpebral) gland
   H. Trichilemmoma
3. Metaplasia or hyperplasia
   A. Trichoepithelioma
   B. Syringoma
   *C. Sebaceous adenoma
   *D. Papilloma-smooth, rounded, or pedunculated elevation
   *E. Nevus—usually pigmented, raised, and smooth surfaced; however, may be papillomatous or contain hair
   F. Benign calcifying epithelioma
   G. Inverted follicular keratosis
   H. Blue nevus—blue-black and velvet-like in appearance
4. Cyst
   *A. Sebaceous
   B. Sudoriferous
   C. Traumatic
   D. Congenital inclusion
5. Lipoid proteinosis—wax-like, pearly nodules

6. Pseudotumor of lid-encysted contact lens

7. Amyloidosis (Lubarsch-Pick syndrome)

Fett, D.R., and Putterman, A.M.: Primary localized amyloidosis presenting as an eyelid margin tumor. Arch. Ophthalmol., 104:584–585, 1986.

Hidayat, A.A., and Font, R.L.: Trichilemmoma of eyelid and eyebrow. Arch. Ophthalmol., 98:844, 1980.

Jakobiec, F.A., et al.: Syringocystadenoma papilliferum of the eyelid. Ophthalmology, 87:1175, 1982.

Older, J.J.: Encysted corneal contact lens presenting an eyelid mass. Ann. Ophthal., 11:1393, 1979.

Pau, H.: Differential Diagnosis of Eye Diseases. 2nd ed. New York, Thieme Med. Pub., 1988.

Perlman, E., and McMahon, R.T.: Sebaceous gland carcinoma of the eyelid. Am. J. Ophthalmol., 86:699–703, 1978.

Rosenbaum, P.S., et al.: Phakomatous Choristoma of the Eyelid. Ophthalmology., 99:1779–1784, 1993.

Saxe, S.J., et al.: Glomus Cell Tumor of the Eyelid. Ophthalmology, 100:139–143, 1993.

Tumors of Eyelids

	Molluscum Contagiosum*	Neoplasm as Basal Cell*	Metaplasia/Hyperplasia as Trichoepithelioma	Cyst as Sebacemon*	Lipoid Proteinosis	Pseudotumor of Lids
History						
1. Foreign body history						U
2. Hereditary			S	U		
3. Malignancy previously		U				
4. More frequent lower lid		U				
5. Viral etiology	U					
Physical Findings						
1. A rise in hair-bearing skin		U				
2. Bead-like excrescences with loss of cilia at lid margins					U	
3. Chalazion		U				
4. Chronic blepharitis		U			U	
5. Conjunctivitis	U					
6. Cystic nodules filled with sebaceous/serious material				U		
7. Ectropion		S				
8. Encysted contact lens						U
9. Entropion		S				
10. Flesh-colored, rounded papules—some pigmented			U			
11. Foreign body sensation						U
12. Keratitis	U					
13. Lid notching		U				
14. Lid retraction		U				
15. Madarosis		U			U	
16. Nodular hyperemic lid lesion						U
17. Nodular/nodular ulcerative lid lesion		U				
18. Small umbilicated tumor	U					
19. Yellow-white nodule				U	U	
Laboratory Data						
Histopathology						
Epithelial cyst walls have serous/sebaceous material				U		
Granuloma	U					
Granulomatous infiltrates with micro-organisms						U
Large, nuclear forms, including multinucleated cells and monstrous cellular forms				U		
Lower lipid content					U	
Narrow strand of basaloid cells like adenoid basal cell carcinomas, keratinizing cysts with pilar differentiation			U			
Tumor cells in nests, cords, sheets; peripheral cells may palisade		U		S		

R = rarely; S = sometimes; and U = usually.

Xanthelasma (Smooth Yellow Deposits in the Eyelid, Especially the Superior Nasal and Inferior Nasal Areas)

1. Xanthelasma with hyperlipemia (primary or secondary)

    *A. Type II-familial hyper-B-lipoproteinemia (familial hypercholesterolemia)

    *B. Type III-familial hyper-B- and hyper-pre-B-lipoproteinemia (familial hyper-lipemia with hypercholesterolemia)

    C. Other types infrequent, including type I, familial fat-induced hyperlipopro-teinemia (hyperchylomicronemia); type IV, familial hyper-pre-B-lipopro-teinemia (carbohydrate-induced hyperlipemia); type V, familial hyperchy-lomicronemia with hyper-pre-B-lipoproteinemia (mixed hyperlipemia), lichen sclerosis et atrophicus.

2. Xanthelasma without hyperlipemia

    A. Generalized

    B. Histiocytosis X (Eosinophilic granuloma, Hand Schüller-Christian disease, and Letterer-Siwe disease)

    C. Local (no systemic disease)

    D. Reticulohistiocytoma cutis

    E. Xanthoma disseminatum

Depot, M.J., et al.: Bilateral and extensive xanthelasma palpebrarum in a young man. Ophthalmol-ogy, 91:522–527, 1984.

Roy, F.H.: Ocular Syndromes and Systemic Diseases. 2nd ed. Philadelphia, W.B. Saunders, 1989.

Chronic Blepharitis (Inflammation of Lids)

*1. Seborrheic—lid margin covered with small, white or gray scales

    A. Associated with seborrheic dermatitis of the scalp

    B. Aggravated by chemical fumes, smoke, and smog

    C. May be associated with uncorrected refractive errors (especially hyperopia)

    D. May be due to Pityrosporon ovale

    E. Aspergillus fumigatus may be its cause

    F. Associated with systemic diseases

        (1) Acne rosacea

        (2) Acinetobacter Iwoffi

        (3) Acrodermatitis chronica atrophicans

        (4) Aspergillosis

        (5) Candidiasis

        (6) Cretinism (hypothyroidism)

        (7) Demodicosis

        (8) Dermatophytosis

        (9) Diphtheria

        (10) Erysipelas

        (11) Herpes simplex

* = most important

(12) Hypocalcemia

(13) Hypoparathyroidism

(14) Listerellosis

(15) Malaria

(16) Moraxella lacunata

(17) Pellagra (avitaminosis B_2)

*(18) Seborrheic dermatitis

(19) Sporotrichosis

(20) Staphylococcus

(21) Streptococcus

(22) Syphilis (acquired lues)

(23) Scleroderma (systemic scleroderma)

(24) Tuberculosis

(25) Vaccinia

(26) Xeroderma pigmentosum

G. Associated with syndromes

(1) Danbolt-Closs syndrome (acrodermatitis enteropathica)

(2) Down syndrome (mongolism)

(3) Goldscheider syndrome (epidermolysis bullosa)

(4) Hand-Schüller-Christian syndrome (lipoid granuloma syndrome)

(5) Lyell syndrome (toxic epidermal necrolysis)

(6) Myotonic dystrophy syndrome (Curschmann-Steinert syndrome)

(7) Parkinson syndrome (paralysis agitans)

(8) Sezary syndrome (mycosis fungoides syndrome)

(9) Siemens syndrome (hereditary ectodermal dysplasia syndrome)

(10) Syndrome of Beal (acute follicular conjunctivitis)

(11) Wernicke syndrome

(12) Thiamine deficiency

(13) Wiskott-Aldrich syndrome

(14) Zinsser-Engman-Cole syndrome (dyskeratosis congenita with pigmentation)

H. Drugs including:

acyclovir	meperidine	thimerosal
benzalkonium	mercuric oxide	trifluridine
F3T idoxuridine	nitromersol	vidarabine
isosorbide	phenylmercuric acetate	
mannitol	phenylmercuric nitrate	

2. Ulcerative—suppurative inflammation of the follicles of the lashes and the associated glands of Zeis and Moll

A. Staphylococcus aureus or S. albus may be responsible

B. Due to mixed infection of a staphylococcus and P. ovale

C. Associated with vaccinia

D. Due to blastomyces dermatitidis

E. Herpes simplex—vesicles at lash line then ulceration

*3. Angular—inflammation of the angles of the lids, usually associated with an angular conjunctivitis

    A. Candida albicans

    B. Moraxella lacunata

    C. Stannus cerebellar syndrome (riboflavin deficiency)

    D. Staphylococcus aureus

4. Exfoliative dermatitis owing to drugs, including:

acetohexamide	busulfan	chlorambucil
acetophenazine	butabarbital	chloroprocaine
acid bismuth sodium tartrate	butalbital	chloroquine
adiphenine	butallylonal	chlorpromazine
allobarbital	butaperazine	chlorpropamide
allopurinol	butethal	chlorprothixene
ambutonium	carbamazepine	cimetidine
aminosalicylate(?)	carbenicillin	clidinium
aminosalicylic acid	carbimazole	clindamycin
amithiozone	carisoprodol	cloxacillin
amobarbital	carphenazine	codeine
amodiaquine	cefaclor	cyclobarbital
amoxicillin	cefadroxil	cyclopentobarbital
ampicillin	cefamandole	cyclophosphamide
anisindione	cefazolin	dapsone
anisotropine	cefonicid	dicloxacillin
aprobarbital	cefoperazone	dicyclomine
atropine methylnitrate	ceforanide	diethazine
auranofin	cefotaxime	diltiazem
aurothioglucose	cefotetan	diphemanil
aurothioglycanide	cefoxitin	diphenadione
barbital	cefsulodin	diphenylhydantoin
bismuth carbonate	ceftazidime	droperidol
bismuth oxychloride	ceftizoxime	enalapril
bismuth salicylate	ceftriaxone	erythrityl tetranitrate
bismuth sodium tartrate	cefuroxime	erythromycin
bismuth sodium thioglycollate	cephalexin	ethionamide
bismuth sodium triglycollamate	cephaloglycin	ethopropazine
	cephaloridine	ethosuximide
bismuth subcarbonate	cephalothin	ethotoin
bismuth subsalicylate	cephapirin	etidocaine
bupivacaine	cephradine	fenoprofen

flecainide
fluphenazine
furosemide
glutethimide
glyburide
glycopyrrolate
gold Au 198
gold sodium thiomalate
gold sodium thiosulfate
griseofulvin
haloperidol
heptabarbital
hetacillin
hexethal
hexobarbital
hexocyclium
hydroxychloroquine
indomethacin
iodide and iodine solutions
   and compounds
isoniazid
isopropamide
isosorbide dinitrate
ketoprofen
lidocaine
lincomycin
mannitol hexanitrate
mechlorethamine
melphalan
mepenzolate
mephenytoin
mephobarbital
mepivacaine
meprobamate
mesoridazine
methantheline
metharbital
methdilazine
methicillin
methimazole
methitural
methixene
methohexital

methotrimeprazine
methsuximide
methylatropine nitrate
methylphenidate
methylthiouracil
methyprylon
moxalactam
nafcillin
naltrexone
naproxen(?)
nitroglycerin
oxacillin
oxyphenbutazone
oxyphencyclimine
oxyphenonium
paramethadione
pentaerythritol tetranitrate
pentobarbital
perazine
pericyazine
perphenazine
phenindione
phenobarbital
phensuximide
phenylbutazone
phenytoin
pimozide
pipenzolate
piperacetazine
piperidolate
piroxicam
poldine
practolol
prilocaine
primidone
probarbital
procaine
procarbazine
prochlorperazine
promazine
promethazine
propantheline
propiomazine

propoxycainepropoxyphene
propranolol
propylthiouracil
quinacrine
quinidine
radioactive iodides
rifampin
secobarbital
streptomycin
sulfacetamide
sulfachlorpyridazine
sulfacytine
sulfadiazine
sulfadimethoxine
sulfamerazine
sulfameter
sulfamethazine
sulfamethizole
sulfamethoxazole
sulfamethoxy-pyridazine
sulfanilamide
sulfaphenazole
sulfapyridine
sulfasalazine
sulfathiazole
sulfisoxazole
sulindac
talbutal
thiabendazole
thiamylal
thiethylperazine
thiopental
thiopropazate
thioproperazine
thioridazine
thiothixene
tolazamide
tolbutamide
trichloroethylene
tridihexethyl
triethylenemelamine
trifluoperazine
trifluperidol

triflupromazine   trolnitrate   vinbarbital
trimeprazine   uracil mustard   vitamin A
trimethadione   vancomycin

5. Other types
     A. Due to mites (Demodex folliculorum)
     B. Due to pubic lice (Phthirus pubis)
6. Erythema due to drugs, including:

acebutolol   cefoperazone   danazol
acetaminophen   ceforanide   dactinomycin
acetanilid   cefotaxime   daunorubicin
acetazolamide   cefotetan   deferoxamine
acyclovir   cefoxitin   demeclocycline
albuterol   cefsulodin   desipramine
allopurinol   ceftazidime   dexamethasone
alprazolam   ceftizoxime   dexbrompheniramine
amitriptyline   ceftriaxone   dexchlorpheniramine
amoxapine   cefuroxime   dextran
antazoline   cephalexin   diacetylmorphine
atenolol   cephaloglycin   diatrizoate
auranofin   cephaloridine   meglumine and sodium
aurothioglucose   cephalothin   diazepam
aurothioglycanide   cephapirin   diazoxide
azatadine   cephradine   dichlorphenamide
BCG vaccine   chlorambucil   diethylcarbamazine
benzalkonium   chlordiazepoxide   diethylpropion
benzathine penicillin G chlorpheniramine   diltiazem
benzphetamine   chlorphentermine   dimethindene
betamethasone   chlorphtermine   dimethyl sulfoxide
betaxolol   chlortetracycline   diphenhydramine
bleomycin   cimetidine   diphenylpyraline
bromide   cisplatin   diphtheria and tetanus toxoids
brompheniramine   clemastine   (adsorbed)
busulfan   clofibrate   diphtheria and tetanus toxoids
cactinomycin   clomipramine   and pertussis vaccine
captopril   clonazepam   (adsorbed)
carbinoxamine   clorazepate   diphtheria toxoid (adsorbed)
carmustine   cortisone   disopyramide
cefaclor   cyclophosphamide   disulfiram
cefadroxil   cyclosporin   doxepin
cefamandole   cyproheptadine   doxorubicin
cefazolin   cytarabine   doxycycline
cefonicid   dacarbazine   doxylamine
                                              enalapril

ergonovine

ergotamine

ethionamide

ethoxzolamide

etretinate

fenfluramine

fenoprofen

flecainide

floxuridine

fluorometholone

fluorouracil

flurazepam

flurbiprofen

framycetin

gold Au 198

gold sodium thiomalate

gold sodium thiosulfate

halazepam

hexachlorophene

hydrabamine penicillin V

hydralazine

hydrocortisone

hydroxyurea

ibuprofen

imipramine

influenza virus vaccine

insulin

iodipamide meglumine

iothalamate meglumine and
   sodium

iothalamic acid

iron dextran

isotretinoin

ketoprofen

labetalol

levallorphan

levobunolol

lomustine

lorazepam

maprotiline

measles and rubella virus
   vaccine (live)

measles, mumps, and rubella
   virus vaccine (live)

measles virus vaccine (live)

mechlorethamine

medrysone

melphalan

meperidine

mercuric oxide

methacycline

methazolamide

methocarbamol

methotrexate

methoxsalen

methylergonovine

methysergide

metocurine iodide

metoprolol

metronidazole

mexiletine

mianserin

midazolam

minocycline

minoxidil

mitotane

mitomycin

moxalactam

mumps virus vaccine (live)

nadolol

nalorphine

naloxone

naltrexone

naproxen

neomycin

neostigmine

nifedipine

nitrazepam

nitromersol

nortriptyline

oxazepam

oxprenolol

oxytetracycline

pentazocine

phenacetin

phendimetrazine

pheniramine

phentermine

phenylephrine

phenylmercuric acetate

phenylmercuric nitrate

pindolol

piroxicam

poliovirus vaccine

potassium penicillin G

potassium penicillin V

potassium phenethicillin

practolol

prazepam

prazosin

prednisolone

procaine penicillin G

procarbazine

propranolol

protriptyline

pyrilamine

rabies immune globulin

rabies vaccine

ranitidine

rifampin

rubella and mumps virus
   vaccine (live)

semustine

smallpox vaccine

spironolactone

streptomycin

streptozocin

succinylcholine

sulindac

temazepam

tetanus immune globulin

tetanus toxoid

tetracycline

thimerosal

thiotepa

timolol

tocainide

trazodone

triazolam

triethylenemelamine	tripelennamine	uracil mustard
trimipramine	triprolidine	verapamil
trioxsalen	tubocurarine	

Fedukowicz, H.B.: External Infections of the Eye. 3rd Ed. New York, Appleton-Century-Crofts, 1984.

Fraunfelder, F.T.: Drug-Induced Ocular Side Effects and Drug Interactions. 4th Ed. Philadelphia, Williams & Wilkins, 1996.

McCulley, J.P., et al.: Classification of chronic blepharitis. Ophthalmol., 89:1173, 1982.

Roy, F.H.: Ocular Syndromes and Systemic Diseases. 2nd Ed. Philadelphia, W.B. Saunders, 1989.

Scheie, H.G.: Textbook of Ophthalmology. 10th Ed. Philadelphia, W.B. Saunders, 1986.

Acute Blepharitis (Inflammation of Lids with Rapid Onset)

1. Usual allergy to drugs, including:

acenocoumarin	atropine	carisoprodol
acetaminophen	atropine methylnitrate	carmustine
acetanilid	auranofin	carphenazine
acetazolamide	aurothioglucose	cefaclor
acetohexamide	aurothioglycanide	cefadroxil
acetophenazine	bacitracin	cefamandole
acetyldigitoxin	barbital belladonna	cefazolin
actinomycin C	bendroflumethiazide	cefonicid
acyclovir	benoxinate	cefoperazone
adenine arabinoside	benzalkonium	ceforanide
adiphenine	benzathine penicillin G	cefotaxime
allobarbital allopurinol	benzphetamine	cefotetan
alprazolam	benzthiazide	cefoxitin
aluminum nicotinate	betamethasone	cefsulodin
ambutonium(?)	betaxolol	ceftazidime
aminopterin	bishydroxycoumarin	ceftizoxime
aminosalicylate(?)	bleomycin	ceftriaxone
aminosalicylic acid(?)	bromide	cefuroxime
amithiozone	bupivacaine	cephalexin
amobarbital	busulfan	cephapirin
amodiaquine	butabarbital	cephaloglycin
amoxicillin	butacaine	cephaloridine
amphotericin B	butalbital	cephalothin
ampicillin	butallylonal	cephradine
amyl nitrite	butaperazine	chloral hydrate
anisindione	butethal	chlorambucil chloramphenicol
anisotropine	cactinomycin	chlordiazepoxide
antazoline	carbachol	chloroprocaine
antipyrine	carbamazepine	chloroquine
aprobarbital	carbenicillin	chlorothiazide
aspirin	carbimazole	chlorphentermine

chlorpromazine	digitalis	gentamicin
chlorpropamide	digitoxin	gitalin
chlorprothixene	digoxin	glutethimide
chlortetracycline	dimercaprol	glyburide
chlorthalidone	dimethyl sulfoxide	glycopyrrolate
chrysarobin	diphenamil	gold Au 198
clidinium	diphenadione	gold sodium thiomalate
clindamycin	diphenylhydantoin	gold sodium thiosulfate
clomiphene	diphtheria and tetanus toxoids	griseofulvin
clonazepam	(adsorbed)	halazepam
clorazepate	diphtheria and tetanus toxoids	haloperidol
cloxacillin	and pertussis vaccine	heparin
cobalt	(adsorbed)	heptabarbital
cocaine	diphtheria toxoid adsorbed	hetacillin
colistin	dipivefrin	hexethal
colloidal silver	disulfiram	hexobarbital
cortisone	doxorubicin	hexocyclium
cyclobarbital	dromostanolone	homatropine
cyclopentobarbital	droperidol	hyaluronidase
cyclopentolate	dyclonine	hydrabamine penicillin V
cyclophosphamide	echothiophate	hydralazine
cycloserine	edrophonium emetine	hydrochlorothiazide
cyclothiazide	ephedrine	hydrocortisone
cytarabine	epinephrine	hydroflumethiazide
dacarbazine	ergonovine	hydromorphone
dactinomycin	ergotamine	hydroxyamphetamine
daunorubicin	erythromycin	hydroxychloroquine
deferoxamine	ethionamide	idoxuridine
demecarium	ethopropazine	indapamide
deslanoside	ethosuximide	influenza virus vaccine
dexamethasone	ethotoin	insulin
diatrizoate meglumine	ethoxzolamide	iodide and iodine solutions
and sodium	ethyl biscoumacetate	and compounds
diazepam	etidocaine	iodipamide meglumine
diazoxide	fenfluramine	iothalamate meglumine and
dibucaine	fluorescein	sodium
dichlorphenamide	fluorometholone	iothalamic acid
dicloxacillin	fluorouracil	isoflurophate
dicumarol	fluoxymesterone	isoniazid
dicyclomine	fluphenazine	isopropamide
diethazine	flurazepam	kanamycin
diethylcarbamazine	framycetin	Lanatoside C
diethylpropion	F3T	levallorphan
	furosemide	

levobunolol
levodopa
lidocaine
lincomycin
lomustine
lorazepam
measles and rubella virus vaccine (live)
measles, mumps, and rubella virus vaccine (live)
measles virus vaccine (live)
mechlorethamine
medrysone
melphalan
mepenzolate
meperidine
mephenytoin
mephobarbital
mepivacaine
meprobamate
mercuric oxide
mesoridazine
methacholine
methantheline
metharbital
methazolamide
methdilazine
methicillin
methimazole
methitural
methixene
methohexital
methotrexate
methotrimeprazine
methsuximide
methyclothiazide
methylatropine nitrate
methyldopa
methylergonovine
methylprednisolone
methysergide
methylthiouracil methyprylon
metolazone

metrizamide
midazolam
mild silver protein
mitomycin
morphine
moxalactam
mumps virus vaccine (live)
nafcillin
nalorphine
naloxone
naltrexone
naphazoline
naproxen
neomycin
neostigmine
niacinamide
nicotinic acid
nicotinyl alcohol
nitrazepam
nitrofurantoin
nitromersol
nystatin
opium
oral contraceptives
ouabain
oxacillin
oxprenolol
oxymorphone
oxyphenbutazone
oxyphencyclimine
oxyphenonium
paramethadione
pentobarbital
perazine
pericyazine
perphenazine
phenacaine
phenacetin
phendimetrazine
phenindione
phenobarbital
phenprocoumon
phensuximide

phentermine
phenylbutazone
phenylephrine
phenylmercuric acetate
phenylmercuric nitrate
phenytoin
physostigmine
pilocarpine
pipenzolate
piperacetazine
piperazine
piperidolate
piperocaine
pipobroman
poldine
polymyxin B
polythiazide
potassium penicillin G
potassium penicillin V
potassium phenethicillin
potassium phenoxymethyl penicillin
prazepam
prednisolone
prilocaine
primidone
probarbital
procaine
procaine penicillin G
prochlorperazine
promazine
promethazine
propantheline
proparacaine
propiomazine
propoxycaine
propranolol
propylthiouracil
quinethazone
quinidine
quinine
rabies immune globulin
rabies vaccine

~~radioactive iodides~~	sulfapyridine	thiothixene
scopolamine	sulfasalazine	timolol
secobarbital	sulfathiazole	tolazamide
semustine	sulfisoxazole	tolbutamide
silver nitrate	talbutal	trazodone
silver protein	temazepam	triazolam
sodium salicylate	testolactone	trichlormethiazide
streptomycin	testosterone	tridihexethyl
streptozocin	tetanus immune globulin	triethylenemelamine
succinylcholine	tetanus toxoid	trifluoperazine
sulfacetamide	tetracaine	trifluorothymidine
sulfachlorpyridazine	tetracycline	trifluperidol
sulfadiazine	tetrahydrozoline	triflupromazine
sulfadimethoxine	thiabendazole	trifluridine
sulfamerazine	thiamylal	trimeprazine
sulfameter	thiethylperazine	trimethadione
sulfamethazine	thimerosal	tropicamide
sulfamethizole	thiopental	uracil mustard
sulfamethoxazole	thiopropazate	vancomycin
sulfamethoxypyridazine	thioproperazine	vidarabine
sulfanilamide	thioridazine	vinbarbital
sulfaphenazole	thiotepa	warfarin

*2. Infections, such as bacterial, fungal, and viral

Tasman, W., and Jaeger, E., eds.: Duane's Clinical Ophthalmology. Philadelphia, J.B. Lippincott, 1990.

Fraunfelder, F.T.: Drug-Induced Ocular Side Effects and Drug Interactions. 4th Ed. Philadelphia, Williams & Wilkins, 1996.

Thickened Eyelids

1. Trachoma

2. Multiple chalazia

*3. Chronic conjunctivitis

*4. Blepharitis—lid margins thickened

5. Tarsitis—rare, such as in syphilis or tuberculosis

6. Trisomy (E syndrome)

7. Congenital hypothyroidism

8. Pheochromocytoma, medullary thyroid carcinoma, and neurofibromatosis

Baum, J.L., and Adler, M.E.: Pheochromocytoma, medullary thyroid carcinoma and multiple mucosal neuroma. Arch. Ophthalmol., 87:574–584, 1972.

Gellis, S.S., and Feingold, M.: Atlas of Mental Retardation. Washington, D.C., U.S. Government Printing Office, 1968.

Blepharophimosis (Short Palpebral Fissure)

1. Blepharochalasis
2. Blepharofacioskeletal syndrome
3. Blepharophimosis-amenorrhea syndrome (Blepharophimosis, ptosis, epicanthus inversus syndrome)
4. Carpenter syndrome (acrocephalopolysyndactyly II)
5. Clefting syndrome with anterior chamber and lid anomalies
6. Craniocarpotarsal syndrome (Freeman-Sheldon syndrome; whistling face syndrome)
7. Down syndrome (trisomy 21, mongolism)
8. Dubowitz syndrome
9. Freeman-Sheldon syndrome (whistling face syndrome)
10. Kaufman oculocerbrofacial syndrome
11. Klein-Waardenburg syndrome
12. Komoto syndrome (congenital eyelid tetrad)
13. Marden-Walker syndrome
14. Meyer-Schwickerath and Weyers syndrome
15. Michel's syndrome
*16. Microphthalmos
17. Mohr syndrome (orofaciodigital syndrome II)
18. Myhre syndrome
19. Oculopalatoskeletal syndrome
20. Ohdo blepharophimosis syndrome
21. Pena-Shokeir type II syndrome
22. Progeria (Hutchinson-Gilford syndrome)
23. Rieger syndrome (dysgenesis mesostromalis)
24. Ring chromosome in the D group (13–15) (ring D syndrome)
25. Schonenberg syndrome (dwarf cardiopathy syndrome)
26. Schwartz-Jampel syndrome (osteochondromuscular dystrophy)
27. Simosa syndrome
28. Syndrome of blepharophimosis with myopathy
*29. Traumatic
30. Trisomy (E syndrome) (Edward syndrome)
31. Waardenburg syndrome (embryonic fixation syndrome)
32. Young-Simpson syndrome
33. X-linked mental retardation syndrome
34. 3p- syndrome
35. 10q- syndrome

Bonthron, D.T., et al.: Parental consanguinity in the blepharophimosis, heart defect, hypothyroidism, mental retardation syndrome (Young-Simpson syndrome). J. Medical Genetics, 30:255–256, 1993.

Isenberg, S.J.: The Eye in Infancy. Chicago, Year Book Medical Publishers, 1989.

* = most important

Melnyk, A.R.: Blepharophimosis, ptosis and mental retardation: further delineation of Ohdo syndrome. Clinical Dysmorphology, 3:121–124, 1994.

Roy, F.H.: Ocular Syndromes and Systemic Diseases. 2nd Ed. Philadelphia, W.B. Saunders, 1989.

Suri, M., et al.: Blepharophimosis, telecanthus, microstomia, and unusual ear anomaly Simosa syndrome in an infant. Amer. J. Medical. Genetics, 51: 222–223, 1994.

Euryblepharon (Horizontally Elongated Palpebral Aperture [Normal, to mm]. May Be Associated with Ectropion and Present in Other Family Members)

1. Excessive tension of skin
2. Defective separation of the lids
3. Excessive pull of the platysma
*4. Localized displacement of the lateral canthi
5. Hypoplasia of tarsus

Feldman, E., et al.: Euryblepharon: A case report with photographs documenting the condition from infancy to adulthood. J. Pediatr. Ophthalmol. Strabismus, 17:307–309, 1980.

Gupta, A.K., et al.: Euryblepharon. J. Pediatr. Ophthalmol., 9:173–174, 1972.

McCord, C.D., et al.: Congenital euryblepharon. Ann. Ophthalmol., 11:1217–1224, 1979.

Lid Coloboma

1. Amniogenic band syndrome (amniotic bands-Streeter anomaly)
2. Epidermal nevus syndrome
3. Facial clefting syndrome (Tessier syndromes)
4. Fraser's syndrome
5. Frontonasal dysplasia syndrome
6. Goldenhar syndrome (oculoauriculovertebral dysplasia)
7. Miller syndrome
8. Nager syndrome
9. Nevus sebaceous of Jadassohn (linear sebaceous nevus syndrome)
10. Palpebral coloboma-lipoma syndrome
*11. Traumatic
12. Treacher Collins-Francheschetti syndrome (mandibulofacial dysostosis)

Braude, L. L., et al.: Ocular abnormalities in the amniogenic band syndrome. Br. J. Ophthalmol., 65:299–303, 1981.

Burch, J.V., et al.: Ichthyosis hystrix (epidermal nevus syndrome) and Coats' disease. Am. J. Opthalmol., 89:25–30, 1980.

Isenberg, S.J.: The Eye of Infancy. Chicago, Year Book Medical Publishers, 1989.

Roy, F.H.: Ocular Syndromes and Systemic Diseases. 2nd Ed. Philadelphia, W.B. Saunders, 1989.

Necrosis of Eyelids

1. Drugs including:

acenocoumarol	diphenadione	phenprocoumon
amphotericin B	ethyl biscoumacetate	warfarin
anisindione	nafcillin	
dicumarol	phenindione	

*2. Mechanical, electrical, or thermal trauma

3. Periorbital cellulitis-periorbital necrotizing cellulitis

4. Secondary to infection

Fraunfelder, F.T.: Drug-Induced Ocular Side Effects and Drug Interactions. 4th Ed. Philadelphia, Williams & Wilkins, 1996.

Scott, P.M., and Bloome, M.A.: Lid necrosis secondary to streptococcal periorbital cellulitis. Ann. Ophthalmol., 13:461, 1981.

Poliosis (Whitening of Hair, Eyebrows, and Eyelashes)

1. Albino

2. Alopecia areata

*3. Aging

4. Drugs including:

amodiaquine	fluorometholone
betamethasone	hydrocortisone
chloroquine	hydroxychloroquine
cortisone	medrysone
cyclosporin A	prednisolone
dexamethasone	thiotepa
epinephrine	

5. Leprosy (Hansen disease)

6. Radiation therapy

7. Rubinstein-Taybi syndrome

8. Severe dermatitis

9. Stress

*10. Unknown etiology

11. Vitiligo

12. Vogt-Koyanagi-Harada syndrome (uveitis-vitiligo-alopecia-poliosis syndrome)

13. Waardenburg syndrome (embryonic fixation syndrome)

14. Werner syndrome (progeria of adults)

Fraunfelder, F.T.: Drug-Induced Ocular Side Effects and Drug Interactions. 4th Ed. Philadelphia, Williams & Wilkins, 1996.

Pau, H.: Differential Diagnosis of Eye Diseases. 2nd Ed. New York, Thieme Med. Pub., 1988.

Rosner, F.: Can hair turn white overnight? J.A.M.A., 246:2324, 1981.

Roy, F.H.: Ocular Syndromes and Systemic Diseases. 2nd Ed. Philadelphia, W.B. Saunders, 1989.

Walsh, F.B., and Hoyt, W.F.: Clinical Neuro-ophthalmology. 4th Ed. Baltimore, Williams & Wilkins, 1985.

Trichomegaly (Long Lashes)

1. Associated with cataract and hereditary spherocytosis

2. Congenital with pigmentary retinal degeneration, dwarfism, and mental retardation

3. Cyclosporine induced

* = most important

4. De Lange syndrome (congenital muscular hypertrophy—cerebral syndrome)

5. Ectodermal dysplasia (Curtius syndrome)

6. HIV (human immunodeficiency virus)

7. Hypertrichosis (hirsutism)

8. Isolated adrenal malfunction and ovarian atrophy

9. Noonan syndrome (male Turner syndrome)

*10. Normal

11. Oliver-McFarlane syndrome

12. Rubinstein-Taybi syndrome (broad thumbs syndrome)

13. Schwartz syndrome

Chang, T.S., et al.: Congenital trichomegaly, pigmentary degeneration of the retina and growth retardation Oliver-McFarlane syndrome year follow-up of the first reported case. Cand. J. Ophthal., 28:191–193, 1993.

Isenberg, S.J.: The Eye in Infancy. Chicago, Year Book Medical Publishers, 1989.

Kaplan, M.H. et al.: Acquired trichomegaly of the eyelashes: a cutaneous marker of immunodeficiency syndrome. J. Am. Acad. Dermatol., 25:801–804, 1991.

McKusick, V.A.: Mendelian Inheritance in Man. 9th Ed. Baltimore, Johns Hopkins University Press, 1994.

Roy, F.H.: Ocular Syndromes and Systemic Diseases. 2nd Ed. Philadelphia, W.B. Saunders, 1989.

Weaver, D.T., and Bartley, G.B.: Cyclosporine-induced trichomegaly. Amer. J. Ophthal., 109:239, 1990.

Madarosis (Loss of Eyelashes)

1. Chronic skin diseases, including psoriasis, neurodermatitis, exfoliative dermatitis, ichthyosis, alopecia areata, acne, lichen planus, epidermolysis bullosa, lupus erythematosus, acanthosis nigricans, dermatophytosis, hereditary ectodermal dysplasia syndrome and acrodermatitis

2. Congenital atrichia

3. Cryptophthalmos

4. Cutaneous t cell lymphoma

5. Demodicosis

6. Drugs, including:

acebutolol(?)	aminosalicylate(?)	aspirin(?)
acenocoumarin(?)	aminosalicylic acid(?)	atenolol(?)
acetazolamide(?)	amiodarone(?)	auranofin(?)
acetohexamide(?)	amithiozone(?)	aurothioglucose(?)
acid bismuth sodium tartrate	aminopterin(?)	aurothioglycanide(?)
actinomycin C(?)	amitriptyline(?)	azathioprine(?)
alcohol(?)	amodiaquine(?)	benzphetamine(?)
allopurinol(?)	amoxapine(?)	betaxolol
aluminum bicotinate(?)	amphetamine(?)	bismuth oxychloride(?)
amantadine(?)	anisindione(?)	bismuth sodium tartrate(?)

bismuth sodium
  thioglycollate(?)

bismuth sodium
  triglycollamate(?)

bismuth subcarbonate(?)

bismuth subsalicylate(?)

bishydroxycoumarin(?)

bleomycin(?)

broxyquinoline(?)

busulfan(?)

cactinomycin

captopril(?)

carbamazepine(?)

carbimazole(?)

carmustine

chlorambucil(?)

chloroquine(?)

chlorphentermine(?)

chlorpropamide(?)

cimetidine(?)

cisplatin

clofibrate(?)

clomiphene(?)

clonazepam(?)

colchicine(?)

cyclophosphamide(?)

cytarabine(?)

dacarbazine

dactinomycin(?)

danazol(?)

daunorubicin

desipramine(?)

dextroamphetamine(?)

dextrothyroxine(?)

diacetylmorphine(?)

dichlorphenamide(?)

dicumarol(?)

diethylcarbamazine

diethylpropion(?)

diltiazem(?)

diphenadione(?)

divalproex sodium(?)

doxepin(?)

doxorubicin

dromostanolone(?)

droperidol(?)

enalapril(?)

epinephrine

ergonovine(?)

ergotamine(?)

ethionamide(?)

ethotoin(?)

ethoxzolamide(?)

ethyl biscoumacetate(?)

etretinate(?)

fenfluramine(?)

fenoprofen(?)

flecainide(?)

floxuridine(?)

fluorouracil(?)

fluoxymesterone(?)

gentamicin

glyburide

glycopyrrolate(?)

gold au 198

gold sodium thiomalate(?)

gold sodium thiosulfate(?)

guanethidine(?)

haloperidol(?)

heparin(?)

hydroxychloroquine(?)

hydroxyurea(?)

ibuprofen(?)

imipramine(?)

indomethacin(?)

interferon(?)

iodochlorhydroxyquin(?)

iodoquinol(?)

isotretinoin(?)

ketoprofen(?)

labetalol(?)

levobunolol

levodopa(?)

lithium carbonate(?)

lomustine

maprotiline(?)

mechlorethamine(?)

melphalan(?)

mephenytoin(?)

methimazole(?)

methamphetamine(?)

methazolamide(?)

methotrexate(?)

methylergonovine(?)

methylthiouracil(?)

methysergide(?)

metoprolol(?)

mexiletine(?)

mianserin(?)

minocycline(?)

minoxidil(?)

mitomycin

mitotane(?)

morphine(?)

nadolol(?)

naltrexone(?)

naproxen(?)

niacin(?)

niacinamide(?)

nicotinyl alcohol(?)

nifedipine(?)

nitrofurantoin(?)

nortriptyline(?)

opium(?)

oral contraceptives(?)

oxprenolol(?)

paramethadione(?)

penicillamine(?)

phendimetrazine(?)

phenindione(?)

phenmetrazine(?)

phenprocoumon(?)

phentermine(?)

pindolol(?)

pipobroman(?)

prazosin(?)

* = most important

piroxicam	sulfamerazine(?)	tetracycline(?)
procarbazine(?)	sulfameter(?)	thiotepa
propranolol(?)	sulfamethazine(?)	tocainide(?)
propylthiouracil(?)	sulfamethizole(?)	tolazamide(?)
protriptyline(?)	sulfamethoxazole	tolbutamide(?)
pyridostigmine(?)	sulfamethoxypyridazine(?)	triethylenemelamine(?)
ranitidine	sulfanilamide(?)	trifluperidol(?)
semustine	sulfaphenazole(?)	trimethadione(?)
sodium salicylate(?)	sulfapyridine(?)	uracil mustard(?)
streptomycin(?)	sulfasalazine(?)	valproate sodium(?)
streptozocin	sulfathiazole(?)	valproic acid(?)
sulfacetamide(?)	sulfisoxazole	verapamil(?)
sulfachlorpyridazine(?)	sulindac(?)	vinblastine(?)
sulfacytine(?)	tamoxifen(?)	vincristine(?)
sulfadiazine(?)	testolactone(?)	vitamin A
sulfadimethoxine(?)	testosterone(?)	warfarin(?)

7. Ehlers-Danlos syndrome, unspecified type

*8. Endocrine disease, including hypothyroidism, hyperthyroidism, pituitary insufficiency, hypoparathyroidism, and pituitary necrosis syndrome (Simmonds-Sheehan syndrome)

9. Following eyelid tattooing

10. Generalized hypotrichosis

11. HIV (human immunodeficiency virus)

12. Hypocalcemia

13. Hypothermal injury

*14. Idiopathic

15. Inflammation and infection of the lids, including seborrheic blepharitis, squamous blepharitis, herpes zoster, sebaceous gland carcinoma, vaccinia, mycotic infection, furuncles, and erysipelas

16. Intoxication with arsenic, bismuth, thallium, gold, quinine and vitamin A

17. Isolated madarosis

18. Keratosis decalvans

19. Keratosis follicularis

20. Keratosis spinulosa

21. Lid colobomas

22. Leprosy

23. Lipoid proteinosis (Urbach-Wiethe syndrome)

24. Polymorphous light eruption

25. Pseudoprogeria syndrome

26. Radiation

27. Severe debilitating systemic diseases, including tuberculosis, syphilis, sickle cell anemia, cholera, and Hansen disease (leprosy)

28. Trauma

29. Vogt-Koyanagi-Harada disease (uveitis-vitiligo-alopecia-poliosis syndrome)

Dana, M.R., et al.: Ocular manifestations of leprosy in a noninstitutionalized community in the United States. Arch. Ophthal., 112:626–629, 1994.

Fraunfelder, F.T.: Drug-Induced Ocular Side Effects and Drug Interactions. 4th Ed. Philadelphia, Williams & Wilkins, 1996.

Isenberg, S.J.: The Eye in Infancy. Chicago, Year Book Medical Publishers, 1989.

Roy, F.H.: Ocular Syndromes and Systemic Diseases. 2nd Ed. Philadelphia, W.B. Saunders, 1989.

* = most important

Madarosis (Loss of Eyelashes)

	Drugs as Thiotepa	Vogt-Koyanagi Harada Disease	Endocrine Diseases (e.g., Hypothyroidism)	Inflammation and Infection (e.g., Blepharitis)	Radiation	Severe Systemic Diseases (e.g., Tuberculosis)	Chronic Skin Diseases (e.g., Psoriasis)
History							
1. Common in females							U
2. Common in whites							U
3. Congenital			S				
4. Hereditary							U
5. Japanese and Italian extraction		U					
6. Onset, 10 to 35 years							U
7. Seborrheic disease					U		
8. Thiotepa eyedrop usage	U						
9. Thyroidectomy/hypophysectomy			S				
10. Young adults		U					
Physical Findings							
1. Blepharitis				U	U	S	
2. Cataract		S	S			S	
3. Chalazion						S	S
4. Choroiditis		U					
5. Chronic dacryoadenitis and dacryocystitis						S	
6. Conjunctivitis, exudative				U			
7. Conjunctivitis, mucopurulent				U		S	
8. Conjunctival phlyctenules				S		U	
9. Corneal ulcer				S	S	S	
10. Decreased tear secretion			S	U	U		
11. Ectropion						S	S
12. Entropion						S	
13. Epiphora	U						
14. Excised pterygium	U						
15. Exophthalmos			R				
16. Exudative retinitis with periphlebitis						S	
17. Glaucoma		S				S	
18. Gray-white appearance of sclera			U				
19. Hypopyon						S	
20. Keratitis				S	S	S	
21. Lid abscess				S			
22. Lid carcinoma						S	
23. Lid collarettes/granuloma						S	S
24. Lid concretions				U			
25. Lid scaling						S	U
26. Lid thickening				S			
27. Loss of eyebrow hairs			U				
28. Lupus tuberculosis lids						S	
29. Meibomianitis				S		S	
30. Optic nerve atrophy						S	

Madarosis (Loss of Eyelashes)

	Drugs as Thiotepa	Vogt-Koyanagi Harada Disease	Endocrine Diseases (e.g., Hypothyroidism)	Inflammation and Infection (e.g., Blepharitis)	Radiation	Severe Systemic Diseases (e.g., Tuberculosis)	Chronic Skin Diseases (e.g., Psoriasis)
Physical Findings							
31. Optic neuritis						S	
32. Panophthalmitis						S	
33. Pannus				S	S	S	S
34. Plaque-like lesions in lids/conjunctiva/cornea							U
35. Pruritus				S			
36. Retinal detachment		S					
37. Retinal hemorrhage		R					
38. Scleritis						S	
39. Sebaceous cyst lid				S			
40. Subconjunctival nodules (tuberculomas)						S	
41. Symblepharon					S		
42. Trichiasis				S			S
43. Tylosis ciliaris				S			
44. Uveitis		U			S	S	
45. Vitreous opacity		S					
46. White lashes (poliosis)		S		S	S		
Laboratory Data							
1. Fluorescein angiography		U				S	
2. Cerebrospinal fluid abnormal		U					
3. Red blood count, white blood count, hemoglobin, hematocrit	U						
4. Radioactive iodine uptake test			U				
5. T3 and T4 serum test			U				
6. Purified protein derivative and ELISA test						U	
7. Chest roentgenogram						U	

R = rarely; S = sometimes; and U = usually.

Distichiasis (Accessory Row of Lashes Growing from Openings of Meibomian Gland)

1. Acquired
    A. Chemical
    B. Immunologic
    C. Physical
*2. Congenital
    A. Anodontia-hypotrichosis syndrome
    B. Distichiasis, lymphedema syndrome
    C. Ectropion and distichiasis
    D. Idiopathic eyelid edema
    E. Pierre Robin syndrome
    F. Tristichiasis
3. Hereditary—autosomal dominant

Fraunfelder, F.T., and Roy, F.H.: Current Ocular Therapy. 4th Ed. Philadelphia, W.B. Saunders, 1995.

Isenberg, S.J.: The Eye in Infancy. Chicago, Year Book Medical Publishers, 1989.

Kolin, T., et al.: Hereditary Lymphedema and Distichiasis. Arch. Ophthalmol., 109:980–982, 1991.

Temple, I.K., and Collin, J.R.: Distichiasis-lymphoedema syndrome: a family report. Clinical Dysmorphology, 3:139–142, 1994.

Coarse Eyebrows

1. Congenital hypothyroidism (cretinism)
2. CPD syndrome (chorioretinopathy and pituitary dysfunction)
3. Hunter syndrome (MPS II)
4. Hurler syndrome (MPS I)
*5. Normal variation
6. Rubinstein-Taybi syndrome (broad thumbs syndrome)
7. Sanfilippo syndrome (MPS III)

Roy, F.H.: Ocular Syndromes and Systemic Diseases. 2nd Ed. Philadelphia, W.B. Saunders, 1989.

Synophrys (Confluent Eyebrows Extending to Midline)

1. Basal cell nevus syndrome (Gorlin syndrome)
2. Cornelia De Lange syndrome (congenital muscular hypertrophy-cerebral syndrome)
3. Del (3p) syndrome
4. Duplication 3q syndrome
5. Frontometaphyseal dysplasia
6. Hirschhorn-Cooper syndrome (chromosome partial deletion syndrome)
7. Labard syndrome
*8. Normal variation
9. Partial trisomy chromosome 15
10. Smith-Lemli-Opitz syndrome (cerebrohepatorenal syndrome)

11. Thirteen trisomy syndrome (Patau syndrome)

12. Waardenburg syndrome (interoculoiridodermatoauditive dysplasia)

Roy, F.H.: Ocular Syndromes and Systemic Diseases. 2nd Ed. Philadelphia, W.B. Saunders, 1989.

Smith, D.W.: Recognizable Patterns of Human Malformation. Philadelphia, W.B. Saunders, 1970.

Hertogh Sign (Lack of Outer Third of Eyebrows)

1. Autonomic nervous system dysfunction

2. Diphtheria

*3. Endocrinopathies

4. Hypogonadism

5. Hypothyroidism

6. Neurodermatitis

7. Scleroderma (systemic scleroderma)

Pau, H.: Differential Diagnoses of Eye Diseases. 2nd Ed. New York, Thieme Med. Pub., 1988.

Roy, F.H.: Ocular Syndromes and Systemic Diseases. 2nd Ed. Philadelphia, W.B. Saunders, 1989.

Lid Myokymia (Spontaneous Fascicular Eyelid Tremor without Muscular Atrophy or Weakness)

*1. Not associated with organic disease

    A. Fatigue

    B. Lack of sleep

    C. Bright light dazzle

    D. Irritative corneal or conjunctival lesions

    E. Debility or anemia

    F. Excessive alcohol or smoking

    G. Overwork

2. Followed by spastic paretic facial contracture—in dorsal pons in adult and children

3. Multiple sclerosis (disseminated sclerosis)

4. Trigeminal neuralgia

5. Myasthenia gravis (pseudoparalytic syndrome)

Fraunfelder, F.T., and Roy, F.H.: Current Ocular Therapy. Philadelphia, W.B. Saunders, 4th ed. 1995.

Preseptal Cellulitis of Eyelid

1. Eczema

*2. Hordeolum

3. Neonatal conjunctivitis

4. Otitis media

5. Sinusitis

6. Staphylococcus aureus

7. Toxic shock syndrome

* = most important

8. Trauma

9. Upper respiratory tract

10. Varicella

Brower, M.F., et al.: Preseptal Cellulitis Complicated by Toxic Shock Syndrome. Arch. Ophthalmol., 105:1631–1632, 1987.

Weiss, A., et al.: Bacterial Periorbital and Orbital Cellulitis in Childhood. Ophthalmology, 90:195–203, 1983.

Telecanthus (Disproportionate Increase in Distance Between Medial Canthi; Measurements in Infants are Eighteen to Twenty-two Millimeters)

*1. Primary

2. Secondary—may occur secondarily to an increased distance between the bony orbits (see hypertelorism)

    A. Aarskog syndrome

    B. Blepharonasofacial syndrome

    C. Blepharophimosis syndrome

    D. Camptomelic dysplasia

    E. Carpenter syndrome

    F. Cerebro-facio-articular syndrome of van Maldegem

    G. Coffin-Lowry syndrome

    H. de Lange syndrome

    I. Deletion 5g syndrome

    J. Duborvitz syndrome

    K. Facial-renal acromesomelic syndrome

    L. Facio-oculoacousticorenal syndrome

    M. Fetal alcohol syndrome

    N. Fetal hydantoin syndrome

    O. Frontonasal dysplasia

    P. Lambotte syndrome

    Q. KBG syndrome (initials of family studied)

    R. Michel's syndrome

    S. Nasopalpebral lipoma-coloboma syndrome

    T. Oculodentodigital syndrome

    Q. Orofaciodigital (OFD) type I and type II (Mohr syndrome)

    R. Prader-Willi syndrome

    S. Rieger syndrome

    T. Simosa syndrome

    U. Tetra-X syndrome

    V. Trisomy syndrome

    W. Toriello-Carey syndrome

    X. Trauma

    Z. Waardenburg syndrome

AA. Williams syndrome

BB. 5p- syndrome (Cri-du-chat)

CC. 10q- syndrome

DD. Fetal hydantoin syndrome

Isenberg, S.J.: The Eye in Infancy. Chicago. Year Book Medical Publishers, 1989.

Suri,M., et al.: Blepharophimosis, telecanthus, microstomia, and unusual ear anomaly (Simosa syndrome) in an infant. Amer. J. Medical Genetics. 51: 222–223, 1994.

Tasman, W., and Jaeger, E., eds.: Duane's Clinical Ophthalmology. Philadelphia, J.B. Lippincott, 1990.

Ankyloblepharon (Partial or Complete Fusion of Upper to Lower Eyelids)

*1. Ablepharon, macrostomia syndrome

2. Ankyloblepharon ectodermal dysplasia, cleft lip and palate

3. Curly Hair, Ankyloblepharon, Nail Dysplasia Syndrome (CHANDS)

4. Cryptophthalmos (complete fusion of lids)

5. Diphtheritic conjunctivitis

6. Ectodermal syndrome

7. Edward's syndrome

8. Fraser syndrome

9. Gastrointestinal anomalies

10. Hay-Wells ectodermal pterygium syndrome

11. Popliteal pterygium syndrome

12. Smallpox

13. Trachoma

14. Trisomy 18

15. Ulcerative blepharitis

Isenberg, S.J.: The Eye in Infancy. Chicago, Year Book Medical Publishers, 1989.

Roy, F.H.: Ophthalmic Surgery: Approaches by the Masters. Philadelphia, Lea & Febiger, 1995.

Flaring of Nasal Part of Eyebrow

1. Blepharonasofacial syndrome

2. Partial trisomy 10q syndrome

*3. Waardenburg syndrome

4. Williams syndrome

Isenberg, S.J.: The Eye in Infancy. Chicago, Year Book Medical Publishers, 1989.

High Arched Brow

1. Kabuki makeup syndrome

2. Shprintzen-Goldberg syndrome

Isenberg, S.J.: The Eye in Infancy. Chicago, Year Book Medical Publishers, 1989.

* = most important

Absent Brow Hair

1. Cryptophthalmos
2. Pseudoprogeria syndrome

Isenberg, S.J.: The Eye in Infancy. Chicago, Year Book Medical Publishers, 1989.

Trichiasis (Inward turning lashes)

*1. Inflammation/infection

     A. Chronic blepharitis

     B. Herpes simplex or zoster

     C. Trachoma

2. Lid Tumors

     A. Basal cell carcinoma

     B. Capillary hemangioma

     C. Conjunctiva amyloidosis

3. Medications

     A. Epinephrine

     B. Idoxuridine

     C. Phospholine iodide

     D. Pilocarpine

     E. Practolol

     F. Trifluridine

     G. Vidarabine

4. Systemic/Immunologic Disorders

     A. Erythema multiforme

     B. Ocular cicatricial pemphigoid

     C. Steven's Johnson syndrome

     D. Toxic epidermal necrolysis

5. Trauma

     A. Chemical injury (lye)

     B. Mechanical injury or repair of injury

     C. Surgery

Byrnes, G.A.: Congenital Distichiasis. Arch. Ophthalmol., 109:1752–1753, 1991.

Foster, C.S.: Cicatricial Pemphigoid. Trans. Am. Ophthalmol. Soc., 84:527–663, 1986.

Roy, F.H.: Ophthalmic Surgery: Approaches by the Masters. Philadelphia, Lea & Febiger, 1995.

Udell, I.J.: Trifluridine-associated Conjunctival Cicatrization. Amer. J. Ophthalmology, 82:117–121, 1976.

Lacrimal System

DAVID TSE MD

Contents

Dacryoadenitis (Inflammation of Lacrimal Gland)

1. Acute dacryoadenitis—rare catarrhal inflammation of the lacrimal gland that usually accompanies systemic disease

    A. In children—*mumps, measles, influenza, scarlet fever, erysipelas, typhoid fever

    B. In adults—gonorrhea, endogenous conjunctivitis and uveitis, infectious mononucleosis, typhoid fever, Crohn's disease

    C. Secondary to inflammation from lids or conjunctiva, to include klebsiella pneumoniae, coliform organisms, *staphylococcus, *streptococcus, Aedes ae-gypti, *diplococcus pneumoniae, and *neisseria gonorrhea

2. Chronic dacryoadenitis—proliferative inflammation of the lacrimal gland, usually because of specific granulomatous disease

    A. Boeck sarcoid (Schaumann syndrome)

    B. Heerfordt disease—chronic bilateral parotitis and uveitis, often associated with paresis of the cranial nerves, usually the seventh nerve, and other general symptoms

        *(1) Sarcoidosis syndrome (Schaumann syndrome)

        (2) Tuberculosis

    C. Mikulicz syndrome—dacryoadenitis and parotitis manifested by chronic bilateral swelling of the lacrimal and salivary glands

        (1) Bang disease (brucellosis)

        (2) Hodgkin disease

        (3) Leukemia

        (4) Lymphoma

        (5) Lymphosarcoma (Brill-Symmers disease)

        (6) Reticuloendothelial disease

        (7) Mumps

        *(8) Sarcoidosis syndrome (Schaumann syndrome)

        (9) Syphilis

        (10) Tuberculosis

        (11) Waldenstroms' macroglobulinemia

    D. Miliary tuberculosis

    E. Pseudotumor

    F. Syphilis (gumma)

3. Painless enlargement of lacrimal gland

    A. Leukemia

    B. Mumps

4. Painful enlargement of lacrimal gland

    A. Lymphomatous disease (25%)

    B. Chronic enlargement arising from sarcoid or orbital pseudotumor (25%)

    C. Lacrimal gland neoplasm (50%)

        (1) Benign

           a. Adenoma

           b. Mixed tumor

        (2) Malignant

           a. Carcinoma unrelated to mixed tumor

              1) Adenocarcinoma (adenoid cystic carcinoma)

              2) Mucoepidermoid carcinoma

3) Squamous cell carcinoma

b. Mixed tumor

Divine, R.D., et al.: Metastatic carcinoid unresponsive radiation therapy presenting as a lacrimal fossa mass. Ophthalmology, 89:516, 1982.

Harris, G.J., et al.: Sarcoidosis of the lacrimal sac. Arch. Ophthalmol., 99:1198, 1981.

Newell, F.W.: Ophthalmology, Principles and Concepts. 7th ed. St. Louis, C.V. Mosby, 1992.

Roy, F.H.: Ocular Syndrome and Systemic Diseases. 2nd ed. Philadelphia, W.B. Saunders, 1989.

Shields, C.L., et al.: Clinicopathologic Review of Cases of Lacrimal Gland Lesions. Ophthalmology, 96:431–435, 1989.

* = most important

Acute Dacryoadenitis (Inflammation of Lacrimal Gland)

	Children (e.g., Mumps)	Adult (e.g., Typhoid Fever)	Inflammation of Lids/Conjunctiva (e.g., Staphylococcus)
History			
1. Affects all ages			U
2. Contagious disease	U	U	
3. Virus infection	U		
Physical Findings			
1. Central retinal artery emboli		S	
2. Central scotoma		S	
3. Congenital punctal occlusion	R		
4. Conjunctivitis	U	U	U
5. Corneal ulcer	S	S	S
6. Cortical blindness	R		
7. Dacryocystitis		S	S
8. Ectropion			S
9. Endophthalmitis		S	S
10. Entropion			S
11. Exophthalmos	R		
12. Granuloma in lids			S
13. Hordeolum			S
14. Hypopyon		S	S
15. Keratitis	U		S
16. Lid abscess/cellulitis			S
17. Madarosis			S
18. Microphthalmos	R		
19. Optic atrophy	R		
20. Optic neuritis	S	S	
21. Panophthalmitis		S	S
22. Orbital vein thrombosis		S	
23. Paralysis of extraocular muscles	S	S	
24. Phlyctenules in conjunctiva			S
25. Ptosis			S
26. Retinal detachment		S	
27. Scleritis	S		
28. Tenonitis	U	U	
29. Uveitis	U	S	R
30. Dacryoadenitis	S	U	S
31. Vitreous hemorrhages	R	S	
Laboratory Data			
1. Stain and culture			
Gram-negative bacillus		U	
Gram-positive cocci			U

R = rarely; S = sometimes; and U = usually.

Mikulicz Syndrome—Chronic Dacryoadenitis and Parotitis

	Tuberculosis	Leukemia	Lymphosarcoma	Hodgkin Disease	Sarcoidosis	Lymphoma
History						
1. Children, young adults, and middle age		U	S	U		
2. Greater in blacks					U	
3. Greater in females					S	
4. Greater in males		S	U			
5. Infants, small children						
6. Malignant lymphoma association					U	
7. Occurs 20 to 40 years					U	
Physical Findings						
1. Blepharitis	U	U				
2. Cataract					U	
3. Central serous retinopathy		S				
4. Chronic dacryocystitis	U					
5. Cranial nerve paralysis (usually facial)					S	
6. Exophthalmos			U			U
7. Extraocular muscle paralysis					S	
8. Firm, elastic, orbital mass	S	U				U
9. Follicular, hypertropic granulomatous, papillary or purulent conjunctivitis	U				S	
10. Granulomatous uveitis, posterior synechiae	U	U			U	U
11. Hemorrhage in conjunctiva, choroid, sclera, orbital tissue, retina, and/or optic disc		U				
12. Hypopyon	U					
13. Keratitis					U	
14. Keratoconjunctivitis sicca					S	
15. Painless lid swelling			U		S	
16. Papilledema		S			S	S
17. Peripheral retinal neovascularization		S				
18. Perivascular retinal white lines		S				
19. Posterior synechiae	U			U		
20. Retinal detachment		S				
21. Soft retinal exudates		U				
22. Subconjunctival nodules	U				U	
23. Lids: nodules (milia), ptosis					S	S
24. Optic-nerve; optic atrophy	S				S	S
Laboratory Data						
1. Angiotensin-converting enzyme test					U	
2. Aqueous cytology		U				
3. Biopsy of gland	U	U	U	U	U	U
4. Blood count		U	U	U		
5. Bone marrow		U				S
6. Chest roentgenogram	U		S	S		
7. Gallium scan test					U	
8. Kveim test					U	
9. Orbit/skull roentgenogram						U
10. Peripheral blood smear		U				
11. Tuberculin skin test	U					
12. HIV	U					

R = rarely; S = sometimes; and U = usually.

Bloody Tears

1. Conjunctiva
    A. Application of a drug such as silver nitrate
    B. Cachectic conjunctivitis
    C. Focal dermal hypoplasia syndrome (Goltz syndrome)
    D. Fibroma
    *E. Giant papillary conjunctivitis secondary to contact lens wear or prosthesis wear
    F. Gross disturbance of autonomic nervous system
    G. Hemangioma
    H. Hereditary hemorrhagic telangiectasis
    I. Inflammatory granuloma
    J. Malignant melanoma
    K. Metastatic carcinoid tumor
    *L. Severe conjunctivitis with marked hyperemia
    *M. Subconjunctival hemorrhage following sudden venous congestion of head from stooping, coughing, choking, valsalva trauma, hemophilia or advanced athrombia
    N. Vicarious menstruation with ectopic tissue
2. Corneal vascular lesion or pannus
3. Lid
    A. Pubic lice and nits on the lashes
    B. Trauma
4. Other
    A. Familial telangiectasis
    B. Hemophilia
    C. Hysteria
    D. Jaundice
    E. Osler-Weber-Render
    F. Pathologic process of lacrimal gland
    G. Severe anemia
    H. Severe epistaxis with regurgitation through the lacrimal passages

Dutt, S., et al.: Acute dacryoadenitis and Crohn's disease: findings and management. Ophthalmic Plastic & Reconstructive Surgery, 8: 295–299, 1992.

Gritz, D.C., and Rao, N.A.: Metastatic Carcinoid Tumor Diagnosis from a Caruncular Mass. Amer. J. Ophthalmol., 112:468–469, 1991.

Hornblass, A., et al.: The management of epithelial tumors of the lacrimal sac. Ophthalmology, 7:476, 1982.

Krohel, G.B., et al.: Bloody Tears Associated with Familial Telangiectasis. Arch. Ophthalmol., 105:1489–1490, 1987.

Bloody Tears

	Systemic Disease as Hemophilia	Local Trauma	Lid Disease as Pubic Lice/Nits on Lashes	Conjunctival Tumor as Granuloma	Subconjunctival Hemorrhage	Corneal Vascular Lesion
History						
1. Associated with systemic and local diseases						S
2. Hereditary	S					
3. Inflammation				U		
4. Skin disease			U			
5. Spontaneous appearance					U	
6. Trauma history	S	U			U	S
7. Aspirin intake					U	
Physical Findings						
1. Associated with sarcoid				U		
2. Conjunctival hemorrhage	S	S			U	U
3. Conjunctival keratinization		S			S	
4. Conjunctival necrosis		S				
5. Conjunctival nodules		S			S	
6. Corneal edema						S
7. Corneal opacity						S
8. Chemosis of conjunctiva		U		S	S	S
9. Epithelial inclusion cysts		S			S	
10. Exophthalmos	S	S				
11. Faulty closure of conjunctival surgical incisions				U		
12. Follicular conjunctivitis			U			
13. Glaucoma	S					
14. Infestation of lids (adult lice/nits on hair shifts)			U			
15. Leukoma of cornea						S
16. Lid hemorrhage	S	S	S			
17. Lid laceration		U			S	
18. Lid scaling			S			
19. Loss of vision	S	S				S
20. Low intraocular pressure		S			S	R
21. Madarosis			S			
22. Marginal keratitis			S	S		
23. Penetration/perforation of sclera		U			U	
24. Perforation/laceration of bulbar conjunctiva		U			U	
25. Pseudomembranous conjunctivitis		S		R		
26. Retained foreign bodies						
27. Retinal hemorrhages posttrauma	U	S				
28. Retinitis proliferans	S	R				
29. Retrobulbar hemorrhages	S	S				
30. Secondary to retinal/strabismus surgery				U	S	
31. Small rust-colored specks of excreta on the skin of the lids			U			
32. Superficial/deep corneal vessels						S
33. Vessels into old corneal lesion						S
34. Vitreous hemorrhage	S	U				
Laboratory Data						
1. Pulse transmission time and factor 8 assay	U					
2. Microscopic exam lid lice/nits			U			

R = rarely; S = sometimes; and U = usually.

* = most important

Excessive Tears

1. Hypersecretion of tears—may be due to basic secretors (mucin, lacrimal, including secretion from glands of Kraus and Wolfring and oil, including secretion from Zeis, Moll, and Meibomian palpebral glands) or reflex secretors (main lacrimal glands and accessory palpebral glands)

    A. Primary (disturbance of lacrimal gland)

    B. Central or psychic

      (1) Central nervous system lues

      (2) Corticomeningeal lesions

      (3) Emotional states

      (4) Hysteria

      (5) Physical pain

      (6) Voluntary lacrimation, such as when acting

    C. Neurogenic

      (1) Ametropia, tropia, phoria, and eyestrain or fatigue

      (2) Caloric, lacrimal, and reflex tearing—bilateral lacrimation when syringing the ear with warm or cold water and during Tensilon testing

      (3) Crocodile or alligator tears—unilateral profuse tearing when eating

        a. Congenital, often associated with ipsilateral paresis of lateral rectus muscle

        b. Acquired with onset in early stage of facial palsy (Bell's palsy) or sequela with parasympathetic fibers to the otic ganglion growing back into superficial petrosal nerve

        c. Duane's retraction syndrome

          1) Bell palsy (idiopathic facial paralysis)

          2) Marin-Amat syndrome (inverted Marcus Gunn Jaw-wink phenomenon)

          3) Melkersson-Rosenthal syndrome (Melkersson idiopathic fibro edema)

        d. Section of the greater superficial petrosal nerve

      (4) Drugs, including:

acetophenazine	ether	nalorphine
acetylcholine	ethopropazine	naloxone
alcohol	fluphenazine	opium
ambenonium	heparin	pentazocine
bishydroxycoumarin	indomethacin(?)	perazine
butaperazine	ketamine	pericyazine
carphenazine	levallorphan	perphenazine
chloral hydrate	mesoridazine	piperacetazine
chlorpromazine	methacholine	prochlorperazine
diazoxide	methaqualone	promazine
diethazine	methdilazine	promethazine
edrophonium	methotrimeprazine	propiomazine
epinephrine	morphine	pyridostigmine

rifampin

thiethylperazine

thiopropazate

thioproperazine

thioridazine

trifluoperazine

triflupromazine

trimeprazine

warfarin

(5) Exposure to wind, cold, or bright light; photosensitivity and sunburn

(6) Glaucoma

(7) Horner syndrome (see p. 64) (cervical sympathetic paralysis syndrome)

(8) Inflammation or infection of the conjunctiva, uvea, cornea, orbit, lids, sinuses, teeth, or ears

   a. Acute hemorrhagic conjunctivitis

   b. Avitaminosis B (pellagra, niacin deficiency)

   c. Conjunctivochalasis

   d. Elschnig syndrome (I) (meibomian conjunctivitis)

   e. Epidemic keratoconjunctivitis

   f. Feer syndrome (acrodynia)

   g. Hanhart syndrome (recessive keratosis palmoplantaris)

   h. Keratodermia palmaris et plantaris

   i. Reiter syndrome (polyarthritis enteric)

   j. Stannus cerebellar syndrome (riboflavin deficiency)

   k. Thelaziasis

(9) Lesions affecting the lids

   a. Acrodermatitis chronic atrophicans

   b. Blepharoptosis

   c. Congenital distichiasis

  *d. Ectropion

  *e. Entropion

   f. Epiblepharon

   g. Eyelid retraction

  *h. Facial paralysis

   i. Lid imbrication syndrome

   j. Papilloma

   k. Punctal apposition

   l. Trachoma

  *m. Trichiasis

(10) Morquio-Brailsford syndrome (MPS IV)

(11) Myasthenia gravis—afternoon ectropion (Erb-Goldflam syndrome)

(12) Ophthalmorhinostomatohygrosis syndrome

(13) Parkinson's disease-facial akinesia

(14) Reflex, such as vomiting or laughing

(15) Sjögren syndrome (secretoinhibitor syndrome)

* = most important

    (16) Stimulation of some cortical areas—thalamus, hypothalamus, cervical sympa-
        thetic ganglia, or the lacrimal nucleus

        a. Diencephalic epilepsy syndrome (Penfield syndrome)

        b. Encephalitis

          1) acute

          2) hemorrhagica superior

          3) lethargia

          4) periaxialis diffusa

        c. Engelmann syndrome (diaphyseal dysplasia)

        d. Giant-cell arteritis (temporal arteritis)

        e. Hypothalamic tumors

        f. Meningitis

        g. Page syndrome (hypertensive diencephalic syndrome)

        h. Pseudobulbar palsy from Parkinson syndrome (shaking palsy)

        i. Sluder syndrome (lower facial neuralgia syndrome)

        j. Tic douloureux (trigeminal neuralgia syndrome)

        k. Various senile dementias

    (17) Gradenigo syndrome (temporal syndrome)

    (18) Raeder syndrome (paratrigeminal paralysis, cluster headache)

    (19) Retroparotid space syndrome (Villaret syndrome)

    (20) Rhabdomyosarcoma

    (21) Rothmund syndrome (telangiectasia-pigmentation-cataract syndrome)

    (22) Thermal burns

  D. Symptomatic

    (1) Bee sting of cornea

    (2) Tabes

    (3) Thyrotoxicosis (Basedow syndrome)

2. Inadequacy of lacrimal drainage system

  A. Congenital anomalies of lacrimal apparatus

    (1) Absence or atresia including ectrodactyly-ectodermal dysplasia-clefting syndrome

    (2) Amniotocele

   *(3) Fistulas of lacrimal sac and nasolacrimal duct

    (4) Lateral displacement of medial canthi with lateral displacement of puncta and
        lengthening of canaliculi as in Waardenburg syndrome (interoculoiridoderma-
        toauditive dysplasia)

    (5) Obstruction of nasolacrimal drainage system, including Walker-Clodius syn-
        drome (lobster claw deformity with nasolacrimal obstruction)

   *(6) Unformed puncta (punctal atresia)

  B. Complications from diseases such as pemphigus and Stevens-Johnson syn-
    drome (dermatostomatitis)

*C. Dacryocystitis

*D. Distended canaliculi with obstruction, such as from Actinomyces israeli (Streptothrix foersteri), papilloma, or dacryolith

E. Because of drugs, including:

adenine arabinoside

demecarium

echothiophate

epinephrine

floxuridine

fluorouracil

idoxuridine

isoflurophate

neostigmine

physostigmine

quinacrine

silver nitrate

silver protein

thiotepa

trifluorothymidine (including Fuchs-Lyell syndrome) (allergic reaction due to drugs causing nasolacrimal obstruction)

*F. Eversion of inferior lacrimal punctum, including involutional ectropion (horizontal lid laxity and retractors disinsertion)

G. Eversion of inferior lacrimal punctum secondary to ichthyosis or scleroderma

H. Goltz syndrome (focal dermal hypoplasia syndrome)

I. Inadequacy of physiologic lacrimal pump

J. Traumatic lesions of lacrimal drainage system

K. Tumor obstruction, including polyps, papillary hypertrophy, and neurofibromas

   (1) Botulinum toxin usage

   (2) Dyskeratosis congenita (Zinsser-Engman-Cole syndrome)

   (3) Gravity inversion

   (4) Irritation from dust and gases

   (5) Inflammation or destruction of turbinates

   (6) Inhalation cocaine abuse

   (7) Leprosy (Hansen disease)

   (8) Leukemia

   (9) Rhinosporidiosis

  (10) Tuberculosis

  (11) Tumors

L. Primary neoplasms

   (1) Fibroma

   (2) Hemangiopericytoma

   (3) Melanoma

   (4) Papilloma

   (5) Squamous cell carcinoma

M. Secondary involvement by neoplasms

   (1) Basal cell carcinoma

   (2) Lethal midline granuloma

   (3) Leukemia

   (4) Lymphoma

   (5) Maxillary sinus tumors

* = most important

(6) Neurofibroma

(7) Wegener's granulomatosis

3. Pseudoepiphora, such as wound fistula following intraocular operation with leak of aqueous

Baron, E.M., et al.: Rhabdomyosarcoma Manifesting as Acquired Nasolacrimal Duct Obstruction. Amer. J. Ophthal., 115:239–242, 1993.

Friberg, T.R., and Weinreb, R.N.: Ocular manifestations of gravity inversion. JAMA, 253:1755–1758, 1985.

Fraunfelder, F.T.: Drug-Induced Ocular Side Effects and Drug Interactions. 4th Ed. Philadelphia, Williams & Wilkins, 1996.

Glatt, H.J.: Epiphora Caused by Blepharoptosis. Amer. J. Ophthalmol., 111:649–650, 1991.

Harris, G.J., and Diclementi, D.: Congenital dacryocystocele. Arch. Ophthalmol., 100:1763, 1982.

Horniblass, A., et al.: The diagnosis and management of epithelial tumors of the lacrimal sac. Ophthalmology, 87:476, 1982.

Isenberg, S.J.: The Eye in Infancy. Chicago, Year Book of Medical Publishers, 1989.

Karesh, J.W., et al.: Eyelid imbrication: an unrecognized cause of chronic ocular irritation. Ophthal., 100: 883, 1993.

Kohn, R., et al.: Rapid recurrence of papillary squamous cell carcinoma of the canaliculus. Amer. J. Ophthalmol., 92:363–367, 1981.

Linberg, J.V., and McCormick, S.A.: Primary acquired nasolacrimal duct obstruction. Ophthal., 93:1055–1063, 1986.

Perman, K.I., et al.: The use of botulinum toxin in the medical management of benign essential blepharospasm. Ophthalmology, 93:1–3, 1986.

Richards, W.W.: Actinomycotic lacrimal canaliculitis. Am. J. Ophthalmol., 75:155–157, 1973.

Roy, F.H.: Ocular Syndromes and Systemic Diseases. 2nd Ed. Philadelphia, W.B. Saunders, 1989.

Wojno, T.H.: Allergic Lacrimal Obstruction. Amer. J. Ophthalmol., 106:48–52, 1988.

Woog, J.J., et al.: The role of aminocaproic acid in lacrimal surgery in dyskeratosis congenita. Am. J. Ophthalmol., 100:728–732, 1985.

Excessive Tears

	Psychic as Hysteria	Neurogenic as Glaucoma	Hyperthyroidism	Congenital Lesion Drainage as Unformed Puncta	Dacryocystitis	Traumatic Lesion as Cut Canaliculi	Obstruction by Actinomyces Israeli	Drugs as Idoxuridine	Eversion—Lower Punctum as Ectropion
History									
1. Anxiety state	U								
2. Bilateral	U	U	U	S				U	S
3. Common 30 to 50 years			U						
4. Common in females			U		U				
5. Common in males						U			S
6. Common in rural midwest United States							U		
7. Common in whites					U				
8. Congenital		S		U					S
9. Dyschromatopsia	S								
10. Exaggeration of symptoms without physical cause	U								
11. Familial		U				S			
12. Night blindiness	S								
13. Onset at 2 weeks					U				
14. Topical idoxuridine during 2 weeks								U	
15. Trauma						U			S
Physical Findings									
1. Accommodative spasm	S								
2. Amaurosis fugax	S								
3. Angioneurotic lid edema	S								
4. Anisocoria	S	S							
5. Optic neuritis	S								
6. Avulsion of medial canthal tendon						U			
7. Canaliculitis					S	S	U		
8. Cataract		S							
9. Central serous retinopathy	S								
10. Closed anterior chamber angle		U							
11. Conjunctivitis						S	U		U
12. Conjunctivitis, self-induced	S								
13. Contact dermatitis	S								
14. Corneal abscess				S					
15. Corneal edema		U							
16. Corneal filaments								U	
17. Corneal hypesthesia	S	U							
18. Corneal superficial neovascularization								S	
19. Corneal ulcer						S	S	S	
20. Creamy pus from punctum often with sulfur granules							U		
21. Cyst of lacrimal gland						S			
22. Lid/lacrimal sac tenderness						U	U		S
23. Turbid tear					U	S	U		S
24. Dye clearance delay				U	U	U	U	S	U
25. Lid imbrication									S
26. Dacryocystitis					U	U	U	R	
27. Disc hemorrhage		S							
28. Ectropion of puncta							U		

Excessive Tears *Continued*

Physical Findings	Psychic as Hysteria	Neurogenic as Glaucoma	Hyperthyroidism	Congenital Lesion Drainage as Unformed Puncta	Dacryocystitis	Traumatic Lesion as Cut Canaliculi	Obstruction by Actinomyces Israeli	Drugs as Idoxuridine	Eversion—Lower Punctum as Ectropion
29. Edema/hyperemia/pain of surrounding lacrimal sac					U				
30. Exposure keratopathy			S						
31. Extraocular muscles involvement			U						
32. Fine punctate keratopathy								U	
33. Fistula of lacrimal sac/gland						U			
34. Folds in Descemet membrane		U							
35. Follicular conjunctivitis								S	
36. Glaucomatous disc cupping		S							
37. Herpetic keratitis	S								
38. Hypopyon							U		
39. Increased intraocular pressure	S	U	S						
40. Lacrimal gland enlargement			S						
41. Lid abscess							S		
42. Lid cicatrization inner canthus						U			S
43. Lid lag			U						
44. Lid retraction			U						
45. Mild dilated and fixed pupil		S							
46. Mucopurulent material from the sac at pressure					U				
47. Nystagmus	S								
48. Optic nerve atrophy		U	S						
49. Orbital cellulitis						S			
50. Panophthalmitis				S					
51. Papilledema			S						
52. Peripheral anterior synechiae		U							
53. Pouting of the punctum							U		
54. Proptosis (axial)			U						
55. Ptosis	S							S	
56. Stenosis of lacrimal punctum							U	S	
57. Strabismus	S								
58. Traumatic corneal epithelial erosions	U								
59. Uveitis							S		
60. Visual field defects		U	S						

R = rarely; S = sometimes; and U = usually.

Drugs Found in Tears

Drugs include:

alcian blue	fluorouracil	sodium salicylate
amodiaquine	hydroxychloroquine	trypan blue
aspirin	methotrexate	vitamin A
chloroquine	minocycline	
fluorescein	rose bengal	

Fraunfelder, F.T.: Drug-Induced Ocular Side Effects and Drug Interactions. 4th Ed. Philadelphia, Williams & Wilkins, 1996.

Tabbara, K.F., and Cooper, H.: Minocycline levels in tears of patients with active trachoma. Arch Ophthal., 107: 93–95, 1989.

Dry Eye (Paucity or Absence of Tears)

1. Xerosis—local tissue changes

    A. Cicatricial degeneration of conjunctiva and mucous tissues

        (1) General: diphtheria

        (2) Upper lid: trachoma

        (3) Lower lid

            a. Avitaminosis A

            b. Chemical irritation (especially due to alkali)

            c. Dermatitis herpetiformis (Duhring-Brocq disease)

            d. Epidermolysis bullosa (Weber-Cockayne syndrome)

            e. Erythema multiforme (Stevens—Johnson syndrome)

            f. Ocular pemphigoid

            g. Plummer-Vinson syndrome (sideropenic dysphagia syndrome)

            h. Radium burns

            i. Reiter syndrome (conjunctivourethrosynovial syndrome)

            j. Sjögren syndrome (secretoinhibitor syndrome)

            k. Uyemura syndrome (fundus albipunctatus with hemeralopia and xerosis)

    B. Exposure keratitis

        (1) Anterior lamella shortage secondary to trauma or facial burn

        *(2) Deficient lid closure as part of facial palsy

        *(3) Ectropion (see p. 91)

        (4) Eyelid retraction-Graves' ophthalmopathy (incomplete blink)

        (5) Exophthalmos

        (6) Following botulism

        *(7) Infrequent blinking, such as with progressive supranuclear palsy

        (8) Lack of blinking as during coma

        (9) Levator spasm

        (9) Melkersson-Rosenthal syndrome (Melkersson idiopathic fibro edema)

* = most important

(10) Methylmalonic aciduria

(11) Ocular proptosis

(12) Rapid evaporation in hot, dry areas

(13) Stiff, immobile, retracted lids, such as those occurring secondary to tuberculoid leprosy (Hansen disease)

2. Keratoconjunctivitis sicca—primary tear diminution of main and accessory lacrimal glands

  A. Congenital

   (1) Congenital absence of lacrimal gland as in Bonnevie-Ullrich syndrome

   (2) Neurogenic

   (3) Associated with generalized disturbance

     a. Anhidrotic type of ectodermal dysplasia

     b. Familial dysautonomia (Riley-Day syndrome)

     c. Cri du chat syndrome (crying cat syndrome)

     d. Cystic fibrosis syndrome (fibrocystic disease of pancreas)

  B. Neurogenic hyposecretion

   (1) Central—aplasia of lacrimal nucleus or lesion of seventh nerve between nucleus and geniculate ganglion

     a. Pontine lesions

     b. Basal fractures

     c. Otitis media

   (2) Peripheral—greater superficial petrosal nerve, sphenopalatine ganglion, or lacrimal branch

     a. Skull fractures

     b. Associated with neoplasms

     c. Neurologic lesion of fifth nerve (neuroparalytic keratitis)

   (3) Herpes zoster of the geniculate ganglion (Ramsey-Hunt syndrome)

   (4) Parasympathetic blocking drugs, such as atropine and scopolamine, may decrease an already barely adequate secretion

   (5) Botulism

   (6) Deep anesthesia

   (7) Debilitating disease such as typhus and cholera, and high temperature

   (8) Allergy

  C. Systemic disease

   (1) AIDS

   (2) Amyotrophic lateral sclerosis

   (3) Danbolt-Closs syndrome (acrodermatitis enteropathica)

   (4) Disseminated lupus erythematosus (Kaposi-Libman-Sacks syndrome)

   (5) Drugs, including:

acebutolol	albuterol	amitriptyline
acetophenazine	aluminum nicotinate(?)	antazoline

astemizole
atenolol
atropine
azatadine
belladonna
bendroflumethiazide
benzalkonium
benzthiazide
brompheniramine
busulfan
butaperazine
carbinoxamine
carphenazine
chlorisondamine
chlorothiazide
chlorpheniramine
chlorpromazine
chlorthalidone
cimetidine(?)
clemastine
clonidine
cyclothiazide
cyproheptadine
desipramine
dexbrompheniramine
dexchlorpheniramine
diethazine
dimethindene
diphenhydramine
diphenylpyraline
disopyramide
doxylamine
dronabinol

ether
ethopropazine
etretinate
fluphenazine
hashish
hexamethonium
homatropine
hydrochlorothiazide
hydroflumethiazide
imipramine
indapamide
isotretinoin
labetolol
marijuana
mesoridazine
methdilazine
methotrexate
methotrimeprazine
methoxsalen
methscopolamine
methyclothiazide
methyldopa
methylthiouracil
metolazone
metoprolol
morphine
nadolol
niacin(?)
niacinamide(?)
nicotinyl alcohol(?)
nitrous oxide
nortriptyline
opium

oxprenolol
perazine
periciazine
perphenazine
pheniramine
pimozide
pindolol
piperacetazine
polythiazide
practolol
prochlorperazine
promazine
promethazine
propiomazine
propranolol
protriptyline
pyrilamine
quinethazone
scopolamine
tetrahydrocannabinol
thiethylperazine
thiopropazate
thioproperazine
thioridazine
timolol
trichlormethiazide
trichloroethylene
trifluoperazine
triflupromazine
trimeprazine
trioxsalen
tripelennamine
triprolidine

(6) Felty syndrome (uveitis-rheumatoid arthritis syndrome)

(7) Gougerot-Sjögren syndrome (oligophrenia-ichthyosis-spastic diplegia syndrome)

(8) Heerfordt syndrome (uveoparotitis)

(9) Lubarsch-Pick syndrome (primary amyloidosis)

(10) Mikulicz syndrome—acryoadenitis and parotitis

    a. Hodgkin disease

    b. Leukemia

    c. Lymphoma

        d. Lymphosarcoma

        e. Mumps

        f. Sarcoidosis syndrome (Schaumann syndrome)

        g. Syphilis

        h. Tuberculosis

        i Waldenstrom's macraglobulinemia

   (11) Pancreatitis

   (12) Pheochromocytoma, medullary thyroid carcinoma, and multiple mucosal neuromas

   (13) Polyarteritis nodosa (Kussmaul disease)

   (14) Relapsing polychondritis

   (15) Rheumatoid arthritis (adult)

   (16) Scleroderma (progressive systemic sclerosis)

Fraunfelder, F.T.: Drug-Induced Ocular Side Effects and Drug Interactions. 4th Ed. Philadelphia, Williams & Wilkins, 1996.

Geier, S.A.: Sicca Syndrome in Patients Infected with the Human Immunodeficiency Virus. Ophthal. 102:1319–1324, 1995.

Isenberg, S.J.: The Eye in Infancy. Chicago, Year Book Medical Publishers, 1989.

Mathers, W.D: Ocular Evaporation in Meibomian Gland Dysfunction and Dry Eye. Ophthalmology, 100:347–351, 1993.

Newell, F.W.: Ophthalmology, Principles and Concepts. 7th Ed. St. Louis, C.V. Mosby, 1992.

Roy, F.H.: Ocular Syndromes and Systemic Diseases. 2nd Ed. Philadelphia, W.B. Saunders, 1989.

Dacryocystitis (Infection of the Lacrimal Sac)

  1. Acute dacryocystitis

     *A. Beta-hemolytic streptococcus

      B. Corynebacterium diphtheriae

      C. Dacryolith

      D. Erysipelothrix insidiosa

      E. Friedlander bacillus

      F. Fusobacterium (canaliculitis and dacryocystis)

      G. Granulomatous 'pseudotumor'

     *H. Haemophilus aegyptius (Koch-Weeks bacillus)

      I. Infectious mononucleosis

      J. Influenza

      K. Lymphocytic neoplasia

      L. Neisseria catarrhalis

     M. Pasteurella multocida

    *N. Pneumococcus

    *O. Pseudomonas aeruginosa

     P. Rhinosporidiosis

     Q. Rubeola (measles)

R. Serratia marcescens—gram-negative coccobacillus

*S. Staphylococcus

T. Streptococcus

U. Tularemia

V. Variola

2. Chronic dacryocystitis

A. Associated with osteopoikilosis

B. Actinomyces israeli

C. Aspergillus

D. Bacillus fusiformis

E. Candida albicans

F. Escherichia coli

G. Lymphoma of the lacrimal sac

H. Mycobacterium fortuitum and mycobacterium cholonei

I. Nocardia asteroides

J. Francisella tularensis

K. Mycobacterium leprae

L. Proteus vulgaris

M. Sporotrichosis

N. Syphilis (acquired lues)

O. Systemic sarcoidosis

P. Thermal burns

Q. Trachoma

R. Treponema vincenti

S. Tuberculosis (mycobacterium tuberculosis)

T. Wegener's granulomatosis

Atkinson, P.L., et al.: Infectious mononucleosis presenting as bilateral acute dacryocystitis. Brit J. Ophthal., 74: 750, 1990.

Artenstein, A.W., et al.: Chronic dacryocystitis caused by Mycobacterium fortuitum. Ophthalmology, 100:666–668, 1993.

Gunal, I., et al.: Dacryocystitis associated with osteopoikilosis. Clinical Genetics, 44:211–213, 1993.

Haynes, B.F., et al.: The ocular manifestations of Wegener's granulomatosis: fifteen year's experience and review of the literature. Amer. J. Med., 63:131, 1977.

Karesh, J.W., et al.: Dacryocystitis associated with malignant lymphoma of the lacrimal sac. Ophthalmology, 100:669–673, 1993.

Kheterpal, S., et al.: Arch. Ophthal., 112:519–520, 1994.

Meyer, D.R., and Wobig, J.L.: Acute dacryocystitis caused by Pasteurella multocida. American J. Ophthal., 110:444–445, 1990.

Roy, F.H.: Ocular Syndrome and Systemic Diseases. 2nd Ed. Philadelphia, W.B. Saunders, 1989.

* = most important

Extraocular Muscles

EDWARD G. BUCKLEY MD

Contents

* = most important

Pseudoesotropia (Ocular Appearance of Esotropia When No Manifest Deviation of Visual Axis is Present)

*1. Abnormal shape of skull or abnormal thickness of skin surrounding the orbits

2. Enophthalmos

3. Entropion (see p. 92)

4. Hypotelorism with narrow interpupillary distance

5. Lateral displacement of the concavity of the upper eyelid margin from the center of the pupil

*6. Negative angle kappa—pupillary light reflex displaced temporally (see decentered pupillary light reflex, p. 407)

*7. Prominent epicanthal fold

8. Telecanthus—the orbits are normally placed, but the medial canthi are far apart secondary to lateral displacement of the soft tissues

Shaterian, E.T., and Weismann, I.L.: An unusual case of pseudostrabismus. Am. Orthopt. J., 23:68–70, 1973.

Urist, M.J.: Pseudostrabismus caused by abnormal configuration of the upper eyelid margins. Am. J. Ophthalmol., 75:455–456, 1973.

Esophoria and Esotropia (Visual Axis Deviated Inward; May Be Latent or Manifest)

1. Comitant (nonparalytic)—angle of deviation is constant in all directions of gaze

   A. Accommodative—hyperopic refractive error

   B. Nonaccommodative—refractive error not cause of deviation

       (1) Anomalous insertion of horizontally acting muscles

       (2) Abnormal check ligaments

       (3) Faulty innervational development

       (4) Autosomal recessive trait

       (5) Idiopathic

       (6) Tumor of brain

           a. cerebellar astrocytoma

           b. pontine glioma

2. Noncomitant—the angle of deviation varies in different directions of gaze

   A. Abducens palsy (p. 186)

   B. Accommodative spasm

   C. Blow-out fracture

   D. Divergence paralysis

   E. Drug usage (marijuana)

   F. Duane's syndrome

   G. Myasthenia gravis

   H. Thyroid myopathy

3. "V" pattern esotropia—deviation greater in downward gaze

   A. Underaction—superior oblique muscles

* = most important

B. Overaction-inferior oblique muscles

4. "A" pattern esotropia

    A. Underaction—inferior oblique muscles

5. Monocular esotropia—one eye may be used to the exclusion of the other; amblyopia is usual in the deviating eye

6. Esotropia—near/distance disparity

    A. High AC/A ratio—greater convergence for near than for distance, causing greater esodeviation for near than for distance

    B. Convergence excess—greater esodeviation for near than for distance

    C. Divergence insufficiency—greater esodeviation for distance than for near

Helveston, E.M.: The origins of congenital esotropia. J. Ped. Ophthal. and Strab., 30:215–232, 1993.

Mazow, M.L., et al.: Intermittent esotropia secondary to marijuana smoking. Binocular Vision, 3:219, 1988.

von Noorden, G.K.: Binocular vision and ocular motility: theory and management of strabismus. St Louis, Mo., Mosby, 1995.

Wright, K.W.: Pediatric ophthalmology and strabismus. St. Louis, Mo., Mosby, 1995.

Williams, A.S., and Hoyt, C.S.: Acute comitant esotropia in children with brain tumors. Arch. Ophthal., 107:376, 1989.

Pseudoexotropia (Ocular Appearance of Exotropia When No Manifest Deviation of Visual Axis is Present)

1. Displaced macula (heterotopia of the macula; see p. 506)

2. Heterochromia when the lighter colored eye appears to diverge (see p. 417)

3. Hypertelorism with wide interpupillary distance

4. Exophthalmos

5. Positive-angle kappa—pupillary light reflex displaced nasally (see decentered pupillary light reflex, p. 407)

6. Narrow lateral canthus

7. Wide palpebral fissure

Beyer-Machule, C., and Noorden, G.K., von: Atlas of Ophthalmic Surgery: Vol 1: Lids, Orbits, Extraocular Muscles. New York, Thieme Med. Pub., 1984.

Shaterian, E.T., and Weissman, I.L.: An unusual case of pseudostrabismus. Am. Orthopt. J., 23:68–70, 1973.

Exophoria and Exotropia (Visual Axis Deviated Outward; May Be Latent or Manifest)

1. Comitant

    A. Refractive—myopic refractive error cause of deviation(low AC/A ratio)

    B. Nonrefractive—refractive error not cause of deviation

    C. Anomalous insertion of horizontally acting muscles

    D. Abnormal check ligaments

    E. Faulty innervational development

    F. Autosomal dominant trait

    G. Idiopathic
2. Noncomitant
    A. Convergence insufficiency
    B. Divergence excess
    C. Duane's type II,III
    D. Internuclear ophthalmoplegia
    E. Myasthenia gravis
    F. Third nerve palsy
    G. Thyroid myopathy
3. Pattern exotropia
    A. V exotropia—deviation greater in upward than in downward gaze
        (1) Underaction superior oblique
        (2) Overaction inferior oblique
    B. A exotropia—deviation greater in downward than in upward gaze
        (1) Underaction inferior oblique muscle
        (2) Overaction superior oblique muscle

von Noorden, G.K.: Binocular vision and ocular motility: theory and management of strabismus. St. Louis, Mo., Mosby.
Wright, K.W.: Pediatric ophthalmology and strabismus. St. Louis, Mosby, 1995.

Pseudohypertropia

    1. Facial asymmetry with one eye placed higher than the other
    2. Unilateral coloboma of lid
    3. Unilateral ptosis

Shaterian, E.T., and Weissman, I.L.: An unusual case of pseudostrabismus. Am. Orthopt. J., 23:68–70, 1973.
Wright, D.W.: Pediatric ophthalmology and strabismus. St. Louis, Mosby, 1995.

Hyperphoria and Hypertropia (Visual Axis Deviated Upward; May Be Manifest or Latent)

    1. Nonparalytic hypertropia
        A. Abnormal insertion of muscles
        B. Abnormal fascial attachments
        C. Complications of systemic diseases, such as myasthenia gravis, thyrotoxicosis, and orbital tumors
    2. Paralytic hypertropia—isolated cyclovertical muscle palsy
        A. Brain stem disease
        B. Fourth nerve palsy
        C. Multiple sclerosis
        D. Skew deviation
        E. Third nerve palsy

Three Step Test

Greater Vertical		Head Tilt	Paretic Muscle
Right Hypertropia	Right Gaze	Right greater	LIO
		Left greater	RIR
	Left Gaze	Right greater	RSO
		Left greater	LSR
Left Hypertropia	Right Gaze	Right greater	RSR
		Left greater	LSO
	Left Gaze	Right greater	LIR
		Left greater	RIO

3. Double hyperphoria (alternating circumduction)—fuses, but cover test shows alternating hyperphoria
4. Apparent paralysis of elevation of one eye
    A. Local neuromuscular and orbital causes
        (1) Dysthyroid ophthalmoplegia (noncongestive and congestive form)
        (2) Myasthenia gravis (Erb-Goldflam syndrome)
        (3) Orbital floor fracture
        (4) Progressive supra nuclear ophthalmoplegia
        (5) Oculomotor nerve paresis superior division
        (6) Unilateral double elevator palsy, congenital dysfunction of superior rectus and inferior oblique muscles
        (7) Myositis
            a. "Collagen diseases"
            b. Infectious myositis
            c. Trichinosis
        (8) Orbital tumors
            a. Dermoid cyst
            b. Hemangioma
            c. Lymphoma
            d. Meningioma
            e. Optic nerve glioma
            f. Previous strabismus surgery
            g. Rhabdomyosarcoma
        (9) Systemic amyloidosis with ocular muscle infiltration

      (10) Vertical retraction syndrome (Parinaud's syndrome)

      (11) Superior oblique tendon sheath syndrome (Brown syndrome)

B. Skew deviation due to a central nervous system lesion—one eye is above the other; may be the same for all directions of gaze or vary in different directions of gaze

      (1) Unilateral labyrinthine disease

      (2) Cerebellar tumors, such as astrocytomas and medulloblastomas

      (3) Acoustic neuromas

      (4) Vascular accidents of pons and cerebellum, such as thrombosis of cerebellar and pontine arteries

      (5) Unilateral internuclear ophthalmoplegia and less frequently bilateral internuclear ophthalmoplegia

      (6) Compressive lesions, such as platybasia and Arnold-Chiari malformation

      (7) Brain-stem arteriovenous malformations

      (8) Aberrant regeneration of third nerve

C. Central nervous system lesions

      (1) Arteriosclerosis, thrombosis, arteritis (syphilitic), or embolus of fine vessels to midbrain

5. Apparent paralysis of elevation of both eyes

    A. Physiologic in older individuals

    B. Parinaud syndrome (divergence paralysis)

    C. CPEO

    D. Progressive supranuclear palsy

    E. Myasthenia gravis

    F. Midbrain lesion

      (1) Upgaze center

      (2) Bilateral third nerve palsy

    G. Congenital fibrous syndrome

    H. Thyroid myopathy

    I. Metastatic tumor (breast cancer)

6. Paralysis of downward gaze

    A. Reverse Parinaud syndrome

    B. Associated with choreoathetotic syndromes

    C. Parkinsonoid syndromes

    D. Myasthenia gravis

    E. Miscellaneous

Jampel, R.S., and Fells, P.: Monocular elevation paresis caused by a central nervous system lesion. Arch. Ophthal., 80:45, 1968.

Keane, J.R.: Ocular skew deviation. Arch. Neurol., 32:185, 1975.

Metz, H.S.: Double elevator palsy. J. Ped. Ophthal. and Strab., 18:31–36, 1981.

Kushner, B.J.: Errors in the three-step test in the diagnosis of vertical strabismus. Ophthalmology, 96:127–132, 1989.

Scott, W.E., and Thalacker, J.A.: Diagnosis and treatment of thyroid myopathy. Ophthalmology, 88:493, 1981.

Walsh, F.B., and Hoyt, W.F.: Clinical Neuro-ophthalmology. 4th Ed. Baltimore, Williams & Wilkins, 1985.

Brown's Superior Oblique Tendon Sheath Syndrome (Limitation of Elevation in Adduction that Resembles an Underaction of Inferior Oblique Muscle)

1. Congenital abnormality of the superior oblique tendon medial to the superior rectus muscle which restricts ocular movement
    A. Anomalous insertion of the superior oblique muscle
    B. Shortening of the tendon of the superior oblique so that the thickened superior oblique muscle is closer to the trochlea and acts as a ball and socket. Being unable to pass through the trochlea.
    C. Thickening of the tendon, resulting in impaired slippage through the trochlea
2. Juvenile or adult rheumatoid arthritis
3. Localized abscess
4. Sleral buckling bands
5. Sinusitis
6. Trauma
    A. Canine tooth syndrome
    B. Sinus surgery

Kaban, J.T., et al.: Natural history of presumed congenital Brown's syndrome. Arch. Ophthal., 111:102, 1993.

Tien, R.D., et al.: Superior oblique tendon sheath syndrome (Brown syndrome). Amer. J. of Neuroradiology, 11:1210, 1990.

Wang, F.M., et al.: Brown's syndrome in children with juvenile rheumatoid arthritis. Ophthal., 91:23–26, 1984.

Wilson, M.E., et al.: Brown's syndrome. Survey Ophthal., 34:153, 1989.

Oculomotor Apraxia-Defective or Absent Horizontal Voluntary Eye Movements; Head Thrusting to Look at Objects to the Side

1. Ataxia-telangiectasia syndrome
2. Brain tumor
    A. Astrocytoma
    B. Lipoma
3. Isolated
4. Male predominance
5. Neurofibromatosis
6. Oral-facial-digital syndrome type II
7. Post cardiac surgery

Isenberg, S.J.: The Eye in Infancy. Chicago, Year Book Medical Publishers, 1989.

Moschner, C., et al.: Comparison of oculomotor findings in the progressive ataxia syndromes. Brain, 117:15–25, 1995.

Zackon, D.H., and Noel, L.: Ocular motor apraxia following cardiac surgery. Can. J. Ophthal., 26:102, 1991.

Zaret, C., et al.: Congenital ocular motor apraxia and brainstem tumor. Arch. Ophthal., 98:328–330, 1980.

Monocular Limitation of Elevation of the Adducted Eye with Forced DuctionTest (in Elevation and Adduction)

Restricted	Unrestricted
A. Brown syndrome of superior oblique tendon sheath: congenitally short superior oblique tendon sheath	A. Paresis of inferior oblique muscle such as impaired innervation (nuclear or infranuclear) or contractility of inferior oblique
B. Simulated Brown syndrome 1. Congenital anomalous insertion of the superior oblique tendon	B. Pseudoparesis of inferior oblique muscle
2. Congenital anomalous check ligament from lateral orbit to insertion of inferior oblique	1. Subtle mechanical restriction affecting superior oblique tendon or sheath, or affecting infeior orbital tissues
3. Swelling of the superior oblique tendon restricting passage through the trochlea	2. Supranucleaer innervation defect
4. Infection in the region of the trochlea	
5. Shortening of the superior oblique tendon by a tuck procedure	
6. Scar produced by superior nasal quadrant operation	
7. Congenital or acquired restrictions affecting inferior orbital tissues, such as a blowout fracture	

Monocular Limitation of Elevation of the Adducted Eye with Forced Duction Test (in Elevation and Adduction [see chart] Strabismus with Restricted Motility)

1. Acquired
    A. Thyroid myopathy
    *B. Excessive recession or resection of muscle
    C. Orbital fracture
    D. Retinal detachment operation
    E. Strabismus surgery complicated by adhesions
    F. CPEO
2. Congenital
    A. Congenital fibrous syndrome
    B. Neurogenic paralysis with secondary contracture of antagonist muscle
    C. Duane's retraction syndrome
    D. Brown's superior oblique tendon sheath syndrome
    E. Strabismus fixus

Harley, R.D., et al.: Congenital fibrosis of the extraocular muscles. Tran. Am. Ophthal. Soc., 76:197, 1978.

Wright, K.W.: Pediatric Ophthalmology and Strabismus. St. Louis, Mosby, 1995.

Cyclic, Recurrent, Repetitive, Episodic Disorders of Extraocular Muscles

1. Cyclic strabismus
    A. Associated with fronto-orbital fibrous dysplasia
    B Associated with Graves disease
    C. Associated with optic atrophy
    D. Cyclic superior oblique palsy
    E. Cyclic third nerve palsy
    F. Esotropia, vertical
        (1) Comitant
        (2) Noncomitant
2. Cyclic vertical deviation
3. Diabetic nerve palsies
4. Myasthenia gravis
5. Oculogyric crisis (see p. 176)
6. Periodic alternating gaze deviation
7. Periodic alternating nystagmus
8. Periodic vertical nystagmus
    A. Associated with potassium abnormality
    B. Familial
9. Petit mal epilepsy
    A. Exotropia
    B. Upward deviation

10. Ping pong gaze

11. Recurrent sixth nerve paralysis in children (see p. 186)

12. Spasmus nutans

13. Twitch of lids (orbicularis)

Hamed, L.: Cyclic periodic disorders in diagnostic problems in clinical ophthalmology. Margo, C.L. ed. Philadelphia, Saunders, 1994.

Hoyt, W.F., and Keane, J.R.: Superior Oblique Myokymia. Arch. Ophthalmol., 84:461–467, 1970.

Windsor, C.E., and Berg, E.F.: Circadian heterotropia. Am. J. Ophthalmol., 67:565–571, 1969.

Syndromes and Diseases Associated with Strabismus

1. A esotropia syndrome

2. A exotropia syndrome

3. Aarskog syndrome (facial-digital-genital syndrome)

4. Aberfeld syndrome (congenital blepharophimosis associated with generalized myopathy)

5. Achondroplasia

6. Addison pernicious anemia

7. African eyeworm disease

8. Albinism

9. Albright hereditary osteodystrophy (pseudohypoparathyroidism)

10. Amyloidosis

11. Apert syndrome (acrocephalosyndactylism syndrome)

12. Arnold-Chiari syndrome (platybasia syndrome)

13. Arylsulfatase A deficiency syndrome

14. Aspergillosis

15. Axenfeld-Schurenberg syndrome (cyclic oculomotor paralysis)

16. Bacterial endocarditis

17. Bang disease (brucellosis)

18. Behçet syndrome (oculobuccogenital syndrome)

19. Benedikt syndrome (tegmental syndrome)

20. Best disease (vitelliform dystrophy)

21. Bielschowsky-Lutz-Cogan syndrome (internuclear ophthalmoplegia)

22. Bing-Neel syndrome (associated with macroglobulinemia and central nervous system symptoms)

23. Bloch-Sulzberger disease (incontinentia pigmenti)

24. Blocked nystagmus syndrome (Nystagmus blockage syndrome)

25. Bonnet-Dechaume-Blanc syndrome (neuroretinoangiomatosis syndrome)

26. Bonnevie-Ullrich syndrome (pterygolymphangiectasia)

27. Botulism

28. Brown-Marie syndrome (hereditary ataxia syndrome)

29. Canine tooth syndrome (class VII superior oblique palsy)

* = most important

30. Cerebral palsy

31. Chediak-Higashi syndrome (anomalous leukocytic inclusions with constitutional stigmata)

32. Chromosome partial deletion (short-arm) syndrome (Wolf syndrome)

33. Chromosome 13q partial deletion (long-arm) syndrome (Thirteen Q syndrome)

34. Chromosome partial deletion (long-arm) syndrome (DeGrouchy syndrome)

35. Chromosome partial (short-arm) partial deletion syndrome

36. Congenital syphilis

37. Convergence insufficiency syndrome

38. Craniocarpotarsal dysplasia (Freeman-Sheldon syndrome; whistling face syndrome)

39. Craniostenosis

40. Cri du chat syndrome (crying cat syndrome)

41. Crohn disease (granulomatous ileocolitis)

42. Crouzon disease (craniofacial dysostosis)

43. Cushing syndrome (II) (cerebellopontine angle syndrome)

44. Cysticercosis

45. Cytomegalic inclusion disease, congenital

46. Dawson disease (subacute sclerosing panencephalitis)

47. De Lange syndrome (congenital muscular hypertrophy—cerebral syndrome)

48. Dengue fever

49. Devic syndrome (ophthalmoencephalomyelopathy)

50. Diabetes mellitus

51. Diphtheria

52. Down disease (mongolism, trisomy 21)

53. Drugs including:

alcohol
baclofen
calcitriol
chloramphenicol(?)
chloroform
cholecalciferol
ergocalciferol
insulin
iothalamate meglumine and sodium iothalamic acid
isocarboxazid
measles and rubella virus vaccine (live)
measles, mumps, and rubella virus vaccine (live)
measles virus vaccine (live)
metoclopramide
metrizamide
mumps virus vaccine (live)
nialamide
pemoline
pentylenetetrazol
phenelzine
rubella and mumps virus vaccine (live)
rubella virus vaccine (live)
tranylcypromine
tripelennamine
vitamin A
vitamin D_2
vitamin D_3

54. Drummond syndrome (idiopathic hypercalcemia)
55. Duane's syndrome (retraction syndrome)
56. Ectrodactyly-ectodermal dysplasia-clefting syndrome (EEC syndrome)
57. Ehlers-Danlos disease (fibrodysplasia elastica generalisata)
58. Electrical injury
59. Ellis-van Creveld syndrome (chondroectodermal dysplasia)
60. Encephalitis, acute
61. Engelmann syndrome (osteopathia hyperostotica scleroticans multiplex infantalis)
62. Epidermal nevus syndrome (ichthyosis hystrix)
63. Erb-Goldflam disease
64. Fetal alcohol syndrome
65. Fibrosarcoma
66. Francois dyscephalic syndrome
67. Gaucher syndrome (glucocerebroside storage disease)
68. Gangliosidosis
    A. Infantile (GM1)
    B. Juvenile (GM2)
69. Goltz syndrome (focal dermal hypoplasia syndrome)
70. Gorlin-Goltz syndrome (multiple basal cell nevi syndrome)
71. Greig syndrome (ocular hypertelorism syndrome)
72. Grönblad-Strandberg syndrome (systemic elastodystrophy)
73. Hemangiomas
74. Hemifacial hyperplasia with strabismus (Bencze syndrome—autosomal dominant)
75. Hemifacial microsomia (otomandibular dysostosis)
76. Homocystinuria
77. Hurler disease (mucopolysaccharidoses type I)
78. Hutchinson syndrome (adrenal cortex neuroblastoma with orbital metastasis)
79. Hydrocephalus, congenital
80. Hydrophobia (rabies)
81. Hyperthyroidism
82. Hypocalcemia
83. Hypomelanosis of Ito syndrome (incontinentia pigmenti achromians)
84. Hypothermal injury
85. Hysteria
86. Infectious mononucleosis
87. Influenza
88. Jacobs syndrome (triple X syndrome)
89. Johnson syndrome (adherence syndrome)
90. Klippel-Feil syndrome (congenital brevicollis)
91. Koerber-Salus-Elschnig syndrome (nystagmus retractorius syndrome)

92. Kohn-Romano syndrome (telecanthus, ptosis, epicanthus inversus, blepharophimosis)
93. Krause syndrome (congenital encephalo-ophthalmic dysplasia)
94. Kugelberg-Welander syndrome (progressive muscle atrophy)
95. Kussmaul disease (necrotizing angiitis)
96. Larsen syndrome (hypertelorism, microtia, and facial clefting)
97. Laurence-Moon-Bardet-Biedl syndrome (retinitis pigmentosa-polydactyly-adiposogenital syndrome)
98. Leigh disease (subacute necrotizing encephalomyelopathy)
99. Leukemia
100. Linear nevus sebaceous of Jadassohn
101. Lowe syndrome (oculocerebrorenal syndrome)
102. Lymphangioma
103. Lymphedema
104. Lymphoid hyperplasia (Burkitt lymphoma)
105. Malaria
106. Malignant hyperpyrexia syndrome
107. Malignant hyperthermia syndrome
108. Maple syrup urine disease
109. Marcus Gunn syndrome (jaw winking syndrome)
110. Marfan syndrome (arachnodactyly-dystrophia mesodermalis congenita)
111. Measles
112. Melnick-Needles syndrome (osteodysplasty)
113. Mieten syndrome (corneal opacity, nystagmus, flexion contracture, growth failure)
114. Millard-Gubler syndrome (abducens—facial hemiplegia alternans)
115. Mobius syndrome (congenital paralysis of 6th or 7th nerves)
116. Monofixation syndrome (blind spot syndrome)
117. Morning glory syndrome (hereditary central glial anomaly of the optic disk)
118. Mucocele
119. Mucormycosis
120. Mulibrey nanism syndrome (Perheentupa syndrome)
121. Multiple lentigines syndrome (leopard syndrome)
122. Multiple sclerosis
123. Mumps
124. Myasthenia gravis (Erb-Goldflam syndrome)
125. Naegeli syndrome (melanophoric nevus syndrome)
126. Nematode ophthalmia syndrome (toxocariasis)
127. Neonatal hemolytic disease of hyperbilirubinemia
128. Neuroblastoma
129. Nevus sebaceous of Jadassohn
130. Nevoid basal cell carcinoma syndrome

131. Nielsen syndrome (exhaustive psychosis syndrome)
132. Noonan syndrome (male Turner syndrome)
133. Noone-Milroy-Meige disease (congenital trophedema)
134. Nothnagel syndrome (ophthalmoplegia cerebellar ataxia syndrome)
135. Nystagmus compensation syndrome
136. Obesity—cerebralocular-skeletal anomalies syndrome
137. Ocular vaccinia
138. Oculocerebellar tegmental syndrome
139. Oculo-oto-ororenoerythropoietic syndrome
140. Ophthalmoplegic retinal degeneration syndrome
141. Orbital floor syndrome (Dejean syndrome)
142. Paget syndrome (osteitis deformans)
143. Papillon-Leage and Psaume syndrome (orodigital facial syndrome)
144. Parkinson syndrome
145. Parry-Romberg disease (progressive facial hemiatrophy)
146. Periocular and ocular metastatic tumors
147. Pertussis (whooping cough)
148. Pierre Robin syndrome (micrognathia-glossoptosis syndrome)
149. Polymyalgia rheumatica
150. Postvaccinial ocular syndrome
151. Pseudo-ophthalmoplegia syndrome (Roth-Bielschowsky syndrome)
152. Prader-Willi syndrome (hypotonia-obesity syndrome)
153. Pseudohypoparathyroidism (Seabright-Bantam syndrome)
154. Reiter syndrome (conjunctivourethrosynovial syndrome)
155. Relapsing fever
156. Retinoblastoma
157. Ring chromosome 18
158. Ring D chromosome
159. Ring dermoid syndrome
160. Rocky mountain spotted fever
161. Rubella, congenital
162. Rubinstein-Taybi syndrome (broad thumb syndrome)
163. Sabin-Feldman syndrome
164. Sandifer syndrome (hiatus hernia-torticollis syndrome)
165. Schilder syndrome (encephalitis periaxialis diffusa)
166. Seckel bird-headed dwarfism
167. Skew deviation syndrome
168. Smallpox
169. Smith-Lemli-Opitz syndrome (cerebrohepatorenal syndrome)
170. Spongy degeneration of the white matter

171. Streptococcus

172. Superior oblique tendon sheath syndrome (Brown's syndrome)

173. Supravalvular aortic stenosis syndrome (infantile hypercalcemia with mental retardation)

174. Tay-Sachs syndrome (familial amaurotic idiocy)

175. Temporal arteritis syndrome (cranial arteritis syndrome)

176. Terson syndrome (subarachnoid hemorrhage syndrome)

177. Thomsen syndrome (congenital myotonia syndrome)

178. Trichinosis

Fraunfelder, F.T.: Drug-Induced Ocular Side Effects and Drug Interactions. 4th Ed. Philadelphia, Williams & Wilkins, 1996.

McKusick, V.A.: Mendelian Inheritance in Man. 9th Ed. Baltimore, Johns Hopkins University Press, 1994.

Roy, F.H.: Ocular Syndromes and Systemic Diseases. 2nd Ed. Philadelphia, W.B. Saunders, 1989.

Horizontal Gaze Palsy (Inability to Look Horizontally in a Given Direction; Analysis Includes Optically Induced Movement, Voluntary or Command Movement, Pursuit Movement, or Vestibular Movement)

1. Horizontal palsy of voluntary and command movement—frontal lobe gaze center (second frontal gyrus, Brodmann's area 8) or in the corresponding internal capsule gaze palsy of side opposite lesion; may be associated with facial palsy as well as hemiparesis or hemiplegia toward the side of the gaze palsy, caloric ocular movement intact, doll's head intact.

2. Horizontal palsy of command and pursuit movements, optically induced movements, and vestibular movements—pons and posterior longitudinal bundle; the gaze palsy is toward the side of the lesion, facial palsy often present, caloric and doll's head responses absent.

Huber, A.: Eye Symptoms in Brain Tumors. 2nd Ed. St. Louis, C.V. Mosby, 1971, pp. 44–47.

Oscillations of Eyes (Involuntary, Rapid, To-and-Fro Movement of Eyes Having No Rhythm or Regularity)

1. Ocular dysmetria—"overshooting" of the eyes with attempted fixation; horizontal ocular dysmetria is associated with lesions of the cerebellum or its pathways as in Friedreich ataxia, Huntington chorea, spinocerebellar degeneration, internuclear ophthalmoplegia, manic-depression, alcoholism, schizophrenia, severe diffuse brain damage, cerebellopontine angle tumors, hereditary ectodermal dysplasia with olivoponto-cerebellar degeneration, Fabry disease (glycosphingolipid lipidosis), vestibulocerebellar ataxia, and toluene abuse

2. Ocular flutter—flutter-like oscillations, which are intermittent, rapid, to-and-fro motions, or motions of equal amplitude, interrupt maintained fixation; horizontal ocular flutter is associated with lesions of the cerebellum or its pathways as in limb ataxia, multiple sclerosis, poliomyelitis, neoplasms, or vascular accident

3. Opsoclonus—irregular, hyperkinetic, multidirectional, spontaneous eye movement that persists in sleep

    A. Infections

        (1) Coxsackie B3

(2) Encephalitis—mild, severe, viral, or postinfections (including St. Louis encephalitis)

(3) Hemophilus influenzae

(4) Meningitis

(5) Paratyphi A

(6) Psittacosis

(7) Salmonella

B. Tumors

(1) Breast malignancy

(2) Bronchogenic carcinoma

(3) Glioblastoma

(4) Neuroblastoma

(5) Thyroid carcinoma

(6) Uterine carcinoma

C. Toxins and drugs

(1) Amitriptyline

(2) Chlordecone

(3) Lithium-Haldol

(4) Thallium

(5) Toluene abuse

D. Other

(1) Acute cerebellar ataxia

(2) Friedreich ataxia

(3) Multiple sclerosis (disseminated sclerosis) (rare)

(4) Nonketotic coma

(5) Sign of 'myoclonic encephalopathy of infancy'

(6) Vascular accidents

(7) Vertebrobasilar insufficiency

4. Lightning eye movements (ocular myoclonus)—rapid, to-and-fro movements of small conjugate saccades; probably because of bilateral abnormality of a pontine paramedial zone and pretectal lesions, such as vascular, inflammatory, neoplastic, demyelinating, or trauma of tegmentum as thyroid, lung or uterus carcinoma, neuroblastoma, Menzel hereditary ataxia, pontine myelinolysis, coxsackie B infection, cherry-red spot myoclonus syndrome, Ramsay-Hunt syndrome, and L-tryptophan

Bollen, E., et al.: Horizontal and vertical saccadic eye movement abnormalities in Huntington's chorea. J. Neurol. Sci., 71:11–22, 1986.

Dropcho, E., and Payne, R.: Paraneoplastic opsoclonus myoclonus: Association with medullary thyroid carcinoma and review of the literature. Arch. Neurol., 43:410–415, 1986.

Farris, B.K., et al.: Neuro-ophthalmologic findings in vestibulocerebellar ataxia. Arch. Neurol., 43:1050–1053, 1986.

Lazar, R.B., et al.: Multifocal central nervous system damage caused by toluene abuse. Neurology, 33:1337–1340, 1983.

Matsumura, K., et al.: Syndrome of opsoclonus-myoclonus in hyperosmolar nonketotic coma. Ann. Neurol., 18:623–624, 1985.

Mattyns, A., and Veres, E.: Multiple sclerosis in childhood. Acta. Paediatr. Hung., 26:193–204, 1985.

Monday, L., et al.: Follow-up study of electro-nystagmographic findings in Friedreich's ataxia patients and evaluation of their relatives. Can. J. Neurol. Sci., 11:57–573, 1984.

Wang, P.Y.: Acute cerebellitis with ocular flutter and truncal ataxia: a case report. Chinese Medical Journal, 50: 169–171, 1992.

Cogwheel Eye Movements (Jerky Inaccurate Pursuit Movements)

1. Basal ganglia disease

   A. Anoxia

   B. Carbon disulfide poisoning

   C. Carbon monoxide poisoning

   D. Drugs including:

acetophenazine	etidocaine	prazepam
alcohol	fluphenazine	prilocaine
allobarbital	flurazepam	primidone
alprazolam	halazepam	probarbital
alseroxylon	heptabarbital	procaine
amitriptyline	hexethal	prochlorperazine
amobarbital	hexobarbital	promazine
aprobarbital	imipramine	promethazine
barbital	lidocaine	propiomazine
bromide	lithium carbonate	propoxycaine
bupivacaine	lorazepam	protriptyline
butabarbital	mephobarbital	rauwolfia serpentina
butalbital	mepivacaine	rescinnamine
butallylonal	mesoridazine	reserpine
butaperazine	metharbital	secobarbital
butethal	methdilazine	syrosingopine
carphenazine	methitural	talbutal
chloral hydrate	methohexital	temazepam
chlordiazepoxide	methotrimeprazine	thiamylal
chloroprocaine	midazolam	thiethylperazine
chlorpromazine	nitrazepam	thiopental
clonazepam	nortriptyline	thiopropazate
clorazepate	oxazepam	thioproperazine
cyclobarbital	pentobarbital	thioridazine
cyclopentobarbital	perazine	triazolam
deserpidine	pericazine	trifluoperazine
desipramine	perphenazine	triflupromazine
diazepam	phencyclidine	trimeprazine
diethazine	phenobarbital	vinbarbital
ethopropazine	pipercetazine	

   E. Exposure to manganese

   F. Idiopathic

G. Parkinsonism (shaking palsy)

H. Trauma

2. Cerebellar tumors

A. Astrocytomas

B. Hemangioblastomas

C. Medulloblastomas

3. With homonymous hemianopia, indicates parietal or occipital lobe involvement

Fraunfelder, F.T.: Drug-Induced Ocular Side Effects and Drug Interactions. 4th Ed. Philadelphia, Williams & Wilkins, 1996.

Huber, A.: Eye Symptoms in Brain Tumors. 2nd Ed. St. Louis, C.V. Mosby, 1971.

Walsh, F.B., and Hoyt, W.F.: Clinical Neuro-ophthalmology. 4th Ed. Baltimore, Williams & Wilkins, 1985.

Pendular Nystagmus (Oscillations that Are Approximately Equal in Rate in Two Directions; May Be Horizontal or Vertical)

1. Albinism in which the macula does not develop

2. Aniridia (see p. 408)

3. Bilateral chorioretinal lesions involving the macula in early infancy (congenital toxoplasmosis)

*4. Congenital—cause unknown, may be inherited as autosomal dominant recessive or X-linked recessive trait; not infrequently associated with astigmatism and convergent strabismus

*5. Congenital cataracts

6. Congenital glaucoma

7. Corneal scars

8. High myopia of early life

9. Laurence-Moon-Bardet-Biedl syndrome (retinitis pigmentosa-polydactyly-adiposogenital syndrome)

10. Leber's congenital amaurosis

11. Optic nerve hypoplasia, coloboma

*12. Total color blindness (monochromatism)

13. Work in poor illuminations (e.g., mining) (rare)

Cogan, D.G.: Neurology of the Ocular Muscles. 4th Ed. Springfield, Ill., Charles C Thomas, 1978.

Walsh, F.B., and Hoyt, W.F.: Clinical Neuro-ophthalmology. 4th Ed. Baltimore, Williams & Wilkins, 1985.

Horizontal Jerk Nystagmus (Horizontal Oscillatory Movement of Eyes with a fast and slow phase)

1. Albinism

2. Amblyopia (manifest latent nystagmus)

3. Cerebellar disease, acute or chronic; fast component to side of lesion

* = most important

4. Chediak-Higashi syndrome (anomalous leukocytic inclusions with constitutional stigmata)

5. Congenital achromatopsia

6. Congenital cataracts

7. Congenital stationary nightblindness

8. Congenital X-linked, dominant, recessive

9. Leber's congenital amaurosis

10. Lesions of labyrinth (e.g., Meniere syndrome) or when one labyrinth has been removed

11. Neoplastic angioendotheliomatosis

12. Optic nerve hypoplasia, coloboma

13. Vestibular nuclei involvement as in persons with multiple sclerosis

Barton, J.J., and Sharpe, J.A.: Oscillopsia and horizonal nystagmus with accelerating slow phases following lumbar puncture in the Arnold-Chiari malformation. Ann. of Neurology, 33:418–421, 1993.

Cogan, D.G.: Neurology of the Ocular Muscles. 4th Ed. Springfield, Ill., Charles C Thomas, 1978.

Elner, V.M., et al.: Neoplastic angioendotheliomatosis. Ophthalmology, 93:1237–1245, 1986.

Spaeth, G. L.: Ocular manifestations of the lipidoses. In Tasman, W. C. (ed.): Retinal Disease in Children. New York, Harper & Row, 1971, pp. 187–188.

Vertical Nystagmus (Spontaneous Vertical Oscillations of Eyes)

1. Up-beat nystagmus—nystagmus in which the fast component is upward and usually most marked when the gaze is directed upward; usually due to a lesion in the posterior fossa

    A. Brain stem lesion, such as that of the vestibular nuclei

    B. Cerebellar disease—acute or chronic, especially in the vermis

    C. Cerebellar degeneration

    D. Drugs—barbiturates and Dilantin

    E. Encephalitis

    F. Labyrinth disease—rare; has no lateralizing value

    G. Multiple sclerosis

    H. Idiopathic

2. Down-beat nystagmus—nystagmus in which the fast component is downward and usually most marked when the gaze is directed downward; probably due to a lesion in the lower end of the brain stem or cerebellum

    A. Alcoholic cerebellar disease

    B. Aneurysm of the supraclinoid part of left carotid siphon

    C. Arnold-Chiari malformation—herniation of cerebellar tonsils and part of medulla through foramen Magnum

    D. Cerebellar atrophy/degeneration

    E. Carbamazepine

    F. Deformities of cervical spine

G. Diabetes mellitus

H. Encephalopathy

 I. Ependymoma of posterior part of the fourth ventricle

J. Idiopathic

K. Insufficiency of basilar artery

L. Klippel-Feil anomaly—upward displacement of odontoid process into foramen magnum

M. Meningioma extending into pontine cistern

N. Morphine poisoning

O. Multiple sclerosis (disseminated sclerosis)

P. Neurogenic muscular atrophy

Q. Platybasia (cerebellomedullary malformation syndrome)

Burde, R.M., and Henkind, P.: Downbeat nystagmus. Surv. Ophthalmol., 25:263, 1981.

Chrousos, G.A.: Downbeat nystagmus and oscillopsia associated with carbamazepine. Am. J. Ophthalmol., 103:221–224, 1957.

Holmes, G. L., et al.: Primary position upbeat nystagmus following meningitis. Ann. Ophthalmol., 13:935, 1981.

Lessell, S., et al.: Prolonged vertical nystagmus after pentobarbital sodium administration. Am. J. Ophthalmol., 30:151–152, 1975.

Monteiro, M.L., and Sampaio, C.M.: Lithium-induced downbeat nystagmus in a patient with Arnold-Chiari malformation. Amer J. Ophthal., 116:648–649, 1993.

Rotary Nystagmus (Rotary Oscillatory Movement of Eyes)

1. Benign paroxysmal positional nystagmus—fast component toward lower ear

*2. Cerebellar disease—acute or chronic

3. Cerebrotendinous xanthomatosis

4. Encephalitis

5. Lesion of vestibular nuclei in floor of fourth ventricle associated with multiple sclerosis, syringobulbia, or thrombosis of postero-inferior cerebellar artery or its branches

*6. Superior oblique myokymia—benign, intermittent, uniocular

7. Vestibular involvement (e.g., labyrinthitis, Meniere syndrome)

Leigh, R.J., et al.: Loss of ipsidirectional quick phases of torsional nystagmus with a unilateral midbrain lesion. J. of Vestibular Research, 3:115–121, 1993.

Rosengart, A., et al.: Intermittent downbeat nystagmus due to vertebral artery compression. Neurology, 43:216–218, 1993.

See-Saw Nystagmus (One Eye Moves Up As Other Eye Moves Down; in Addition, There Is Torsion of Eyes—Eye Moving Up Intorts, and Eye Moving Down Extorts). This nystagmus probably is due to lesions located in mesodiencephalic region, hypothalamus, and thalamus; it may be associated with bitemporal hemianopsia and reduced vertical optokinetic nystagmus

1. Brain stem vascular disease

*2. Chiasmal glioma

* = most important

*3. Chromophobe adenoma of the pituitary gland, involving the optic chiasm and third ventricle

4. Congenital

*5. Craniopharyngioma, involving the optic chiasm and hypothalamus

6. Head injury with fracture of frontal

7. Idiopathic

8. Multiple sclerosis

9. Oligodendroglioma involving the pons and third ventricle

10. Post operative after strabismus surgery

11. Retinitis pigmentosa

12. Septo-optico dysplasia

13. Suprasellar epidermoid tumor involving optic chiasm and hypothalamus

14. Syringomyelia and syringobulbia

15. Toxoplasmosis of the brain stem

Fein, J.M., and Williams, R.D.B.: See-saw nystagmus. J. Neurol. Neurosurg. Psychiatry, 32:202–207, 1969.

Walsh, F.B., and Hoyt, W.F.: Clinical Neuro-ophthalmology. 4th Ed. Baltimore, Williams & Wilkins, 1985.

Retraction Nystagmus (Spasmodic Retraction of Eyes When an Attempt Is Made to Move Them in Any Direction; Caused by Lesions of Midbrain, Especially Lesions in Vicinity of Aqueduct of Sylvius)

1. Arteriovenous aneurysm

2. Brucellosis (Bang disease)

3. Cysticercus cyst

4. Ependymoma

5. Koerber-Salus-Elschnig syndrome (sylvian aqueduct syndrome)

*6. Parinaud syndrome (paralysis of vertical movement)

7. Vascular lesions

Duke-Elder, S., and Scott, G.I.: System of Ophthalmology. Vol. XII. St. Louis, C.V. Mosby, 1971.

Huber, A.: Eye Symptoms in Brain Tumors. 2nd Ed. St. Louis, C.V. Mosby, 1971.

Monocular Nystagmus

1. Horizontal

   A. Lesions of optic nerve, chiasm, midbrain, or brain stem

   B. Nervous system disease, such as multiple sclerosis, epidemic meningitis, and congenital syphilis

   C. Seizures

   D. Superior oblique myokymia—benign, intermittent, uniocular

   E. Spasmus nutans—most common cause in children

   F. Tumors of brain stem

   G. Unilateral amblyopia

      H. Unilateral astigmatism or high refractive error

      I. Unilateral opacity of the ocular media

  2. Vertical

      A. Multiple sclerosis

      B. Myokymia of lower eyelid

      C. Sleep

      D. Spasmus nutans

      E. Unilateral amblyopia

Farmer, J., and Hoyt, C.S.: Monocular nystagmus in infancy and early childhood. Am. J. Ophthalmol., 98:504–509, 1984.

Gottlob, I., et al.: Signs distinguishing spasmus nutans from infantile nystagmus. Ophthal., 97:1166, 1990.

Jacome, D.E., and Fitzgerald, R.: Monocular ictal nystagmus. Arch. Neurol., 39:653, 1982.

Smith, J.L., et al.: Monocular vertical oscillations of amblyopia. J. Clin. Neurol., 39:653, 1982.

Periodic Alternating Nystagmus (Central Vestibular Nystagmus with Rhythmic Jerk Type of Nystagmus that Undergoes Phasic or Cyclic Changes in Amplitude and Direction)

  1. Cerebral trauma or fractured skull

  2. Chiasmal lesion such as craniopharyngioma

  3. Chronic otitis media

  4. Congenital

  5. Diabetes mellitus

  6. Encephalitis

  7. Friedreich hereditary ataxia

  8. Meningioma of tentorium cerebelli, cerebellar glioma, and cholesteatoma of the cerebellopontine angle

  9. Mesencephalic brain stem and cerebellar disease

 10. Multiple sclerosis (disseminated sclerosis)

 11. Syringobulbia (Passow syndrome)

 12. Syphilitic optic atrophy

 13. Tumor of the corpus callosum

 14. Vertebrobasilar artery insufficiency

 15. von Recklinghausen syndrome (neurofibromatosis)

Davis, D.G., and Smith, J.L.: Periodic alternating nystagmus. Am. J. Ophthalmol., 72:757–762, 1971.

Walsh, F.B., and Hoyt, W.F.: Clinical Neuro-ophthalmology. 4th Ed. Baltimore, Williams & Wilkins, 1985.

Positional Nystagmus (Nystagmus that Appears or Changes in Form or Intensity after Certain Positional Changes of the Head Indicate Vestibular Stimulation)

  1. After general anesthesia

  2. After head injury

* = most important

3. Drugs, including:

acetophenazine
alcohol
allobarbital
alprazolam
amiodarone
amitriptyline
amobarbital
amodiaquine
amoxapine
aprobarbital
aspirin
auranofin
aurothioglucose
aurothioglycanide
baclofen
barbital
BCG vaccine
bleomyin(?)
bromide
bromisovalum
broxyquinolin
bupivacaine
butabarbital
butalbital
butallylonal
butaperazine
butethal
calcitriol
carbamazepine
carbinoxamine
carbon monoxide
carbromal
carisoprodol
carphenazine
cefaclor
cefadroxil
cefamandole
cefazolin
cefonicid
cefoperazone
ceforanide

cefotaime
cefotetan
cefoxitin
cefsulodin
ceftazidime
ceftizoxime
ceftriaxone
cefuroxime
cephalexin
cephaloglycin
cephaloridine
cephalothin
cephapirin
cephadrine
chloral hydrate
chloramphenicol(?)
chlordiazepoxide
chloroform
chloroprocaine
chloroquine
chlorpromazine
cholecalciferol
clemastine
clomipramine
clonazepam
clorazepate
colistimethate
colistin
cyclobarbital
cyclopentobarbital
cytarabine
desipramine
diazepam
diethazine
digitalis(?)
diiodohydroxyquin
dimethyl tubocurarine iodide
diphenhydramine
diphenylhydantoin
diphenylpyraline
disulfiram

divalproex sodium
doxepin
doxylamine
dronabinol
ergocalciferol
ergot(?)
ethacrynic acid
ethchlorvynol
ethopropazine
ethotoin
etidocaine
fenfluramine
flecainide
floxuridine
fluorouracil
fluphenazine
flurazepam
glutethimide
gold Au 198
gold sodium thiomalate
gold sodium thiosulfate
halazepam
hashish
heptabarbital
hexethal
hexobarbital
hydroxychloroquine
ibuprofen
imipramine
influenza virus vaccine(?)
insulin
iodochlorhydroxyquin
iodoquinol
iophendylate
isoniazid
ketamine
lidocaine
lithium carbonate
lorazepam
marijuana
meperidine

mephenesin
mephentermine
mephenytoin
mephobarbital
mepivacaine
meprobamate
mesoridazine
metaraminol
methaqualone
metharbital
methdilazine
methitural
methocarbamol
methohexital
methoxamine
methotrimeprazine
methyl alcohol
methylpentynol
methylthiouracil
methyprylon
metoclopramide
methocurine iodide
metrizamide
mexiletine
midazolam
nalidixic acid
nifedipine
nitrazepam
nitrofurantoin
norepinephrine
nortriptyline
oral contraceptives
oxazepam
paramethadione

pemoline
penicillamine
pentazocine
pentobarbital
perhexilene
pericyazine
perphenazine
pencyclidine
phenelzine
phenobarbital
phenylpropanolamine
phenytoin
piperacetazine
piperazine
polymyxin B
prazepam
prilocaine
primidone
probarbital
procaine
procarbazine
prochlorperazine
promazine
promethazine
propiomazine
propoxycaine
protriptyline
quinine
scopolamine
secobarbital
sodium salicylate
streptomycin
talbutal
temazepam

tetanus immune globulin
tetanus toxoid
tetrahydrocannabinol
thiamylal
thiethylperazine
thiopental
thioperazine
thiopropazate
thioproperazine
thioridazine
tobramycin
tocainide
tranylcypromine
triazolam
trichloroethylene
trifluoperazine
triflupromazine
trimeprazine
trimethadione
trimipramine
tripelennamine
tubocurarine
urea(?)
urethan
valproate sodium
valproic acid
verapamil
vinbarbital
vinblastine(?)
vincristine(?)
vitamin A
vitamin D
vitamin D_2
vitamin D_3

4. Inner ear pathologic changes, including hemorrhage, inflammation, thrombosis, emboli, circulatory and secretory conditions

5. Normal individuals

6. Other causes include neuritis, meningitis, tumors, vascular anomalies, degeneration, atrophy, syphilis, arteriosclerosis, hypertonia, vasomotor disturbance, allergic and toxic conditions, cranial trauma, hemorrhage, emboli, or thrombosis

Fraunfelder, F.T.: Drug-Induced Ocular Side Effects and Drug Interactions. 4th Ed. Philadelphia, Williams & Wilkins, 1996.

Fuijimoto, M., et al.: A study into the phenomenon of head-shaking nystagmus: its presence in a dizzy population. J. of Otolaryngology, 22:376–379, 1993.

Solmon, S.D.: Positional nystagmus. Arch. Otolaryngol., 90:58–63, 1969.

Optokinetic Nystagmus (Normal Physiologic Nystagmus Obtained by Watching Moving Targets; Slow Component in Direction Targets are Moving, and Fast Component in Opposite Direction). Abnormal Optokinetic Nystagmus can be seen in the following.

1. Aberrant regeneration of third nerve—absent vertical optokinetic nystagmus, normal horizontal optokinetic nystagmus

2. Internuclear palsies—horizontal targets bring out dissociation of ocular response movements

3. Lesions of optic tract, geniculate body, temporal and occipital lobes show no asymmetry of horizontal optokinetic responses

4. Lesions of parietal lobe give asymmetrical horizontal optokinetic responses

5. Occipital lobe lesions with homonymous hemianopia and asymmetrical horizontal optokinetic responses suggests a mass lesion extending into parietal lobe rather than a vascular lesion

6. Parinaud syndrome—vertical optokinetic nystagmus with targets moving downward enhances the retraction nystagmus seen on attempted upgaze.

7. Parkinsonism (shaking palsy)—vertical optokinetic nystagmus may be reduced

8. See-saw nystagmus—vertical optokinetic nystagmus may be reduced either upward or downward (see p. 167)

9. Test for malingering in "blind" eye or eyes with normal optokinetic responses

Smith, J.L.: Optokinetic Nystagmus: Its Use in Topical Neuro-ophthalmologic Diagnosis. Springfield, Ill., Charles C Thomas, 1963.

Walsh, F.B., and Hoyt, W.F.: Clinical Neuro-ophthalmology. 4th Ed. Baltimore, Williams & Wilkins, 1985.

Syndromes and Diseases Associated with Nystagmus

1. African eye-worm disease

2. Albers-Schonberg syndrome (osteosclerosis fragilis generalisata)

3. Albinism, ocular

4. Anterior spinal artery syndrome

5. Apert syndrome (acrocephalosyndactylism syndrome)

6. Arnold-Chiari syndrome (platybasia syndrome)

7. Arylsulfatase A deficiency syndrome

8. Babinski-Nageotte syndrome (medullary tegmental syndrome)

9. Bacterial endocarditis

10. Bassen-Kornzweig syndrome (abetalipoproteinemia)

11. Behçet syndrome (dermatostomato-ophthalmic syndrome)

12. Behr disease (optic atrophy-ataxia syndrome)

13. Bielschowsky-Lutz-Cogan syndrome (internuclear ophthalmoplegia)

14. Bloch-Sulzberger disease (incontinentia pigmenti)*

15. Blocked nystagmus syndrome (Nystagmus blockage syndrome)

16. Bonnet-Dechaume-Blanc syndrome (neuroretinoangiomatosis syndrome)

17. Botulism

18. Brown-Marie syndrome (hereditary ataxia syndrome)

19. Caisson syndrome (bends)

20. Canavan disease (spongy degeneration of the white matter)

21. Cerebral palsy

22. Cestan-Chenais syndrome (combination of Babinski-Nageotte and Avellis syndrome)

23. Charcot-Marie-Tooth disease (progressive peroneal muscular atrophy)

24. CHARGE syndrome (optic nerve, Coloboma, Heart defects, coAnal atresia, Gu abnormalities, Ear anomalies, Retardation)

25. Chediak-Higashi syndrome (anomalous leukocytic inclusions with constitutional stigmata)

26. Cherry-red spot myoclonus syndrome

27. Chromosome 18, partial deletion (long-arm) syndrome

28. Cockayne syndrome (dwarfism with retinal atrophy and deafness)

29. Cogan syndrome (II) (oculomotor apraxia syndrome)

* 30. Cone dysfunction syndrome (achromatopsia)

31. Costen syndrome (temporomandibular joint syndrome)

32. Craniocervical syndrome (whiplash syndrome)

33. Craniopharyngioma

34. Craniostenosis

35. Creutzfeldt—Jakob syndrome (spastic pseudosclerosis)

36. Crouzon disease (craniofacial dysostosis)

37. Curtius syndrome (ectodermal dysplasia with ocular malformations)

38. Cushing syndrome (II) (angle tumor syndrome)

39. Cytomegalic inclusion disease, congenital

40. Dawson disease (subacute sclerosing panencephalitis)

41. de Lange syndrome (congenital muscular hypertrophy-cerebral syndrome)

42. Diencephalic syndrome (autonomic epilepsy syndrome) (Russell syndrome)

43. Disseminated lupus erythematosus (Kaposi-Libman-Sacks syndrome)

*44. Disseminated sclerosis (multiple sclerosis)

45. Down disease (mongolism, trisomy 21)

46. Drummond syndrome (idiopathic hypercalcemia)

47. Eclampsia and pre-eclampsia

48. Electrical injury

49. Encephalitis, acute

50. Epidermal nevus syndrome (ichthyosis hystrix)

* = most important

51. Epiphysial dysplasia, microcephaly, and nystagmus—autosomal recessive
52. Extreme hydrocephalus syndrome
53. Fanconi-Turler syndrome (familial ataxic diplegia)
54. Forsius-Eriksson syndrome (Aland disease)
55. Francois dyscephalic syndrome
56. Gangliosidosis (generalized gangliosidosis, infantile)
57. General fibrosis syndrome
58. Goltz syndrome (focal dermal hypoplasia syndrome)
59. Gorlin-Chaudhry-Moss syndrome
60. Guillain-Barré syndrome (acute infectious neuritis)
61. Hallervorden-Spatz syndrome (pigmentary degeneration of globus pallidus)
62. Hallgren syndrome (retinitis pigmentosa-deafness-ataxia syndrome)
63. Hand-Schüller-Christian syndrome (histiocytosis X)
64. Hanhart syndrome (recessive keratosis palmoplantaris)
65. Hartnup syndrome (niacin deficiency)
66. Hennebert syndrome (luetic-otitic-nystagmus syndrome)
67. Hermansky-Pudlak syndrome (oculocutaneous albinism and hemorrhagic diathesis)
68. Hurler syndrome (mucopolysaccharidoses I-H)
69. Hypervitaminosis D
70. Hypomelanosis of Ito syndrome (incontinentia pigmenti achronians)
71. Hypothyroidism (cretinism)
72. Hysteria
73. Infantile globoid cell leukodystrophy (Krabbe disease)
74. Infantile neuroaxonal dystrophy
75. Infectious mononucleosis
76. Japanese river fever (typhus)
77. Jeune disease (asphyxiating thoracic dystrophy)
78. Kernicterus—high levels of bilirubin in the blood
79. Klippel-Feil syndrome (congenital brevicollis)
80. Koerber-Salus Elschnig syndrome (sylvian aqueduct syndrome)
81. Kohn-Romano syndrome (blepharophimosis, ptosis, epicanthus inversus, telecanthus) (Blepharophimosis syndrome)
82. Kugelberg-Welander syndrome (progressive proximal muscle atrophy)
83. Laurence-Moon-Bardet-Biedl syndrome (retinitis pigmentosa-polydactyly-adiposogenital syndrome)*
84. Leber's congenital amaurosis syndrome (retinal aplasia)
85. Leigh disease (subacute necrotizing encephalomyelopathy)
86. Lenoble-Aubineau syndrome (nystagmus-myoclonia syndrome)
87. Lermoyez syndrome (form of Meniere's disease)
88. Linear nevus sebaceous of Jadassohn

89. Lockjaw (tetanus)
90. Louis-Bar syndrome (ataxia-telangiectasia syndrome)
91. Lowe disease (oculocerebrorenal syndrome)
92. Malignant hyperthermia syndrome
93. Maple syrup urine disease
94. Marfan syndrome (acrachnadactyly-dystrophia mesodermalis congenita)
95. Marinesco-Sjögren syndrome (congenital spirocerebellar ataxia-congenital cataract-oligophrenia syndrome)
96. Meniere syndrome (vertigo, tinnitus, nystagmus)
97. Meningococcemia (meningitis)
98. Mietens syndrome
99. Morning glory syndrome (optic nervie dysplasi, encephalocele)
100. Moyamoya disease (multiple progressive intracranial arterial occlusion)
101. Multiple lentigines syndrome (Leopard syndrome)
102. Naegeli syndrome (melanophoric nevus syndrome)
*103. Nystagmus, congenital
104. O'Donnell-Pappas syndrome (dominant foveal hypoplasia and presenile cataracts)* Optic nerve hypoplasia, coloboma
106. Papillon-Lefèvre syndrome (hyperkeratosis palmoplantaris with periodontosis)
107. Parkinson disease
108. Passow syndrome (status dysraphicus syndrome)
109. Pelizaeus-Merzbacher disease (aplasia axialis extracorticalis congenita)—x-linked
110. Photomyoclonus, diabetes mellitus, deafness, neuropathy, and cerebellar dysfunction—autosomal dominant
111. Poliomyelitis
112. Posthypoxic encephalopathy syndrome
113. Pyle disease (familial metaphyseal dysplasia)
114. Quincke disease (angioedema)
115. Rubella, congenital
116. Reimann syndrome (hyperviscosity syndrome)
117. Relapsing polychondritis
118. Scaphocephaly syndrome
119. Schilder disease (encephalitis periaxialis diffusa)
120. Seckel syndrome (bird-headed dwarf syndrome)*
121. Septo-optic dysplasia (de Morsier syndrome)
122. Smith-Lemli-Opitz syndrome (cerebrohepatorenal syndrome)
123. Sorsby syndrome (hereditary macular coloboma syndrome)
124. Spastic paraplegia—x-linked
125. Split hand with congenital nystagmus, fundal changes, cataracts—autosomal dominant
126. Stannus cerebellar syndrome (riboflavin deficiency)

* = most important

127. Subclavian steal syndrome
128. Tay-Sachs disease (familial amaurotic idiocy)
129. Traumatic encephalopathy syndrome (punch drunk syndrome)
130. Tremor, nystagmus, and duodenal ulcer—autosomal dominant
131. Tuomaala-Haapanen syndrome (similar to pseudohypoparathyroidism)
132. Vermis syndrome
133. Vertebral basilar artery syndrome
134. von Economo syndrome (encephalitis lethargica)
135. von Reuss syndrome (galactosemic syndrome)
136. Wagner syndrome (hyaloideoretinal degeneration)
137. Wallenberg syndrome (lateral bulbar syndrome)
138. Werner syndrome (progeria of adults)
139. Wernicke syndrome (superior hemorrhagic polioencephalopathic syndrome)
140. Wildervanck syndrome (cervico-oculoacoustic syndrome)
141. Wilson disease (hepatolenticular degeneration)
142. Wolf syndrome (monosomy partial syndrome)
143. Zellweger syndrome (cerebrohepatorenal syndrome of Zellweger)

McKusick, V.A.: Mendelian Inheritance in Man. 9th Ed. Baltimore, Johns Hopkins University Press, 1994.

Roy, F.H.: Ocular Syndromes and Systemic Diseases. 2nd Ed. Philadelphia, W.B. Saunders, 1989.

Oculogyric Crisis (Spasmodic and Involuntary Deviation of Eyes, Usually Upward, Lasting from a Few Minutes to Several Hours)

1. Cerebellar disease
2. Drugs, including:

acetophenazine	desipramine	mesoridazine
alprazolam	diazepam	methdilazine
alseroxylon	diethazine	methotrimeprazine
amantadine	doxepin	metoclopramide
amitriptyline	droperidol	metronidazole
amodiaquine	ethopropazine	midazolam
butaperazine	fluphenazine	nitrazepam
carbamazepine	flurazepam	nortriptyline
carphenazine	halazepam	oxazepam
chlordiazepoxide	haloperidol	pemoline
chloroquine	hydroxychloroquine	pentazocine
chlorpromazine	imipramine	perazine
chlorprothixene	influenza virus vaccine	pericyazine
cisplatin	levodopa	perphenazine
clonazepam	lithium carbonate	phencyclidine
clorazepate	lorazepam	pimozide
deserpidine	loxapine	piperacetazine

prazepam	rescinnamine	thioridazine
prochlorperazine	reserpine	thiothixene
promazine	syrosingopine	triazolam
promethazine	temazepam	trifluoperazine
propiomazine	thiethylperazine	trifluperidol
protriptyline	thiopropazate	triflupromazine
rauwolfia serpentina	thioproperazine	trimeprazine

3. Late manifestations of encephalitis

4. Lesions of fourth ventricle and cerebellum, especially lesions of the flocculus

5. Multiple sclerosis (disseminated sclerosis)

6. Parkinsonism syndrome (shaking palsy)

7. Syphilis (acquired lues)

8. Trauma

Burstein, A.H., and Fullerton, T.: Oculogyric crisis possibly related to pentazocine. Ann. of Pharmacotherapy, 27:874–876, 1993.

Fraunfelder, F.T.: Drug-Induced Ocular Side Effects and Drug Interactions. Ed. Philadelphia, Williams & Wilkins, 1996.

Ocular Bobbing (Both Globes Move Synchronously in Vertical Plane by Spontaneously and Intermittently Dipping Downward Through an Arc of a Few Millimeters and Then Return to Primary Position; Reverse Ocular Bobbing Has Also Been Described). Ocular bobbing differs from vertical nystagmus by virtue of absence of a fast and a slow component in movements; it is due to advanced pontine disease.

1. Acute organophosphate poisoning (Diazinon)

2. Associated with palatal myoclonus

*3. Encephalitis

4. Fibrocartilaginous embolism to the anterior spinal artery

5. Hypertensive pontine hemorrhage

6. Leigh encephalopathy (Gangliosidosis GM type 3)

7. Locked-in syndrome

8. Phenothiazine and benzodiazepine poisoning (combined) (reverse)

9. Ruptured giant distal posterior inferior cerebellar artery aneurysm

10. Thrombosis of basilar, middle cerebral, or vertebral arteries with posterior fossa infarction

Hata, S., et al.: Atypical ocular bobbing in acute organophosphate poisoning. Arch. Neurol., 43:185–186, 1986.

Kase, C.S., et al.: Medial medullary infarction from fibrocartilaginous embolism to the anterior spinal artery. Stroke, 14:413–418, 1983.

Larmoude, P., et al.: Ocular bobbing: Abnormal eye movement. Ophthalmology, 187:161–165, 1983.

Lennox, G.: Reverse ocular bobbing due to combined phenothiazine and bezodiazepine poisoning. J. of Neurology, Neurosurgery & Psychiatry, 56:1136–1137, 1993.

Osenbach, R.K., et al.: Ocular bobbing with ruptured giant distal posterior interior cerebellar artery aneurysm. Surg. Neurol., 25:149–152, 1986.

* = most important

Tijssen, C.C., and Terbruggen, J.P.: Locked-in syndrome associated with ocular bobbing. Acta. Neurol. Scand., 73:444–446, 1986.

Zegers, B.D., et al.: Ocular bobbing and myoclonus in central pontine myelinolysis. J. Neurol. Neurosurg. Psychiatry, 46:564–565, 1983.

Paralysis of Third Nerve (Oculomotor Nerve) (Ptosis; Inability to Rotate Eye Upward, or Inward; A Dilated Unreactive Pupil [Iridoplegia] and Paralysis of Accommodation [Cycloplegia])

1. Intracerebral

   A. Lesion of red nucleus (Benedikt syndrome)—homolateral oculomotor paralysis with contralateral intention tremor

   B. Nuclear types—pareses of a single or a few extraocular muscles supplied by the oculomotor nerve in one or both eyes; there may or may not be pupillary disturbances (mydriasis, sluggish pupillary reaction) and paresis of accommodation; in tumors within or near the midbrain (pinealomas), there is a combination of isolated muscle pareses with vertical gaze palsy, possibly a disturbance of convergence, and nystagmus retractorius (Parinaud syndrome, Sylvian aqueduct syndrome, pineal syndrome); includes Axenfeld-Schurenberg syndrome (cyclic oculomotor paralysis), Bruns syndrome (postural change syndrome), Claude syndrome (inferior nucleus ruber syndrome), congenital vertical retraction syndrome, and Nothnagel syndrome (ophthalmoplegia-cerebellar ataxia syndrome)

   C. Occlusion of basilar artery—due to emboli especially but also to hemorrhage or aneurysm

   D. Recurrent third nerve palsy secondary to vascular spasm of migraine

   E. Syndrome of cerebral peduncle (Weber syndrome)—homolateral oculomotor paralysis and cross-hemiplegia

   F. Tumors

2. Intracranial

   A. Amebic dysentery

   B. Aneurysm rupture at base of brain—third nerve paralysis, pain around the face (fifth nerve), and headache

   C. Botulism

   D. Chickenpox

   E. Craniopharyngioma

   F. Dengue fever

   G. Devic syndrome (optical myelitis)

   H. Diphtheria

   I. Encephalitis, acute

   J. Hepatic failure

   K. Hepatitis

   L. Influenza

   M. Lockjaw (tetanus)

   N. Lymphoma

O. Malaria

P. Measles immunization

Q. Meningococcal meningitis

R. Multiple sclerosis (disseminated sclerosis)

S. Ophthalmic migraine

T. Periarteritis nodosa

U. Poliomyelitis

V. Polyneuritis because of toxins such as alcohol, lead, arsenic, and carbon monoxide; dinitrophenol or carbon disulfide poisoning; or diabetes mellitus, herpes zoster, or mumps

W. Rabies

X. Relapsing polychondritis

Y. Smallpox vaccination

Z. Subdural hematoma

AA. Syphilis (acquired lues)

BB. Temporal arteritis syndrome (Hutchinson-Horton-Magrath-Brown syndrome)

CC. Tuberculosis

3. Lesions affecting exit from cranial cavity

A. Cavernous sinus syndrome—paralysis of third, fourth, and sixth nerves with proptosis

   (1) Aneurysm (arteriovenous fistula syndrome)

   (2) Carotid-cavernous fistula

   (3) Cavernous sinus thrombosis

   (4) Extension from lateral sinus thrombosis

   (5) Extension of nasopharyngeal tumor

   (6) Pituitary adenoma—lateral extension

   (7) Tolosa-Hunt syndrome (painful ophthalmoplegia)

B. Superior orbital fissure syndrome—same as for cavernous sinus syndrome except exophthalmos is less likely to occur and optic nerve involvement and miotic pupil are more likely

   (1) Aneurysm of internal carotid artery syndrome (foramen lacerum syndrome)

   (2) Occlusion of superior ophthalmic vein

   (3) Skull fractures or hemorrhage

   (4) Sphenoid sinus suppuration (sphenocavernous syndrome)

   (5) Temporal syndrome (Gradenigo syndrome)

   (6) Tumors, such as sphenoid ridge meningioma (Rochon-Duvigneaud syndrome), nasopharyngeal tumor, metastatic carcinoma, rhabdomyosarcoma, chordoma, and sarcoma

C. Orbital apex—involvement of III, IV, VI, first division of V cranial nerves, and optic nerve proptosis is common

4. Other

    A. Alber-Schönberg syndrome (marble bone disease, osteopetrosis)

    B. Associated with aspirin poisoning

    C. Congenital

    D. Hodgkin disease

    E. Lupus erythematosus (Kaposi-Libman-Sacks syndrome)

    F. Myasthenia gravis (masquerade)

    G. Passow syndrome (status dysraphicus syndrome)

    H. Porphyria cutanea tarda

    I. Sarcoid (Schaumann syndrome)

Galetta, S.L., et al.: Spontaneous remission of third-nerve palsy in meningeal lymphoma. Annals of Neurology., 32:100–102, 1992.

Getenet J.C., et al.: Isolated bilateral third nerve palsy caused by a mesencephalic hematoma. Neurology, 44:981–982, 1994.

Ing, E.B., et al.: Oculomotor nerve palsies in children. J. Pediat. Ophthal. Strabismus, 29:331–336, 1992.

Kirkali, P., et al.: Third nerve palsy and internuclear ophthalmoplegia in periarteritis nodosa. J. of Pediatric Ophthal. and Strabismus, 28:45–46, 1991.

Patel, C.K., et al.: Congenital third nerve palsy associated with mid-trimester amniocentesis. Brit. J. Ophthal., 77:530–533, 1993.

Purvin, V.: Third cranial nerve palsy. In: Diagnostic Problems in Clinical Ophthalmology. Margo, C.E. (ed) Philadelphia, Saunders, 678, 1994.

Roy, F.H.: Ocular Syndromes and Systemic Diseases. 2nd Ed. Philadelphia, W.B. Saunders, 1989.

Paralysis of Third Nerve

	Intracerebral							Intracranial					Cranial Cavity Exit					
	Benedikt Syndrome	Weber Syndrome	Basilar Artery Emboli	Migraine	Tumors as Pinealoma	Parinaud Syndrome	Aneurysm Rupture Base Brain	Neuritis as Diabetes Mellitus	Poliomyelitis	Meningitis	Multiple Sclerosis	Temporal Arteritis	Post Coronary Artery Aneurysm	Post Viral	Cavernous Sinus Syndrome as Carotid-Cavernous Fistula	Superior Orbital Fissure Syndrome as Sphenoid Ridge Meningioma	Orbital Apex Syndrome	Isolated
History																		
1. All age groups				U									U					U
2. Children, 2 to 8 years				S										U				
3. Common—seventh decade	S	S						S				U				U		
4. Congenital							S											
5. Familial				U														
6. Head trauma	U	U	U				U								S		S	S
7. Hemorrhage/neoplasm/inflammation	U	U	U		U	U	U						U	U	U	U	U	
8. Unilateral	U	U	U	U			U						U	U				U
9. Unilateral transient visual loss				U														
10. Usually more than 40 years	U	U	U				U	U				U				U		
11. Viral infection									U					U				
12. Visual loss			S				S			S		S				S		R
Physical Findings																		
1. Acute decreased intraocular pressure				U								S						
2. Anterior ischemic optic neuropathy								S				S						
3. Cataract								U										
4. Central retinal artery occlusion												U						
5. Central retinal vein occlusion					S													
6. Convergence abnormal	U				U	U	S											U
7. Corneal anesthesia												S			S	S	S	
8. Corneal opacity															S			
9. Corneal ulcer															S			
10. Cotton wool exudates								U										
11. Disk hemorrhage													U					
12. Elevation and depression of eyes limited	U		U				S											R
13. Fixed/dilated pupil	U	U	U	S	U	U	S	S				U	U	U	U	U	U	U
14. Glaucoma												S						
15. Hard exudates								U										
16. Horner syndrome															S	S		R
17. Keratitis														U	S			
18. Lid edema															U	U		
19. Macular edema								S		S								
20. Microaneurysms of retina								S										
21. Miosis															R			
22. Nystagmus		S									U							
23. Ocular bruit															U			

Paralysis of Third Nerve *Continued*

	Intracerebral							Intracranial							Cranial Cavity Exit			
	Benedikt Syndrome	Weber Syndrome	Basilar Artery Emboli	Migraine	Tumors as Pinealoma	Parinaud Syndrome	Aneurysm Rupture Base Brain	Neuritis as Diabetes Mellitus	Poliomyelitis	Meningitis	Multiple Sclerosis	Temporal Arteritis	Post Coronary Artery Aneurysm	Post Viral	Cavernous Sinus Syndrome as Carotid-Cavernous Fistula	Superior Orbital Fissure Syndrome as Sphenoid Ridge Meningioma	Orbital Apex Syndrome	Isolated
Physical Findings																		
24. Ocular pain			U				U					S	S	S	U	U		S
25. Optic nerve atrophy								S				U	R	R	S	S	S	
26. Optic neuritis									S	S	U				S		S	
27. Orbital hemorrhage							R									S		S
28. Papilledema						U	R	S		R					S	U	S	
29. Proptosis															U	S	S	
30. Ptosis		U									U	S	U				S	
31. Retinal hemorrhage							S	U		R					S			
32. Uveitis										U					S			
33. Visual field defects					S	S					S					S		
34. Vitreous hemorrhage							S	S										
Laboratory Data																		
1. Cerebrospinal fluid abnormal				S			S							S				
2. Computed tomographic scan/MRI	U	U	U		U	U	U				U				U	U	U	
3. Elevated blood sugar								U										
4. Erythrocyte sedimentation rate elevated												U						
5. Red blood cell count, white blood cell count, hemoglobin, and hematocrit									U	U			U	U				
6. Selective cerebral angiography	S	S	U			S	U									U		

R = rarely; S = sometimes; and U = usually.

Paralysis of Fourth Nerve (Trochlear Nerve) (Produces Palsy of Superior Oblique Muscle Resulting in Limitation of Downward Movement of Eye When It Is in Adducted Position—Frequently Associated Third Cranial Nerve Palsy)

1. Intracerebral

    A. Thrombosis of nutrient vessels, including median penetrating branch of basilar artery to fourth nucleus

    B. Hemorrhage in the roof of the midbrain

    C. Aneurysm, including direct involvement by posterior cerebral and superior cerebellar arteries

    D. Tumors (rare if isolated 4th palsy)

        (1) Primary

            a. Gliomas, such as astrocytomas, ependymomas, and medulloblastomas

            b. Other primary tumors, including meningiomas, pinealomas, craniopharyngiomas, and hemangiomas

    E. Metastatic lesions, such as those from the nasopharynx, rhabdomyosarcomas, and neuroblastomas

    F. Neonatal hypoxia

    G. Nuclear type—trochlear paresis combined with a homolateral oculomotor paresis, occasionally in association with vertical gaze palsies, convergence spasm or convergence palsy, and pupillary disturbances seen in tumors of the roof of the midbrain or pinealomas (pineal syndrome)

    H. Claude syndrome (inferior nucleus ruber syndrome)

    I. Passow syndrome (syringomyelia)

    J. Inflammatory lesions, such as meningoencephalitis, cerebellitis, and abscess

2. Intracranial

    A. Aneurysms, such as that of the posterior communicating artery or foramen lacerum syndrome (aneurysm of internal carotid artery syndrome)

    B. Hematomas, traumatic

    C. Hydrocephalus

    D. Meningitis, encephalitis, polyneuritis—diabetes mellitus, herpes zoster, multiple sclerosis, myasthenia gravis, chickenpox, diphtheria, hydrophobia, Gradenigo syndrome, influenza, malaria, poliomyelitis

    E. Trauma

    F. Tumors, including cerebellopontine angle tumor

3. Lesions affecting exit from cranial cavity

    A. Cavernous sinus syndrome (Foix syndrome)

    B. Superior orbital fissure syndrome (Rochon-Duvigneaud syndrome)

    C. Orbital apex syndrome (Rollet syndrome)

4. Orbital lesions

    A. Fracture of superior orbital rim

    B. Sinusitis

    C. Operations on the frontal sinus in which there is trochlear displacement

   D. Trochlear disturbance, such as in Paget disease or hypertrophic arthritis

   E. Adherence syndrome—adhesions between the superior rectus and superior oblique muscles

   F. Abnormal insertion of superior oblique muscle or abnormal fascial attachments

   G. Rochon-Duvigneaud syndrome (superior orbital fissure syndrome)

   H. Idiopathic

Celli, P., et al.: Neurinoma of third, fourth, and sixth cranial nerves; a survey and report of a new fourth nerve case. Surgical Neurology, 38:216–224, 1992.

Elliot, D., et al.: Fourth nerve paresis and ipsilateral relative afferent pupillary defect without visual sensory disturbance. A sign of contralateral dorsal midbrain disease. J. of Clinical Neuro-Ophthalmology, 11:169–172, 1991.

Keane, J.R.: Fourth nerve palsy: historical review and study of inpatients. Neurology, 43:2439–2433, 1993.

Peatfield, R.C.: Recurrent VI nerve palsy in cluster headache. Headache, 25:325–327, 1985.

Roy, F.H.: Ocular Syndromes and Systemic Diseases. 2nd Ed. Philadelphia, W.B. Saunders, 1989.

Paralysis of Fourth Nerve

	Intracerebral			Intracranial			Exit from Cranial Cavity		Orbital		
	Thrombosis Basilar Artery	Aneurysm Posterior Cerebral/Superior Cerebellar Arteries	Tumor as Pinealoma	Aneurysm Posterior Communicating Artery	Tumor as Cerebellopontine Angle	Polyneuritis	Cavernous Sinus Syndrome	Orbital Apex Syndrome	Superior Orbital Rim Fracture	Isolated	Isolated Congenital
History											
1. Bacterial infection							S	S			
2. Hemorrhagic, neoplasic, or inflammation cause						U	U	U			
3. Metabolic disorder											
4. More than 40 years						U					
5. Rare incidence	R	R	R	R	R	S	R	S	R	U	U
6. Bilateral										S	
Physical Findings											
1. Conjunctival hemorrhage							S		S		
2. Convergence insufficiency			U		R						
3. Cotton-wool spots						S					
4. Fixed and dilated pupil	S			U		R		U		R	R
5. Keratitis							S				
6. Limitation of adduction	S	U	S	U	R	S			S	R	R
7. Limitation of downward/upward gaze	S	U	U	U	R	S		S	U	R	R
8. Ocular/periocular pain	U	R		S		S	U	U	S	R	R
9. Ophthalmoplegia, third and sixth nerves	U	S		S			S	S	S	R	R
10. Optic nerve atrophy						R	S	S	S		
11. Optic neuritis								S	S		
12. Palsy—fifth, sixth, seventh, eighth, ninth, and tenth cranial nerves					U						
13. Papilledema							S	S	S		
14. Progressive proptosis											
15. Ptosis				U				U	S		
16. Pupil afferent defect	S		U					U	S		
17. Retinal hemorrhages							S		S		
18. Retinal neovascularization/microaneurysms						U					
19. Subdural/orbital bleeding									U		
20. Temporary homonymus field defect		S									
Laboratory Data											
1. Blood sugar elevated/SED rates						U					
2. Cerebral arteriography	U	U		U			U				
3. Cerebrospinal fluid abnormal			U	U					S		
4. Computed tomographic brain scan	U	U	U	U	U		U	U	U	S	
5. Magnetic resonance imaging		S								S	
6. Orbit roentgenogram									U		
7. Skull roentgenogram	U	S	S		U		S	U	S		
8. Visual field test		S									

R = rarely; S = sometimes; and U = usually.

Pseudoabducens Palsy

1. Accommodative spasm
2. Blowout fracture (medial rectus entrapment)
3. Cross fixation (congenital esotropia)
4. Duane syndrome (retraction syndrome)
5. Fibrosis of medial rectus
6. Horizontal gaze palsy (bilateral)—with or without contraction
7. Lack of effort involved in abducting a habitually adducted eye—patch on other eye differentiates from abducens palsy
8. Myasthenia gravis
9. Myositis
10. Orbital cellulitis (abscess)
11. Overambitious (large) resection of medial rectus
12. Thyroid myopathy (Graves disease, hyperthyroidism)
13. Unwillingness to co-operate—doll's head phenomenon (sudden passive turning of head) differentiates from abducens palsy

Beyer-Machule, C., and von Noorden, G.K.: Atlas of Ophthalmic Surgery. Vol. 1: Lids, Orbits, Extraocular Muscles. New York, Thieme Med. Pub., 1984.

Goldhammer, Y.: Pseudopalsy of the abducens nerve. In: Neuro-Ophthalmology Update. J.L. Smith (ed), New York. Masson Pub. 1977.

Paralysis of Sixth Nerve (Abducens Palsy) (Produces Palsy of Lateral Rectus Muscle with Esotropia Increasing When Eye Is Moved Laterally). The course of the sixth nerve makes it more vulnerable than other cranial nerves to injury

1. Intracerebral
    A. Foville syndrome (Foville peduncular syndrome)
    B. Gaucher disease (cerebroside lipidosis)
    C. Hydrocephalus
    D. Inflammatory lesions, such as meningoencephalitis, cerebellitis, and abscess
    E. Lateral ventricular cyst
    F. Leukemia
    G. Millard-Gubler syndrome (abducens-facial hemiplegia alternans)
    H. Mycoplasma pneumoniae
    I. Nuclear aplasia—autosomal dominant
    J. Platybasia (cerebellomedullary malformation syndrome)
    K. Spontaneous subdural hematoma
    L. Thrombosis or aneurysm of nutrient vessels to sixth nucleus—basilar artery
    M. Tumors—intracranial, pontine glioma, or metastatic tumor from breast, thyroid glands, or nasopharynx
        (1) Primary
            a. Gliomas, such as astrocytomas, ependymomas, and medulloblastomas

      b. Other primary tumors, including meningiomas, pinealomas, craniopharyngiomas, and hemangiomas

    (2) Metastatic lesions, such as those from the nasopharynx, rhabdomyosarcomas, and neuroblastomas

  N. Wernicke encephalopathy—thiamine deficiency in alcoholics with sixth nerve palsy, paresis of horizontal conjugate gaze, nystagmus, ataxia, and Korsakoff psychosis

2. Intracranial

  A. Carotid artery aneurysm (foramen lacerum syndrome)

  B. Cerebellopontine angle tumor, such as acoustic neuroma, producing unilateral deafness, facial paralysis, diplopia, and papilledema

  C. Chickenpox

  D. Coccidioidomycosis

  E. Congenital absence of sixth nerve

  F. Cushing syndrome (II) (angle tumor syndrome)

  G. Dandy-Walker syndrome (artresia of the foramen magendie)

  H. Diphtheria

  I. Gradenigo syndrome—osteitis of petrous tip of pyramid following homolateral mastoid or middle ear infection; facial pain (fifth nerve involvement)

  J. Greig syndrome (ocular hypertelorism syndrome)

  K. Hydrophobia (rabies)

  L. Hydrocephalus (decreased intracranial pressure)

  M. Increased intracranial pressure

  N. Malaria

  O. Massive pituitary adenoma

  P. Measles

  Q. Meningitis

  R. Mobius syndrome (congenital paralysis of 6th and 7th nerves)

  S. Neuritis because of diseases such as diabetes mellitus, herpes zoster, poliomyelitis, lead or arsenic poisoning, multiple sclerosis, syphilis, brucellosis

  T. Ophthalmoplegic migraine syndrome

  U. Osteosarcoma

  V. Passow syndrome (status dysraphicus syndrome)

  W. Pseudotumor cerebri (Symonds syndrome)

  X. Raymond syndrome (pontine syndrome)

  Y. Relapsing polychondritis

  Z. Skeletal dysplasia (mental retardation, abducens palsy)—x-linked

  AA. Skull fractures—usually crush injury

  BB. Spontaneous dissection of the internal carotid artery

  CC. Subdural hematoma

  DD. Trichinellosis

    EE. Tumor extension as chordoma

    FF. Vascular lesions, because of congenital aneurysm, arteriovenous fistulas, diabetes, hypertension

    GG. Water-soluble contrast myelography

3. Lesions affecting exit of sixth nerve from cranial cavity

    A. Cavernous sinus syndrome (Foix syndrome)

    B. Le Fort I maxillary osteotomy

    C. Optic nerve sheath fenestration

    D. Orbital apex lesion

    E. Percutaneous thermal ablation of trigeminal nerve rootlet

    F. Sphenocavernous syndrome

    G. Sphenopalatine fossa lesion—loss of tearing and paresis of second division of fifth nerve, most frequently because of malignant tumor

    H. Superior orbital fissure syndrome

    I. Tolosa-Hunt syndrome (painful ophthalmoplegia)

    J. Transient in newborns

4. Other

    A. Cluster headache

    B. Cretinism (hypothyroid goiter)

    C. Duane syndrome (retraction syndrome)

    D. Engelmann syndrome (hereditary multiple diaphyseal sclerosis)

    E. Following lumbar puncture, lumbar anesthesia, or Pantopaque injection for myelography

    F. Kahler disease (multiple myeloma)

    G. Lupus erythematosus (Kaposi-Libman-Sacks syndrome)

    H. Myasthenia gravis

    I. Optic nerve sheath fenestration (rare)

    J. Preeclampsia

    K. Sarcoidosis

    L. Secondary to immunization or viral illness

    M. Toxic substances, such as arsenic, carbon tetrachloride, dichloroacetylene, Dilantin, gold salts, isoniazide, nitrofuran, thalidomide, trichloroethylene, furaltadone (Altafur), lithium

Paralysis of Sixth Nerve

	Intracerebral					Intracranial					Cranial Cavity Exit					
	Basilar Artery Aneurysm	Wernicke Encephalopathy	Millard-Grubler Syndrome	Foville Syndrome	Cerebellomedullary Malformation Syndrome	Meningitis	Carotid Artery Aneurysm	Gradenigo Syndrome	Cerebellopontine Angle Tumor as Acoustic Neuroma	Neuritis as Diabetes Mellitus	Myasthenia Gravis	Cavernous Sinus Syndrome	Superior Orbital Fissure Syndrome	Orbital Apex Syndrome	Isolated	Pseudo Tumor Cerebai
History																
1. Bilateral					U											S
2. Children								U							U	S
3. Common in alcoholics		U														
4. Common—20 to 40 years												U				S
5. Common—more than 40 years	U		U	U						U						R
6. Common—more than 60 years	U						U							U	R	
7. Extradural abscess of petrous portion temporal bone								U								
8. Lack of vitamin B$_1$ (thiamine)		U														
9. More in females												U				U
10. More in males							U									
11. Pain, periocular												U	S	S		
12. Severe pain in ophthalmic branch of fifth cranial nerve								U								
13. Vascular/infectious/tumor at the pons base			U													
14. Vascular/inflammatory/tumor in cranial cavity												U	U	U		
15. Vascular/thrombosis/tumor of pyramidal tract				U												
16. Vestibular nerve tumor									U							
Physical Findings																
1. Anesthesia of face				U												
2. Associated hydrocephalus	S				S				S							U
3. Blepharitis		S														
4. Cataract										U						
5. Central scotoma		S														S
6. Conjunctivitis		S				U										
7. Cortical blindness						S										
8. Cotton-wool spots										U						
9. Deviation of eyes to the side opposite lesion and inability to move toward side lesion when unilateral			U													
10. Esotropia	U	S	U	U	S	S	S	S	S	S	S	U	U	U	U	
11. Hard exudates										S						
12. Involvement—other cranial nerves	S		U	U					U	U	S	R	U	U	U	S
13. Keratitis					U	U							S			
14. Lacrimation								U								
15. Nystagmus		S				S			S							
16. Ophthalmoplegia		S											S			

Paralysis of Sixth Nerve *Continued*

	Intracerebral						Intracranial					Cranial Cavity Exit				
	Basilar Artery Aneurysm	Wernicke Encephalopathy	Millard-Grubler Syndrome	Foville Syndrome	Cerebellomedullary Malformation Syndrome	Meningitis	Carotid Artery Aneurysm	Gradenigo Syndrome	Cerebellopontine Angle Tumor as Acoustic Neuroma	Neuritis as Diabetes Mellitus	Myasthenia Gravis	Cavernous Sinus Syndrome	Superior Orbital Fissure Syndrome	Orbital Apex Syndrome	Isolated	Pseudo Tumor Cerebri
Physical Findings																
17. Optic nerve atrophy		S					U			R		S	S	S		S
18. Optic neuritis		S				S	S	R					S			
19. Papilledema		S			U		S		S				U	S		U
20. Paralysis lateral conjugate gaze			U													
21. Ptosis		S										U		U		
22. Pupillary afferent defects		S											U	U		S
23. Pupillary paralysis		S														
24. Reduced corneal sensitivity								S								
25. Retinal hemorrhages		S								S						
26. Retinal microaneurysms										U						
27. Retinal neovascularization										U						
28. Uveitis							U									
29. Vertical nystagmus in upgaze and downgaze					U											
30. Visual field defects							U					S	S	S		U
Laboratory Data																
1. Cerebral arteriography												U	S			
2. Cerebrospinal fluid abnormalities			U	U												U
3. Computed tomographic scan	U		U	U			U	U	U			U	U	U		U
4. Blood sugar (glycemia)										U						
5. MRI	U		U	U	U		U	U	U			U	U			U
6. Red blood cell count, white blood cell count, hemoglobin, and hematocrit						U					U					
7. Tensilon test			U	U							U					
8. Twenty-four-hour urine—thiamine		U														
9. Ultrasonography (oculorbital)													U	U		

R = rarely; S = sometimes; and U = usually.

Paralysis of Third, Fourth, and Sixth Cranial Nerves

	Cavernous Sinus Thrombosis	Pituitary Adenoma	Aneurysm	Carotid-Cavernous Fistula	Nasopharyngeal Tumor	Lateral Sinus Thrombosis	Skull Fracture	Tumor as Sphenoid Ridge Meningioma	Superior Ophthalmic Vein Occlusion	Orbital Mass
History										
1. Common during fourth to seventh decades		U	S	S	U			U		
2. Common in females				S					U	
3. Common in males					U		S			
4. Congenital			S	R						S
5. Following head trauma	R		S	U			U			
6. Infectious etiology (septic thrombus)	U								U	S
7. Ocular pain			S	S		U				S
8. Unilateral	U		U	S		U			U	U
9. Visual loss		S	S	R		S				S
Physical Findings										
1. Anisocoria	U		U						U	
2. Central retinal vein occlusion			S							
3. Corneal ulcer	S		S							S
4. Choroidal folds	S			S			S			S
5. Dilated conjunctival vessels	S			U			S			S
6. Dilation of episcleral veins	U			U					S	
7. Facial nerve involvement							U			
8. Glaucomatous cupping	S			S						
9. Hyperopia								S		
10. Increased intraocular pressure	S			U						S
11. Infections face/nose/forehead									U	
12. Ipsilateral horizontal gaze paresis						U				
13. Ischemic neuritis	S								S	
14. Keratopathy	U							U		
15. Leakage of blood/spinal fluid from external ear canal							U			
16. Lid edema	U					U				S
17. Mastoid ecchymosis (Battle sign)							U			
18. Miosis		S								
19. Nasolacrimal obstruction						U	S			
20. Ocular bruit				U						
21. Ocular hypotony		S								
22. Optic nerve atrophy		S	S			S		S		
23. Orbital hemorrhage			R			R				S
24. Papilledema	S	R	R				S	S		S
25. Pulsating exophthalmos				U						
26. Pupil, afferent defect	U			U				U	U	S
27. Proptosis	U	S		S		U		S		U
28. Ptosis	S	S								S
29. Retinal hemorrhages	S			S			S		S	
30. Trigeminal aesthesia		S				U				
31. Visual field defects		U	S					S	U	

Paralysis of Third, Fourth, and Sixth Cranial Nerves *Continued*

	Cavernous Sinus Thrombosis	Pituitary Adenoma	Aneurysm	Carotid-Cavernous Fistula	Nasopharyngeal Tumor	Lateral Sinus Thrombosis	Skull Fracture	Tumor as Sphenoid Ridge Meningioma	Superior Ophthalmic Vein Occlusion	Orbital Mass
Laboratory Data										
1. Arteriography, cerebral			U	U			S			
2. Biopsy/culture of paranasal sinus	S									S
3. Biopsy nasopharynx lesions					U					
4. Blood culture	U								S	S
5. Cerebrospinal fluid abnormal			U							
6. Computed tomographic orbit scan				U						U
7. Culture lesions face/nose/forehead	U								U	S
8. Paranasal sinus roentgenogram	U				S					S
9. Pituitary panel—serum prolactin, growth hormone, adrenocorticotropic hormone, follicle-stimulating hormone, luteinizing hormone, thyroid-stimulating hormone		S								
10. Selective catheterization of external carotid arteries					U					
11. Selective cerebral angiography			U	U						
12. Visual field test		U						S		

R = rarely; S = sometimes; and U = usually.

Barry-Kinsella, C., et al.: Sixth nerve palsy: an unusual manifestation of preeclampsia. Obstetrics & Gynecology, 83:849–851, 1994.

Glaser, J.S.: Neuro-Ophthalmology. 2nd Ed. Philadelphia, J.B. Lippincott Co., 1989.

McKusick, V.A.: Mendelian Inheritance in Man. 9th Ed. Baltimore, Johns Hopkins University Press, 1994.

O'Boyle, J.E., et al.: Sixth nerve palsy as the initial presenting sign of metastatic prostate cancer. A case report and review of literature. J. of Clinical Neuro-Ophthalmology, 12:149–153, 1992.

Roy, F.H.: Ocular Syndromes and Systemic Diseases. 2nd Ed. Philadelphia, W.B. Saunders, 1989.

Rucker, C.W.: The causes of paralysis of the third, fourth, and sixth cranial nerves. Am. J. Ophthalmol., 61:1293, 1966.

Sachs R., et al.: Sixth nerve palsy as the initial manifestation of sarcoidosis. Am J. Ophthalmol., 110: 438–440, 1990.

Smith, K.H., et al.: Combined third and sixth nerve paresis following optic nerve sheath fenestration. J. of Clinical Neuro-Ophthalmology, 12:85–87, 1992.

Acute Ophthalmoplegia (acute onset of extraocular muscle palsy)

1. Infranuclear

    A. Aneurysm of internal carotid artery or circle of Willis

    B. Trauma

        (1) Orbital fracture

        (2) Orbital hematoma

    C. Orbital cellulitis secondary to acute paranasal sinusitis including mucormycosis in a diabetic

    D. Ophthalmoplegic migraine

    E. Myasthenia gravis

    F. Orbital pseudotumor

    G. Orbital tumors

        (1) Lymphoma

        (2) Metastatic

        (3) Rhabdomyosarcoma

2. Nuclear

    A. Acute and subacute infections

        (1) Infectious encephalitis

            a. Viral encephalitis

                1) Anterior poliomyelitis

                2) Encephalitis lethargica and other epidemic viral encephalitides

                3) Fisher syndrome (ophthalmoplegia, ataxia, areflexia)

                4) Rabies

                5) Vaccinal encephalitis

                6) Varicella, variola, measles, mumps, influenza, infectious mononucleosis

                7) Zoster

            b. Organismal encephalitic infections

                1) Typhoid

        2) Scarlet fever

        3) Whooping cough

        4) Gas gangrene

        5) Septicemia

        6) Pneumonia

        7) Typhus

        8) Malaria

   c. Acute central nervous system diseases

      1) Acute demyelinating diseases—acute disseminated encephalomyelitis, acute multiple sclerosis

      2) Neuritic infections

         a) Polyradiculoneuritis

         b) Epidemic paralyzing vertigo

         c) Acute infectious (rheumatic) polyneuritis

         d) Interstitial neuritis—meningitis, cranial sinusitis, petrositis, nasal sinusitis, orbital periostitis, orbital abscess

      3) Widespread infections

         a) Meningovascular syphilis

         b) Mucormycosis (diabetes, immunosuppressed, AIDS)

         c) Tuberculosis

         d) Torula and cryptococcosis

      4) Toxic conditions

         a) Diphtheria

         b) Tetanus

         c) Botulism

      5) Allergic conditions

         a) Sarcoidosis syndrome (Schaumann syndrome)

         b) Recurrent multiple cranial nerve palsies

B. Metabolic diseases

  (1) Deficiency diseases

    a. Thiamine deficiency (Wernicke-Korsakoff syndrome)

    b. Nicotinic acid deficiency—pellagra

    c. Ascorbic acid deficiency—scurvy

  (2) Diabetes

  (3) Anemias

    a. Primary anemia—leukemia

    b. Secondary anemia (loss of blood)

  (4) Exophthalmic ophthalmoplegia

  (5) Porphyria

C. Poisoning such as lead, carbon monoxide, snake poisons, wasp stings, ergot, sulfuric acid, phosphorus, triorthoceresylphosphate, and dichloroacetylene

D. Drugs, including:

acetohexamide
adrenal cortex injection
alcohol
aldosterone
allobarbital
amitriptyline
amobarbital
amoxapine
amphotericin B
aprobarbital
aspirin
aurothioglucose
aurothioglycanide
barbital
betamethasone
bupivacaine
butalbital
butallylonal
butethal
calcitriol(?)
carbamazepine
carisoprodol
chloral hydrate
chloroform
chloroprocaine
chloroquine
chlorpropamide
colchicine
cortisone
cyclobarbital
cyclopentobarbital
cytarabine
desipramine
desoxycorticosterone
dexamethasone
diazepam(?)
dibucaine
digitalis
digitoxin
diphtheria and tetanus toxoids (adsorbed)
diphtheria and tetanus toxoids and pertussis
  vaccine (adsorbed)

diphtheria toxoid (adsorbed)
dimethyl tubocurarine iodide
diphenydramine
diphenylhydantoin
disulfiram
doxepin
DPT vaccine
ergocalciferol(?)
ethambutol
fludrocortisone
fluprednisolone
gold Au 198
gold sodium thiomalate
griseofulvin
heptabarbital
hexethal
hexobarbital
hydrocortisone
hydroxychloroquine
imipramine
iodide and iodine solutions and compounds(?)
insulin
iophendylate
isoniazid
ketoprofen
levodopa
lidocaine
measles and rubella virus vaccine (live)
measles, mumps, and rubella virus vaccine
  (live)
measles virus vaccine
mephenesin
mephobarbital
mepivacaine
meprobamate
metharbital
methitural
methohexital
methylene blue
metoclopramide
metocurine iodide
metrizamide

midazolam

mumps virus vaccine (live)

methylprednisolone

nalidixic acid

naproxen

nitrazepam

nitrofurantoin

nortriptyline

oral contraceptives

oxazepam

oxyphenbutazone

paramethasone

pentobarbital

phenobarbital

phenylbutazone

piperazine

piperocaine

poliovirus vaccine

prazepam

prednisolone

prednisone

prilocaine

procaine

propoxycaine

protriptyline

radioactive iodides(?)

rubella and mumps virus vaccine (live)

rubella virus vaccine (live)

secobarbital

sodium salicylate

succinylcholine

talbutal

temazepam

tetracaine

thiamylal

thiopental

tolazamide

tolbutamide

triamcinolone

trichloroethylene

tubocurarine

vinbarbital

vinblastine

vincristine

vitamin A

vitamin D

vitamin D_2

vitamin D_3

E. Neoplasms and cysts

F. Trauma affecting the midbrain, base of the skull, and orbit

G. Vascular lesions as arteriosclerosis, hemorrhage and thrombosis in the midbrain, subarachnoid, hemorrhage, aneurysms, congenitally dilated arteries, giant-cell arteritis

H. Idiopathic—etiologic basis undetermined

Fraunfelder, F.T.: Drug-Induced Ocular Side Effects and Drug Interactions. 4th Ed. Philadelphia, Williams & Wilkins, 1996.

Pacifici, L., et al.: Acute third cranial nerve ophthalmoplegia: possible pathogenesis from alpha-II-interferon treatment. Italian J. Neurological Sciences, 14:579–580, 1993.

Roy, F.H.: Ocular Syndromes and Systemic Diseases. 2nd Ed. Philadelphia, W.B. Saunders, 1989.

Chronic Ophthalmoplegia (Slow Onset of Extraocular Muscle Palsy)

1. Degenerative conditions

   A. Amyotrophic lateral sclerosis—progressive bulbar palsy

   B. Chronic progressive external ophthalmoplegia

   C. Hereditary ataxias—Friedreich ataxia, Sanger-Brown ataxia

   D. Progressive supranuclear palsy

     E. Syringomyelia (syringobulbia)

     F. Thyroid myopathy (Graves disease)

  2. Infective conditions

     A. Diffuse sclerosis

     B. Disseminated sclerosis (multiple sclerosis)

     C. Syphilis

Duke-Elder, S., and Scott, G.I.: System of Ophthalmology. Vol. XII. St. Louis, C.V. Mosby, 1971.

Roy, F.H.: Ocular Syndromes and Systemic Diseases. 2nd Ed. Philadelphia, W.B. Saunders, 1989.

Bilateral Complete Ophthalmoplegia (Bilateral Palsy of Ocular Muscles, Ptosis, with Pupil and Accommodation Involvement)

  1. Arteriosclerotic hemorrhage and occlusion

  2. Cerebellopontine angle tumors (Cushing syndrome II)

  3. Encephalitis, acute

  4. Fisher syndrome (ophthalmoplegia-ataxia areflexia syndrome)

  5. Giant-cell arteritis (Hutchinson-Horton-Magath-Brown syndrome)

  6. Kiloh-Nevin syndrome (ocular myeomyopathy)

  7. Midbrain tumors

  8. Multiple sclerosis (rare)

  9. Mucormycosis

  10. Ohaha syndrome (ophthalmoplegia, hypotonia, ataxia hypacusis, athetosis)

  11. Orbital abscess

  12. Parinaud syndrome (conjunctiva-adenitis syndrome)

  13. Retrobulbar block complication

  14. Rochon-Duvigneaud syndrome (superior orbital fissure syndrome)

  15. Rollet syndrome (orbital apex-sphenoidal syndrome)

  16. Syphilis (acquired lues)

  17. Trauma

  18. Wernicke encephalopathies (thiamine deficiency)

  19. Whipple disease (intestinal lipodystrophy)

Brookshire, G.L., et al.: Life-threatening complication of retrobulbar block. Ophthalmology, 93:1476–1478, 1986.

Kaufman, L.M., et al.: Invasive sinonasal polyps causing ophthalmoplegia, exophthalmos, and visual field loss. Ophthalmology, 96:1667–1672, 1989.

McKusick, V.A.: Mendelian Inheritance in Man. 9th Ed. Baltimore, Johns Hopkins Hospital Press, 1994.

Roy, F.H.: Ocular Syndromes and Systemic Diseases. 2nd Ed. Philadelphia, W.B. Saunders, 1989.

Sergott, R.C., et al.: Simultaneous, bilateral diabetic ophthalmoplegia. Ophthalmology, 91:18–22, 1984.

External Ophthalmoplegia (Paralysis of Ocular Muscles Including Ptosis with Sparing of Pupil and Accommodation)

  1. Abiotrophy—specific for one particular tissue, bilateral, symmetric

  2. Amyloidosis (Lubarsch-Pick syndrome)

3. Aneurysm of internal carotid artery (foramen lacerum syndrome)

4. Bassen-Kornzweig syndrome (familial hypolipoproteinemia)

5. Bee sting

6. Chronic progressive external ophthalmoplegia

7. Congenital and familial

8. Diabetes mellitus (Willis disease)

9. Diphtheria

10. Epidemic encephalitis

11. Friedreich ataxia

12. Garcin syndrome (Schmincke tumor unilateral cranial paralysis)

13. Graves disease (hyperthyroidism)

14. Jacod syndrome (petrosphenoidal space syndrome)

15. Kearns-Sayre syndrome (ophthalmoplegic retinal degeneration syndrome)

16. Mumps

17. Myasthenia gravis (Erb-Goldflam syndrome)

18. Myotonic dystrophy (Curschmann-Steinert syndrome)

19. Myositis

20. Nevus sebaceous of Jadassohn

21. Nothnagel syndrome (ophthalmoplegia-cerebellar ataxia syndrome)

22. Oculopharyngeal syndrome (progressive muscular dystrophy with ptosis and dysphagia)

23. Olivopontocerebellar atrophy III (with retinal degeneration)—dominant

24. Ophthalmoplegia, progressive external, and scoliosis (horizontal gaze paralysis, familial)—recessive

25. Pernicious anemia

26. Polyradiculoneuronitis (Guillain-Barré and Fisher syndromes)

27. Progressive facial hemiatrophy (Parry-Romberg syndrome)

28. Pseudotumor (orbital)

29. Refsum syndrome (heredopathia atactica polyneuritiformis syndrome)

30. Scleroderma (progressive systemic sclerosis)

31. Shy-Drager syndrome (orthostatic hypotension syndrome)

32. Shy-Gonatas syndrome (accumulation of lipids in muscles simulates gargoylism)

33. Tick paralysis (Lyme disease, Rocky mountain spotted fever)

34. Vincristine—may have fifth and seventh nerve and peripheral neuropathies

35. Wernicke encephalopathies (beriberi, thiamine deficiency)

Fassati, A, et al.: Chronic progressive external ophthalmoplegia: a correlative study of quantitative molecular data and histochemical and biochemical profile. J. Neurological Sciences, 123:140–146, 1994.

Marsch, S.C., and Schaefer, H.G.: External ophthalmoplegia after total intravenous anaesthesia. Anaesthesia, 49:525–527, 1994.

McKusick, V.A.: Mendelian Inheritance in Man. 9th Ed. Baltimore, Johns Hopkins Hospital Press, 1994.

Roy, F.H.: Ocular Syndromes and Systemic Diseases. 2nd Ed. Philadelphia, W.B. Saunders, 1989.

Internuclear Ophthalmoplegia (Paralysis of Medial Rectus Muscles on Attempted Conjugate Lateral Gaze without Other Evidence of Third-Nerve Paralysis due to Involvement of Medial Longitudinal Fasciculus: Jerk Nystagmus of Abducting Eye and Vertical Nystagmus, Usually on Upward Gaze, May Be Present)

1. Bilateral
    A. Arnold-Chiari malformation (cerebellomedullary malformation syndrome)
    B. "Crack" cocaine
    C. Fabry disease (glycosphingolipid lipidosis)
    D. Inflammation, such as upper respiratory infection
    E. Midbrain infarction
    *F. Multiple sclerosis (disseminated sclerosis)
    G. Myasthenia gravis (Erb-Goldflam syndrome)
    H. Occlusive vascular disease
    I. Oculocerebellar tegmental syndrome
    J. Pontine hematoma
    K. Syphilis (acquired lues)
    L. Temporal arteritis
    M. Vertebral basilar artery syndrome (whiplash injury)
    N. Webino syndrome (wall-eyed exotropia bilateral internuclear ophthalmoplegia)
    O. Wernicke's encephalopathy
2. Unilateral
    A. Bielschowsky-Lutz-Cogan syndrome (internuclear ophthalmoplegia)
    B. Cryptococcosis (torulosis)
    C. Multiple sclerosis (disseminated sclerosis)
    D. Myasthenia gravis (Erb-Goldflam syndrome)
    E. Tumors of the brain stem
    *F. Vascular lesion—infarct of small branch of basilar artery

Internuclear Ophthalmoplegia

	Multiple Sclerosis	Inflammation as Upper Respiratory Infection	Neoplasm as Medulloblastoma	Myasthenia Gravis	Arnold Chiari Malformation	Fabry Disease	Ischemia (Vasolar)
History							
1. Age 20 to 40 years	U			U	S		
2. Over 60							U
3. First decade of life		U	U				
4. Hereditary						U	
5. More in females				U			
6. More in males			U				
7. Usually viral infection		U					
Physical Findings							
1. Associated hydrocephalus			S		S		
2. Central retinal artery occlusion						U	
3. Cogan lid twitch				U			
4. Conjunctivitis		U					
5. Cornea verticillata						U	
6. Corneal opacities						U	
7. Corneal ulcer		S					
8. Dacryoadenitis		S					
9. Dacryocystitis		S					
10. Esotropia, sudden onset			U				
11. Keratitis		S					
12. Lid edema						U	
13. Myokimia of lids	S						
14. Nystagmus	U		S		U		
15. Optic nerve atrophy	S						S
16. Optic neuritis	U	S					
17. Oscillopsia	S						
18. Panophthalmitis		S					
19. Papilledema			U		U	U	
20. Ptosis	S			U			
21. Pupillary afferent defect	U						S
22. Reduced visual acuity with exercise/hyperthermia	S						
23. Uveitis	S	S					
24. Varicosities palpebral/bulbar conjunctiva						U	
25. Visual field defects	S		S				S
Laboratory Data							
1. Cerebral anteriography						S	
2. Chest roentgenogram		S					
3. Cerebrospinal fluid abnormal	U	S	S		S		
4. Computed tomographic scan			U	U	U	U	
5. MRI	U	S	U	R	U	U	U
6. Peripheral blood test (Sadate, CBC, etc)		S					U
7. Throat culture		U					

R = rarely; S = sometimes; and U = usually.

Atabay, C., et al.: Eales disease with internuclear ophthalmoplegia. Annals of Ophthal., 24:267–269, 1992.

De La Paz, M.A., et al.: Bilateral internuclear ophthalmoplegia in a patient with Wernicke's encephalopathy. J Clinical Neuro-Ophthal., 12:116–120, 1992.

Diaz-Calderon, E., et al.: Bilateral internuclear ophthalmoplegia after smoking "crack" cocaine. J. Clinical Neuro-Ophthal., 11:297–299, 1991.

Glaser, J.S.: Neuro-Ophthalmology. 3rd Ed. Philadelphia. J.B. Lippincott Co., 1990.

Okuda, B., et al.: Bilateral internuclear ophthalmoplegia, ataxia, and tremor from a midbrain infarction. Stroke, 24:481–482, 1993.

Zee, D.S.: Internuclear ophthalmoplegia: pathophysiology and diagnosis. Baillieres Clinical Neurology, 1:455–470, 1992.

Painful Ophthalmoplegia (Palsy of Ocular Muscles with Pain)

1. Adenocarcinoma metastatic to the orbit
2. Atypical facial neuralgia
3. Cavernous sinus syndrome (Foix syndrome)
4. Collier sphenoidal palsy
5. Diabetic ophthalmoplegia
6. Intracavernous carotid aneurysm
7. Myositis (orbital)
8. Nasopharyngeal tumor
9. Ophthalmoplegic migraine
10. Orbital abscess (mucormycosis-diabetes, immunosuppressed, AIDS)
11. Orbital apex sphenoidal syndrome (Rollet syndrome)
12. Orbital periostitis
13. Postherpetic neuralgia
14. Pseudotumor of orbit
15. Superior orbital fissure syndrome (Rochon-Duvigneaud syndrome, including superior orbital fissuritis)
16. Temporal arteritis
17. Tic douloureux of the first trigeminal division
18. Tolosa-Hunt syndrome (inflammatory lesion of cavernous sinus)

Roy, F.H.: Ocular Syndromes and Systemic Diseases. 2nd Ed. Philadelphia, W.B. Saunders, 1989.

Sananman, M.L., and Weintroub, M.I.: Remitting ophthalmoplegia due to rhabdomyosarcoma. Arch. Ophthalmol., 86:6:459–461, 1971.

Painful Ophthalmoplegia

	Rhabdomyosarcoma	Thyroid Myopathy	Diabetes Mellitus (Third in Palsy)	Myositis	Orbital Cellulitis	Tolosa-Hunt Syndrome	Superior Orbital Fissure Syndrome	Nasopharyngeal Tumor	Pseudotumor (orbital)	Metastatic Adenocarcinoma	Neuralgia as Tic Doloreaux of First Division Trigeminal	Cavernous-Sinus Syndrome	Carotid/Dural Sinus Fistula
History													
1. Bilateral	R	S		S	R				R	U			S
2. Chronic inflammatory disease						U							
3. Familial			U										
4. Idiopathic inflammation				U		U			U				
5. Inflammatory, traumatic, tumor, or vascular lesion							U					U	
6. Ipsilateral lacrimation during pain											U		
7. Loss of vision	S	S	S	R	S	R			S	S		S	S
8. More in females											U		
9. More in males								U					
10. More than 40 years old		S											U
11. Only in children	U				U								
12. Periorbital pain	S	S		S		U			U		U		U
13. Scintillating scotoma						U							
Physical Findings													
1. Cataract			U										
2. Central retinal artery thrombosis										R			
3. Cotton-wool spots			U										
4. Chemosis, conjunctiva		S	S		S							U	U
5. Diminished corneal sensitivity							U	U	S			S	
6. Glaucoma			U						U	R			
7. Hard exudates			U										
8. Intraorbital bleeding										U			
9. Keratitis		S	S									U	S
10. Lid edema		S			U		U	S	U				U
11. Mild conjunctivitis					U			S	U				
12. Nasolacrimal obstruction					R			U					
13. Ocular bruit												U	U
14. Optic neuritis						U			S	R			
15. Optic nerve atrophy			R					U	S			S	
16. Papilledema			S					U	S				
17. Periorbital edema and tenderness	S	S			U				S				S
18. Proptosis	U	U	S	S	U		U	S	U	U		U	U
19. Ptosis			U				U		S				
20. Sluggish pupil reaction to light			S			U	U						
21. Uveitis											S		
Laboratory Data													
1. Arteriography, cerebral												U	U
2. Biopsy								U	U	S			
3. Blood sugar elevated			U										
4. Computed tomographic scan of orbit	U	U		U	U	U	S	U	U	U		U	R
5. MRI	R	R	U	R	R	S	R	S	R	S	S		R
6. Ultrasonography (oculo-oribital)		S		S	S			U	U	U		S	S

Transient Ophthalmoplegia (Extraocular Muscle Paralysis of Short Duration)

1. Cranial irradiation and intrathecal chemotherapy
2. Cyclic esotropia
3. Cyclic oculomotor palsy
4. Following internal carotid artery ligation for treatment of intracavernous giant aneurysm
5. Lethargic encephalitis
6. Multiple sclerosis (disseminated sclerosis—usually the lateral rectus)
7. Myasthenia gravis (ocular, early)
8. Oculomotor nuclear complex infarction
9. Ophthalmoplegia migraine
10. Post lumbar puncture abducens palsy
11. Syphilis (acquired lues)
12. Tabes doralis
13. Treatment of arteriovenous fistulas with Debrun balloon technique
14. Wilson's disease (hepatolenticular degeneration)

Gadoth, N., and Liel, Y.: Transient external ophthalmoplegia in Wilson's disease. Metab. Pediatr. Ophthalmol., 4:71–72, 1980.

Lepore, F.E., and Nissenblatt, M.J.: Bilateral internuclear ophthalmoplegia after intrathecal chemotherapy and cranial irradiation. Am. J. Ophthalmol., 92:851–853, 1981.

Nakao, S., et al.: Transient ophthalmoplegia following internal carotid artery ligation for treatment of intracavernous giant aneurysm. Surg. Neurol., 17:458–463, 1982.

Painful Ocular Movements (Pain with Movement of the Eyes)

1. Bone-break fever (dengue fever) (rare)
2. Influenza
3. Myositis
    A. "Collagen diseases"
    B. Infectious myositis
    C. Trichinosis
4. Orbital cellulitis
5. Orbital periostitis
6. Retrobulbar neuritis

Jampel, R.S., and Fells, P.: Monocular elevation paresis caused by a central nervous system lesion. Arch. Ophthalmol., 80:45, 1968.

Poor Convergence (Inability of Both Eyes to Fixate Simultaneously on a Near Object)

1. Functional
    A. Convergence insufficiency
    B. Exophoria
    C. Exotropia

      D. Hysteria

      E. Poor attention span of patient

2. Organic

    A. Brain lesion, to include bilateral occipital lobe lesions, superior colliculi, and anterior internuclear ophthalmoplegia, such as in hemorrhage, trauma, or tumors

    B. Encephalitis

    C. Exophthalmic goiter—Mobius sign

    D. Exophthalmos

    E. Multiple sclerosis

    F. Myotonic dystrophy

    G. Narcolepsy

    H. Poor visual acuity in one or both eyes

    I. Postencephalitis

    J. Syphilis and tabes

    K. Third nerve paralysis (see p. 176)

    L. Whiplash injury

3. Drugs, including:

alcohol	cyclopentobarbital	morphine
allobarbital	dextroamphetamine	opium
amobarbital	dimethyl tubocurarine iodide	penicillamine
amphetamine	diphenylhydantoin	pentobarbital
aprobarbital	floxuridine	phenmetrazine
barbital	fluorouracil	phenobarbital
bromide	heptabarbital	phenytoin
bromisovalum	hexethal	primidone
butabarbital	hexobarbital	probarbital
butalbital	mephobarbital	secobarbital
butallylonal	methamphetamine	talbutal
butethal	metocurine iodide	thiamylal
carbon dioxide	metharbital	thiopental
chloral hydrate	methitural	tubocurarine
cyclobarbital	methohexital	vinbarbital

Fraunfelder, F.T.: Drug-Induced Ocular Side Effects and Drug Interactions. 4th Ed. Philadelphia, Williams & Wilkins, 1996. Walsh, F.B., and Hoyt, W.F.: Clinical Neuro-ophthalmology, 4th ed. Baltimore, Williams & Wilkins, 1985.

Spasm of Convergence (Occurs with Spasm of Accommodation and Miosis, i.e., Spasm of the Near Reflex)

1. Encephalitis—accompanied with nystagmus

2. Hysteria—may be confused with lateral rectus palsy

3. Labyrinthine fistulas

4. Kenny syndrome

5. Oculogyric crisis in myasthenia gravis

6. Paralysis of horizontal gaze with compensatory spasm of near reflex

7. Parinaud syndrome (divergence paralysis)

8. Tabes dorsalis

9. Trauma

10. Wernicke syndrome (avitaminosis B_1)

Thompson, R.A., and Zynde, R.H.: Convergence spasm associated with Wernicke's encephalopathy. Neurology, 19:711–712, 1969.

Feiler-Ofry, V., et al.: Lipoid protcinosis (Urbach-Wiethe Syndrome). Br. J. Ophthalmol., 63:694–698, 1979.

Divergence Paralysis (Supranuclear Cause with Sudden Onset of Comitant Esotropia and Uncrossed Diplopia at Distance, Fusion at Near [Usually One to Two Meters], Normal Ductions and Versions, and Gross Impairment of Fusional Amplitudes of Divergence)

*1. Brain stem lesions

    A. Cerebellar cyst

    B. Hemangioma

    C. Tumors, such as cerebellar and acoustic neuromas

2. Cerebral hemorrhage

3. Diazepam

4. Diphtheria

5. Epidemic encephalitis

6. Functional

7. Head injuries

8. Increased intracranial pressure

9. Influenza

10. Lead poisoning

11. Multiple sclerosis (disseminated sclerosis)

12. Poliomyelitis

13. Syphilis

14. Unknown

15. Vascular disease

    A. Diabetes mellitus

    B. Hypertension

    C. Occlusion of subclavian artery with reversal of flow in vertebral artery

    D. Vertebral basilar insufficiency

Arai, M., and Fujii, S.: Divergence Paralysis Neurol., 237:45–46, 1990.

Krohel, G.B., et al.: Divergence Paralysis. Am. J. Ophthalmol., 94:506, 1982.

* = most important

Walsh, F.B., and Hoyt, W.F.: Clinical Neuro-ophthalmology. 4th Ed. Baltimore, Williams & Wilkins, 1985.

Oculocardiac Reflex (Bradycardia, Nausea, and Faintness Dependent on Trigeminal Sensory Stimulation Evoked by Pressure on or within the Eyeball or From Sensory Impulses by Stretching of Ocular Muscles)

1. Acute glaucoma
2. Anophthalmic socket
3. During ophthalmoscopy examination of premature infants
4. Exaggerated in epidemic encephalitis
5. Intermittent exophthalmos due to congenital venous malformations of the orbit
6. Intraocular injections
7. Orbital hematoma
*8. Pressure on globe
9. Retinal detachment operation
10. Severe injury to eye or orbit
*11. Traction on extraocular muscles including levator palpebrae superioris

Arnold, R.W., et al.: Lack of global vagal propensity in patients with oculocardiac reflex. Ophthal., 101:1347–1352, 1994.

Clarke, W.N., et al.: The oculocardiac reflex during ophthalmoscopy in premature infants. Am. J. Ophthalmol., 99:649–651, 1985.

Ginsburg, R.M, et al.: Oculocardiac reflex in the anophthalmic socket. Ophthalmic Surgery. 23:35–137, 1992.

Walsh, F.B., and Hoyt, W.F.: Clinical Neuro-ophthalmology. 4th Ed. Baltimore, Williams & Wilkins, 1985.

Retraction of the Globe (on Horizontal Conjugate Gaze)

*1. Duane syndrome (retraction syndrome)—co-contraction of horizontal rectus muscles, lateral rectus, and both vertical muscles, or medial and inferior rectus muscles or fibrotic lateral rectus
    A. Acroreno-ocular syndrome
    B. Goldenhar syndrome
    C. Hanhart syndrome
    D. Isolated
    E. Okihiro syndrome
    F. Wildervanck syndrome (Klippel-Feil anomaly with Duane syndrome)
2. Fibrosis secondary to strabismus surgery
3. Medial wall fracture with incarceration of orbit contents—retraction of globe with attempted abduction
4. Orbital mass
    A. Dermoid cyst
    B. Hemiangioma
    C. Lymphangioma
    D. Osteofibroma

5. Retraction of convergent nonfixating eye associated with loss of conjugate lateral gaze and occurrence of the near reflex on attempted lateral gaze

6. Thyroid myopathy

Holtz, S.J.: Congenital ocular anomalies associated with Duane's retraction syndrome, the nevus of ota, and axial anisometropia. Am. J. Ophthalmol., 74:729–731, 1974.

Isenberg, S.J.: The Eye in Infancy. Chicago, Year Book Medical Publishers, 1989.

Forced Duction Test (The Eyeball Is Moved Away from Muscle Being Tested by Grasping with a Forceps the Conjunctiva and Episclera Close to the Limbus)

1. Supraduction-infraduction

   A. Resistance

      (1) Abnormal fascial or muscle attachments

      (2) Congenital fibrosis syndrome

      (3) Double elevator palsy

      (4) Orbital floor fracture

      (5) Orbital mass

      (6) Thyroid myopathy of inferior rectus muscle

   B. Unrestricted

      (1) Elevator paresis

      (2) Paresis of inferior superior rectus muscle

2. Supraduction in adduction

   A. Brown superior oblique tendon sheath syndrome—resistance (see p. 154)

   B. Paresis of inferior oblique muscle—unrestricted

3. Adduction

   A. Resistance

      (1) Chronic third nerve palsy with contracture lateral rectus

      (2) Congenital fibrosis syndrome

      (3) Duane retraction syndrome because of fibrosis of lateral rectus muscle

      (4) Orbital mass

      (5) Tight lateral rectus following excessive resection operation

      (6) Thyroid myopathy

   B. Unrestricted

      (1) Extensive medial rectus recession

      (2) Duane retraction syndrome because of central or peripheral co-contraction of medial and lateral rectus on attempted adduction

4. Abduction

   A. Resistance

      (1) Abnormal fascial or muscle attachments including strabismus fixus

      (2) Blowout fracture

      (3) Chronic sixth nerve palsy with contracture medial rectus

      (4) Myositis

* = most important

(5) Orbital mass

(6) Thyroid myopathy

Tight medial rectus following excessive resection operation

    B. Unrestricted

        (1) Extensive lateral rectus recession

        (2) Paralysis of lateral rectus muscle

Beyer-Machule, C., and Noorden, G.K., von: Atlas of Ophthalmic Surgery: Vol. 1: Lids, Orbits, Extraocular Muscles, New York, Thieme Med. Pub., 1984.

Double Elevator Palsy (Apparent Paralysis of Globe Elevators, i.e., Superior Rectus and Inferior Oblique Muscles)

1. Inferior rectus muscles restriction

    A. Anomalous insertion of inferior rectus muscle

    B. Blow-out fracture

    C. Congenital orbital fibrosis syndrome

    D. Thyroid ophthalmopathy

2. Monocular elevation paresis secondary to CNS lesions

    A. Monocular elevation paresis

    B. Skew deviation

3. Neurogenic or myogenic superior rectus muscle weakness

    A. Myasthenia gravis (Erb-Goldflam syndrome)

    B. Postoperative Berke-Motais surgery

    C. Superior oblique tendon sheath syndrome (see p. 154)

    D. Third cranial nerve palsy (see p. 178)

    E. Trauma

Callahan, M.A.: Surgically mismanaged ptosis associated with double elevator palsy. Arch. Ophthalmol., 99:108, 1981.

Ocular Neuromyotonia (Paroxysmal Monocular Deviations Ascribable to Involuntary Contraction of Muscles Innervated by the Third, Fourth, or Sixth Cranial Nerves)

1. Aneurysmal compression of third nerve

2. Chondrosarcoma

3. Cystic craniopharyngioma

4. Following radiation therapy

5. Rhabdomyosarcoma

Bateman, D.E., and Saunders, M.: Cyclic oculomotor palsy. J. Neurol. Neurosurg. Psychiatry, 46:451, 1983.

Lessell, S., et al.: Ocular neuromyotonia alter radiation therapy. Am. J. Ophthalmol., 102:766–770, 1986.

Extraocular Muscle Enlargement On Orbital Computerized and Tomographic Scan

1. Diffuse

    A. Acromegaly

B. Amyloidosis

*C. Graves disease as thyroid ophthalmopathy

*D. Infection

E. Parasitic infiltration

F. Trauma

G. Tumors including pseudotumor

H. Vascular abnormalities as arterio-venous fistula

I. Collagen vascular disease

2. Focal

A. Cysticercosis

B. Hemorrhagic cyst

C. Primary or metastatic carcinoma

D. Trichinella

Albert, D.M., and Jakobiec, F.A.: Principles and Practice of Ophthalmology. Philadelphia, W.B. Saunders, Co., 1881–2095, 1994.

Howard, G.R., et al.: Orbital dermoid located within lateral rectus muscle. Ophthal., 101:767–778, 1994.

Kaltreider, S.A., et al.: Destructive cysts of the maxillary sinus affecting the orbit. Arch. Ophthal., 106:1398–1402, 1988.

Maurrello, J.A., and Flanagan, J.C.: Management of orbital inflammatory disease. A protocol. Surv. Ophthalmol., 29:104–116, 1984.

* = most important

Conjunctiva

FERNANDO MURILLO, M.D.

Contents

Cellular responses

1. Basophilic reaction—significant only when seen in large numbers; Ig-E mediated allergic conditions; key role in asthma, atopy and hypersensitivity responses; present in vernal (. eosinophils) and GPC conjunctivitis.

2. Eosinophilic reaction—giant papillary conjunctivitis; Charcot-Leyden crystals more prominent than intact eosinophils in chronic allergy; parasitic conjunctivitis.

   *A. Vernal conjunctivitis—characteristic with fragmentation of eosinophil

   B. Hay fever conjunctivitis—rarely fragmentation of eosinophil

   C. Allergic conjunctivitis due to various drugs, cosmetics, and other antigens

   D. Atropine sensitivity—not present when eserine or pilocarpine is employed

3. Mononuclear reaction

   A. Viral disease—100% without secondary infection; usually lymphocytic

      *(1) Epidemic keratoconjunctivitis—adenovirus type 8

      (2) Pharyngoconjunctival fever—adenovirus type 3

      *(3) Herpetic keratoconjunctivitis

      (4) Acute follicular conjunctivitis of Beal

   B. Chronic ocular infections

4. Neutrophilic reaction—early stage of severe viral conjunctivitis

   A. All bacteria but two—Neisseria catarrhalis and Haemophilus duplex (Morax-Axenfeld diplobacillus)

   B. Viruses of the family Chlamydiaceae (TRIC agent)

      (1) Trachoma

      *(2) Inclusion conjunctivitis

      (3) Lymphogranuloma venereum

   C. Fungal disease

      (1) Streptothrix conjunctivitis secondary to canaliculitis

* = most important

      (2) Nocardial corneal ulcers

      (3) Monilial corneal ulcers

   D. Unknown cause

     *(1) Erythema multiforme (Stevens-Johnson syndrome)

     (2) Conjunctivitis of Reiter disease

   E. Vernal conjunctivitis—eosinophilic and neutrophilic reaction

   F. Epidemic keratoconjunctivitis and herpetic keratoconjunctivitis have a shift from mononuclear to polymorphonuclear reaction when a membrane is formed

5. Plasma-cell reaction—Trachoma—especially with spontaneous rupturing of follicles; chlamydial conjunctivitis.

6. Epithelial changes

   A. Keratinization of conjunctival epithelial cells

     *(1) Vitamin A deficiency

     (2) Exposure

     (3) Cicatrization (such as pemphigold and Stevens Johnson syndrome)

     (4) Keratoconjunctivitis sicca—partially keratinized epithelial cells, specific

     (5) Epithelial plaque

   B. Large, multipointed epithelial cells

     (1) Characteristic of viral infection

     *(2) Most often found in herpetic keratitis

   C. Intracellular granules

     (1) Pseudoinclusion bodies—extension of nuclear material into cytoplasm

     (2) Intracellular-free green pigment in cytoplasm—present in persons with dark complexion

     (3) Intracellular-free blue granules—present in cytoplasm in about 12% of normal individuals

     (4) Sex chromatin—present in nuclei only of female

7. Cellular inclusions

   A. Trachoma and inclusion conjunctivitis have identical inclusions—basophilic, cytoplasmic (Halberstadter-Prowazek)

  *B. Molluscum contagiosum—eosinophilic, cytoplasmic

   C. Lymphogranuloma venereum—eosinophilic

  *D. Herpes simplex and herpes zoster—eosinophilic, internuclear (Lipshutz)

   E. Measles—multinucleated giant cells with eosinophilic internuclear inclusion bodies and cytoplasmic, eosinophilic masses

  *F. Chickenpox—eosinophilic, internuclear

   G. Smallpox—eosinophilic, cytoplasmic

Brinser, J.H., and Burd, E.M.: Principles of diagnosis ocular microbiology. In Tabbara K.F., Hyndiuk, R.A. (eds): Infections of the Eye. Boston, Little Brown and Co., 1986, 73–92.

Fedukowicz, H.B.: External Infections of the Eye: Bacterial, Viral, Mycotic. 3rd Ed. New York, Appleton-Century-Crofts, 1984.

Spencer, W.H.: Ophthalmic Pathology Vol. 1, Philadelphia, W.B. Saunders, 1985.

Purulent Conjunctivitis (Violent Acute Conjunctival Inflammation, Great Swelling of Lids, Copious Secretion of Pus, and a Marked Tendency to Corneal Involvement and Even Possible Loss of Eye)

1. Gram-positive group

    A. Bacillus of Doderlein (Lactobacillus sp.)

    B. Listeria monocytogenes

    *C. Pneumococcus

    D. Staphylococcus

    *E. Streptococcus

2. Gram-negative group

    A. Aerobacter aerogenes

    B. Enterobacteriaceae

    C. Escherichia coli

    *D. Haemophilus influenzae biotype III

    E. Klebsiella pneumoniae

    F. Moraxella lacunata

    *G. Neisseria gonorrhoeae

    H. Neisseria meningitidis

    I. Proteus species

    J. Pseudomonas

    K. Serratia marcescens

3. Vaccinia virus

4. Fungus

    A. Actinomyces

    B. Candida

    *C. Nocardia

5. Wiskott-Aldrich syndrome—x-linked

Fedukowicz, H.B.: External Infections of the Eye: Bacterial, Viral, Mycotic. 3rd Ed. New York, Appleton-Century-Crofts, 1984.

Roy, F.H.: Ocular Syndromes and Systemic Diseases. 2nd Ed. Philadelphia, W.B. Saunders, 1989.

Snead, J.W., et al.: Listeria monocytogenes endophthalmitis. Am. J. Ophthalmol., 84:337–344, 1977.

Acute Mucopurulent Conjunctivitis (Epidemic Pink Eye—Marked Hyperemia and a Mucopurulent Discharge, Which Tends Toward Spontaneous Recovery)

1. Gram-positive group

    *A. Pneumococcus

    B. Staphylococcus—eyelid lesions and punctate staining of the lower cornea may occur

2. Gram-negative group

    *A. Haemophilus aegyptius (Koch-Weeks bacillus)

    B. Haemophilus influenzae

* = most important

3. Associated with exanthems and viral infections
    A. German measles (Gregg syndrome)
    B. Measles (rubeola)
    C. Mumps
   *D. Reiter syndrome (conjunctivourethrosynovial syndrome)
    E. Scarlet fever

4. Fungus
    A. Candida albicans
    B. Leptothrix

5. Lyell disease—toxic epidermal necrolysis or scalded skin syndrome

6. Relapsing polychondritis

7. Sjögren syndrome (secretoinhibitor syndrome)

8. Etiology obscure in many cases

Fedukowicz, H.B.: External Infections of the Eye: Bacterial, Viral and Mycotic. 3rd Ed. New York, Appleton-Century-Crofts, 1984.

Okumoto, M., and Smolin, G.: Pneumococcal infections of the eye. Am. J. Ophthalmol., 77:346–352, 1974.

Roy, F.H.: Ocular Syndromes and Systemic Diseases. 2nd Ed. Philadelphia, W.B. Saunders, 1989.

Chronic Mucopurulent Conjunctivitis (Mucopurulent Discharge, Moderate Hyperemia with a Chronic Course)

1. Infective element-lids or lacrimal apparatus
    A. Monilia
    B. Morax-Axenfeld diplobacillus (angular conjunctivitis)
   *C. Pneumococcus
    D. Pubic lice
    E. Staphylococcus
    F. Streptothrix foersteri

2. Allergic—cosmetic

3. Irritative
    A. Associated infections or irritation of lids, lacrimal apparatus, nose, or skin
    B. Deficiency of lacrimal secretions
    C. Direct irritants—foreign body, mascara, dust, wind, smog, insecticides, chlorinated water, and many others
    D. Exposure—ectropion, facial paralysis, exophthalmos, and others
    E. Eyestrain
    F. Metabolic conditions—gout, alcoholism, or prolonged digestive disturbances
    G. Overtreatment by drugs—antibiotics, miotics, mydriatics

Fedukowicz, H.B.: External Infections of the Eye: Bacterial, Viral and Mycotic. 3rd Ed. New York, Appleton-Century-Crofts, 1984.

Geyer, O., et al.: Phenylephrine prodrug. Ophthal., 98:1483, 1991.

Okumoto, M., and Smolin, G.: Pneumococcal infections of the eye. Am. J. Ophthalmol., 77:346–352, 1974.

Roy, F.H.: Ocular Syndromes and Systemic Diseases. 2nd Ed. Philadelphia, W.B. Saunders, 1989.

Membranous Conjunctivitis (Exudate Permeates Epithelium to Such an Extent That Removal of Membrane is Difficult and a Raw Bleeding Surface Results). Membranous conjunctivitis may lead to symblepharon, ankyloblepharon, and entropion with trichiasis.

1. Chemical irritants

    A. Acids, such as acetic or lactic

    *B. Alkalis, such as ammonia or lime

    C. Metallic salts, such as silver nitrate or copper sulfate

2. Corynebacterium diphtheriae

3. Ligneous conjunctivitis—chronic, cause unknown

4. Pneumococcus

5. Streptococcus

6. Uncommon—Actinomyces, glandular fever, measles, Neisseria catarrhalis, variola, Pseudomonas aeruginosa, herpes simplex, Leptothrix, and epidemic keratoconjunctivitis (type adenovirus)

Fedukowicz, H. B.: External Infections of the Eye: Bacterial, Viral and Mycotic. 3rd Ed. New York, Appleton-Century-Crofts, 1984.

Roy, F.H.: Ocular Syndromes and Systemic Diseases. 2nd Ed. Philadelphia, W.B. Saunders, 1989.

Pseudomembranous Conjunctivitis (Fibrin Network—Easily Peeled Off Leaving the Conjunctiva Intact, Forms on Conjunctiva)

1. Bacteria

    A. Corynebacterium diphtheriae

    *B. Gonococcus

    *C. Meningococcus

    D. Pneumococcus

    E. Staphylococcus

    *F. Streptococcus

    G. Uncommon—Haemophilus aegyptius, Haemophilus influenzae, Neisseria catarrhalis, Pseudomonas aeruginosa, Escherichia coli, Bacillus subtilis, Shigella, Bacillus faecalis alcaligenes, Salmonella paratyphi B, Mycobacterium tuberculosis, and Treponema pallidum

2. Viral

    *A. Epidemic keratoconjunctivitis (type adenovirus)

    *B. Herpes simplex

    C. Herpes zoster

    D. Reiter syndrome (conjunctivourethrosynovial syndrome)

    E. Vaccina

3. Fungal—Candida albicans

*4. Allergic—vernal conjunctivitis

5. Toxic

    *A. Stevens-Johnson syndrome can be caused by drugs, including:

* = most important

acetaminophen	cefonicid
acetanilid	cefoperazone
acetazolamide	ceforanide
acetohexamide	cefotaxime
acetophenazine	cefotetan
allobarbital	cefoxitin
allopurinol	cefsulodin
aminosalicylate(?)	ceftazimide
aminosalicylic acid(?)	ceftizoxime
amidarone	ceftriaxone
amithiozone	cefuroxime
amobarbital	cephalexin
amodiaquine	cephaloglycin
amoxicillin	cephaloridine
ampicillin	cephalothin
antipyrine	cephapirin
aprobarbital	cephradine
aspirin	chloroquine
auranofin	chlorothiazide
aurothioglucose	chlorpromazine
aurothioglycanide	chlorpropamide
barbital	chlortetracycline
bella donna	chlorthalidone
bendroflumethiazide	cimetidine
benzathine penicillin G	clindamycin
benzthiazide	cloxacillin
bromide	cyclobarbital
bromisovalum	cyclopentobarbital
butabarbital	cyclothiazide
butalbital	danazol
butallylonal	demeclocycline
butaperazine	dichlorphenamide
butethal	dicloxacillin
captopril	diethazine
carbamazepine	diphenylhydantoin
carbenicillin	doxycycline
carbromal	enalapril
carisoprodol	erythromycin
carphenazine	ethopropazine
cefaclor	ethosuximide
cefadroxil	ethotoin
cefamandole	ethoxzolamide
cefazolin	fenoprofen

fluphenazine
furosemide
glyburide
gold Au 198
gold sodium thiomalate
gold sodium thiosulfate
heptabarbital
hetacillin
hexethal
hexobarbital
hydrabamine penicillin V
phenoxymethyl penicillin
hydrochlorothiazide
hydroflumethiazide
hydroxychloroquine
ibuprofen
indapamide
indomethacin
isoniazid
lincomycin
mephenytoin
mephobarbital
meprobamate
mesoridazine
methacycline
metharbital
methazolamide
methdilazine
methicillin
methitural
methohexital
methotrimeprazine
methsuximide
methyclothiazide
methylphenidate
metolazone
minocycline
minoxidil
moxalactam
nafcillin
naproxen
oxacillin
oxyphenbutazone

oxytetracycline
paramethadione
pentobarbital
perazine
pericyazine
perphenazine
phenacetin
phenobarbital
phenoxymethyl penicillin
phensuximide
phenylbutazone
phenytoin
piperacetazine
piperoxicam
polythiazide
potassium penicillin G
potassium penicillin V
potassium phenethicillin
potassium phenoxymethyl penicillin
primidone
probarbital
procaine penicillin G
prochlorperazine
promazine
promethazine
proparacaine
propiomazine
propranolol
quinethazone
quinine
rifampin
secobarbital
smallpox vaccine
sodium salicylate
sulfacetamide
sulfachlorpyridazine
sulfacytine
sulfadiazine
sulfadimethoxine
sulfamerazine
sulfameter
sulfamethazine
sulfamethizole

sulfamethoxazole	thiethylperazine
sulfamethoxypyridazine	thiopental
sulfanilamide	thiopropazate
sulfaphenazole	thioproperazine
sulfapyridine	thioridazine
sulfasalazine	tolazamide
sulfathiazole	tolbutamide
sulfisoxazole	trichlormethiazide
sulindac	trifluoperazine
sulthiame	triflupromazine
talbutal	trimeprazine
tetracycline	trimethadione
thiabendazole	vancomycin
thiamylal	vinbarbital

*B. Benign mucous membrane pemphigoid can be caused by drugs, including:

carbamazepine	methsuximide
carbimazole	methylthiouracil
diphenylhydantoin	paramethadione
ethosuximide	phensuximide
griseofulvin	practolol
hydralazine	propylthiouracil
isoniazid	streptomycin
methimazole	trimethadione

C. Lyell disease (toxic epidermal necrolysis or scalded skin syndrome) can be caused by drugs, including:

acetaminophen	bendroflumethiazide
acetanilid	benzthiazide
acetazolamide	benzathine penicillin G
acid bismuth sodium tartrate	betamethasone
adrenal cortex injection	bismuth oxychloride
aldosterone	bismuth sodium tartrate
allobarbital	bismuth sodium thioglycollate
amoxipine	bismuth sodium triglycollamate
amoxicillin	busulfan
amobarbital	butabarbital
ampicillin	butalbital
antipyrine	butallylonal
aprobarbital	butethal
aurothioglucose	carbamazepine
aurothioglycanide	carbenicillin
barbital	carbimazole

chlorambucil
chlorothiazide
chlortetracycline
chlorthalidone
clomipramine
cloxacillin
cortisone
cyclobarbital
cyclopentobarbital
cyclothiazide
cyclophosphamide
dapsone
demeclocycline
desoxycorticosterone
dexamethasone
dichlorphenamide
dicloxacillin
diltiazem
diphenylhydantoin
doxepin
doxycycline
erythromycin
ethambutol
ethotoin
ethoxzolamide
fludrocortisone
fluprednisolone
gold Au 198
gold sodium thiomalate
heptabarbital
hetacillin
hexethal
hexobarbital
hydrabamine penicillin V
hydrochlorothiazide
hydrocortisone
ibuprofen
indapamide
indomethacin
isoniazid
kanamycin
mechlorethamine
melphalan

mephenytoin
mephobarbital
meprednisone
methacycline
metharbital
methazolamide
methicillin
methitural
methohexital
methotrexate
methyclothiazide
methylprednisolone
metolazone
minocycline
nafcillin
nitrofurantoin
oxacillin
oxyphenbutazone
oxytetracycline
paramethadione
paramethasone
penicillamine
pentobarbital
phenobarbital
phenylbutazone
phenytoin
piroxicam
poliovirus vaccine
polythiazide
phenoxymethyl penicillin
phenylbutazone
potassium penicillin G
potassium penicillin V
potassium phenethicillin
prednisolone
prednisone
primidone
probarbital
procaine penicillin G
procarbazine
quinethazone
secobarbital
smallpox vaccine

* = most important

sodium salicylate	sulfisoxazole
streptomycin	sulindac
sulfacetamide	talbutal
sulfachlorpyridazine	tetracycline
sulfadiazine	thiabendazole
sulfadimethoxine	thiamylal
sulfamerazine	thiopental
sulfameter	triamcinolone
sulfamethazine	trichlormethiazide
sulfamethizole	triethylene-melamine
sulfamethoxazole	trimethadione
sulfamethoxypyridazine	trimipramine
sulfanilamide	uracil mustard
sulfaphenazole	vinbarbital
sulfapyridine	
sulfasalazine	
sulfathiazole	

    D. Pemphigus vulgaris

    E. Hereditary epidermolysis bullosa

6. Chemical irritants

    A. Acids, such as acetic or lactic

    *B. Alkalis, such as ammonia or lime

    C. Metallic salts, such as silver nitrate or copper sulfate

    D. Vegetable and animal irritants

7. Acute graft-versus-host disease

8. Foot and mouth disease

9. Koch-Weeks bacillus

10. Ligneous conjunctivitis—chronic, cause unknown

11. Lipoid proteinosis (Urbach-Wiethe syndrome)

*12. Superior limbic keratoconjunctivitis

13. Traumatic or operative healing of wounds

14. Wegner granulomatosis

Barthelemy, H., et al.: Lipoid proteinosis with pseudomembranous conjunctivitis. J. Am. Acad. Dermatol., 14:367–371, 1986.

Fraunfelder, F.T.: Drug-Induced Ocular Side Effects and Drug Interactions. 4th Ed. Philadelphia, Lea & Febiger, 1996.

Hirst, L.W., et al.: The eye in bone marrow transplantation. Arch. Ophthalmol., 101:580–584, 1983.

Pau, H.: Differential Diagnosis of Eye Diseases. 2nd Ed. New York, Thieme Medical Publishers, 1988.

Ophthalmia Neonatorum (Conjunctivitis Occurring in Newborns)

1. Acinetobacter Sp

2. Branhamella catarrhalis

3. Candida albicans

*4. Chemical conjunctivitis, such as from silver nitrate instillation

*5. Chlamydia trachomatis

6. Citrobacter feundi

7. Clostridium perfringes

8. Coliform bacillus, such as Escherichia coli

9. Coxsackie A

10. Corynebacterium diphtheriae

11. Enterobacter cloacae

12. Hemophitius influenzae

13. Hemophilus influenzae

14. Hemophilus parainfluenzae

*15. Herpes simplex

16. Inclusion blennorrhea

17. Klebsiella pneumoniae

18. Listeriosis (Listeria monocytogenes)

*19. Meningococcus

20. Mima polymorpha-gram negative

21. Moraxella

22. Mycoplasma

*23. Neisseria gonorrhoeae and N. catarrhalis

24. Neisseria sp

25. Peptococcus prevotii

26. Pneumococcus

27. Proprionbacter

28. Proteus mirabilis

29. Pseudomonas aeruginosa

30. Pseudomonas pyocyanca

31. Serratia marcescens

32. Staphylococcus aureus

33. Staphylococcus epidermidis

34. Streptococcus Group D

35. Streptococcus pneumoniae

36. Streptococcus viridans

37. Trichomonas vaginalis

38. Tric virus

Cohen, K.L., and McCarthy, L.R.: Haemophilus influenzae ophthalmia neonatorum. Arch. Ophthalmol., 98:1214, 1980.

Isenberg, S.J.: The Eye in Infancy. Chicago, Year Book Medical Publishers, 1989.

Rapoza, P.A., et al.: Epidemiology of neonatal conjunctivitis. Ophthalmology, 94:461, 1986.

Stenson, S., et al.: Conjunctivitis in the newborn: Observations on incidence, cause, and prophylaxis. Ann. Ophthalmol., 13:329, 1981.

* = most important

Acute Follicular Conjunctivitis (Lymphoid Follicles [Cobblestoning] of Conjunctiva with Rapid Onset)

*1. Inclusion conjunctivitis—adult inclusion conjunctivitis (AIC) (begins 2 days after exposure to organism, may be bilateral, no systemic symptoms, a unilateral or bilateral preauricular node is often present).

*2. Adenovirus conjunctivitis—EKC has been reported worldwide from virus serotypes (the most common: 8,11,19); pharynconjunctival fever (PCF) is usually caused by serotypes 3, 4, and 7.

   A. Pharyngoconjunctival fever—usually because of type adenovirus; common in swimming-pool epidemics in summer and fall

   B. Epidemic keratoconjunctivitis because of adenovirus type (rarely occurs in children)

*3. Primary herpetic keratoconjunctivitis—conjunctival reaction may be follicular or pseudomembranous

4. Newcastle disease (fowlpox) conjunctivitis—usually seen in poultry handlers, veterinarians (caused by a paramyxovirus: single-stranded RNA virus that causes respiratory infections)

5. Influenza virus A

6. Herpes zoster

*7. Cat-scratch fever (Parinaud oculoglandular syndrome)—fever caused by two types of rickettsia: Rochalimaea henselae and afipia felis)

8. Trachoma (sometimes)

9. Bacterial (rare)—streptococcus, moraxella and treponema

10. Mesantoin use

11. Chlamydia epizootic (feline pneumonitis)

12. Ophthalmomyiasis

13. Unknown types—a case that resists etiologic classification is encountered occasionally; it is probable that other viruses can occasionally produce acute follicular conjunctivitis

14. Associated with regional adenitis

   A. Angelucci syndrome (critical allergic conjunctivitis syndrome)

   B. Anoxic overwear syndrome

   C. Benjamin-Allen syndrome (brachial arch syndrome)

   D. Floppy eyelid syndrome

   *E. Giant papillary conjunctivitis syndrome

   *F. Inclusion conjunctivitis in adults—acute mucopurulent follicular inflammation, persisting as long as several months, sometimes with scarring

   G. Syndrome of Beal—transient unilateral disease, usually resolving in weeks

Allansmith, M.R.: The Eye and Immunology. St. Louis, C.V. Mosby, 1982.

Kowalski, R.P., and Harwick, J.C.: Incidence of Moraxella Conjunctival Infection. Am. J. Ophthalmol., 101:437–440, 1986.

Roy, F.H.: Ocular Syndromes and Systemic Diseases. 2nd Ed. Philadelphia, W.B. Saunders, 1989.

Chronic Follicular Conjunctivitis (Lymphoid Follicles [Cobblestoning] of Conjunctiva with Long-Term Course)

1. Chronic follicular conjunctivitis—Axenfeld's type (orphan's) frequently found in institutionalized children; almost asymptomatic; long duration (to months or longer); no keratitis; cause unknown

*2. Chronic follicular conjunctivitis, toxic type

    A. Bacterial origin, such as that due to a diplobacillus or other microorganism

    B. Drugs, including:

acyclovir	homatropine
adenine arabinoside	hyaluronidase
amphotericin B	idoxuridine
atropine	isoflurophate
carbachol	neomycin
demecarium	neostigmine
diatrizoate meglumine and sodium	physostigmine
diisopropyl fluorophosphate	pilocarpine
dipivefrin	scopolamine
echothiophate	sulfacetamide
eserine	sulfamethizole
framycetin	sulfisoxazole
F3T	trifluorothymidine
gentamicin	trifluridine

3. Chronic follicular conjunctivitis with epithelial keratitis; differentiated from Axenfeld type by shorter duration (to months) and by epithelial keratitis involving upper third of cornea; epidemic in schools; can be transmitted by mascara pencil; cause unknown

4. Ectodermal syndrome (Rothmund syndrome)

5. Folliculosis—associated general lymphoid hypertrophy

*6. Molluscum contagiosum conjunctivitis

7. Neurocutaneous syndrome (ectodermal dysgenesis)

*8. Postoperative penetrating keratoplasty or cataract surgery sutures

9. Trachoma—stages to 3

10. Use of hard and soft contact lens

*11. Use of ocular prostheses

12. With generalized lymphadenopathy

Albert, D.M., and Jakobiec, F.A.: Principles and practice of Ophthalmology. Vol. 1, Philadelphia, W.B. Saunders, 1994.

Fedukowicz, H.B.: External Infections of the Eye: Bacterial, Viral and Mycotic. 3rd Ed. New York, Appleton-Century-Crofts, 1984.

Fraunfelder, F.T.: Drug-Induced Ocular Side Effects and Drug Interactions. 4th Ed. Philadelphia, Williams & Wilkins, 1996.

* = most important

Meisler, D.M., et al.: An immunopathologic study of giant papillary conjunctivitis associated with an ocular prosthesis. Am. J. Ophthalmol., 92:368–371, 1981.

Mondino, B.J., et al.: Allergic and toxic reactions in soft contact lens wearers. Surv. Ophthalmol., 26:337, 1982.

Roy, F.H.: Ocular Syndromes and Systemic Diseases. 2nd Ed. Philadelphia, W.B. Saunders, 1989.

Cicatricial Conjunctivitis (Scarring of Conjunctiva)

*1. General: a post-infectious type of membranous conjunctivitis such as corynebacterium diphtheriae, streptococcal conjunctivitis, autoimmune or presumably autoimmune, sarcoidosis, scleroderma, lichen planus, atopic blepharoconjunctivitis, miscellaneous causes and linear IgA dermatosis.

2. Upper lid

   A. Trachoma

3. Lower lid

   *A. Acne rosacea (ocular rosacea)

   B. Chemical (especially alkali)

   C. Chlamydia (psittacosis-lymphogranuloma group)

   D. Chronic cicatricial conjunctivitis—occurs in the elderly; has a chronic course; may have concurrent skin and mucous membrane lesions

   *E. Congenital syphilis

   F. Dermatitis herpetiformis

   G. Epidemic keratoconjunctivitis

   H. Epidermolysis acuta toxica (Lyell syndrome)

   I. Epidermolysis bullosa

   *J. Erythema multiforme (Stevens-Johnson disease)

   K. Erythroderma ichthyosiforme

   L. Exfoliative dermatitis

   M. Fuchs-Lyell syndrome

   N. Hydroa vacciniforme

   O. Impetigo

   *P. Ocular pemphigoid

   Q. Radium burns

   R. Reiter syndrome (conjunctivourethosynovial syndrome)

   S. Sjögren syndrome (secretoinhibitor syndrome)

   T. Staphylococcal granuloma

   U. Syphilis (acquired lues)

   V. Systemic scleroderma (progressive systemic sclerosis)

   W. Vaccinia

*4. Drugs

   A. Demecarium bromide

   *B. Echothiophate iodide

   C. Idoxuridine

D. Penicillamine

E. Pilocarpine

F. Practolol

G. Thiabendazole

H. Timolol

*I. Topical ocular epinephrine

Chan, L.S., et al.: Ocular cicatricial pemphigoid occurring as a sequela of Stevens-Johnson syndrome. JAMA 266:1543–1546, 1991.

Fiore P.M., et al.: Drug-induced pemphigoid. A spectrum of diseases. Arch Ophthalmol. 105:1660–1663, 1987.

Fraunfelder, F.T.: Interim report: National registry of possible drug-induced ocular side effects. Ophthalmology, 87:88–89, 1982.

Mondino, B.J., and Brown, S. I.: Ocular cicatricial pemphigoid. Ophthalmology, 88:95, 1981.

Newell, F.W.: Ophthalmology, Principles and Concepts. 7th Ed. St. Louis, C.V. Mosby, 1991.

Angular Conjunctivitis (Inflammation at Angle of Eye, Usually Lateral)

1. Candida albicans

*2. Moraxella lacunata (Morax-Axenfeld diplobacillus)

3. Stannus cerebellar syndrome (riboflavin deficiency)

4. Staphylococcus aureus

Fedukowicz, H.B.: External Infections of the Eye: Bacterial, Viral and Mycotic. 3rd Ed. New York, Appleton-Century-Crofts, 1984.

Scheie, H.G.: Textbook of Ophthalmology. 10th Ed. Philadelphia, W.B. Saunders, 1986.

Conjunctival Disorders Associated with Dermatologic Disorders

1. Dermatoses

A. Acanthosis nigricans

B. Acne rosacea

C. Acrodermatitis chronica atrophica

D. Acrodermatitis enteropathica

*E. Atopic eczema dermatitis

F. Diffuse cutaneous mastocytosis

G. Erythroderma exfoliativa (Wilson-Brocq disease)

H. Ichthyosis

I. Keratosis follicularis

J. Keratosis follicularis spinulosa decalvans

K. Lichen planus

L. Pityriasis rubra pilaris; lichen acuminatus

M. Porokeratosis

N. Psoriasis vulgaris

O. Seborrhea

P. Xeroderma pigmentosum

* = most important

2. Mucocutaneous eruptions

    *A. Behçet disease (dermatostomato-ophthalmic syndrome)

    B. Benign mucous membrane pemphigoid

    C. Dermatitis herpetiformis (Duhring-Brocq disease)

    *D. Erythema multiforme (Stevens-Johnson disease)

    E. Epidermolysis bullosa

    F. Hydroa vacciniforme (recurrent summer eruption)

    G. Pemphigus-vulgaris, vegetans, foliaceus

    H. Pyostomatitis vegetans

    I. Reiter's disease (polyarthritis enterica)

Roy, F.H.: Ocular Syndromes and Systemic Diseases. 2nd Ed. Philadelphia, W.B. Saunders, 1989.
Wilson, L.A.: External Diseases of the Eye. Philadelphia, Harper and Row, 1979.

Conjunctival Disorders Associated With Genital Disorders

1. Bacteria

    A. Bacteroides species

    B. Calymmatobacterium granulomatis (granuloma inguinale)

    C. Escherichia coli

    D. Haemophilus ducreyi

    E. Haemophilus vaginalis

    F. Mimeae species

    G. Mycobacterium leprae

    H. Mycobacterium tuberculosis

    *I. Neisseria gonorrhoeae

    J. Proteus species

    *K. Pseudomonas aeruginosa

    L. Staphylococcus species

    M. Streptococcus species

2. Fungi

    A. Candida species

    B. Other

3. Viruses

    A. Cytomegalovirus

    *B. Herpes virus hominis 2

    *C. Molluscum contagiosum virus

    D. Rubella

    E. Varicella zoster

    F. Verruca virus

4. Spirochetes

    A. Treponema pallidum

5. Chlamydiae

    A. Chlamydia lymphogranulomatis

    *B. Chlamydia oculogenitalis

    C. Unclassified Chlamydia from Reiter disease

6. Parasites

    A. Beetles

    B. Fly larvae

    C. Moths

    D. Phthirus pubis

    E. Trichomonas vaginalis

Roy, F.H.: Ocular Syndromes and Systemic Diseases. 2nd Ed. Philadelphia, W.B. Saunders, 1989.

Vergnami, R.J., and Smith, R.S.: Reiter syndrome in a child. Arch. Ophthalmology, 91:165–166, 1974.

Congestion of Conjunctiva (Noninfectious Hyperemia of the Conjunctiva)

  *1. Acute lupus erythematosus (Kaposi-Libman-Sacks syndrome)

   2. Alcoholism

  *3. Allergic conjunctivitis such as contact with cosmetics or plastic

   4. Avitaminosis

   5. Carcinoid syndrome

  *6. Carotid-cavernous fistula or arteriovenous aneurysm

   7. Cavernous sinus thrombosis (Foix syndrome)

   8. Conjunctivitis caused by air pollution (smog, dust, and/or smoke)

  *9. Drugs causing conjunctival hyperemia, including:

acetohexamide	benzalkonium	cefoxitin
acetylcholine	benzthiazide	cefsulodin
adrenal cortex injection	betamethasone	ceftazidime
aldosterone	bupivacaine	ceftizoxime
allobarbital	butalbital	ceftriaxone
allopurinol	butallylonal	cefuroxime
alprazolam	butethal	cephalexin
alseroxylon	carbachol	cephaloglycin
amithiozone	carmustine	cephaloridine
amobarbital	cefaclor	cephalothin
antazoline	cefadroxil	cephapirin
aprobarbital	cefamandole	cephradine
aspirin	cefazolin	chloral hydrate
auranofin	cefonicid	chloramphenicol
aurothioglucose	cefoperazone	chlordiazepoxide
aurothioglycanide	ceforanide	chloroprocaine
barbital	cefotaxime	chlorothiazide
bendroflumethiazide	cefotetan	chlorpropamide

* = most important

chlortetracycline
chlorthalidone
chrysarobin
cimetidine
cisplatin
clofibrate
clonazepam
clorazepate
clindamycin
colchicine
colloidal silver
cortisone
cyclobarbital
cyclopentobarbital
cycloserine
cyclosporine
cyclothiazide
cytarabine
deferoxamine
deserpidine
desoxycorticosterone
dexamethasone
dextran
dextrothyroxine
diazepam
diacetylmorphine
diatrizoate meglumine and
    sodium
dicumarol
diethylcarbamazine
diltiazem
dimercaprol
diphenadione
diphtheria and tetanus toxoids
    and pertussis vaccine
    adsorbed
disopyramide
doxorubicin
emetine
ephedrine
erythromycin
ether
ethotoin
ethyl biscoumacetate

etidocaine
fenoprofen
fludrocortisone
fluorescein
fluprednisolone
flurazepam
flurbiprofen
glyburide
gold Au
gold sodium thiomalate
gold sodium thiosulfate
griseofulvin
halazepam
heparin
heptabarbital
hexethal
hexobarbital
hydralazine
hydrochlorothiazide
hydrocortisone
hydroflumethiazide
ibuprofen
idoxurindine
indapamide
indomethacin
interferon
iodide and iodine solutions
iothalamate meglumine and
    sodium
iothalamic acid
ketoprofen
levothyroxine
lidocaine
lincomycin
liothyronine
liotrix
lithium carbonate
lorazepam
maprotiline
measles and rubella virus
    vaccine (live)
measles virus vaccine (live)
meperidine
mephenytoin

mephobarbital
mepivacaine
meprednisone
mercuric oxide
methacholine
metharbital
methimazole
methitural
methocarbamol
methohexital
methyclothiazide
methyldopa
methylprednisolone
methylthiouracil
metolazone
metronidazole
mianserin
midazolam
minoxidil
morphine
moxalactam
mumps virus vaccine (live)
naproxen
nifedipine
nitrazepam
nitromersol
norepinephrine
opium
oxazepam
oxprenolol
oxyphenbutazone
oxyphenonium
pentazocine
pentobarbital
phenacetin
phenindione
phenobarbital
phenprocoumon
phenylbutazone
phenylephrine
phenylmercuric acetate
phenylmercuric nitrate
pilocarpine

piroxicam
polythiazide
practolol
prazepam
prazosin
prednisolone
prednisone
prilocaine
primidone
probarbital
procaine
propoxycaine
propranolol
propylthiouracil
quinethazone
radioactive iodides
ranitidine
rauwolfia serpentina
rescinnamine
reserpine
rifampin
rubella and mumps virus vaccine (live)
rubella virus vaccine (live)
secobarbital

silver nitrate
silver protein
sodium chloride
sodium salicylate
streptomycin
sulfacetamide
sulfachlorpyridazine
sulfacytine
sulfadiazine
sulfadimethoxine
sulfamerazine
sulfameter
sulfamethazine
sulfamethizole
sulfamethoxazole
sulfamethoxypyridazine
sulfanilamide
sulfaphenazole
sulfapyridine
sulfasalazine
sulfathiazole
sulfisoxazole
syrosingopine
talbutal
tamazepam

tetanus immune globulin
tetanus toxoid
tetracycline
thiamylal
thiopental
thiotepa
thimerosal
thyroglobulin
thyroid
tolazamide
tolazoline
tolbutamide
triamcinolone
triazolam
trichlormethiazide
trichloroethylene
trifluridine
vancomycin
verapamil
vidarabine
vinbarbital
vitamin A

10. Gout (hyperuricemia)

11. Hormone deficiency (estrogenic)

12. Hypothyroidism

13. Irritative follicular conjunctivitis (see p. 222)

*A. Chemical conjunctivitis because of drugs, including:

acenocoumarol
acetaminophen
acetanilid
acetohexamide
allobarbital
allopurinol
alprazolam
amobarbital
anisindione
antazoline
antipyrine
aprobarbital

aspirin
barbital
bendroflumethiazide
benzalkonium
benzthiazide
butabarbital
butalbital
butallylonal
butethal
carbamazepine
carbimazole
cefaclor

cefadroxil
cefamandole
cefazolin
cefonicid
cefoperazone
ceforanide
cefotaxime
cefotetan
cefoxitin
cefsulodin
ceftazidime
ceftizoxime

* = most important

ceftriaxone	flurazepam	moxalactam
cefuroxime	flurbiprofen	mumps virus vaccine (live)
cephalexin	halazepam	naproxen
cephaloglycin	heparin	nifedipine
cephaloridine	heptabarbital	nitrazepam
cephalothin	hexethal	opium
cephapirin	hexobarbital	oxazepam
cephradine	hydralazine	oxprenolol
chloramphenicol	hydrochlorothiazide	oxyphenbutazone
chlordiazepoxide	hydroflumethiazide	oxyphenonium
chlorothiazide	ibuprofen	pentazocine
chlorpropamide	indapamide	pentobarbital
chlortetracycline	indomethacin	phenacetin
chlorthalidone	interferon	phenindione
chrysarobin	iodide and iodine solutions	phenobarbital
cimetidine	and compounds	phenprocoumon
cisplatin	iothalamate	phenylbutazone
clofibrate	meglumine and sodium	phenylephrine
clonazepam	iothalamic acid	piroxicam
clorazepate	ketoprofen	polythiazide
colloidal silver	lithium carbonate	practolcol
cyclobarbital	lorazepam	prazepam
cyclopentobarbital	maprotiline	prazosin
cycloserine	measles and rubella virus	primidone
cyclosporine	vaccine (live)	probarbital
cyclothiazide	measles virus vaccine (live)	propranolol
cytarabine	meperidine	propylthiouracil
dextran	mephenytoin	quinethazone
diazepam	mephobarbital	radioactive iodides
dicumarol	metharbital	ranitidine
diethylcarbamazine	methimazole	rubella and mumps virus
diltiazem	methitural	vaccine (live)
dimercaprol	methocarbamol	rubella virus vaccine (live)
diphenadione	methohexital	secobarbital
diphtherian and tetanus	methyclothiazide	silver nitrate
toxoids and pertussis vaccine	methyldopa	silver protein
disopyramide	methylthiouracil	sodium salicylate
doxorubicin	metolazone	streptomycin
emetine	metronidazole	sulfacetamide
ephedrine	mianserin	sulfachlorpyridazine
ethotoin	midazolam	sulfacytine
ethyl biscoumacetate	minoxidil	sulfadiazine
fenoprofen	morphine	sulfadimethoxine

sulfamerazine	sulfathiazole	tolazamide
sulfameter	sulfisoxazole	tolbutamide
sulfamethazine	talbutal	triazolam trichlormethiazide
sulfamethizole	temezapam	trichloroethylene
sulfamethoxazole	tetanus immune globulin	verapamil
sulfamethoxypyridazine	tetanus toxoid	vinbarbital
sulfanilamide	tetracycline	vitamin A
sulfaphenazole	thiamylal	warfarin
sulfapyridine	thiopental	
sulfasalazine	thiotepa	

   B. Topical drugs that are hypotonic, hypertonic, or in which the pH is above or below 6.9, or a drug degradation causing chemical irritation

   C. Toxic conjunctivitis because of drugs, such as miotics or cycloplegics

   D. Vegetable irritants (e.g., caster bean)

*14. Malignant lymphoma

15. Ophthalmic vein thrombosis

16. Photosensitive conjunctivitis

*17. Polycythemia vera (Vaquez disease)

18. Sjögren syndrome (Secretoinhibitor syndrome)

19. Vascular changes

   A. Facial paralysis (see p. 75)

   *B. Hereditary hemorrhagic telangiectasis (Rendu-Osler-Weber disease)

   C. Petechial hemorrhage of conjunctiva (see p. 238)

Collins, J.F.: Handbook of Clinical Ophthalmol, New York, Masson, 1982.

Fraunfelder, F.T.: Drug-Induced Ocular Side Effects and Drug Interactions. 4th Ed. Philadelphia, Williams & Wilkins, 1996.

Ciliary Flush (Circumcorneal Congestion) (Congestion of Ciliary Vessels Immediately Surrounding the Cornea; Individual Vessels Are Not Seen; Color Is Violaceous; Redness Fades toward the Fornices; and Vessels Do Not Move with Conjunctiva)

   1. Corneal disease, such as with inflammations and erosions

   2. Glaucoma, especially acute glaucoma

   3. Iridocyclitis

   4. Iris irritation, such as with corneal foreign bodies

   5. Iritis

Vaughan, D., et al.: General Ophthalmology. 14th Ed. Los Altos, Ca., Lange Medical Publishers, 1995.

Conjunctival Aneurysms, Varicosities, Tortuosities, and Telangiectasis

   1. Local causes

      *A. Acne rosacea

       B. Chronic congestive glaucoma

       C. Delayed mustard gas keratitis

    D. Idiopathic anomaly

    E. Irradiation of the eye

    F. Long-standing ocular inflammation

  *G. Metastatic primary tumor

  *H. Pterygium

  *I. Underlying choroidal or ciliary body melanomas

2. Systemic causes

    A. AIDS

    B. Arteriosclerosis

    C. Associated with familial amyloidotic polyneuropathy, type 1

    D. Ataxic telangiectasia (Louis-Bar syndrome)

  *E. Degos syndrome (malignant atrophic papulosis)

    F. Diabetes

    G. Dysproteinemia as Waldenstrom macroglobulinemia, cryoglobulinemia, and multiple myeloma

    H. Endangitis obliterans

    I. Fabry disease (diffuse angiokeratosis)

    J. Hereditary hemorrhagic telangiectasia (Rendu-Osler-Weber disease)

    K. Hypertension

    L. Klippel-Trenaunay-Weber syndrome (angioosteohypertrophy syndrome)

    M. Normal individuals

  *N. Pulmonary insufficiency

    O. Reimann syndrome (hyperviscosity syndrome)

    P. Renal failure

    Q. Rheumatic fever or rheumatic heart disease

    R. Scleroderma (progressive systemic sclerosis)

    S. Sturge-Weber syndrome (meningocutaneous syndrome)

  *T. Syphilis (acquired lues)

    U. Varicose veins—generalized

Ando, E., et al.: Ocular microangiopathy in familial amyloidotic polyneuropathy, type 1. Graefes Archive for Clinical and Experimental Ophthalmol 230: 1–5, 1992.

Baumann, S., et al.: Conjunctival microvasculopathy and Kaposi's sarcoma in patients with AIDS. AIDS, 8:134–135, 1994.

Roy, F.H.: Ocular Syndromes and Systemic Diseases. 2nd Ed. Philadelphia, W.B. Saunders, 1989.

Conjunctival Sludging and Segmentation

1. Local

    A. Aging

    B. Hypothermia

    C. Sympathetic irritation

    D. Vasodilator drugs that are applied locally

2. Systemic or hyperviscosity with increase in serum proteins—erythrocyte sedimentation rate is usually above mm in first hour

    A. Cryoglobulinemia

    B. Hyperglobulinemia

    C. Hypertension

    D. Macroglobulinemia (Waldenström syndrome)

    *E. Multiple myeloma (Kahler disease)

    *F. Sickle-cell disease (Herrick syndrome)

Lu, L.M., et al.: Sjögren's Syndrome and Benign Hyperglobulinemic Purpura of Waldenstrom. Ann. Ophthalmol., 13:1285–1287, 1981.

Maisel, J.M., et al.: Multiple Myeloma Presenting with Ocular Inflammation. Ann. Ophthalmol., 19:170–174, 1987.

Roy, F.H.: Ocular Syndromes and Systemic Diseases. 2nd Ed. Philadelphia, W.B. Saunders, 1989.

Conjunctival Edema (Chemosis)

1. Acquired blockage of orbital lymphatics following orbital surgery (lateral orbitotomy) or because of erysipelas or lymphogranuloma venereum

*2. Chronic hereditary lymphedema (Nonne-Milroy-Meige disease)

*3. Drugs, including:

acetohexamide	bleomycin
acetophenazine	bupivacaine
actinomycin C	butabarbital
adrenal cortex injection	butalbital
albuterol	butallylonal
aldosterone	butaperazine
allobarbital	butethal
aminopterin	cactinomycin
aminosalicylate	captopril
aminosalicylic acid	carbamazepine
amobarbital	carbenicillin
antimony lithium thiomalate	carphenazine
antimony potassium tartrate	cefaclor
antimony sodium tartrate	cefadroxil
antimony sodium thioglycollate	cefamandole
antipyrine	cefazolin
aprobarbital	cefonicid
aspirin	cefoperazone
auranofin	ceforanide
aurothioglucose	cefotaxime
aurothioglycanide	cefotetan
barbital	cefoxitin
betamethasone	cefsulodin

* = most important

ceftazidime	doxepin
ceftizoxime	doxorubicin
ceftriaxone	doxycycline
cefuroxime	dromostanolone
cephalexin	echothiophate
cephaloglycin	emetine
cephaloridine	enalapril
cephalothin	ergonovine
cephapirin	ergotamine
cephradine	ethopropazine
chlorisondamine	etidocaine
chloral hydrate	etretinate
chlorambucil	floxuridine
chloroprocaine	fludrocortisone
chlorpromazine	fluorouracil
chlorpropamide	fluoxymesterone
chlortetracycline	fluphenazine
chrysarobin	fluprednisolone
cisplatin	F3T
clofibrate	glyburide
clomipramine	gold Au 198
cloxacillin	gold sodium thiomalate
colloidal silver	griseofulvin
cortisone	heptabarbital
cyclobarbital	hetacillin
cyclopentobarbital	hexamethonium
cyproheptadine	hexethal
dactinomycin	hexobarbital
danazol	hydrabamine penicillin
dapsone	hydralazine
daunorubicin	hydrocortisone
demecarium	ibuprofen
demeclocycline	idoxuridine
desipramine	imipramine
desoxycorticosterone	iodide and iodine solutions and compounds
dexamethasone	iron dextran
dextrothyroxine	isoflurophate
diacetylmorphine	isosorbide
diatrizoate meglumine and sodium	isotretinoin
dicloxacillin	ketoprofen
diethazine	levodopa
diethylcarbamazine	levothyroxine
dionin	lidocaine

lithium carbonate
mannitol
maprotiline
mecamylamine
medrysone
mephobarbital
mepivacaine
meprednisone
mercuric oxide
mesoridazine
metharbital
methdilazine
methitural
methohexital
methotrimeprazine
methyldopa
methylergonovine
methylpentynol
methylprednisolone
methysergide
metoclopramide
metrizamide
metronidazole
mianserin
minocycline
mitomycin
moxalactam
mild silver protein
nafcillin
naproxen
nitromersol
nortriptyline
oral contraceptives
oxacillin
oxprenolol
oxyphenbutazone
oxytetracycline
paramethasone
pentobarbital
pentolinium
perazine
pericyazine
perphenazine

phenazine
phenobarbital
phenylbutazone
piperacetazine
piperazine
pipobroman
poliovirus vaccine
potassium penicillin G
potassium penicillin V
potassium phenethicillin
practolol
prazosin
prednisolone
prednisone
prilocaine
primidone
procaine
probarbital
prochlorperazine
promazine
promethazine
propiomazine
propoxycaine
protriptyline
quinacrine
radioactive iodides
rifampin
rubella virus vaccine (live)
sanguinarine
secobarbital
silver nitrate
silver protein
sodium antimonylgluconate
sodium salicylate
stibocaptate
stibophen
streptomycin
succinylcholine
sulindac
suramin
talbutal
tetracycline
testolactone

testosterone	tolbutamide
tetraethylammonium	triamcinolone
thiamylal	trifluoperazine
thiethylperazine	triflupromazine
thiopental	trimeprazine
thiopropazate	trimethaphan
thioproperazine	trimethidinium
thioridazine	vidarabine
thyroid	vinbarbital
tolazamide	

4. Glandular fever

5. Hypersensitivity—local topical allergies

*6. Increased bulk of orbital contents—orbital tumors, cysts, or endocrine exophthalmos

7. Local inflammatory conditions

    *A. Cerebral cavity—acute meningitis

    *B. Eye—viral conjunctivitis, corneal ulcer, fulminating iritis, or panophthalmitis

    C. Lacrimal passages—dacryocystitis

    D. Lids—styes, vaccinia, acute meibomitis, insect bites, or vaccinal pocks

    E. Nasal cavity—sinusitis

    *F. Orbit—cellulitis, periostitis, dacryoadenitis, tenonitis

8. Myxedema—infiltration with mucopolysaccharides

9. Reduced plasma protein level—nephrotic state

10. Systemic lupus erythematosus

*11. Vasomotor instability—angioneurotic edema or premenstrual phase of water retention

12. Venous congestion—local obstruction of orbital apex, carotid—cavernous fistula, thrombosis of cavernous sinus, or right-sided heart failure

13. Whipple's disease

Disdier, P., et al.: Chemosis associated with Whipple's disease. Am J Ophthalmol. 112:217–219, 1991.

Fraunfelder, F.T.: Drug-Induced Ocular Side Effects and Drug Interactions. 4th Ed. Philadelphia, Williams & Wilkins. 1996.

Leahey, A.B., et al.: Chemosis as a presenting sign of systemic lupus erythematosus. Arch Ophthalmol. 110:609–610, 1992.

Conjunctival Xerosis (Dryness of Conjunctiva)

1. Absence of blinking

2. Drugs including:

acebutolol(?)	chlorambucil	ketoprofen
amiodarone	clonidine(?)	labetalol(?)
atenolol(?)	cyclophosphamide	levobunolol
betaxolol	doxepin	methyldopa
busulfan	ibuprofen	metoprolol(?)

nadolol(?)	practolol	sulindac
naproxen(?)	primidone	thiabendazole
oxprenolol(?)	propoxyphene	timolol
perhexiline	propanolol(?)	vinblastine(?)
pindolol(?)	quinidine	

3. Following cicatricial conjunctivitis (see p. 224)

4. Illness or coma

*5. Lack of closure of lids in sleep

6. Result of exposure of conjunctiva to air

    A. Deficient closure of lids, such as with paralysis of orbicularis, as part of facial palsy, spasms of the levator or ectropion

    B. Excessive proptosis, such as in exophthalmic goiter or orbital tumor

*7. Vitamin A deficiency

    A. Dietary deficiencies, including malnutrition, cystic fibrosis, anorexia nervosa and bulimia

    B. Digestive tract disorders

      (1) Colitis and enteritis

     *(2) In pancreas—chronic pancreatitis

      (3) In stomach—achlorhydria, chronic gastritis or diarrhea, peptic ulcer

    C. Hookworm disease

   *D. Liver disease, such as chronic cirrhosis

    E. Malaria

    F. Pregnancy

    G. Pulmonary tuberculosis

    H. Skin disorders, such as pityriasis rubra pilaris

   *I. Thyroid gland disorder, such as hyperthyroidism

    J. Uyemura syndrome (fundus albipunctatus with hemeralopia and xerosis)

8. Decrease tear production

    A. Congenital alacrima

    B. Keratoconjunctivitis sicca

    C. Riley-Day syndrome (familial dysautonomia)

    D. Sjögren's syndrome

    E. Surgical excision of the lacrimal and accessory lacrimal glands

    F. X-irradiation of the lacrimal gland

9. Following x-irradiation of the conjunctiva

Fraunfelder, F.T.: Drug-Induced Ocular Side Effects and Drug Interactions. 4th Ed. Philadelphia, Williams & Wilkins, 1996.

Gilbert, J.M., et al.: Ocular manifestations and impression cytology of anorexia nervosa. Ophthalmology, 97:1001, 1990.

Newell, F.W.: Ophthalmology, Principles and Concepts. 7th Ed. St. Louis, C.V. Mosby, 1991.

Roy, F.H.: Ocular Syndromes and Systemic Diseases. 2nd Ed. Philadelphia, W.B. Saunders, 1989.

* = most important

Bitot Spots (Small Gray or White Sharply Outlined Areas, Cheeselike or Foamy, Occurring on Either Side of Limbus but Especially in Temporal Area)

1. Associated with coloboma of lid (see p. 114)
2. Associated with corectopia, nystagmus, and absent foveal reflexes
3. Associated with Rieger anomaly
4. Congenital anomaly
5. Corneal snowflake dystrophy
6. Exposure
7. Idiopathic
*8. Keratosis follicularis (Darier-White disease) associated with retinitis pigmentosa
9. Pellagra or other poor nutritional states
10. Vitamin A deficiency

Daicker, B.: Ocular involvement in keratosis follicularis associated with retinitis pigmentosa. Ophthalmologica, 209:47–51, 1995.

de Keizer, R.J.: Conjunctival xerosis, arcus lipoides and Rieger's disease. Documenta Ophthalmologica, 78:365–371, 1991.

Subconjunctival Hemorrhage (Blood under Conjunctiva)

1. Acute febrile systemic infections
   A. Bacteria, such as those responsible for meningococcal septicemia, subacute bacterial endocarditis, scarlet fever, diphtheria, typhoid fever, or cholera
   B. Parasites, such as plasmodia (malaria)
   C. Rickettsia, such as those causing typhus fever
   D. Unknown infective agents, such as those causing glandular fever
   E. Viruses, such as those responsible for influenza, smallpox, measles, yellow fever, or sandfly fever
2. Associated with use of drugs, including:

acetylcholine	bismuth subcarbonate
acid bismuth sodium tartrate	bismuth subsalicylate
adrenal cortex injection	butacaine
aldosterone	cobalt(?)
allopurinol	cocaine
alseroxylon	cortisone
aspirin	deserpidine
benoxinate	desoxycorticosterone
betamethasone	dexamethasone
bismuth carbonate	dibucaine
bismuth oxychloride	dyclonine
bismuth salicylate	epinephrine
bismuth sodium tartrate	ethambutol
bismuth sodium thioglycollate	fludrocortisone
bismuth sodium triglycollamate	fluorometholone

fluorouracil

fluprednisolone

glycerin

heparin

hexachlorophene

hydrocortisone

indomethacin(?)

iodide and iodine solutions and compounds(?)

isosorbide

ketoprofen

lincomycin

mannitol

medrysone

meprednisone

methaqualone

methylphenidate

methylprednisolone

mithramycin

mitotane

oxyphenbutazone

paramethasone

penicillamine

phenacaine

phenylbutazone

piperocaine

plicamycin

pralidoxime

prednisolone

prednisone

proparacaine

radioactive iodides(?)

rauwolfia serpentina

rescinnamine

reserpine

sodium chloride

sodium salicylate

sulfacetamide

sulfachlorpyridazine

sulfadiazine

sulfadimethoxine

sulfamerazine

sulfameter

sulfamethazine

sulfamethizole

sulfamethoxazole

sulfamethoxypyridazine

sulfanilamide

sulfaphenazole

sulfapyridine

sulfasalazine

sulfathiazole

sulfisoxazole

sulindac

syrosingopine

tamoxifen

tetracaine

triamcinolone

trichloroethylene

urea

urokinase(?)

3. Blood dyscrasias

    A. Associated with thrombocytopenia

        *(1) Anemias, especially, aplastic anemia

        *(2) Drugs, including:

acenocoumarin

acetaminophen

acetanilid

acetazolamide

acetohexamide

acetophenazine

actinomycin C

allobarbital

allopurinol

aminopterin

aminosalicylic acid(?)

amithiozone

amitriptyline

amobarbital

* = most important

amodiaquine

amphotericin B

ampicillin

anisindione

antimony lithium thiomalate

antimony potassium tartrate

antimony sodium thioglycollate

antipyrine

aprobarbital

aurothioglucose

aurothioglycanide

azathioprine

barbital

bendroflumethiazide

benzathine penicillin G

benzthiazide

bishydroxycoumarin

bleomycin

brompheniramine

busulfan

butabarbital

butalbital

butallylonal

butaperazine

butethal

carbamazepine

carbenicillin

carbimazole

carbinoxamine

carisoprodol

carphenazine

cefazolin

cephalexin

cephaloglycin

cephaloridine

cephalothin

chlorambucil

chloramphenicol

chlordiazepoxide

chloroquine

chlorothiazide

chlorpheniramine

chlorpromazine

chlorpropamide

chlorprothixene

chlortetracycline

chlorthalidone

clindamycin

cloxacillin

colchicine

cyclobarbital

cyclophosphamide

cycloserine

cyclothiazide

cyproheptadine

cytarabine

dactinomycin

deferoxamine

demeclocycline

desipramine

dexbrompheniramine

dexchlorpheniramine

diazepam

dichlorphenamide

dicloxacillin

diethazine

dimethindene

diphenadione

diphenhydramine

diphenylhydantoin

diphenylpyraline

doxycycline

dromostanolone

droperidol

erythromycin

ethacrynic acid

ethopropazine

ethosuximide

ethotoin

ethoxzolamide

floxuridine

fluorouracil

fluoxymesterone

fluphenazine

flurazepam

furosemide

gentamicin

glutethimide

gold Au 198

gold sodium thiomalate

griseofulvin

guanethidine

haloperidol

heparin

heptabarbital

hetacillin

hexethal

hexobarbital

hydralazine

hydrabamine phenoxymethyl penicillin

hydrochlorothiazide

hydroflumethiazide

hydroxychloroquine

hydroxyurea

imipramine

indomethacin

isoniazid

levodopa

lincomycin

measles virus vaccine

mechlorethamine

mefenamic acid

melphalan

mephenytoin

mephobarbital

meprobamate

mercaptopurine

mesoridazine

methacycline

methaqualone

metharbital

methazolamide

methdilazine

methicillin

methimazole

methitural

methohexital

methotrimeprazine

methotrexate

methsuximide

methyclothiazide

methyldopa

methylene blue

methylphenidate

methylthiouracil

methyprylon

minocycline

nafcillin

nalidixic acid

nitrofurantoin

nitroglycerin

nortriptyline

oral contraceptives

orphenadrine

oxacillin

oxyphenbutazone

oxytetracycline

paramethadione

penicillamine

pentobarbital

perazine

pericyazine

perphenazine

phenacetin

phenformin

phenindione

phenobarbital

phenoxymethyl

penicillin

phenprocoumon

phensuximide	tetracycline
phenylbutazone	thiabendazole
piperacetazine	thiamylal
pipobroman	thiethylperazine
polythiazide	thioguanine
potassium penicillin G	thiopental
potassium penicillin V	thiopropazate
potassium phenethicillin	thioproperazine
potassium phenoxymethyl penicillin	thioridazine
primidone	thiotepa
probarbital	thiothixene
procaine penicillin G	tolazamide
procarbazine	tolbutamide
prochlorperazine	trichlormethiazide
promazine	triethylenemelamine
promethazine	trifluoperazine
propiomazine	trifluperidol
propylthiouracil	triflupromazine
protriptyline	trimeprazine
pyrimethamine	trimethadione
quinacrine	tripelennamine
quinidine	uracil mustard
quinine	urethan
secobarbital	vancomycin
sodium antimonylgluconate	vinbarbital
stibocaptate	vinblastine
stibophen	vincristine
streptomycin	vitamin A
sulfonamides	vitamin D
talbutal	vitamin D_2
testolactone	vitamin D_3
testosterone	warfarin

        *(3) Leukemia

        (4) Septicemias

        (5) Splenic disorders, such as Banti or Gaucher disease, Felty syndrome, and hemolytic icterus

        *(6) Systemic lupus erythematosus (Kaposi-Libman-Sacks syndrome)

    B. Ehlers-Danlos syndrome (fibrodysplasia elastica generalisata)

    C. Hemochromatosis

    D. Schomberg disease

E. Scurvy (avitaminosis C)

F. Secondary, such as that because of nephritic, cardiac, or hepatic disease

G. Thrombocytopenia purpura

4. Fragility of vessel walls because of systemic vascular disease

    A. Age

    B. Arteriosclerosis

    C. Diabetes

    D. Hypertension

    E. Nephritis

5. Gravity inversion

6. Injury to orbital or adjacent structures, such as sinus, basal skull fracture, subarachnoid hemorrhage

7. Local acute inflammation, including, acute pneumococcal conjunctivitis, leptospirosis ictero-hemorrhagica, epidemic typhus, and scrub typhus

8. Local trauma, including surgical trauma

9. Remote injury associated with fractured bones and fat emboli following angiography or open heart operation causing "splinter" subconjunctival hemorrhage

10. Spontaneous during menstruation

11. Spontaneous rupture of telangiectasis, varicosities, aneurysm, or angiomatous tumor (see p. 567)

*12. Sudden severe venous congestion of head, including that because of coughing, vomiting, epileptic fit, strangulation, or an orbital tumor (neuroblastoma)

13. Without apparent cause—most common

Fraunfelder, F.T.: Drug-Induced Ocular Side Effects and Drug Interactions. 4th Ed. Philadelphia, Williams & Wilkins, 1996.

Friberg, T.R., and Weinreb, R.N.: Ocular Manifestations of Gravity Inversion. J.A.M.A., 253, 1985.

Tasman, W. and Jaeger, E., eds.: Duane's Clinical Ophthalmology. Philadelphia, J.B. Lippincott, 1990.

Werblin, T.P. and Peiffer, R.L.: Persistent hemorrhage after extracapsular surgery associated with excessive aspirin ingestion. Am. J. Ophthalmol., 104:426, 1987.

Tumors of the Conjunctiva

1. Epithelial tumors

    A. Kerato-acanthoma

    B. Dyskeratosis

        (1) Epithelial plaques—leukoplakia, hereditary benign intraepithelial dyskeratosis

        (2) Intraepithelial epithelioma (Bowen disease)

    *C. Papilloma—including virus type 16

    D. Epithelioma

    E. Adenoma

        (1) Papillary cystadenoma lymphomatosum (Warthin tumor)

        (2) Oncocytoma (oxyphil-cell adenoma)

        (3) Pleomorphic adenoma of Krause glands

* = most important

2. Mesoblastic tumors

    A. Inflammatory hyperplasias

        (1) Granuloma

        (2) Plasmoma

    B. Connective tissue tumors

        (1) Fibroma

        (2) Lipoma

        (3) Myxoma

3. The reticuloses

    *A. Lymphoma

    B. Lymphosarcoma

    *C. Mycosis fungoides

4. Vascular tumors—angiomas

    A. Polymorphous hemangioma, telangiectatic granuloma, granuloma pyo-
genicum

    B. Lymphangioma

    C. Angiosarcoma monomorphous angioma, Kaposi (hemorrhagic) sarcoma

5. Pigmented tumors

    *A. Nevus

    B. Malignant melanoma

    C. Intraepithelial melanoma-precancerous melanosis

6. Peripheral nerve tumors

    A. Neurofibroma

        *(1) Neurilemmoma (neurinoma, schwannoma)

        (2) Malignant schwannoma (neurogenic sarcoma; neurofibrosarcoma)

        (3) Plexiform neurofibromatosis

    B. Tuberous sclerosis (Bourneville disease)

    *C. Intrascleral nerve loops

7. Amyloidosis

Grossniklaus, H.E., et al.: Hemangiopericytoma of the conjunctiva. Ophthalmology, 93:265–267, 1986.

Marsh, W.M., et al.: Localized conjunctival with amyloidosis associated with extranodal lymphoma. Ophthalmology, 94:61–64, 1987.

Odrich, M.G., et al.: A spectrum of bilateral squamous conjunctival tumors associated with the human papillomavirus type 16. Ophthalmology, 98:628–635, 1991.

Peter, J., and Hidayat, A.A.: Myxomas of the conjunctiva. Am. J. Ophthalmol., 102:80–86, 1986.

Sagerman, R.H., and Abramson, D.H.: Tumors of the Eye & Ocular Adnexae. New York, Pergamon Press, 1982.

Winward, K.E., and Curtin, V.T.: Conjunctival squamous cell carcinoma in a patient with human immunodeficiency virus infection. Am. J. Ophthalmol., 554–556, 1989.

Conjunctival Cysts

    1. Congenital corneoscleral cyst (rare)

    2. Epibulbar dermoids with cystic form

*3. Epithelial cyst

    A. Apposition of folds of conjunctival mucosa (common)

    *B. Downgrowth of epithelium—chronic inflammatory conditions, such as that following inflammation of pterygium

    C. Glandular retention—involvement of Krause glands in chronic inflammatory conditions, including trachoma and pemphigus

    D. Pigmented cyst appearing after prolonged topical use of cocaine or epinephrine

4. Limbal wounds with iris prolapse

5. Lymphatic cyst

*6. Muscle inclusion cyst/complication of strabismus surgery

7. Parasitic cyst such as filarial cyst

8. Traumatic cyst (epithelial implantation)

Cibis, G.W., and Waeltermann, J.M.: Muscle inclusion cyst as a complication of strabismus surgery. Am. J. Ophthalmol., 100:740–741, 1985.

Jahnle, R.L., et al.: Conjunctival inclusion cyst simulating malignant melanoma. Am. I. Ophthalmol., 100:483–484, 1985.

Soong, H. K., et al.: Corneal astigmatism from conjunctival cysts. Am. J. Ophthalmol., 93:118, 1982.

Limbal Mass

1. Allergic reaction

    *A. Phlyctenules

    B. Vernal limbal lesions

2. Amyloid—perilimbal

3. Associated with skin disease

    *A. Acne rosacea (ocular rosacea)

    B. Hereditary benign intraepithelial dyskeratosis

    *C. Hodgkin disease

    D. Limbal squamous carcinoma in xeroderma pigmentosa

    E. Pityriasis rubra pilaris

    F. Psoriasis (psoriasis vulgaris)

    *G. Reticulum cell sarcoma—raised, pink, smooth lesions

4. Benign nodular fascitis

*5. Dermoids

6. Ectopic lacrimal gland tissue

7. Epithelial hyperplasia

8. Fibrous histiocytoma

9. Granulomas

10. Hemangioma

11. Intraepithelial epitheliomas (Bowen disease)

12. Lymphomas

13. Malignant melanomas

* = most important

14. Mononucleosis (infectious)

*15. Nevi

16. Papillomas

17. Pterygia

18. Sarcomas

19. Salmon patch associated with relapsing polychondritis

20. Squamous cell carcinoma

21. Subconjunctival nodules associated with Crohn's disease

22. Synthetic fiber granuloma

Ferry, A.P.: Synthetic fiber granuloma 'Teddy Bear' granuloma of the conjunctiva. Arch. Ophthalmol. 112:1339–1341, 1994.

Grewal, R.K., et al.: Subconjunctival nodules: an unusual ocular complication of Crohn's disease. Cand J Ophthalmol. 29:238–239, 1994.

Tucker, S.M., et al.: Relapsing polychondritis, another cause for a "salmon patch." Ann. Ophthalmol. 25:338–391, 1993.

Urback, S.F.: Infectious mononucleosis presenting as a unilateral conjunctival tumor. Acta Ophthalmologica, 72:133–135, 1993.

Large, Flat, Fleshy Lesions of Palpebral Conjunctiva

1. Accidental or surgical injuries

2. Carthy disease (pyorhinoblepharostomatitis vegetans)

*3. Chalazion

*4. Embryonal rhabdomyosarcoma of children

*5. Granuloma pyogenicum

6. Ligneous conjunctivitis

7. Lymphogranuloma venerun

8. Myopic infection

9. Papillary hyperplasia of vernal conjunctivitis

*10. Syphilis

11. Tuberculosis

12. Tularemia

Friedman, A.H., and Henkind, P.: Granuloma pyogenicum of the palpebral conjunctiva. Am. J. Ophthalmol., 71:868–872, 1971.

Pau, H.: Differential Diagnosis of Eye Diseases. 2nd Ed. New York, Thieme Med. Pub., 1988.

Chronic or Recurrent Ulcers of the Conjunctiva

1. Behcet's disease

2. Crohn's disease

3. Drugs including:

allopurinol	ferrous fumarate
amphotericin B	ferrous gluconate
ferrocholinate	ferrous succinate

ferrous sulfate   iron sorbitex

floxuridine   phenytoin

fluorouracil   polysaccharide-iron complex

iron dextran

4. Fungi

*5. Herpes simplex

6. Mucous membrane pemphigoid

7. Pseudomonas ulcer in patients with AIDS

8. Soft chancre

*9. Syphilis (acquired lues)

10. Tuberculosis

11. Wegener's granulomatosis

Fraunfelder, F.T.: Drug-Induced Ocular Side Effects and Drug Interactions. 4th Ed. Philadelphia, Williams & Wilkins, 1996.

Fraunfelder, F.T., and Roy, F.H.: Current Ocular Therapy. 4th Ed. Philadelphia, W.B. Saunders, 1995.

Hegab, S.M., et al.: Conjunctival ulcer in patients with Crohn's disease. Ophthalmic Surgery, 25:638–639, 1994.

Jordan, D.R., et al.: Wegener's granulomatosis. Eyelid and conjunctival manifestations as the presenting feature in two individuals. Ophthalmology 101:602–607, 1994.

Phlyctenular Keratoconjunctivitis (Localized Conjunctival, Limbal, or Corneal Nodule about One to Three Millimeters in Size)

*1. Delayed hypersensitivity to bacterial protein, particularly tuberculoprotein and staphylococci; lymphopathia venereum and coccidioidomycosis may also be allergens

2. Malnutrition

3. Secondary infection of the conjunctiva, especially from Staphylococcus aureus, pneumococcus, and Koch-Weeks bacillus

4. Systemic infection

    A. Bang disease (Brucellosis)

    B. Candidiasis

    C. Neurodermatitis

    D. Mikulicz-Radecki syndrome (dacryosialoadenopathy)

    E. Trachoma

    F. Sjögren syndrome (secretoinhibitor syndrome)

Davis, P.L., and Watson, J.I.: Experimental conjunctival phlyctenulosis. Canad. J. Ophthalmol., 4:183–190, 1969.

Newell, F.W.: Ophthalmology, Principles and Concepts. 7th Ed. St. Louis, C.V. Mosby, 1991.

Pigmentation of the Conjunctiva (See Pigment Spots of Sclera and Episclera, p. 269)

1. Blood pigment

    *A. After subconjunctival hemorrhage—red or later fine brown spots (see p. 238)

    B. Yellow tinge of malaria, blackwater fever, or yellow fever

* = most important

C. Pigmentary limbal ring associated with senile, traumatic, or diseased conditions

2. Bile pigments (yellow)—obstructive or hemorrhagic jaundice

3. Melanin pigmentation

    A. Acanthosis nigricans

  *B. Addison disease (adrenal cortical insufficiency)

    C. Chlorpromazine (Thorazine)

    D. Endogenous ochronosis

    E. Keratomalacia

    F. Trachoma

  *G. Use of epinephrine, or epinephrine bitartrate, borate, and hydrochloride

    H. Vernal conjunctivitis

    I. Vitiligo (leukoderma)—increased conjunctival pigmentation

    J. Xeroderma pigmentosum

4. Drugs, including:

acid bismuth sodium tartrate	ferrous gluconate
alcian blue	ferrous succinate
antimony lithium thiomalate	ferrous sulfate
antimony potassium tartrate	fluorescein
antimony sodium tartrate	iron dextran
antimony sodium thioglycollate	iron sorbital
antipyrine	methylene blue
bismuth carbonate(?)	polysaccharide iron complex
bismuth oxychloride(?)	quinacrine
bismuth salicylate(?)	rose bengal
bismuth sodium thioglycollate (?)	sodium antimonylgluconate
bismuth sodium triglycollamate(?)	stibocaptate
chrysarobin	stibophen
ferrocholinate	tetracycline
ferrous fumarate	

5. Foreign substances such as silver (argyrosis), iron (siderosis), copper (chalcosis), arsenic (arsenic melanosis), gold (chrysiasis), quinones, aniline dyes and eye cosmetics containing carbon black

*6. Benign melanosis—overactivity of melanocytes

    A. Epithelial—congenital or acquired, e.g., following radiation or use of chemicals (arsenic); in Addison disease; because of chronic conjunctivitis (trachoma, vernal conjunctivitis, onchocerciasis, keratomalacia)

    B. Subepithelial—congenital or in association with melanosis oculi or nevus of Ota

7. Neoplasms

  *A. Nevus—most common in children, localized stationary, elevated, cystic, may or may not have pigmentation

*B. Malignant melanoma arising from pre-existing nevus, apparently normal conjunctiva, or from an area of acquired pigmentation (intraepithelial melanoma), middle age, diffuse, flat, pigmentation, progressive, no cysts

C. Secondary melanotic tumors

D. Incidentally pigmented tumors, such as a melanocarcinoma

Brothers, D.M., and Hidayat, A. A.: Conjunctival pigmentation associated with tetracycline medication. Ophthalmology, 88:1212, 1980.

Fraunfelder, F.T.: Drug-Induced Ocular Side Effects and Drug Interactions. Philadelphia, Williams & Wilkins 1996.

Roy, F.H.: Ocular Syndromes and Systemic Diseases. 2nd Ed. Philadelphia, W.B. Saunders, 1989.

Verdaguea, J., et al.: Melanocytoma of the conjunctiva. Arch. Ophthalmol., 91:363–366, 1974.

Discoloration of Conjunctiva

1. Red

   A. Subconjunctival hemorrhage

2. Yellow

   A. Bilirubinemia—obstructive or hemorrhagic jaundice

   B. Picric acid

   C. Leptospirosis

   D. Brucellosis (Barg disease or Mediterranean fever)

   E. Aromatic nitro and amino compounds

   F. Conjunctival fat—elderly and negro patients

   G. Blood pigment tinge of malaria, blackwater fever, and yellow fever

3. Gray (black)

   *A. Argyrosis (silver)

   B. Drugs, including:

   atabrine   phenols
   acetyomilid   specifically phenylic acid and carbon disulfide
   nitrochlorobenzine

   C. Chrysiasis (gold)—gray-green effect

   D. Arsenicals—ash-white

   E. Mascara

4. Brown

   A. Subconjunctival hemorrhage—fine brown spots

   B. Pigmentary limbal ring associated with senile traumatic, or diseased conditions

   *C. Benign melanosis—overactivity of melanocytes

      (1) Epithelial—congenital or acquired, following radiation or use of chemicals (arsenic); in Addison disease (adrenal cortical insufficiency); because of chronic conjunctivitis (trachoma, vernal conjunctivitis, onchocerciasis, keratomalacia)

      (2) Subepithelial—congenital or in association with melanosis oculi or nevus of Ota

* = most important

D. Neoplasms

*(1) Nevus—most common in children, localized, stationary, elevated, cystic, may or may not have pigmentation

*(2) Malignant melanoma arising from pre-existing nevus, apparently normal conjunctiva, or from an area of acquired pigmentation (intraepithelial melanoma), middle age, diffuse, flat, pigmentation, progressive, no cysts

E. Drugs, including:

phenothiazines
anilquinoline
combinations (benzoquinone
   paraquinone hydroquinone)
phenol derivatives

aniline dyes
bromides
chromic acid and chromates
sympathomimetics (adrenalin, Eppy)

F. Metabolic or vitamin disturbance, including alkaptonuria

5. Blue pigmentation

A. Ink tattoo from pens

B. Manganese dust

Roy, F.H.: Ocular Syndromes and Systemic Diseases. 2nd Ed. Philadelphia, W.B. Saunders, 1989.

Symblepharon (Fusing of Eyelid to Opposing Surface, Such as Tarsal and Bulbar Conjunctiva)

1. Physical trauma with denuded epithelium, including purulent, membranous, bullous, or ulcerative conjunctivitis and trauma

*2. Chemical burns—especially lime or caustic burns

*3. Inflammation—especially from drug reactions, including:

allobarbital	dipivefrin	penicillamine
amobarbital	echothiophate	pentobarbital
aprobarbital	epinephrine	phenobarbital
auranofin	F3T	phenylbutazone
aurothioglucose	gold Au 198	pilocarpine
aurothioglycanide	gold sodium thiomalate	primidone
barbital	heptabarbital	probarbital
benzalkonium	hexethal	secobarbital
butabarbital	hexobarbital	silver nitrate
butalbital	idoxuridine	silver protein
butallylonal	isoflurophate	sulfacetamide
butethal	mephobarbital	sulfachlorpyridazine
carbachol(?)	metharbital	sulfacytine
clonidine(?)	methitural	sulfadiazine
colloidal silver	methohexital	sulfadimethoxine
cyclobarbital	mild silver protein	sulfamerazine
demecarium	oxyphenbutazone	sulfameter

sulfamethizole   sulfasalazine   timolol
sulfamethoxazole   sulfathiazole   trifluridine
sulfamethoxypyridazine sulfisoxazole   vidarabine
sulfanilamide   talbutal(?)   vinbarbital(?)
sulfaphenazole   thiamylal
sulfapyridine   thiopental(?)

    A. Pemphigus (Cazenave disease)

    B. Stevens-Johnson disease (dermatostomatitis)

4. Longstanding acute inflammation

5. Congenital

6. Associated with cyanoacrylate tissue adhesive

Fraunfelder, F.T.: Drug-Induced Ocular Side Effects and Drug Interactions. 4th Ed. Philadelphia, Williams & Wilkins, 1996.

Leahey, A.B., and Gottsch, J.D.: Symblepharon associated with cyanoacrylate tissue adhesive. Amer. J. Ophthal., 115:46–49, 1993.

Meyer, S.J., et al.: Conjunctival involvement in paraneoplastic pemphigus. Amer. J Ophthal., 114: 621–624, 1992.

Conjunctival Concretions (Small Yellow Spots Most Common in Tarsal Conjunctiva)

1. Chronic inflammatory conditions, including: atopic keratoconjunctivitis, vernal conjunctivitis, and post-trachomatous degenerations

2. Elderly

3. Calcium deposits in patients with chronic renal failure treated with maintenance hemodialysis

Chin, G.N., et al.: Ultrastructural and histochemical studies of conjunctival concretions. Arch. Ophthalmol., 98:720, 1980.

Pahor, D., et al.: Conjunctival and corneal changes in chronic renal failure patients treated with maintenance hemodialysis. Ophthalmologica, 209:14–16, 1995.

Lesions of Caruncle

1. Apocrine hydrocystoma

*2. Basal-cell carcinoma

3. Capillary hemangioma

4. Chronic inflammation

5. Dermoid

6. Ectopic lacrimal gland

7. Epithelial inclusion cyst

8. Foreign-body granuloma

9. Granular cell myeloblastoma

10. Histiocytic lymphoma

11. Lipogranuloma

12. Lymphangiectasis

* = most important

13. Malignant melanoma

14. Nevus

15. Normal caruncle

*16. Oncocytoma

17. Papilloma

18. Pilar cyst

19. Plasmacytoma

20. Pyogenic granuloma

21. Reactive lymphoid hyperplasia

22. Sebaceous gland hyperplasia

* 23. Sebaceous gland adenoma

24. Seborrheic keratosis

25. Squamous-cell carcinoma

Rennie, I.G.: Oncocytomas of the lacrimal caruncle. Br. J. Ophthalmol., 64:935, 1980.

Shields, C. L., et al.: Types and frequency of lesions of the caruncle. Am J Ophthalmol., 102:771–778, 1986.

Shields, C.L., and Shields, J.A.: Tumors of the caruncle. Inter Ophthal Clinics. 33:31–36, 1993.

Globe

NICK MAMALIS, M.D.

Contents

Microphthalmia (Small Globe)

1. Microphthalmia associated with

    A. Cataract—dominant inheritance

    B. Coloboma—dominant and sex-linked inheritance

    C. Congenital spastic diplegia—x-linked

    D. Ectopic pupils—dominant inheritance

    E. Glaucoma—recessive inheritance

    F. Harelip and cleft palate—autosomal recessive

    G. High hypermetropia—recessive inheritance

    H. Malformation of hands and feet—autosomal recessive

    I. Polydactyly—autosomal recessive

    J. Retinitis pigmentosa and glaucoma—dominant inheritance

2. Colobomatous microphthalmia

    A. X-linked

       (1) Aicardi syndrome

    (2) Bloch-Sulzberger syndrome (incontinentia pigmenti)

    (3) Goltz syndrome (focal dermal hypoplasia)

    (4) Lenz microphthalmia syndrome

  B. Autosomal recessive

    (1) Cohen syndrome

    (2) Ellis-van Creveld syndrome

    (3) Hepatic fibrosis, polycystic kidneys, colobomas, and encephalopathy

    (4) Humeroradial synostosis

    (5) Kartagener syndrome

    (6) Laurence-Moon-Biedl syndrome

    (7) Marinesco-Sjögren syndrome

    (8) Meckel syndrome

    (9) Sjögren-Larsson syndrome

    (10) Warburg syndrome

  C. Autosomal dominant

    (1) Basal cell nevus syndrome

    (2) Congenital contractural arachnodactyly

    (3) Crouzon syndrome

    (4) Stickler syndrome

    (5) Treacher Collins syndrome

    (6) Tuberous sclerosis

    (7) Zellweger syndrome

  D. Chromosomal abnormalities

    (1) Deletions 4p, 4r, 11q, 13q, 18q, 18r, XO

    (2) Duplications 3q, 4p, 4q, 7q, 9p, 9q, 13q, 22q

    (3) Ring B Syndrome

    (4) Triploidy

    (5) Trisomy 8, 9, 13, 17, 18, XXX, XYY

  E. Unknown cause

    (1) Amniogenic band syndrome (Streeter dysplasia)

    (2) Cat-eye syndrome (Schmid-Fraccaro syndrome)

    (3) CHARGE syndrome

    (4) Dyscraniopygophalangea (Ullrich syndrome)

    (5) Facial clefting syndromes

    (6) Frontonasal dysplasia (median cleft face syndrome)

    (7) Goldenhar syndrome (oculoauriculovertebral syndrome)

    (8) Hemifacial microsomia syndrome

    (9) Linear sebaceous nevus syndrome

    (10) Rubinstein-Taybi syndrome

3. Noncolobomatous microphthalmia

  A. X-linked

(1) Anderson-Warburg syndrome

(2) Forsius-Eriksson syndrome (Aland disease)

(3) Lowe syndrome (oculocerebrorenal syndrome)

B. Autosomal recessive

(1) Cerebro-oculofacioskeletal syndrome

(2) Conradi syndrome

(3) Cross syndrome

(4) Diamond-Blackfan syndrome

(5) Fanconi

C. Autosomal dominant

(1) Blatt syndrome

(2) Gansslen syndrome

(3) Hypomelanosis of Ito syndrome

(4) Leri syndrome

(5) Myotonic dystrophy

(6) Rieger syndrome

D. Chromosomal abnormalities

(1) Duplication 10q

(2) Chromosome deletion Xp22.1

E. Unknown cause

(1) Arachnoidal cyst

(2) Gorlin-Chaudhry-Moss syndrome

(3) Hallerman-Streff syndrome

(4) Hutchinson-Gilford syndrome (progeria)

(5) Krause syndrome (encephalo-ophthalmic)

(6) Meyer-Schwickerath and Weyers syndrome

(7) Pierre Robin syndrome

(8) Retinal disinsertion syndrome

(9) Sabin-Feldman syndrome

(10) Weyers syndrome

F. Infectious etiology

(1) Congenital rubella (Gregg syndrome)

(2) Congenital spherocytic anemia

(3) Congenital toxoplasmosis

(4) Cytomegalovirus

(5) Epstein-Barr syndrome

(6) Herpes virus

(7) Mumps

(8) Varicella

G. Intoxicants

(1) Fetal alcohol effects

(2) Maternal phenylketonuria fetal effects

4. Idiopathic

5. Nanophthalmos

Eng, A, et al.: Linear facial skin defects associated with microphthalmia and other malformations, with chromosome deletion Xp22.1. J. Amer Acad of Dermatology. 31:680–682, 1994.

Isenberg, S.J.: The Eye in Infancy. Chicago, Year Book Medical Publishers, 1989.

McKusick, V.A.: Mendelian Inheritance in Man. 11th Ed. Baltimore, Johns Hopkins University Press, 1994.

Rodini, E.S., et al.: Ectodermal dysplasia, ectrodactyly, clefting, anophthalmia/microphthalmia and genitourinary anomalies: nosology of Goltz-Gorlin syndrome versus EEC syndrome. Amer. J Medical Genetics, 1992.

Roy, F.H.: Ocular Syndromes and Systemic Diseases. 2nd Ed. Philadelphia, W.B. Saunders, 1989.

Buphthalmos (Large Globe) Usually associated with corneal abnormalities such as opacities and rupture of Descemet membrane; transition from cornea to sclera is unclear and a thin bluish sclera may be present

1. Associated with anterior chamber cleavage syndrome (Reese-Ellsworth syndrome)

2. Autosomal recessive inheritance

3. Cerebrohepatorenal syndrome (Smith-Lemli-Opitz syndrome)

4. Chondrodystrophia calcificans congenita (Conradi syndrome)

5. Congenital glaucoma

6. Congenital rubella syndrome (Gregg syndrome)

7. Cryptophthalmia syndrome (cryptophthalmos-syndactyly)

8. Hurler syndrome

9. Krabbe syndrome

10. Lowe syndrome (oculocerebrorenal syndrome)

11. Milroy disease (chronic hereditary edema; Noone-Milroy-Meige disease)

12. Neurofibromatosis (von Recklinghausen disease)

13. Oculodentodigital dysplasia

14. Rieger syndrome (hypodontia and iris dysgenesis)

15. Sporadic occurrence

16. Sturge-Weber syndrome (encephalotrigeminal syndrome)

McKusick, V.A.: Mendelian Inheritance in Man. 11th Ed. Baltimore, Johns Hopkins University Press, 1994.

Roy, F.H.: Ocular Syndromes and Systemic Diseases. 2nd Ed. Philadelphia, W.B. Saunders, 1989.

Pseudoendophthalmitis (Conditions that Simulate Endophthalmitis)

*1. Chemical reactions from irritating chemicals (irrigating solutions or medications) introduced into the anterior chamber

2. Foreign material in the anterior chamber

3. Metastatic carcinoma

4. Retained lenticular material

5. Severe postoperative iridocyclitis

6. Toxic anterior segment syndrome (TASS)

Levine, R.A., and Williamson, D.E.: Metastatic carcinoma simulating a post-operative endoph-thalmitis. Arch. Ophthalmol., 83:59–60, 1970.

Mamalis, N.: Inflammation. In: Charlton, J.F., and Weinstein, G.W. Ophthalmic Surgery Complica-tions: Prevention and Management. Philadelphia. J.B. Lippincott, 1995, 313–338.

Monson, M.C., et al.: Toxic anterior segment inflammation following cataract surgery. J Cataract Ref Surg. 18:184–189, 1992.

Theodore, F.H.: Complications after cataract surgery. Part I. Int. Ophthalmol. Clin., 4:853–885, 1964.

Endophthalmitis (Intraocular Infection)

1. Bacterial agents

    A. Gram positive

        (1) Bacillus subtilis, megaterium, anthracis, cereus

        (2) Clostridium perfringens (B. welchii)

        (3) Clostridium tetani

        (4) Coryneform bacterium

        (5) Diplococcus pneumoniae (Pneumococcus)

        (6) Diphtheroids

        (7) Listeria monocytogenes

      *(8) Propionibacterium acnes

      *(9) Staphylococcus aureus, albus, and epidermidis

      (10) Streptococcus viridans, hemolytic, pneumoniae, and pyogenes salivarius

    B. Gram negative

        (1) Aerobacter aerogenes

        (2) Enterobacter cloacae

        (3) Escherichia coli

        (4) Fusobacterium

        (5) Klebsiella pneumoniae (Friedlander bacillus)

        (6) Meningococci

        (7) Morganella

        (8) Mycobacterium

        (9) Neisserias catarrhalis

      (10) Pasteurella multocida and tularensis

      (11) Proteus vulgaris (B. proteus) and mirabilis

    *(12) Pseudomonas aeruginosa (B. pyocyaneus)

      (13) Serratia marcescens

      (14) Yersinia enterocolitica or Y. pseudotuberculosis

2. Fungal agents

    A. Actinomyces sp., including Nocardiosis

    B. Aspergillus

    C. Candida sp.

    D. Cephalosporium sp., hyphas

    E. Hormodendrum

* = most important

        F. Hyalopus bogolepofi

        G. Hyalosporus

        H. Mucormycosis

        I. Neurospora sitophila

        J. Sporothrix schenkii

        K. Sporotrichum schenkii

        L. Volutella sp.

3. Viral agents

        A. Behçet syndrome (dermatostomato-ophthalmic syndrome)

        B. Cytomegalovirus

        C. Myxovirus (influenza)

        D. Nocardia asteroides

        E. Vaccinia

        F. Variola

4. Nematode agents

        A. Taenia solium

        B. Toxocara canis and T. cati

5. Other agents

        A. Mycosis fungoides

Driebe, W.T., et al.: Pseudophakic endophthalmitis: Diagnosis and Management. Ophthalmology, 93: 442–448, 1986.

Heidemann, D.G., et al.: Streptococcus salivarius endophthalmitis from contaminated donor cornea after keratoplasty. Am J Ophthalmol., 107:523–527, 1989.

Irvine, W.D., et al.: Endophthalmitis caused by gram-negative organisms. Arch Ophthalmol., 110: 1450–1459, 1992.

Okada, A.A., et al.: Endogenous bacterial endophthalmitis. Report of a ten-year retrospective study. Ophthalmology, 101:832–888, 1994.

Ormerod, L.D., et al.: Endophthalmitis Caused by the Coagulase-negative Staphylococci. Ophthalmology, 100:715–723, 1993.

Patel, A.S., et al.: Endogenous Fusarium endophthalmitis in patient with acute lymphocytic leukemia. Amer J Ophthalmol., 117:363–368, 1994.

Puliafito, C.A., et al.: Infectious endophthalmitis: Review of cases. Ophthalmology, 89:921–929, 1982.

Roy, F.H.: Ocular Syndromes and Systemic Diseases. 2nd Ed. Philadelphia, W.B. Saunders, 1989.

Zimmerman, P.I., et al.: Chronic Nocardia Asteroides Endophthalmitis After Extracapsular Cataract Extraction. Arch Ophthalmol., 111: 837–840, 1993.

Intraocular Cartilage

1. Angiomatosis of the retina

2. Chromosome deletion

3. Chronic inflammation

4. Facial nevus of Jadassohn (linear sebaceous nevus syndrome)

5. Incidental findings in microphthalmic eye, microphthalmus with cyst, microphthalmic eye from a cyclopic orbit, in eyes with coloboma of the choroid and retina or ciliary body

6. Incontinenta pigmenti (Bloch-Sulzberger disease)

7. Persistent hyperplastic primary vitreous

8. Retinal dysplasia

9. Teratoid medulloepithelioma (dictyomas)

10. Trisomy (13-Patau syndrome) (globe less than mm in diameter)

Broughton, W.L., and Zimmerman, L.E.: A clinical pathologic study of cases of intraocular medul-loepitheliomas. Amer J Ophthalmol., 85:407–418, 1978.

Roy, F.H.: Ocular Syndromes and Systemic Diseases. 2nd Ed. Philadelphia, W.B. Saunders, 1989.

Wilkes, S.R., et al.: Ocular malformation in association with ipsilateral facial nevus of Jadassohn. Am. J. Ophthalmol., 92:344–352, 1981.

Intraocular Calcifications

1. Choroidal osteoma

2. Facial nevus of Jadassohn (linear sebaceous nevus syndrome)

3. Intraocular calcifications

    A. Congenital deformity

    B. Recurrent iritis and keratitis

    C. Retinal detachment

    D. Trauma (perforating, nonperforating, or surgical)

4. Intraocular sarcoma

*5. Retinoblastoma

6. Retinopathy of prematurity (end stage)

7. Sites of intraocular calcification

    A. Calcific emboli of retinal and ciliary arteries

    B. Cyclitic membrane

    C. Lens

    D. Peripapillary choroid

    E. Posterior pole to ora serrata in region of choroid and pigment epithelium

    F. Retina

    G. Vitreous

Trimble, S.N., et al.: Spontaneous decalcification of a choroidal osteoma. Ophthalmology, 95:631–634, 1988.

Wilkes, S.R., et al.: Ocular malformation in association with ipsilateral facial nevus of Jadassohn. Am. J. Ophthalmol., 92:344–352, 1981.

Wolter, J.R.: The message of a bony lens. Ophthalmol. Surg., 12:332, 1981.

Intraocular Adipose Tissue

1. Congenital malformations

    A. Dermoid or dermolipoma extending from the cornea or limbus into the globe

    B. Malformed optic nerve

    C. Persistent hyperplastic vitreous (PHPV) and other related ocular malforma-tions, such as microphthalmia, persistent hyaloid vessels, cataract, and abnor-mal differentiation of the angle of the anterior chamber

2. Embolic phenomenon secondary to crush wounds of the thorax and abdomen or fracture of long bones of the extremities

* = most important

3. Formation of fatty tissue within the marrow spaces of metaplastic bone

4. Missile passing through orbit carrying orbital fat into the eye

Font, R.L., et al.: Intraocular adipose tissue and persistent hyperplastic primary vitreous. Arch. Ophthalmol., 82:43–59, 1969.

Willis, R., et al.: Heterotropic adipose tissue and smooth muscle in the optic disc: Association with isolated colobomas. Arch. Ophthalmol., 86:139–146, 1972.

Soft Globe (Decreased Intraocular Pressure)

*1. Fistula from intraocular source, including penetrating intraocular trauma or surgery and ruptured wall of the globe

*2. Laser or cryotherapy ciliodestructive procedure

3. Phthisis bulbi

4. Choroidal detachment

5. Injury to the cervical sympathetic nerve

6. Serous detachment of the retina

7. Myotonic dystrophy (Curschmann-Steinert syndrome)

8. Systemic disturbances

    A. Cardiac edema

    B. Diabetic coma

    C. Extreme or rapid dehydration because of malnutrition, cholera, or diarrhea

    D. Fall in ocular blood pressure due to hypotension, ligation of the carotid artery, carotid occlusion, or pulseless disease (Takayasu syndrome)

    E. Giant-cell arteritis (temporal arteritis syndrome)

    F. Leprosy (Hansen disease)

    G. Parkinson disease (shaking palsy)

    H. Postencephalitic syndrome following severe cerebral trauma, barbiturate poisoning, in deep anesthesia, following leukotomy, or on the paralyzed side in cases of cerebral hemiplegia

    I. Severe abdominal disturbances, such as intestinal perforation or obstruction

    J. Profound anemias

    K. Uremic coma

9. Drugs, including:

asacebutolol	aprobarbital
aceclidine	aspirin
acetazolamide	atenolol
acetylcholine	barbital
acetyldigitoxin	bendroflumethiazide
albuterol	benzthiazide
alcohol	betamethasone
allobarbital	betaxolol
alseroxylon	bupivacaine
amobarbital	butabarbital
amyl nitrite	butalbital

butallylonal

butethal

carbachol

carisoprodol(?)

chlordiazepoxide

chlorisondamine

chloroform

chlorothiazide

chlorthalidone

clofibrate(?)

clonidine

cortisone

cyclobarbital

cyclopentobarbital

cyclothiazide

demecarium

deserpidine

deslanoside

dexamethasone

diacetylmorphine

diazepam

dichlorphenamide

digitoxin

digoxin

dimethyl tubocurarine iodide

diphenylhydantoin

dipivefrin

dronabinol

droperidol

echothiophate

ephedrine

epinephrine

erogovine

ergotamine

erythrityl tetranitrate

ether

ethoxzolamide

etidocaine

fluorometholone

flurazepam

furosemide

gitalin

glycerin

guanethidine

haloperidol

hashish

heparin

heptabarbital

hexamethonium

hexethal

hexobarbital

hydrochlorothiazide

hydrocortisone

hydroflumethiazide

insulin

isoflurophate

isosorbide

isosorbide dinitrate

labetalol

lanatoside C

mannitol

mannitol hexanitrate

marijuana

mecamylamine

medrysone

meperidine

mephenesin

mephobarbital

mepivacaine

meprobamate(?)

methacholine

metharbital

methazolamide

methitural

methohexital

methoxyflurane

methyclothiazide

methyldopa

methylergonovine

methylprednisolone

methysergide

metocurine iodide

metolazone

metoprolol

morphine

nadolol

* = most important

naphazoline

neostigmine

nitroglycerin

nitrous oxide

norepinephrine

opium

oral contraceptives

ouabain

oxprenolol

oxygen

pargyline

pentaerythritol tetranitrate

pentobarbital

pentolinium

phenobarbital

phenoxybenzamine(?)

physostigmine

pilocarpine

polythiazide

practolol

prednisolone

primidone

probarbital

propranolol

protriptyline

quinethazone

rauwolfia serpentina

rescinnamine

reserpine

secobarbital

sodium salicylate

spironolactone

succinylcholine

syrosingopine

talbutal

tetraethylammonium

tetrahydrocannabinol

tetrahydrozoline

thiamylal

thiopental

timolol

tolazoline

trichlormethiazide

trichlorethylene

trifluperidol

trimethaphan

trimethidinium

trolnitrate

tubocurarine

urea

urokinase

vinbarbital

vitamin A

10. Detachment of the ciliary body, planned or inadvertent

11. Hyperosmotic agents, such as mannitol or urea

12. Iritis or iridocyclitis

13. After central retinal vein occlusion

14. Myopia—low scleral rigidity may give false low readings with Schiotz tonometer, but normal readings with applanation intraocular pressure

15. Herpes zoster

16. Following irradiation by roentgenograms or beta rays

17. Congenital lesions, including microphthalmos, aniridia, and coloboma

18. Concussion trauma

19. Necrosis of anterior segment of the eye

20. Idiopathic, including normal variation

Fraunfelder, F.T.: Drug-Induced Ocular Side Effects and Drug Interactions. 4th Ed. Philadelphia, Williams & Wilkins, 1996.

Maus, M., and Katz, J.L.: Choroidal detachment flat anterior chamber and hypotony as complications of YAG laser cyclocoagulation. Ophthalmol, 97:69–71, 1990.

Roy, F.H.: Ocular Syndromes and Systemic Diseases. 2nd Ed. Philadelphia, W.B. Saunders, 1989.

Phthisis Bulbi (Degenerative Shrinkage of Eyeball with Hypotony)

1. Ciliodestructive procedures such as cyclocryotherapy or laser
2. Endophthalmitis
3. Following cataract surgery, especially with rubella syndrome (German measles)
4. Panophthalmitis
5. Severe ocular injury with loss of tissue
6. Severe uveitis
7. Sympathetic ophthalmia
8. Tumor, such as retinoblastoma or malignant melanoma

Boniuk, J., and Boniuk, M.: The incidence of phthisis bulbi as a complication of cataract surgery in the congenital rubella syndrome. Trans. Am. Acad. Ophthalmol. Otolaryngol., 74:360–369, 1970.

Cyclin, M.N., et al.: Ciliodestructive procedures in glaucoma. Clinical signs. Ophthalmol., 12:1–15, 1991.

Newell, F.W.: Ophthalmology, Principles and Concepts. 7th Ed. St. Louis, C.V. Mosby, 1991.

Clinical Anophthalmos (Apparent Absence of Globe)

1. Anencephaly
2. Gross midline facial defects (Median cleft face syndrome)
3. Dyscraniopygophalangea
4. Goldenhar syndrome (oculoauriculovertebral syndrome)
5. Goltz syndrome (focal dermal hypoplasia syndrome)
6. Hallermann-Strieff syndrome (dyscephalic mandibulo-oculofacial syndrome)
7. Hypervitaminosis A
8. Idiopathic
9. Kleinfelter syndrome (gynecomastia-aspermatogenesis)
10. Lanzieri syndrome (craniofacial malformations)
11. Leri syndrome (carpal tunnel syndrome)
12. Meckel syndrome (dysencephalia splanchnocystica syndrome)
13. Oculovertebral dysplasia (Weyers-Thier syndrome)
14. Otocephaly
15. Trisomy 13–15
16. Sex-linked or recessive hereditary
17. Waardenburg anophthalmia syndrome (anophthalmos with limb anomalies)—recessive

Graham, C.A., et al.: X-linked clinical anophthalmos. Localization of the gene to Xq27-Xq28. Ophthal Paediatrics & Genetics, 12:43–48, 1991.

Matsui, H., et al.: Congenital cataract in the right eye and primary clinical anophthalmos of the left eye in a patient with cerebellar hypoplasia.

Roy, F.H.: Ocular Syndromes and Systemic Diseases. 2nd Ed. Philadelphia, W.B. Saunders, 1989.

* = most important

Oculodigital Stimulation (Patient Presses on Globe through Lids with Index Finger or Hand; Poor Visual Acuity)

1. Bilateral congenital cataracts
2. Combined retinal detachment and congenital cataract
3. Congenital glaucoma
4. Congenital rubella syndrome (German measles)
5. Leber amaurosis congenita or other congenital retinal degeneration (Leber tapetoretinal dystrophy syndrome)
6. Norrie disease (fetal iritis syndrome)
7. Total corneal leukomas

Franklin, A.H.: Norrie's disease. Am. J. Ophthalmol., 72:947–948, 1971.

Roy, F.H.: Ocular autostimulation. Am. J. Ophthalmol., 63:1776–1777, 1967.

Anterior Segment Ischemia (Hypoxia with Involvement of Cornea, Iris, Anterior Chamber, Lens, and Ciliary Body)

1. Damage to normal intact anterior vessels
    A. Pressure
        (1) Scleral buckle
        (2) Suture (Jensen procedure)
    B. Thermal
        (1) Cryothermy
        (2) Diathermy
2. Disinsertion of normal vessels (Hummelsheim or Knapp procedure)
3. Fuchs syndrome (I) (heterochromic cyclitis syndrome)
4. Hematologic abnormality
    A. Extreme leukocytosis
    B. Extreme thrombocytosis
    C. Hyperglobulinemia
    D. Red blood cell dysfunction including sickle cell trait
        (1) Hemoglobinopathy
        (2) Polycythemia vera (Vaquez-Osler syndrome)
5. Vessel wall abnormality (arteriosclerosis)
    A. Arteriosclerosis
    B. Giant cell arteritis

Berger, B.B., et al.: Anterior segment of ischemia in Fuchs' heterochromic cyclitis. Arch. Ophthalmol., 98:499, 1980.

Birt, C.M., et al.: Anterior segment ischemia in giant cell arteritis. Canadian J. Ophthal. 29: 93–94, 1994.

Cartwright, M.J., et al.: Anterior segment ischemia: a complication of retinal detachment repair in a patient with sickle cell trait. Ann. of Ophthalmol., 22:333–334, 1990.

Roy, F.H.: Ocular Syndromes and Systemic Diseases. 2nd ed. Philadelphia, W.B. Saunders, 1989.

Saunder, R.A., et al.: Anterior segment ischemia after strabismus surgery. Survey of Ophthalmol., 38: 456–466, 1995

Sclera

FERENC KUHN M.D., TAMAS HALDA PhD, AND
C. DOUGLAS WITHERSPOON M.D.

Contents

Blue Sclera (Localized or Generalized Blue Coloration of Sclera Because of Thinness and Loss of Water Content Allowing Underlying Dark Choroid to Be Seen)

1. Associated with high urine excretion
    A. Folling's syndrome (phenylketonuria)
    B. Hypophosphatasia (phosphoethanolaminuria)
    C. Lowe's syndrome (oculocerebrorenal syndrome; chondroitin-4-sulfate-uria)
2. Associated with skeletal disorders
    A. Brachmann-deLange syndrome
    B. Brittle cornea syndrome (blue sclera syndrome)—recessive
    C. Crouzon disease (craniofacial dysostosis)
    D. Hallermann-Streiff syndrome (dyscephalia mandibulo-oculo-facial syndrome)
  * E. Marfan syndrome (dystrophia mesodermalis congenita)
    F. Marshall-Smith syndrome
    G. McCune-Albright syndrome (fibrosus dysplasia)
    H. Mucopolysaccharidosis VI (Maroteaux-Lamy syndrome)
    I. Osteogenesis imperfecta (van der Hoeve's syndrome)
    J. Paget syndrome (osteitis deformans)
    K. Pierre-Robin syndrome (micrognathia-glossoptosis syndrome)

       L. Robert syndrome

       M. Silver-Russell syndrome

       N. Werner syndrome (progeria of adults)

3. Chromosome disorders

       A. Trisomy syndrome

       B. Turner's syndrome

4. Ocular

      * A. Congenital glaucoma

       B. Myopia

     *C. Repeated surgeries

       D. Scleromalacia (perforans)

     *E. Staphyloma

       F. Trauma

5. Miscellaneous

       A. Ehlers-Danlos syndrome (fibrodysplasia elastica generalisata)

       B. Goltz's syndrome (focal dermal hypoplasia syndrome)

       C. Incontinentia pigmenti (Bloch-Sulzberger syndrome)

       D. Lax ligament syndrome

       E. Oculodermal melanocytosis (nevus of Ota)

       F. Pseudoxanthoma elasticum (Grönblad-Strandberg syndrome)

       G. Relapsing polychondritis

Cameron, J.A., et al.: Epikeratoplasty for keratoglobus associated with blue sclera. Ophthalmology, 98:446–452, 1991.

Howard, F.M.: Lax ligament syndrome in children associated with blue sclera and bat ears. Brit. J. General Practice, 40:233–235, 1990.

Isenberg, S.J.: The Eye in Infancy. Chicago, Year Book Medical Publishers, 1989.

Roy, F.H.: Ocular Syndromes and Systemic Diseases. 2nd Ed. Philadelphia, W.B. Saunders, 1989.

Blue Sclera

	McCune-Albright syndrome	Brittle cornea syndrome	Cruson's syndrome	Brachmann de Lange syndrome	Ehlers-Danlos syndrome	Hallerman-Streiff-François syndrome	Hypophosphatasia	Marfan syndrome	Osteogenesis imperfecta	Turner's syndrome	Werner's syndrome
History											
1. Chromosomal abnormality										U	
2. Common in females	U									U	
3. Familial occurrence and consanguinity						R					S
4. Hereditary	U	U	U	U	U			U	U		U
5. Inborn error of metabolism							U				
6. Male and female equal						U					
7. Occurs during second to third decades											U
8. Present from birth	U		U		U						
Physical Findings											
1. Abnormal deep recess in angle of anterior chamber								U			
2. Absence of eyelashes and scanty eyebrows											U
3. Angioid streaks					S						
4. Aniridia								R			
5. Anisocoria			S								
6. Antimongoloid obliquity (downward displacement of temporal canthus)			U	U		S					
7. Astigmatism											S
8. Bilateral exophthalmos			U	S		S	U			S	
9. Blepharophimosis			S								
10. Bullous keratitis											S
11. Cataract	S		S			S	S	R	U	S	
12. Chorioretinal hemorrhages					S						
13. Conjunctival calcification							S				
14. Corneal dystrophy			R								S
15. Corneal nebulae										S	
16. Corneal spontaneous perforation	S	S									
17. Corneal subepithelial calcification							U				
18. Epicanthal folds										S	
19. Exposure keratitis			S								
20. Extraocular muscles hypotony						S					
21. Glaucoma							S		S	S	
22. High myopia				S	S			U			
23. Hydrophthalmos								R			
24. Hyperelasticity of palpebral skin					U						
25. Hypertelorism	S		U							U	
26. Hypertrichosis of eyebrows				U							
27. Iris atrophy						S					
28. Iris coloboma						S		R			
29. Iris heterochromia								R			
30. Keratitis	S										
31. Keratoglobus						S					
32. Lens coloboma								R			
33. Lens subluxation					S			U			
34. Lid retraction							S				
35. Lid telangiectasia											S

* = most important

Blue Sclera Continued

	McCune-Albright syndrome	Brittle cornea syndrome	Cruson's syndrome	Brachmann-e Lange syndrome	Ehlers-Danlos syndrome	Hallerman-Streiff-François syndrome	Hypophosphatasia	Marfan syndrome	Osteogenesis imperfecta	Turner's syndrome	Werner's syndrome
Physical Findings											
36. Long eyelashes				U							
37. Macula and optic nerve coloboma								R			
38. Macular degeneration					S						
39. Megalocornea								R			
40. Microcornea					S	S					
41. Microphthalmos						U			R		
42. Miosis								U			
43. Nystagmus			S	S		S				S	
44. Optic disc and choroid coloboma						S					
45. Optic nerve atrophy			S	S		S	U				
46. Papilledema	S		S				U				
47. Paramacular retinal degeneration											S
48. Persistent pupillary membrane						S					
49. Pigmentary retinal degeneration								R			
50. Presbyopia, early											S
51. Prominent iris processes								U			
52. Ptosis			S	S	U					S	
53. Retinal detachment					S			U			
54. Retinitis proliferans					S						
55. Sclera and choroidal calcifications	S										
56. Strabismus	S		S	S	S	S					
57. Telecanthus				S							
58. Thinning of cornea with keratoconus					S			R	S		
59. Upper lid easy eversion					U						
60. Uveitis											S
Laboratory Data											
1. Blood phosphate							U				
2. Chromosome studies										U	
3. Hearing test									S		
4. Hyperglycemia											S
5. Skeletal roentgenogram									U	S	
6. Skull roentgenogram			U	S					U		

R = rarely; S = sometimes; and U = usually.

Dilated Episcleral Vessels

1. Carotid-cavernous fistula
2. Cavernous sinus thrombosis (Foix syndrome)
*3. Chronic respiratory diseases
*4. Glaucoma, untreated
5. Increased viscosity of circulating blood
    A. Leukemia (early)
    B. Polycythemia vera (erythremia, Vaquez-Osler syndrome)
6. Occlusion of orbital veins of the apex of the orbit
    A. Endocrine exophthalmos of rapid development
    B. Inflammatory lesions
    C. Orbital thrombophlebitis
    D. Tumor (rare)
7. Ophthalmic vein thrombosis
8. Uveal neoplasm with localized engorgement

Boniuk, M.: The ocular manifestations of ophthalmic vein and aseptic cavernous sinus thrombosis. Trans. Am. Acad. Ophthalmol. Otolaryngol., 76:1519–1534, 1972.

Minas, T.F., and Podos, S.M.: Familial glaucoma associated with elevated episcleral venous pressure. Arch. Ophthalmol., 80:202–213, 1968.

Episcleritis (Benign self-limited nodular or diffuse-disease that usually resolves spontaneously within to weeks, but has a tendency to recur. Inflammation of episcleral tissues causing discomfort rather than pain; not affecting visual acuity. Even recurrent attacks do not produce scleritis. Complications are minimal and include areas of scleral transparency and localized keratitis)

*1. Idiopathic (single, short episode that does not recur)
2. Associated with the following diseases (recurrent attacks)
    A. Addison's syndrome (adrenal cortical insufficiency)
    B. Arthritides
        (1) Involving small and medium size vessels
            a. Necrotizing granulomatous arthritis; Wegener's granulomatosis (Wegener's syndrome)
            b. Polyarteritis nodosa (Kussmaul's disease)
        (2) Involving small, medium, and large vessels
            a. Arteritis in collagen vascular diseases
                i.   Progressive systemic sclerosis (PSS; scleroderma)
                ii. Rheumatoid arthritis
                iii. Rheumatic fever
    C. Cogan's syndrome
    D. Crohn's disease (granulomatous ileocolitis)
    E. Goodpasture's syndrome (pulmonary hemosiderosis)
    F. Heerfordt's disease (uveoparotid fever)

* = most important

G. Inflammatory pseudotumor

H. Initial manifestation of uveal melanoma (ciliary body)

I. Myeloproliferative diseases

    (1) Hodgkin's disease

    (2) T cell leukemia

J. Paraneoplastic syndromes

    (1) Dermatomyositis

    (2) Sweet's syndrome (cutan paraneoplastic syndrome)

K. Paraproteinemia

    (1) Familial Mediterranean fever

    (2) Necrobiotic xanthogranuloma (increased IgG/IgA)

L. Parry-Romberg syndrome (progressive hemifacial atrophy)

M. Relapsing polychondritis

N. Skin diseases

    (1) Chronic cutaneous lupus erythematosus (CCLE)

    (2) Erythema elevatum diutinum

    (3) Lichen planus

    (4) Progressive systemic sclerosis (PSS; scleroderma)

    (5) Psoriasis

    (6) Reiter's syndrome (polyarteritis enterica)

    (7) Wiscott-Aldrich syndrome

O. Terrien's marginal corneal disease

P. Ulcerative colitis (regional enteritis)

Q. Weber-Christian disease (systemic panniculitis)

R. Pseudoepiscleritis (lesions resembling episcleritis)

    (1) Conjunctivitis

    (2) In-growing lash

  *(3) Inflamed pinguecula

    (4) Punctate keratitis

    (5) Sclerosing keratitis

3. Drugs

A. Pamidronate disodium

4. Infectious

A. Brucellosis (Bang disease, undulant fever)

B. Coccidioidomycosis

C. Influenza

D. Leprosy (Hansen disease)

E. Leptospirosis (Weil disease)

F. Lyme disease (borreliosis, relapsing fever)

G. Lymphogranuloma venereum (Nichols-Favre disease)

      H. Nematode (angiostrongylus cantonensis)

      I. Q fever

   5. Trauma

      *A. Episcleral foreign body

      B. Following transscleral fixation of posterior chamber IOL

      C. Insect bite granuloma

      D. Malpositioned (Jones) tube

Aracena, T., et al.: Progressive hemifacial atrophy (Parry-Rombery syndrome): report of two cases. Ann. Ophthal., 11:953–958, 1979.

Bartley, G.B., and Gustafson, R.O.: Complications of malpositioned of Jones tubes. Am J Ophthalmol., 109:66–69, 1990.

Goto, K., et al.: Recurrent episcleritis associated with adult T cell leukaemia. Brit J Ophthal., 77:743–744, 1993.

Hohenleutner, S., et al.: Necrobiotic xanthogranuloma with eye involvement. Overview and case report. Hautarzt., 46:163–173m, 1995.

Knox, D.L., et al.: Primary, secondary and coincidental ocular complications of Crohn's disease. Ophthalmology, 91:163–173, 1984.

Leo, R.J., and Palmer, D.J.: Episcleritis and secondary glaucoma after transscleral fixation of a posterior chamber intraocular lens (letter). Arch Ophthalmol., 109:617, 1991.

Marcarol, V., and Fraunfelder, F.T.: Pamidronate disodium and possible ocular adverse drug reactions. Amer J. Ophthal., 118:220–224, 1994.

Roy, F.H.: Ocular Syndromes and Systemic Diseases. 2nd Ed. Philadelphia, W.B. Saunders, 1989.

Sainz dela Maza, M., et al.: Severity of Scleritis and Episcleritis. Ophthalmology, 101:389–396, 1994.

Pigment Spots of Sclera and Episclera

   *1. Acquired melanosis

   2. Cysts

   3. Drugs, including:

acetophenazine	iron dextran	promethazine
butaperazine	iron sorbitex	propiomazine
carphenazine	mesoridazine	thiethylperazine
chlorpromazine	methdilazine	thiopropazate
diethazine	methotrimeprazine	thioproperazine
ethopropazine	perazine	thioridazine
ferrocholinate	pericyazine	trifluoperazine
ferrous fumarate	perphenazine	triflupromazine
ferrous gluconate	piperacetazine	trimeprazine
ferrous succinate	polysaccharide iron complex	vitamin D
ferrous sulfate	prochlorperazine	vitamin D_2
fluphenazine	promazine	vitamin D_3

   4. Extension of adjacent or underlying malignant melanoma

   5. Foreign body

   6. Intrascleral nerve loops with uveal pigment (painful to touch)

* = most important

*7. Nevus

8. Ochronosis with melanin deposition

*9. Resolving hemorrhage

10. Staphyloma

11. Transscleral migration of pigment following cryotherapy of intraocular tumor or trauma

12. Uveal melanocytes carried by the scleral emissaria into the episclera (most often in eyes with dark irides in superior, inferior temporal, and nasal quadrants in descending frequency; conjunctiva freely movable over them)

Fraunfelder, F.T.: Drug-Induced Ocular Side Effects and Drug Interactions. Philadelphia, Williams & Wilkins, 1996.

Kampik, A., et al.: Ocular ochronosis. Arch. Ophthalmol., 98:1411, 1980.

Shields, J.A., et al.: Uveal pseudomelanoma due to post-traumatic pigmentary migration. Arch. Ophthalmol., 89:519–522, 1973.

Scleritis. (Potentially destructive inflammatory process that may accompany severe systemic disease. Ocular pain occasionally radiates to temple, jaw, or sinuses. Women are more frequently affected. Most cases present with bilateral involvement. Early perforation of sclera is possible. The anterior portion of the eye is affected most severely. Posterior scleritis may be a diagnostic challenge.)

1. Associated with systemic disease

   A. Collagen diseases

      *(1) Dermatomyositis (Wagner-Unverricht syndrome)

      *(2) Felty's syndrome

      *(3) Giant cell (temporal) arteritis

      (4) Juvenile rheumatoid arthritis (Still's disease)

      (5) Polyarteritis nodosa (Kussmaul's disease)

      (6) Progressive systemic sclerosis (PSS; scleroderma)

      (7) Relapsing polychondritis

      (8) Reiter's syndrome (polyarteritis enterica)

      (9) Rheumatoid arthritis

      (10) Sjögren's syndrome

      (11) Systemic lupus erythematosus (SLE)

      (12) Wegener's granulomatosis (Wegener's syndrome)

   B. Metabolic diseases

      (1) Cretinism (hypothyroidism)

      (2) Gout

      (3) Porphyria cutanea tarda

   C. Myeloproliferative diseases

      (1) Hodgkin's disease (lymph node disease)

      (2) Mycosis fungoides syndrome (Sezary's syndrome)

2. Infectious

A. Bacterial

   (1) Leprosy

   (2) Lymphogranuloma venereum (Nichols-Favre disease)

   (3) Syphilis (acquired lues)

   (4) Tuberculosis

B. Viral infections

   (1) Herpes simplex

   (2) Herpes zoster

   (3) Influenza

   (4) Mumps

C. Fungal—aspergillosis

D. Helminth infection—acanthamoeba

E. Protozoan—toxoplasmosis

F. Infections

   (1) Associated with skin disease, or immunosuppressive status

   (2) Spreading directly from conjunctiva, cornea, uvea, periorbital tissues, nose, or sinuses

3. Miscellaneous

A. Cogan's syndrome

B. Crohn's disease (granulomatous ileocolitis)

C. Goodpasture's syndrome (pulmonary hemosiderosis)

D. Erythema nodosum

E. Exogenous infection via penetration through conjunctiva

F. Heerfordt's disease (uveoparotid fever)

G. Necrobiotic xanthogranuloma (increased IgG/IgA)

H. Terrien's marginal corneal disease

4. Drugs

A. Pamidronate disodium

*5. Trauma—following cataract or strabismus surgery

Carlson, A.N., et al.: Fungal scleritis after cataract surgery. Successful outcome using itraconazole. Cornea, 11:151–154, 1992.

Dougherty, P.J., et al.: Acanthamoeba Sclerokeratitis. Amer J Ophthalmol., 117:475–479, 1994.

Frost, N.A., et al.: Posterior scleritis with retinal vasculitis and choroidal and retinal infarction. Brit. J Ophthalmol., 78:410–412, 1994.

Gross, S.A., et al.: Necrotizing scleritis and transient myopia following strabismus surgery. Ophthalmic Surgery, 24:839–841, 1993.

Herbort, C.P.: Uveoscleritis after excessive neodymium: YAG laser posterior capsulotomy J Cataract & Refractive Surgery, 20:80–81, 1994.

Hoang-Xuan, T., et al.: Scleritis in relapsing polychondritis. Ophthalmology, 97:892–898, 1990.

Maskin, S. L.: Infectious Scleritis After a Diabetic Foot Ulcer. Amer J Ophthal., 115:254–255, 1993.

Roy, F.H.: Ocular Syndromes and Systemic Diseases. 2nd Ed. Philadelphia, W.B. Saunders, 1989.

Tuft, S.J., and Shah, P., et al.: Posterior scleritis—an unusual manifestation of Cogan's syndrome. Brit J Rheumatology, 33:774–775, 1994.

* = most important

Watson, P.G.: Progression of scleral disease. Ophthalmology, 98:467–471, 1991.
Yap, E., et al: Scleritis as an Initial Manifestation of Choroidal Malignant Melanoma. Ophthalmology, 99:1693–1697, 1992.

Staphyloma. (Stretching and Thinning of the Sclera with Incarceration of Uveal Tissue)

1. Collagen diseases
    A. Felty's syndrome
    B. Rheumatoid arthritis (adult)
    C. Wegener's syndrome (Wegener's granulomatosis)
2. Following trauma
    A. Beta radiation
    B. Deep scleral resection for episcleral malignancies
    C. Pterygium excision and mitomycin therapy
    *D. Scleral buckle removal
    E. Subconjunctival injection of corticosteroids
    F. Ultrasound treatment for glaucoma
3. Infectious
    A. Aspergillosis
    B. Herpes zoster (rare)
    C. Plague (bubonic plague)
    D. Syphilis
    E. Tuberculosis
4. Ocular cause
    A. Buphthalmos associated with increased intraocular pressure
    B. Corneoscleral ectasia
    C. Myopia with increased anteroposterior diameter
    D. Scleritis, e.g., secondary to rheumatoid arthritis
    E. Uveitis
5. Miscellaneous
    A. Ehler-Danlos syndrome (fibrodysplasia elastica generalisata)
    B. Endarteritis
    C. Epidermolysis bullosa
    D. Hyperparathyroidism
    E. Meckel's syndrome (dysencephalia syndrome)
    F. Oculodental syndrome (Peter's syndrome)
    G. Porphyria cutanea tarda

Dunn, J.P., et al.: Development of scleral ulceration and calcification after pterygium excision and mitomycine therapy. Am. J. Ophthalmol., 112:344, 1991.
Fraunfelder, F.T., and Roy, F.H.: Current Ocular Therapy. 4th Ed. Philadelphia, W.B. Saunders, 1995.
Pope, J., et al.: Mycobacterium chelonae scleral abscess after removal of scleral buckle. Am J Ophthalmol., 107:557–559, 1989.

Roy, F.H.: Ocular Syndromes and Systemic Diseases. 2nd Ed. Philadelphia, W.B. Saunders, 1989.

Wilensky, J.T.: Staphyloma formation as a complication of ultrasound treatment in glaucoma. Arch Ophthalmol., 103:1113, 1985.

Episcleral and Scleral Tumors

1. Carcinomas
2. Choroidal melanomas
*3. Epibulbar tumor
4. Fibromas
5. Hemangiomas
6. Lymphomas
7. Leiomyoma (transscleral)
8. Melanoblastoma (spread from choroid)
9. Retinoblastoma

Pau, H.: Differential Diagnosis of Eye Diseases. 2nd Ed. New York, Thieme Med. Pub., 1988.

Perry, H.D.: Isolated episcleral neurofibroma. Ophthalmology, 89:1095, 1982.

* = most important

Cornea

CHRISTOPHER J. RAPUANO, M.D.

Contents

* = most important

Crystals of the Cornea
(Deposition of Crystalline Substances in the Cornea)

1. Bietti marginal crystalline dystrophy
2. Calcium oxalate—diffenbachia and other plants
3. Cholesterol crystals—primary or secondary with corneal neovascularization
*4. Crystalline dystrophy of Schnyder
5. Crystalline retinopathy
6. Cystinosis syndrome (Lignac-Fanconi syndrome)
    A. Benign adult
    B. Congenital
7. Drugs, such as indomethacin (Indocin), chloroquine, and Mellaril, clofazimine
8. Dysproteinemia
    A. Cryoglobulinemia
    *B. Multiple myeloma
9. Elevated bilirubin with crystalline dystrophy
10. Fine multicolored glittering crystals following successful transplant that later underwent graft rejection and was treated with steroids
11. Gout (hyperuricemia)

12. Hyperparathyroidism

13. IgG K monoclonal gammopathy

*14. Infectious crystalline retinopathy, usually with more indolent streptococcal and staphylococcal species

15. Post-keratoplasty, Kaye's dots

16. Renal failure

17. Uremia

18. Waldenstrom syndrome (macroglobulinemia syndrome)

Font, R.L., et al.: Polychromatic corneal and conjunctival crystals secondary to clofazimine therapy in a leper. Ophthalmology, 96:311–315, 1989.

Ormerod, L.D., et al.: Paraproteinemic crystalline keratopathy. Ophthalmology, 95:202–212, 1988.

Roy, F.H.: Ocular Syndromes and Systemic Diseases. 2nd Ed. Philadelphia, W.B. Saunders, 1989.

Weisenthal, R.W., et al.: Postkeratoplasty crystalline deposits mimicking bacterial infectious crystalline keratopathy. Am J Ophthalmol., 105:70–74, 1988.

* = most important

Crystals of the Cornea (Deposition of Crystalline Substance in the Cornea)

	Cystinosis (i.e., Congenital)	Crystalline Dystrophy of Schnyder	Multiple Myeloma	Bietti Marginal Crystalline Dystrophy	Gout	Drugs (i.e., Chloroquine)	Hyperparathyroidism	Porphyria Cutanea Tarda	Cholesterol Crystals	Infectious Crystalline Keratopathy
History										
1. Amaurosis fungax			S							
2. Between 50 and 70 years			S							
3. Common in 40s								U		
4. Corneal trauma including chemical burns; infections including herpes simplex and zoster; interstitial kerstitis									U	
5. Crystals appear 6 to 24 months	U	U								
6. Disseminated malignancy of plasma cells			U							
7. Excessive alcohol intake								U		
8. Fatal disease	U									
9. Genetic metabolic disease	S			S	U					
10. Glare						U				
11. Hereditary	U	U		U						
12. Thyroid surgery							S			
13. Photophobia	U									
14. Prior Corneal Surgery										U
Physical Findings										
1. Attenutated retinal vessels						S				
2. Bull's eye or doughnut retinal lesion						U				
3. Bushy eyebrows								S		
4. Cicatricial ectropion								S		
5. Conjunctival calcification							S	R		
6. Conjunctivitis					U					S
7. Corneal arcus		S								
8. Corneal neovascularization									S	
9. Corneal infiltrate										U
10. Cotton wool spots			S					S		
11. Crystals in conjunctiva	S		S					S		
12. Crystals in aqueous humor	U									
13. Choroidal detachment			S							
14. Dilated retina veins			S							
15. Episcleritis					S					
16. Lacrimal obstruction									S	
17. Macula edema									S	
18. Occlusion of central artery vein			S							
19. Ocular motor disturbances including sixth nerve palsy			S		S			S		
20. Optic nerve atrophy							U	S		
21. Pigmentary retinopathy	U					S				
22. Posterior scleritis					S					
23. Proptosis			S							
24. Ptosis								S		
25. Retinal hemorrhages			S							
26. Retinal microaneurysms			S							
27. Retinitis punctata albescens				U						
28. Retrobulbar neuritis			S							
29. Scleromalacia							S	R		

Crystals of the Cornea (Deposition of Crystalline Substance in the Cornea) *Continued*

	Cystinosis (i.e., Congenital)	Crystalline Dystrophy of Schnyder	Multiple Myeloma	Bietti Marginal Crystalline Dystrophy	Gout	Drugs (i.e., Chloroquine)	Hyperparathyroidism	Porphyria Cutanea Tarda	Cholesterol Crystals	Infectious Crystalline Keratopathy
Physical Findings										
30. Silverwire or chalky-white arterioles						S				
31. Tumor of orbit			S							
32. Vascular engorgement of retina							S			
33. Vitreous hemorrhage			S							
34. Vogt limbal girdle		S								
35. Xanthelasma		S								
Laboratory Data										
1. Blood hyperviscosity			U							
2. Color vision abnormal						U				
3. Conjunctival biopsy	U								S	
4. Corneal cholesterol		U							U	
5. Electro-oculogram						S	S			
6. Corneal cholesterol		U							U	
7. Corneal scraping										U
8. Electro-oculogram						S	S			
9. Electroretinogram	U					U				
10. Fluorescein angiography	U					U				
11. High porphyria level in urine								U		
12. Hypercalcemia			U				U			
13. Hyperuricemia			S							
14. Hypophosphatemia							U	U		
15. Parathyroid hormone increased							U			
16. Proteinuria			U							
17. Serum lipid elevated									U	
18. Uricemia					U					
19. Visual field abnormal										
(blind spot enlarged and								U		
central scotoma)						U				

R = rarely; S = sometimes; and U = usually.

Anesthesia of the Cornea (Hypesthesia or Diminished Corneal Sensation in Trigeminal Distribution)

1. Cornea
   *A. Cerebellopontine angle tumors
   B. Congenital
   C. Corneal dystrophy granular, lattice, and macular
   D. Dysautonomia
   *E. Infections including herpes zoster, herpes simplex, leprosy, and malaria
   F. Inflammations including after electrocautery of Bowman membrane, stromal edema, vascularized scars, congestive glaucoma, exposure keratitis, radiation damage, and vitamin A deficiency
   G. Trauma including constant wearing of contact lenses and post-operatively including cataract extraction and within corneal transplant, following operation for detached retina—from an encircling band or, less frequently, a circumscribed buckle; from refractive surgery

2. Maxillary division
   A. Interruption of trigeminal nerve or gasserian ganglion, including cerebellopontine angle tumor or other space-occupying lesion in the region of the superior orbital fissure
   B. Maxillary antrum carcinoma
   C. Neoplasm, foramen rotundum, sphenopterygoid fossa
   D. Orbital floor fracture
   E. Perineural spread of skin carcinoma

3. Ophthalmic division
   A. Aneurysm, cavernous sinus
   B. Neoplasm, cavernous sinus
   C. Neoplasm, middle fossa
   D. Neoplasm, orbital apex
   E. Neoplasm, superior orbital fissure

4. Syndromes and diseases
   A. Anhidrotic ectodermal dysplasia
   B. Barré Lieou syndrome (posterior cervical sympathic syndrome)
   C. Diabetes mellitus-youth onset, more marked with age
   D. Eaton-Lambert syndrome (myasthenic syndrome)
   E. Foix syndrome (cavernous sinus syndrome)
   F. Gradenigo syndrome (temporal syndrome)
   G. Hereditary fleck dystrophy of the cornea
   H. Herpes zoster
   I. Hunt syndrome (herpes zoster auricularis)
   J. Hydroa vacciniforme (lower cornea)
   K. Oculoauriculovertebral dysplasia (Goldenhar-Gorlin syndrome)

L. Nephropathic cystinosis

M. Passow syndrome (Bremer status dysraphicus)

N. Psoriasis (lower cornea)

O. Riley-Day syndrome (congenital familial dysautonomia)

P. Rochon-Duvigneaud syndrome (superior orbital fissure syndrome)

Q. Rollet syndrome (orbital apex-sphenoidal syndrome)

R. Scholz subacute cerebral sclerosis (arylsulfatase A deficiency syndrome)

S. Temporal arteritis syndrome (cranial arteritis syndrome)

T. Tolosa-Hunt syndrome (painful ophthalmoplegia)

5. Toxins and drugs including:

amiodarone	chloroquine	levobunolol	propanolol
amitriptyline	clorazepate	meprobamate	steladex
amodiaquine	desipramine	methyprylon	stelazine
atenolol(?)	diazepam	metoprolol(?)	timolol
betaxolol	gentamicin(?)	nadolol(?)	trichloroethylene
bromide	glutethimide	nortriptyline	vinblastine
carbon dioxide	hydrogen sulfide	paraldehyde	vincristine
carbon disulfide	hydroxychloroquine	phencyclidine	
carisoprodol	imipramine	pindolol(?)	

Carpel, E.F.: Congenital corneal anesthesia. Am J Ophthalmol., 85:357–359, 1978.

Deg, J.K., et al.: Delayed corneal wound healing following radial keratotomy. Ophthalmology, 92:734–740, 1986.

Fraunfelder, F.T.: Drug-Induced Ocular Side Effects and Drug Interactions. 4th Ed. Philadelphia, Williams & Wilkins, 1996.

Glaser, J.S.: Neuro-Ophthalmology. 2nd Ed. Philadelphia, J.B. Lippincott Co., 1989.

Katz, B., et al.: Corneal sensitivity in nephropathic cystinosis. Am. J. Ophthalmol., 104:413–416, 1987.

Pau, H.: Differential Diagnosis of Eye Diseases. 2nd Ed. New York, Thieme Med. Pub., 1988.

Roy, F.H.: Ocular Syndromes and Systemic Diseases. 2nd Ed. Philadelphia, W.B. Saunders, 1989.

Hyperplastic Corneal Nerves (Overgrowth of Corneal Nerves up to Twenty Times the Normal Number). This nonspecific change may occur in association with the following:

1. Deep filiform dystrophy of Maeder and Danis

*2. Herpes simplex

*3. Herpes zoster

*4. Multiple endocrine neoplasia—type II B

5. Neurofibromatosis (von Recklinghausen syndrome)

6. Neuroparalytic keratitis

7. Normal eyes at advanced age

8. Ocular pemphigus foliaceus (Cazenave disease)

9. Opaque corneal grafts

* = most important

10. Phthisis bulbi

11. Posterior polymorphous dystrophy

Charlin, R.: Neoplasia endocrina multiple tipo II-B. Arch Chil. de Oftal., 38:21–27, 1981.

Menshen, J.H.: Corneal nerves. Surv. Ophthalmol., 19:1–18, 1974.

Roy, F.H.: Ocular Syndromes and Systemic Diseases. 2nd Ed. Philadelphia, W.B. Saunders, 1989.

Increased Visibility of Corneal Nerves

1. "Colloidin" skin syndrome (bullous ichthyosiform erythroderma)

2. Congenital

3. Ectodermal dysplasia (Rothmund syndrome)

4. Fuchs' dystrophy

5. Ichthyosis

6. Idiopathic

*7. Keratoconus

8. Leprosy (Hansen disease)

9. Neurofibromatosis (von Recklinghausen syndrome)

*10. Neurofibromatosis associated with pheochromocytoma and thyroid carcinoma (Sipple syndrome)

11. Posterior polymorphous dystrophy

12. Primary amyloidosis

13. Refsum syndrome (phytanic acid storage disease)

14. Siemen disease (keratosis follicularis spinulosa decalvans)

Arffa, R.C.: Grayson's Diseases of the Cornea. 3rd Ed. St. Louis, Mosby–Year Book, 1991.

Pau, H.: Differential Diagnosis of Eye Diseases. 2nd Ed. New York, Thieme Med. Pub., 1988.

Roy, F.H.: Ocular Syndromes and Systemic Diseases. 2nd Ed. Philadelphia, W.B. Saunders, 1989.

Pigmentation of Cornea

1. Melanin pigmentation

   A. Epithelial melanosis

   (1) Congenital

   (2) Presence of limbal malignant melanoma

   (3) Sequela of trachoma and other inflammations

   (4) Melanocytic migration in heavily pigmented individuals

   B. Stromal pigmentation such as that in ochronosis

   C. Endothelial melanosis

   (1) Congenital

   (2) Senile

   (3) Degenerative, including: atrophic and inflammatory conditions (such as cornea guttata, herpes simplex, zoster keratitis, myopia, diabetes mellitus, senile cataract, chronic glaucoma, and melanoma)

   *(4) Krukenberg spindle, with or without pigmentary glaucoma, may be present in association with diabetes mellitus

(5) Trauma—from contusions, wounds, or intraocular operations

(6) Turks line—fine vertical line in the lower portion of the cornea

2. Hematogenous pigmentation

   *A. Blood—staining of the cornea, most often because of total hyphema associated with elevated intraocular pressure

   B. Hemorrhage into cornea—following subconjunctival hemorrhage and intra-corneal hemorrhage from newly formed vessels, as in interstitial keratitis or mustard gas keratitis

   C. Epithelial deposit associated with spherocytic anemia

3. Metallic pigmentation

   A. Copper (chalcosis)

      *(1) Kayser-Fleischer ring—limbal ring associated with Wilson's disease

      (2) Copper foreign body in cornea or intraocular region

      (3) Occupational exposure or topical therapeutic use of copper-containing substance

      (4) Advanced cirrhosis of the liver, such as that associated with parasitic infestation (schistosomiasis)

   B. Silver (argyrosis)—from topical, local, or systemic use; also occupational use

   C. Gold (chrysiasis)—from topical, local, or systemic use

   D. Iron (siderosis)

      (1) Foreign body in cornea or intraocular area

      (2) Iron lines

         *a. Fleischer ring—associated with keratoconus around base of the cone

         b. Hudson-Stahli line—horizontal line at the junction of the middle and lower one third of the cornea, believed to be related to exposure, trauma of lid closure, and chronic corneal infection

         c. Stocker line—line running parallel with head of the pterygium

         d. Ferry line—associated with filtering blebs, believed to result from minute, re-peated, localized trauma caused by eyelid striking the elevated bleb

         e. Circular lesion associated with congenital spherocytosis

         f. Iron lines following refractive corneal surgery, such as radial keratotomy and photorefractive keratectomy

   E. Bismuth (bismuthiasis)—from therapeutic use

   F. Arsenic melanosis

4. Drugs, discoloration, including:

acetophenazine	aurothioglucose
acid bismuth sodium tartrate	auranofin
alcohol	aurothioglycanide
amiodarone	bismuth carbonate
amodiaquine	bismuth oxychloride
antimony potassium tartrate	bismuth salicylate
antimony sodium tartrate	bismuth sodium tartrate
antimony sodium thioglycolate	bismuth sodium thioglycollate

* = most important

bismuth sodium triglycollamate   mild silver protein
bismuth subcarbonate   perazine
bismuth subsalicylate   perhexiline
butaperazine   pericyazine
calcitriol   perphenazine
carphenazine   phenylmercuric nitrate
chloroquine   piperacetazine
chlorpromazine   polysaccharide-iron complex
chlorprothixene   prochlorperazine
chlortetracycline   promazine
colloidal silver   promethazine
diethazine   propiomazine
echothiophate   quinacrine
epinephrine   quinidine
ergocalciferol   silver nitrate
ethopropazine   silver protein
ferrocholinate   sodium antimonylgluconate
ferrous fumarate   stibocaptate
ferrous gluconate   stibogluconate
ferrous succinate   stibophen
ferrous sulfate   tetracycline
fluphenazine   thiethylperazine
gold Au 198   thimerosal
gold sodium thiomalate   thiopropazate
gold sodium thiosulfate   thioproperazine
hydroxychloroquine   thioridazine
indomethacin   thiothixene
iron dextran   trifluoperazine
iron sorbitex   triflupromazine
meperidine(?)   trimeprazine
mercuric oxide   vitamin A(?)
mesoridazine   vitamin D
methdilazine   vitamin D_2
methotrimeprazine   vitamin D_3
methylene blue

5. Other color changes

   A. White discoloration—scars, fatty degeneration or infiltration, and calcified areas

   B. Yellow, discoloration—hyaline or colloid degeneration, and Tangier disease
      (familial deficiency of high-density lipoprotein)

   C. Black discoloration—coal powder, dirt, epinephrine, or ink (tattooing)

   D. Yellow-brown discoloration—Kyrle disease (hyperkeratosis follicularis et
      parafollicularis in cutem penetrans)

E. Grey-black discoloration—chronic phenol exposure as carbolic acid

F. Grey-white discoloration—anesthetic cornea

G. Brown discoloration—aniline (amidobenzole), including: benzoquinone and hydroquinine

Brodrick, J.D.: Pigmentation of the cornea. Ann. Ophthalmol., 11:855–861, 1979.

Fraunfelder, F.T.: Drug-Induced Ocular Side Effects and Drug Interactions. 4th Ed. Philadelphia, Williams & Wilkins, 1996.

Grant, W.M.: Toxicology of the Eye. 3rd Ed. Springfield, Ill., Charles C Thomas, 1986.

Pau, H.: Differential Diagnosis of Eye Diseases. 2nd Ed. New York, Thieme Med. Pub., 1988.

Corneal Edema

1. Drugs, including:

acetophenazine

acetylcholine

alpha-chymotrypsin

amodiaquine

amphotericin B

bacitracin

benoxinate

benzalkonium chloride

benzathine penicillin G

butacaine

butaperazine

carbachol

carphenazine

chloramphenicol

chlorhexidine

chloroquine

chlorpromazine

chlortetracycline

cocaine

colistin

deslanoside

dibucaine

diethazine

digitoxin

digoxin

dyclonine

epinephrine

erythromycin

ethopropazine

fluphenazine

hydrabamine penicillin

hydrogen peroxide

hydroxychloroquine

idoxuridine

IDU

lanatoside C

melphalan

mesoridazine

methdilazine

methicillin

methotrimeprazine

neomycin

perazine

pericyazine

perphenazine

phenacaine

phenoxymethyl penicillin

phenylephrine

piperacetazine

piperocaine

polymyxin B

potassium penicillin G

potassium penicillin V

potassium phenethicillin

potassium phenoxymethyl penicillin

procaine penicillin G

prochlorperazine

promazine

promethazine

proparacaine

propiomazine

quinacrine

silicone	thiotepa
streptomycin	trifluoperazine
tetracaine	triflupromazine
tetracycline	trifluridine
thiethylperazine	trimeprazine
thiopropazate	urokinase
thioproperazine	vidarabine
thioridazine	vinblastine

2. Endothelial decompensation

    A. Noninflammatory

        *(1) Acute hydrops with keratoconus

        (2) Congenital

            a. Anhidrotic ectodermal dysplasia

          *b. Birth trauma, typically a forceps injury

            c. Congenital glaucoma

            d. Congenital hereditary endothelial dystrophy

            e. Posterior polymorphous dystrophy

        (3) Environmental cold in trigeminal nerve palsy

        (4) Essential corneal edema

        (5) Failed corneal graft

        (6) Metabolic such as myxedema and hypercholesteremia

        (7) Neuropathic conditions

        (8) Postsurgical

            a. Anterior segment ischemia

            b. Anterior synechiae

            c. Direct mechanical damage to endothelium including argon laser iridotomy

            d. Epithelial or fibrous downgrowth

            e. Osmotic, such as irrigation of cornea or anterior chamber with distilled water

            f. Stripped Descemet membrane

            g. Vitreous touch

        *(9) Primary degenerative—Fuchs' dystrophy

        (10) Traumatic

            a. Anoxia of epithelium, such as from excessive wearing of contact lens (Sattler veil)

            b. Chemical, such as tear gas, hydrogen peroxide and Hibiclens

            c. Exposure as in exophthalmos

            d. Large epithelial defect

            e. Nonpenetrating including after air bag inflation injury

            f. Penetrating

            g. Radiation injury such as from UV, roentgenograms, gamma rays

      h. Retained foreign body-anterior chamber

      i. Trigeminal nerve palsy with cold exposure

  B. Inflammatory

    (1) Any severe iritis

    (2) Acute graft rejection

    (3) Chandler's syndrome (iridocorneal endothelial syndrome)

   *(4) Herpes simplex keratitis or keratouveitis

   *(5) Herpes zoster keratouveitis

    (6) Retinal tacks

3. Increased intraocular pressure

  *A. Acute glaucoma

  B. Chronic glaucoma

    (1) Minimal to moderate pressure elevations in the presence of abnormal endothelium

    (2) Prolonged moderately high elevations in the presence of normal or near-normal endothelium

4. Hypotony

Arffa, R.C.: Grayson's Diseases of the Cornea. 3rd Ed. St. Louis, Mosby—Year Book, 1991.

Fraunfelder, F.T.: Drug-Induced Ocular Side Effects and Drug Interactions. 4th Ed. Philadelphia, Williams & Wilkins, 1996.

Herse, P., and Hooker, B.: Corneal edema recovery dynamics in diabetes: is the alloxan induced diabetic rabbit a useful model? Investigative Ophthal. & Visual Science, 35:310–313, 1994.

Lesher, M.P., et al.: Corneal edema, hyphema, and angle recession after air bag inflation. Archives of Ophthalmol., 111:1320–1322, 1993.

Reed, J.W., et al.: Clinical and pathologic findings of aphakic peripheral corneal edema: Brown-McLean syndrome. Cornea, 11:577–583, 1992.

Wilhelmus, K.R.: Corneal edema following argon laser iridotomy. Ophthal. Surgery, 23:533–537, 1992.

Corneal Hydrops (Ruptures of Descemet's Membrane with Cornea Intralamellar Dissection and Collection of Aqueous Humor)

1. Congenital glaucoma

2. Forceps injury

*3. Keratoconus

4. Pellucid marginal degeneration

5. Terrien marginal degeneration

6. Trauma, blunt

Soong, H.K., et al.: Corneal hydrops in Terrien's marginal degeneration. Ophthalmology, 93:340–343, 1986.

* = most important

Microcornea

	Ehlers-Danlos Syndrome	Meyer-Schnickerath-Weyers Syndrome	Riegler Syndrome	Azenfeld Syndrome	Laurence-Moon-Biedl Syndrome	Weill-Marchesani Syndrome	Rubella*	Gansslen Syndrome	Hallerman-Strieff Syndrome	Hemifacial Microsomia Syndrome	Trisomy 13–15 (Patau Syndrome)
History											
1. Death during first month											U
2. Hereditary	U		U	U	U	R		U	U		U
3. More in males					U						
4. Onset in childhood		U			U		U			S	
Physical Findings											
1. Angioid streaks	S										
2. Aniridia									R		
3. Blue sclera									S		
4. Cataracts					R	S	U		S	S	S
5. Chamber angle iris strands											
6. Choroidal/vitreous hemorrhage	S										
7. Coloboma of iris					S					S	S
8. Corectopia		U									
9. Corneal opacification			S	S				S			S
10. Ectopia lentis	S					S					
11. Epicanthus	S							S			R
12. Exophthalmos	S										
13. Glaucoma		S	U	U		R	U				
14. Hypertelorism				S				S			S
15. Hypoplasia anterior iris stroma		S	U								
16. Iritis								S			
17. Keratoconus	S				S						
18. Lacrimal duct defects	S								R		
19. Lid skin laxity	S										
20. Macular pigment degeneration	S				S	R	S				
21. Microphthalmos	S	S					S	S	U	S	S
22. Microspherophakia						S					
23. Myopia	S	S			S	S		S			
24. Nystagmus						S			S		
25. Optic atrophy					S						
26. Optic nerve hypoplasia											R
27. Persistent hyperplastic primary vitreous											S
28. Ptosis	S				S						
29. Pupillary membrane		S							S		
30. Retinal detachment	S							R			
31. Retinal hemorrhage								S	S		
32. Retinitis pigmentosa					S						
33. Sclerocornea									R		
34. Soft retinal exudate								S			
35. Strabismus					S			S	S	U	
36. Subretinal neovascularization								S			
Laboratory Data											
1. Immunoglobuin M antibody							U				
2. Chromosomal studies											U

R = rarely; S = sometimes; and U = usually.

Microcornea (Cornea Having a Horizontal Diameter of Less than Ten Millimeters)

1. Associated ocular findings
    A. Aniridia and subluxated lenses
    B. Autosomal dominant cataract and myopia
    C. Autosomal dominant cataract, nystagmus and glaucoma
    D. Axenfeld syndrome (posterior embryotoxon)
    E. Colobomatous macrophthalmia
    F. Congenital glaucoma
    G. Corectopia and macular hypoplasia
    H. Hyperopia
    I. Meckel syndrome (dysencephalia splanchnocystica syndrome)
    J. Nanophthalmos
    K. Narrow-angle glaucoma
    L. Sclerocornea
2. Aberfeld syndrome (congenital blepharophimosis associated with generalized myopathy)
3. Autosomal recessive or dominant trait
4. Carpenter syndrome (acrocephalopolysyndactyly II)
5. Cataract microcornea syndrome
6. Chromosome partial deletion (long-arm) syndrome
7. Deafness retardation, arched palate syndrome
8. Ehlers-Danlos syndrome (fibrodysplasia elastica generalisata)
9. Gansslen syndrome (familial hemolytic icterus)
10. Hallermann-Streiff syndrome (dyscephalic mandibulo-oculo-facial syndrome)
11. Hemifacial microsomia syndrome (Francois Haustrate syndrome)
12. Hutchinson-Gilford syndrome (Progeria)
13. Laurence-Moon-Biedl syndrome (retinitis pigmentosa-polydactylyadiposo-genital syndrome)
14. Lenz microphthalmia syndrome
15. Little syndrome (nail patella syndrome)
16. Marchesani syndrome (mesodermal dysmorphodystrophy)
17. Marfan syndrome (arachnodactyly dystrophica mesodermalis congenita)
18. Meckel syndrome (dysencephalia splanchnocystica syndrome)
19. Meyer-Schwickerath-Weyers syndrome (oculodentodigital dysplasia)
20. Microcornea, glaucoma, absent frontal sinuses
21. Micro syndrome
22. Rieger syndrome (hypodontia and iris dysgenesis)
23. Ring chromosome
24. Rubella syndrome (Gregg syndrome)
25. Sabin-Feldman syndrome

* = most important

26. Schwartz syndrome (glaucoma associated with retinal detachment)
27. Triploidy (chromosomes instead of 46)
28. Trisomy 13 (D trisomy, Patau syndrome)
29. Trisomy syndrome
30. Waardenburg syndrome (interoculoiridodermatoauditive dysplasia)

Isenberg, S.J.: The Eye in Infancy. Chicago Medical Publishers, 1989.

Mollica, F., et al.: Autosomal dominant cataract and microcornea associated with myopia in a Sicilian family. Clin. Genet, 28:42–46, 1985.

Roy, F.H.: Ocular Syndromes and Systemic Diseases. 2nd Ed. Philadelphia, W.B. Saunders, 1989.

Warburg, M., et al.: Autosomal recessive microcephaly, microcornea, congenital cataract, mental retardation, optic atrophy, and hypogenitalism. Amer J of Disease of Children, 147:1309–1312, 1993.

Megalocornea (Cornea Having a Horizontal Diameter of More Than Fourteen Millimeters)

	Aarksog Syndrome	Autosomal Dominant or Recessive Trait	Congenital Glaucoma	Marfan Syndrome	Scheie Syndrome (Mucopolysaccharidoses I-S)	Lowe Syndrome	Osteogenesis Imperfecta	Posterior Embryotoxon	Rieger Syndrome	Sex-linked Recessive Trait
History										
1. Autosomal dominant trait		U		U			U	U	U	
2. Autosomal recessive trait		S			U					
3. Congenital			U					U		
4. Early childhood			U							
5. Hereditary	U	U		U	U	U	U		U	U
6. Night blindness					U					
7. Sex-linked recessive	U					U				U
8. Tearing			S							
Physical Findings										
1. Aniridia of iris										
2. Anisocoria					U				U	
3. Anterior displaced Schwalbe line								U	U	
4. Anterior embryotoxon										U
5. Anterior synechiae									U	
6. Antimongoloid lid slants (temporal canthus lower)		U								
7. Blepharoptosis	U									
8. Blue sclera							U			
9. Breaks in Descemet membrane			U							
10. Buphthalmos			U			U				
11. Cataracts			U	U	S	U	U			
12. Coloboma of iris				R						
13. Corneal clouding					U	U			S	
14. Corneal epithelial and stromal edema			U							
15. Epicanthal folds		U								
16. Glaucomatous cupping			U		S					
17. High astigmatism										U
18. Hyperopic astigmatism	S									
19. Hypertelorism	U									
20. Increased intraocular pressure			U		S	U	U		U	
21. Iris hypoplasia		S							U	
22. Keratoconus				U						
23. Krukenberg spindle									R	U
24. Lens dislocation				U						
25. Malformed anterior chamber angle/iris						U				
26. Microphakia						U				
27. Microphthalmos						U				
28. Myopia			S	U						U
29. Nystagmus					S	U				
30. Optic atrophy			S		S				S	
31. Proptosis					S					
32. Pupillary reaction absent						U				
33. Ring scotoma					U					
34. Spherophakia				U						
35. Strabismus	S			S		U				

Megalocornea (Cornea Having a Horizontal Diameter of More Than Fourteen Millimeters) *Continued*

	Aarskog Syndrome	Autosomal Dominant or Recessive Trait	Congenital Glaucoma	Marfan Syndrome	Scheie Syndrome (Mucopolysaccharidoses I-S)	Lowe Syndrome	Osteogenesis Imperfecta	Posterior Embryotoxon	Rieger Syndrome	Sex-linked Recessive Trait
Physical Findings										
36. Tapetoretinal degeneration					S					
37. Telecanthus	U									
Laboratory Data										
1. Bone roentgenogram				U			U			
2. Cardiovascular studies				U						
3. Genetic studies	U	U		U	U	U	U		U	U
4. Urine tests										
Aminoaciduria/phosphaturia						U				
Chondroitin sulfate B elevated						U				
Hematuria/proteinuria						U				
5. Visual field test			U		U				S	

R = rarely; S = sometimes; and U = usually.

Megalocornea (Cornea Having a Horizontal Diameter of More than Fourteen Millimeters)

1. Aarskog syndrome (facial digital genital syndrome)
2. Autosomal dominant or recessive trait
3. Congenital glaucoma (rare)
4. Craniosynostosis
5. Down syndrome
6. Facial hemiatrophy
7. Isolated
8. Marchesani syndrome (brachymorphia with spherophakia)
9. Marfan syndrome (arachnodactyly dystrophia mesodermalis congenita)
10. MMR syndrome (megalocornea-mental retardation)
11. MMMM syndrome (megalocornea, macrocephaly, mental and motor retardation)
12. Mucopolysaccharidoses I-S (Scheie syndrome)
13. Neuhauser syndrome (megalocornea-mental retardation syndrome)
14. Oculocerebrorenal syndrome (Lowe syndrome)
15. Oculodental syndrome (Peter syndrome)
16. Osteogenesis imperfecta (van der Hoeve syndrome)
17. Oxycephaly (dysostosis craniofacialis)
18. Pierre-Robin syndrome (micrognathia-glossoptosis syndrome)
19. Posterior embryotoxon
20. Rieger syndrome (hypodontia and iris syndrome)
21. Rubella syndrome (Gregg syndrome)
22. Sex-linked recessive trait
23. Sturge-Weber syndrome (meningocutaneous syndrome)

Arffa, R.C.: Grayson's Diseases of the Cornea. 3rd Ed. St. Louis, Mosby–Year Book, 1.

Frydman, M., et al.: Megalocornea, macrocephaly, mental and motor retardation (MMMM). Clinical Genetics, 38:149–154, 1990.

Isenberg, S.J.: The Eye in Infancy. Chicago, Year Book Medical Publishers, 1989.

Roy, F.H.: Ocular Syndromes and Systemic Diseases. 2nd Ed. Philadelphia, W.B. Saunders, 1989.

Verloes, A., et al.: Heterogeneity versus variability in megalocornea-mental retardation (MMR) syndromes: report of new cases and delineation of probable types. Am J. Medical Genetics, 46: 132–137, 1993.

Corneal Opacification in Infancy (See Conditions Simulating Congenital Glaucoma, p. 342)

*1. Birth trauma, such as Descemet membrane rupture
2. Chromosomal aberrations
    A. Mongolism (Down syndrome)—trisomy 21
    B. Trisomy 13 (Patau syndrome)
3. Congenital malformations
    A. Amyloidosis (Lubarsch-Pick syndrome)

* = most important

  B. Anterior chamber cleavage syndromes

    (1) Axenfeld's anomaly

    (2) Congenital central anterior synechiae

    (3) Congenital anterior staphyloma

   *(4) Peter's anomaly

    (5) Rieger's anomaly

  C. Bilateral corneal dermis-like choristomas

  D. Congenital glaucoma

 *E. Dermoid tumors

 *F. Sclerocornea

  G. Xanthomas

4. Corneal dystrophy

 *A. congenital hereditary endothelial dystrophy

  B. congenital hereditary stromal dystrophy

  C. posterior polymorphous dystrophy

5. Idiopathic

6. Inborn errors of metabolism

 *A. Mucopolysaccharidoses (MPS)

   (1) Hurler syndrome (MPS IN)

   (2) Maroteaux-Lamy syndrome (MPS VI)

   (3) Morquio-Brailsford syndrome (MPS IV)

   (4) Scheie syndrome (MPS IS)

  B. Lowe syndrome (oculocerebrorenal syndrome)

  C. von Gierke disease (glycogen disease)

  D. Corneal lipoidosis—later

  E. Mucolipidosis

   (1) Generalized gangliosidosis (GM1-gangliosidosis I and II)

   (2) ML I (lipomucopolysaccharidosis)

   (3) ML III (pseudo-Hurler polydystrophy)

  F. Riley-Day syndrome (congenital familial dysautonomia)

7. Inflammatory processes

  A. Corneal ulceration

  B. Herpes simplex and herpes zoster

  C. Interstitial keratitis

  D. Rubella syndrome (German measles)

Kolker, A.E., and Hetherington, I.: Becker-Shaffer's Diagnosis and Therapy of Glaucoma. 6th Ed. St. Louis, C.V. Mosby Co., 1989.

Roy, F.H.: Ocular Syndromes and Systemic Diseases. 2nd Ed. Philadelphia, W.B. Saunders, 1989.

Topilow, H.W., et al.: Bilateral corneal dermis-like choristomas. Arch Ophthalmol., 99:1387, 1981.

Band-shaped Keratopathy (Corneal Opacification Extending Horizontally over the Cornea at the Level of Bowman Membrane in Exposed Part of Palpebral Aperture)

1. Anterior mosaic dystrophy, primary type
    A. Episkopi (sex-linked recessive)
    B. Labrador keratopathy
2. Discoid lupus erythematosus
3. Dysproteinemia
4. Gout (hyperuricemia)
5. High levels of visible electromagnetic radiation such as xenon arc photocoagulation and laser causing acute severe anterior uveitis
6. Hypercalcemia
    A. Excessive vitamin D as with oral intake, Boeck sarcoid with liver involvement, acute osteoporosis, Heerfordt syndrome, and Schaumann syndrome
    B. Hyperparathyroidism
    C. Hypophosphatasia (phosphoethanolaminuria)
    D. Idiopathic hypercalcemia
    E. Milk-alkali syndrome
    F. Paget syndrome (osteitis deformans)
    G. Renal failure, such as that associated with Fanconi syndrome (cystinosis)
7. Ichthyosis vulgaris
*8. Local degenerative diseases, including: chronic uveitis, phthisis bulbi, absolute glaucoma, infantile polyarthritis (Still disease), rheumatoid arthritis, interstitial keratitis, Felty syndrome, and juvenile rheumatoid arthritis
9. Long-term miotic therapy
10. Progressive facial hemiatrophy (Parry-Romberg syndrome)
11. Rothmund syndrome (ectodermal syndrome)
12. Silicone oil in anterior chamber
13. Traumatic—chronic exposure to irritants, such as mercury fumes, calomel, calcium bichromate vapor, and hair
14. Tuberous sclerosis (Bourneville syndrome)
15. Tumoral calcinosis
16. Viscoat usage
17. Wagner syndrome (hyaloideoretinal degeneration)
18. X-linked recessive ocular dystrophy

Arffa, R.C.: Grayson's Diseases of the Cornea. 3rd Ed. St. Louis, Mosby–Year Book, 1991.

Beekhuis, W.H., et al.: Silicone oil in the anterior chamber of the eye. Arch Ophthalmol., 104:793, 1986.

Feist, R.M, et al.: Transient calcific band-shaped keratopathy associated with increased serum calcium. Amer J Ophthal., 113:459–461, 1992.

Grossniklaus, H.E., et al.: Sulfur and calcific keratopathy associated with retinal detachment surgery and vitrectomy. Ophthalmology, 93:260–264, 1986.

* = most important

Gutt, L., et al.: Band keratopathy and calcific lid lesions in tumoral calcinosis. Arch Ophthalmol., 106:725–726, 1988.

Nevyas, A.S., et al.: Acute band keratopathy following intracameral viscoat. Arch Ophthalmol., 105:958–964, 1987.

Roy, F.H.: Ocular Syndromes and Systemic Diseases. 2nd Ed. Philadelphia, W.B. Saunders, 1989.

Corneal Keloids

1. Lowe syndrome (oculocerebrorenal syndrome)
2. Trauma, usually with iris perforation

Cibis, G.W., et al.: Corneal keloid in Lowe's syndrome. Arch. Ophthalmol., 100:1795, 1982.

Punctate Keratitis or Keratopathy

1. Alimentary disorders
    A. Mouth
       *(1) Dry mouth as in Sjôgren syndrome
        (2) Ulcers, such as primary herpes, ocular cicatricial pemphigoid, and erythema multiforme
    B. Lower alimentary tract
        (1) Ulcerative colitis as in Sjôgren disease
        (2) Mild colitis, such as that due to an adenovirus
    C. Stomach
        (1) Indigestion as in Sjôgren syndrome and acne rosacea
2. Articular diseases
    A. Psoriasis arthropathica
    B. Reiter disease (polyarthritis enterica)
    C. Riley-Day syndrome (congenital familial dysautonomia)
    D. Sjôgren syndrome (secretoinhibitor syndrome)
3. Conjunctival discharge
    A. Mucoid
        (1) Other types of keratoconjunctivitis sicca
        (2) Sjôgren disease (secretoinhibitor syndrome)
    B. Mucopurulent (see p. 213)
        (1) Angular blepharoconjunctivitis
        (2) Erythema multiforme (Stevens-Johnson syndrome)
        (3) Gonococcal
        (4) Inclusion conjunctivitis (acute stage)
        (5) Meningococcal
        (6) Reiter disease (polyarthritis enterica)
        (7) Trachoma
        (8) Vernal conjunctivitis
    C. Serous

(1) Adenovirus

(2) Herpes simplex

(3) Herpes zoster

(4) Inclusion conjunctivitis (later)

(5) Molluscum contagiosum

(6) Trachoma (later)

(7) Warts

4. Conjunctival inflammation

A. Cicatrizing (see p. 224)

*(1) Ocular circutricial pemphigoid

(2) Chemical burns

*(3) Erythema multiforme (Stevens-Johnson syndrome)

(4) Diphtheria

(5) Fuchs-Salzmann-Terrien syndrome (allergic reactions from drugs)

(6) Radiation burns

*(7) Sjôgren keratoconjunctivitis sicca

(8) Thermal burns

(9) Trachoma

B. Diffuse catarrhal

(1) Adenovirus

(2) Bacterial conjunctivitis

(3) Erythema multiforme (Stevens-Johnson syndrome)

(4) Onchocerciasis syndrome (river blindness)

(5) Reiter disease (polyarthritis enterica)

(6) Superior limbic keratoconjunctivitis

(7) Vaccinia

C. Follicular (see p. 220)

(1) Adenovirus

(2) Herpes simplex

(3) Herpes zoster

(4) Inclusion conjunctivitis

(5) Molluscum contagiosum

(6) Trachoma

D. Giant papillary, such as in vernal and atopic conjunctivitis, and related to contact users, prosthesis, and exposed sutures

E. Papillary

(1) Sjôgren syndrome (secretoinhibitor syndrome)

(2) Trachoma

5. Corneal conditions

A. Deep keratitis, disciform or irregular

* = most important

~~*(1)   Herpes simplex~~

    (2)   Herpes zoster and other viral diseases

    (3)   Corneal dystrophy, e.g. lattice, superi

B. Thinned facets because of previous ulcerative or other lesions

    (1)   Acne rosacea (ocular rosacea)

    (2)   Erythema multiforme (Stevens-Johnson syndrome)

    (3)   Gorlin-Chaudhry-Moss syndrome

    (4)   Herpes simplex

    (5)   Sjôgren keratoconjunctivitis sicca

C. Vascularization

    (1)   Acne rosacea (ocular rosacea)

    (2)   Molluscum contagiosum

    (3)   Ocular cicatricial pemphigoid

    (4)   Phlyctenular disease (see p. 318)

    (5)   Sjôgren keratoconjunctivitis sicca

    (6)   Trachoma

    (7)   Vaccinia

D. Trauma

    (1)   Chemical injury

    (2)   Contact lens related

    (3)   Foreign body under upper eyelid

    (4)   Mild, such as eye rubbing

    (5)   Ultraviolet photokeratopathy

E. Thygeson's SPK

6. Diseases of the lids

A. Dermatitis

    (1)   Psoriasis

    (2)   Seborrheic blepharitis

B. Ectropion (see p. 91)

    (1)   Exposure keratopathy

    (2)   Neuroparalytic keratopathy

C. Folliculitis (see p. 109)

    (1)   Blepharitis due to Demodex folliculorum

    (2)   Seborrheic blepharitis

    (3)   Staphylococcal blepharitis

D. Lid retraction (see p. 71)

    (1)   Endocrine exophthalmos

    *(2) Exposure keratopathy

E. Madarosis, such as that associated with leprosy (stiff immobile lids)

F. Nodules

        (1) Acne rosacea (ocular rosacea)

        (2) Molluscum contagiosum

        (3) Papilloma

        (4) Warts

    G. Trichiasis or entropion with traumatic keratitis (see p. 295)

    H. Vesicles or ulcers

        (1) Herpes simplex

        (2) Herpes zoster

        (3) Ocular cicatricial pemphigoid

        (4) Vaccinia

    I. Floppy eyelid syndrome

7. Diseases of the skin associated with punctate keratitis

    A. Acne rosacea (ocular rosacea)

    B. CRST syndrome (calcinosis)

    C. Erythema multiforme (Stevens-Johnson syndrome)

    D. Follicular hyperkeratosis of the palms and soles

    E. Hypertrichosis

    F. Ichthyosis

    G. Leprosy (Hansen disease)

    H. Melkersson-Rosenthal syndrome (Melkersson idiopathic fibroedema)

    I. Ocular cicatricial pemphigoid

    J. Psoriasis

8. Genitourinary diseases associated with punctate keratitis

    A. Erythema multiforme (Stevens-Johnson syndrome)

    B. Inclusion blennorrhea

    C. Ocular cicatricial pemphigoid

    D. Reiter disease (polyarthritis enterica)

9. Keratitis, associated with use of drugs, including:

acetophenazine	auranofin
acetyldigitoxin	aurothioglucose
acyclovir	aurothioglycanide
adenine arabinoside	bacitracin
alcohol	benoxinate
allopurinol	benzalkonium
amantadine	betamethasone
amphotericin B	betaxolol
antazoline	brompheniramine
antipyrine	butacaine
aspirin	butaperazine
atenolol	carbimazole

carphenazine
chlorambucil
chloroform
chlorpheniramine
chlorpromazine
chlorprothixene
chlortetracycline
chrysarobin
ciprofloxacin
cocaine
colchicine
cortisone
cyclopentolate
cytarabine
deslanoside
dexamethasone
dexbrompheniramine
dexchlorpheniramine
dextran
dibucaine
diethazine
diethylcarbamazine
digitoxin
digoxin
dimethindene
dipivefrin
dyclonine
emetine
epinephrine
ether
ethopropazine
etretinate
fluorometholone
fluphenazine
flurbiprofen
framycetin
gentamicin
gitalin
gold Au 198
gold sodium thiomalate
guanethidine
hexachlorophene
hydrocortisone

idoxuridine
indomethacin
iodide and iodine solutions and compounds
isoniazid
isotretinoin
lanatoside C
levobunolol
medrysone
mesoridazine
methdilazine
methimazole
methotrexate
methotrimeprazine
methoxsalen
methylthiouracil
metoprolol
nadolol
naphazoline
neomycin
ofloxacin
ouabain
oral contraceptives
oxprenolol
oxyphenbutazone
penicillamine
perazine
pericyazine
perphenazine
phenacaine
pheniramine
phenylbutazone
phenylephrine
pilocarpine
pindolol
piperacetazine
piperocaine
polymyxin B
prednisolone
prochlorperazine
promazine
promethazine
proparacaine
propiomazine

propylthiouracil

radioactive iodides

rubella virus vaccine (live)

smallpox vaccine

sodium salicylate

sulfacetamide

sulfachlorpyridazine

sulfacytine

sulfadiazine

sulfadimethoxine

sulfamerazine

sulfameter

sulfamethazine

sulfamethizole

sulfamethoxazole

sulfamethoxypyridazine

sulfanilamide

sulfaphenazole

sulfapyridine

sulfasalazine

sulfathiazole

sulfisoxazole

sulindac

suramin

tetracaine

tetracycline

tetrahydrozoline

thiethylperazine

thimerosal

thiopropazate

thioproperazine

thioridazine

thiotepa

thiothixene

timolol

tobramycin

trichloroethylene

trifluoperazine

trifluorothymidine

triflupromazine

trimeprazine

trimethoprim

trioxsalen

triprolidine

tropicamide

vidarabine

vinblastine

vidarabine

10. Limbal conditions associated with punctate keratitis

    A. Focal necrotic lesions

        (1) Herpes simplex

        (2) Phlyctenular disease

        (3) Vaccinia

    B. Follicles

        (1) Acne rosacea (ocular rosacea)

        (2) Herpes simplex

        (3) Inclusion conjunctivitis

        (4) Molluscum contagiosum

        (5) Trachoma

        (6) Other viral infections

    C. Nodules and plaques

        (1) Avitaminosis A (Bitot spots)

        (2) Bowen disease (dyskeratosis)

        (3) Intra-epithelial melanoma

        (4) Limbal vernal conjunctivitis

11. Punctate keratitis preceded by lymphadenopathy

    A. Adenovirus

    B. Herpes simplex

    C. Herpes zoster

    D. Inclusion conjunctivitis

    E. Trachoma

    F. Vaccinia

12. Respiratory diseases

    A. Adenovirus infections

    B. Myxovirus infections (influenza, Newcastle disease, mumps)

    C. Recurrent herpes complicating any fever

Dekkers, N.W.H.M.: The Cornea in Measles. The Hague, Dr. Junk, 1981.

Fraunfelder, F.T.: Drug-Induced Ocular Side Effects and Drug Interactions. 4th Ed. Philadelphia, Williams & Wilkins. 1996.

Jones, B.R.: Differential diagnosis of punctate keratitis. Int. Ophthalmol. Clin., 2:591–611, 1962.

Maudgal, P.C., and Missotten, L.: Superficial Keratitis. The Hague, Dr. Junk, 1981.

Roy, F.H.: Ocular Syndromes and Systemic Diseases. 2nd Ed. Philadelphia, W.B. Saunders, 1989.

Sachs, R.: Corneal Complications Associated with the Use of Crack Cocaine. Ophthalmology, 100:187–191, 1993.

Yang, Y.F., et al.: Epidemic hemorrhagic keratoconjunctivitis. Am. J. Ophthalmol., 30:192–197, 1975.

Morphologic Classification of Punctate Corneal Lesions (Classification by Anatomic Location)

1. Punctate epithelial erosions—fine, very slightly depressed spots scarcely visible without staining with fluorescein

    A. Warts

    B. Artificial—silk keratitis

    C. Staphylococcal blepharoconjunctivitis (lower cornea)

    *D. Keratoconjunctivitis sicca (interpalpebral area)

    *E. Exposure keratitis (interpalpebral area)

    F. Neuroparalytic keratitis (see p. 295)

    G. Ocular medications (especially those with preservatives)

    H. Trichiasis

    I. Trauma, mild (e.g. eye rubbing)

2. Punctate epithelial keratitis—very small, whitish flecks on the surface of the epithelium

    A. Fine

        (1) Scattered—staphylococcal blepharitis; viral keratitis, especially trachoma and molluscum contagiosum, sometimes, inclusion conjunctivitis, and not infrequently herpetic keratitis and rubeola and rubella

        (2) Confluent—keratitis sicca, exposure keratitis, vernal conjunctivitis, topical steroid-induced, and early viral keratitis

B. Coarse

   *(1) Thygeson superficial punctate keratitis (characteristic)

   (2) Herpes zoster

   (3) Adenovirus infections

   (4) Early herpes simplex

   (5) Acne rosacea (lower cornea)

   (6) Encephalitozoon hellem

C. Areolar—spots have enlarged to occupy a large area

   (1) Herpes simplex

   (2) Thygeson superficial punctate keratitis

   (3) Herpes zoster

   (4) Vaccinia

3. Filamentary keratitis or keratopathy—formation of fine epithelial filaments that are attached at one end

  *A. Keratoconjunctivitis sicca (frequent)

  B. Infections, such as that due to adenovirus, herpes, vaccinia, acne rosacea, molluscum contagiosum, rubella, rubeola, and staphylococcus

  C. Trauma, such as wounds, abrasions, exposure to shortwave diathermy, and prolonged eye-patching

  D. Edema of cornea, such as that due to recurrent erosions or wearing of contact lens

  E. Sarcoid with infiltration of conjunctiva and lacrimal gland

  F. Heerfordt syndrome and Mikulicz syndrome

  G. After irradiation of the lacrimal gland

  H. Keratoconus (see p. 328)

  I. Neuropathic keratopathy (anesthesia of cornea, p. 282)

  J. Conjunctival cicatrization, such as that associated with ocular cicatricial pemphigoid, erythema multiforme, ocular psoriasis, and advanced trachoma

  K. Degenerative condition of corneal epithelium, such as in advanced glaucoma

  L. Superior limbic keratoconjunctivitis

  M. Hereditary hemorrhagic telangiectasis (Rendu-Osler-Weber disease)

  N. Aerosol keratitis

  O. Diabetes mellitus

  P. Ectodermal dysplasia

  Q. Following cataract or corneal transplant surgery

  R. Following patching

  S. Use of diphenhydramine hydrochloride (Benadryl)

  T. Idiopathic

4. Punctate subepithelial keratitis—punctate epithelial keratitis may progress to combine epithelial and subepithelial lesions followed by healing of the epithelial component, leaving a punctate subepithelial keratitis typical of viral punctate keratitis

* = most important

      A. Areolar or stellate lesions—grayish-white in color

        (1) Herpes simplex (usually)

        (2) Herpes zoster

        (3) Vaccinia

      B. Fine or medium-sized lesions, typically

        (1) Adenovirus, especially types and 7—grayish-white

      C. Yellowish tinge—typical of trachoma, inclusion conjunctivitis, acne rosacea, and marginal "catarrhal infiltrates" associated with staphylococcal blepharitis, Neisseria conjunctivitis, and Reiter disease

   5. Punctate opacifications of Bowman membrane—gray, homogeneous, thickened spots, often having irregular edges

      A. Salzmann's degeneration

      B. Punctate lesion of trachoma, measles, or phlyctenular disease

Jones, B.R.: Differential diagnosis of punctate keratitis. Int. Ophthalmol. Clin., 2:591–611, 1962.

Diesenhouse, M.C., et al.: Treatment of Microsporidial Keratoconjunctivitis with Topical Fumagillin. Amer. J. Ophthal., 115:293–298, 1993.

Roy, F.H.: Ocular Syndromes and Systemic Diseases. 2nd Ed. Philadelphia, W.B. Saunders, 1989.

Seedor, J.A., et al.: Filamentary keratitis associated with diphenhydramine hydrochloride. Am. J. Ophthalmol., 101:376–377, 1986.

Sicca Keratitis (Dry Eye with Secondary Corneal Changes)

   1. Boeck sarcoid (Schaumann syndrome)

   2. Dermatitis herpetiformis

   3. Diabetes mellitus (Willis disease)

   4. Herpes simplex

   5. Lye burns

  *6. Ocular cicatricial pemphigoid

   7. Polychondritis

  *8. Sjôgren syndrome (secretoinhibitor syndrome)

   9. Trachoma

  10. Vitamin A deficiency (xerosis)

  11. Stevens-Johnson syndrome

Arffa, R.C.: Grayson's Diseases of the Cornea. 3rd Ed. St. Louis, Mosby–Year Book, 1991.

White Rings of the Cornea (Coats Disease) (Rings Made Up of a Series of Tiny White Dots that May Coalesce at the Level of Bowman's Membrane or Just Below It)

   1. Congenital

   2. Trauma

     *A. Foreign body usually metal

     B. Occupational—in working with limestone there may be deposition of some of the substance's components, especially calcium oxide, in the cornea

   3. Intraocular disease

   4. Iron deposition

Miller, E.M.: Genesis of white rings of the cornea. Am. J. Ophthalmol., 61:904, 1966.

Nevins, R.C., and Elliott, J.H.: White ring of the cornea. Arch. Ophthalmol., 82:457, 1969.

Dry Spots of the Cornea (Precorneal Tear Film Drying in Spot-wise Fashion). The precorneal tear film is best examined by using fluorescein and cobalt-blue filtered light. Patients may have difficulty in wearing contact lenses or have corneal pain. Normal tear film break-up time is greater than seconds and averages 25 to 30 seconds.

1. Associated with corneal dellen (see p. 320)
2. Chemical burns
3. Chronic bacterial or viral conjunctivitis
4. Congenital alacrima
5. Instillation of topical anesthetic
*6. Keratitis sicca
*7. Ocular cicatricial pemphigoid
8. Ocular pemphigus (chronic cicatricial conjunctivitis)
9. Sometimes in elderly persons without obvious pathology
10. Stevens-Johnson syndrome (erythema multiforme)
11. Vitamin A deficiency

Dohlman, C.H.: The function of the corneal epithelium in health and disease. Invest. Ophthalmol., 10:376–407, 1971.

Lemp, M.A., and Hamill, J.R.: Factors affecting tear film break-up in normal eyes. Arch. Ophthalmol., 89:103–105, 1973.

Anterior Embryotoxon (Arcus) (White or Gray Substance Deposited at Level of Descemet Membrane and Bowman Membrane Initially, Then in Stroma with a Clear Limbal Interval)

*1. Age—may be present normally in a Caucasian older than 40 years of age or in a black older than years of age
2. Alport syndrome (hereditary nephritis)
3. Associated with corneal disease, such as interstitial keratitis
*4. Contralateral carotid occlusive disease–when unilateral
5. Familial hypercholesterolemia (type II, familial beta-lipo-proteins and type III, familial hyper-beta- and pre-beta-lipoproteins [carbohydrate-induced hyperlipemia])
6. Hereditary—autosomal dominant or autosomal recessive inheritance
7. Isolated phenomenon
8. Long exposure to irritating dust or chemicals
9. Ocular anomaly association, such as blue sclera (see p. 265), megalocornea (see p. 295), or aniridia (see p. 410)
10. Secondary to ocular disease, such as large corneal scars, sclerokeratitis, limbal dermoid, nevus, or epithelial cyst
11. Schnyder's crystalline dystrophy

Bagla, S.K., and Golden, R.L.: Unilateral arcus corneae senilis and carotid occlusive disease. J.A.M.A., 233:450, 1975.

* = most important

Chavis, R.M., and Groshong, T.: Corneal arcus in Alport's syndrome. Am. J. Ophthalmol., 75:793–794, 1973.

Bowman Membrane Folds

1. Bullous keratopathy
2. Idiopathic
3. Inflammation
4. Lowering of intraocular pressure, such as occurs in association with phthisis bulbi

Duke-Elder, S., and Leigh, A.G.: Diseases of the Outer Eye. In System of Ophthalmology, Vol. VIII. Part 2. St. Louis, C.V. Mosby, 1965.

Differential Diagnosis of Anterior Corneal Abnormalities

Entity	Distinguishing Features
Cornea verticillata	Corneal pattern, ocular and systemic findings of Fabry disease, drug history
Meesmann dystrophy	Corneal pattern, family history
Reis-Bucklers dystrophy	Family history, histopathology
Keratosis palmaris et plantaris	Dermatologic, systemic findings
Post-traumatic recurrent erosion	History of trauma, localized corneal pathology
Map-dot fingerprint	Corneal pattern, possible family history

Anterior Corneal Abnormalities

	Fabry Disease	Messman Dystrophy	Reis-Buckler Dystrophy	Drug-induced Cornea Vascularization	Post-traumatic Recurrent Erosion	Map-Dot Fingerprint Dystrophy
History						
1. Asymptomatic female carrier	U					
2. Bilateral	U	U	U	U		U
3. Common in adults					S	U
4. Common in women						U
5. Familial	S	U	U			S
6. Hereditary	S	U	U			S
7. History of corneal injury from fingernails, paper, photocoagulation or vitrectomy					U	
8. Ocular pain			S		U	R
9. Onset, first decade		U	U	S		
10. Patient taking chloroquine, amiodarone, phenotidzine, or indomethacin				U		
11. Photophobia		U	U		U	R
12. Recurrent erosions		R	U		U	S
Physical Findings						
1. Corneal bullae					S	
2. Corneal clouding			S			
3. Corneal irregularity		S	S		S	S
4. Decreased corneal sensation		R	S			
5. Diffuse opacities are geographic in nature at level of Bowman layer with peak-like projections into the epithelial layer			U			
6. Dot-like opacities, as gray-white intraepithelial opacities (round, oblong, or comma shaped)					S	U
7. Epithelial filament formation					U	
8. Epithelial loss					U	S
9. Epithelial microcysts					U	S
10. Fingerprint lesions are concentric contoured lines						U
11. Fingerprints are formed by subepithelial sheets						U
12. Foreign body sensation			U		U	R
13. Gray-white interlacing lines resembling the architecture of a map or diffuse gray patches						S
14. Dendritiform lesions of cornea					S	
15. Lack of adherence of sheets of epithelium					U	S
16. Lacrimation		U	S		U	R
17. Pigmented whorl-shaped lines travel in the epithelial and superficial subepithelial tissue	U			U		
18. Small bleb-like lesions in epithelium appears as small white-gray punctate opcities diffusely distributed over corneal surface		U				
19. Subepithelial scarring			S		U	U
20. Superficial reticulated gray-white opacities and epithelial defects			U			
21. Superficial pseudomicrocysts						U
22. Visual acuity decreased with lesion in pupil			S		U	R

R = rarely; S = sometimes; and U = usually.

Delayed Corneal Wound Healing

Delayed corneal wound healing because of drugs, including:

adenine amphotericin B	dexamethasone	phenacaine
arabinoside	dibucaine	phenylephrine(?)
adrenal cortex injection	dyclonine	piperocaine
aldosterone	fludrocortisone	prednisolone
alpha chymotrypsin(?)	fluorometholone	prednisone
azathioprine	fluprednisolone	proparacaine
bacitracin	flurbiprofen	sulfacetamide
benoxinate	F3T	sulfamethizole
benzalkonium	gentamicin	sulfisoxazole
betamethasone	hydrocortisone	tetracaine
butacaine	idoxuridine	thiotepa
chymotrypsin(?)	iodine solution	triamcinolone
cocaine	medrysone	trifluorothymidine
colchicine	meprednisone	trifluridine
cortisone	methylprednisolone	vidarabine
cytarabine	paramethasone	
desoxycorticosterone	penicillamine(?)	

Fraunfelder, F.T.: Drug-Induced Ocular Side Effects and Drug Interactions. 4th Ed. Philadelphia, Williams & Wilkins, 1996.

Anterior Corneal Mosaic (Pattern of Fluorescein Pooling in Corneal Epithelial Grooves that Can be Induced in Any Normal Eye by Pressure on Cornea)

1. Exophthalmos as in dysthyroid eye disease with corneal compression against the eyelids
2. Exposure to a high pressure fire extinguisher jet
3. Pressure on the cornea, either directly on the cornea or indirectly through the lids

Bron, A.J.: Anterior corneal mosaic. Br. J. Ophthalmol., 52:659, 1968.

Frazer, D.G., et al.: Compression keratopathy. Am. J. Ophthalmol., 102:208–210, 1986.

Linear Opacity in Superficial Corneal Stroma

1. Arc like at superior limbus
   A. Poorly fit contact lens
   B. Well fitting soft contact lens with tight eyelids
2. Central
   A. Amiodarone
   B. Chloroquine and hydroxychloroquine
   C. Phenothiazines

Arffa, R.C.: Grayson's Diseases of the Cornea. 3rd Ed. St. Louis, Mosby–Year Book, 1991.

Horowitz, G.S., et al.: An unusual corneal complication of soft contact lens. Am. J. Ophthalmol., 100:794–797, 1985.

Superficial Vertical Corneal Striations—Epithelial Wrinkles Can be Accentuated with Fluorescein

1. Corneal surgery with corneal indentation or low intraocular pressure
2. Graves disease
3. Scarred lids
4. Soft contact lens

Blue, P.W., and Lapiana, F.G.: Superficial vertical corneal striations: A new eye sign of Graves' disease. Ann. Ophthalmol., 12:635, 1980.

Mobilia, E.F., et al.: Corneal wrinkling induced by ultra-thin soft contact lenses. Ann. Ophthalmol., 12:371, 1980.

Dendritic Corneal Lesions (Area of Staining of Cornea in a Branching Pattern)

*1. Corneal erosions, in which the epithelium may become loose
*2. Herpes simplex
*3. Herpes zoster
 4. Use of soft contact lenses
*5. Acanthamoeba keratitis

Linquist, T.D., et al.: Clinical signs and medical therapy of early acanthamoeba keratitis. Arch. Ophthalmol., 106:73–76, 1988.

Margulies, L.J., and Mannis, M.: Dendritic corneal lesions associated with soft contact lenses wear. Arch. Ophthalmol., 101:1551–1553, 1983.

Bullous Keratopathy (Terminal Stages of Severe or Prolonged Epithelial Edema Secondary to Endothelial Damage)

1. Anterior-posterior corneal incisions for myopia
2. Anterior synechiae
3. Associated with progressive facial hemiatrophy (Parry-Romberg syndrome)
4. Birth trauma (forceps injury)
5. Chronic uveitis, especially herpes simplex or herpes zoster
6. Congenital corneal dystrophy
7. Congenital glaucoma
8. Congenital hereditary endothelial dystrophy
9. Corneal hydrops (acute keratoconus)
10. Epithelial downgrowth
*11. Following cataract surgery with or without intraocular implantation
12. Following perforating wounds, especially when the lens capsule or vitreous is adherent to the cornea
*13. Fuchs epithelial-endothelial dystrophy
14. Immunologic reaction after keratoplasty, or endothelial decompensation
15. Iridocorneal endothelial syndrome
16. Long-standing glaucoma
17. Posterior polymorphous dystrophy

* = most important

18. Prolonged inflammation of corneal stroma, such as in disciform or interstitial keratitis (rare)

19. Silicone oil in anterior chamber

Deekhuis, W.H., et al.: Silicone oil in the anterior chamber of the eye. Arch. Ophthalmol., 104:793, 1986.

Grayson, M., and Pieroni, D.: Progressive facial hemiatrophy with bullous and band-shaped keratopathy. Am. J. Ophthalmol., 70:42–44, 1970.

Yamaguchi, T., et al.: Bullous keratopathy after anterior posterior radial keratotomy for myopia and myopic astigmatism. Am. J. Ophthalmol., 93:600–606, 1982.

Nummular Keratitis (Coin-shaped Lesions of Cornea)

1. Brucellosis
2. Dimmers nummular keratitis
3. Epidemic keratoconjunctivitis
4. Herpes zoster
5. Infectious mononucleosis–Epstein-Barr virus
6. Onchocerciasis (River blindness)
7. Varicella
8. Herpes simplex

Arffa, R.C.: Grayson's Diseases of the Cornea. 3rd Ed. St. Louis, Mosby–Year Book, 1991.

Pau, H.: Differential Diagnosis of Eye Diseases. 2nd Ed. New York, Thieme Med. Pub., 1988.

Deep Keratitis

1. Behçet disease (dermatostomato-ophthalmic syndrome)
2. Deep pustular keratitis
3. Disciform keratitis
4. Herpes zoster
5. Keratitis profunda
6. Stromal herpes
7. Vaccinia
8. Varicella

Arffa, R.C.: Grayson's Diseases of the Cornea. 3rd Ed. St. Louis, Mosby–Year Book, 1991.

Interstitial Keratitis (Corneal Stromal Inflammation, not Primarily on Anterior or Posterior Surfaces of Stroma)

1. After burns
    A. Acid
    B. Alkali
2. Deep punctate
    A. Influenza
    B. Local trauma
    C. Mumps
    *D. Ophthalmic zoster

*3. Luetic (syphilis)

4. Non-luetic

    A. Acne rosacea (ocular rosacea)

    B. Brucellosis (Bang disease)

    C. Cogan I syndrome (nonsyphilitic interstitial keratitis)

    D. Filariasis

    E. Herpes simplex

    F. Hodgkin disease (lymph node disease)

    G. Mycosis fungoides

    H. Mumps

    I. Recurrent fever

    J. Sarcoidosis (Schaumann syndrome)

    K. Sleeping sickness (von Economo syndrome)

    L. Steroid therapy

    M. Topical anesthetic abuse

    N. Trypanosomiasis

    O. Tuberculosis (scrofulous keratitis)

    P. Viral as metaherpetic keratitis

    Q. Corneal opacification after forceps delivery

5. Sclerosing keratitis

    A. Scleritis

        (1) Foci or some local process

        (2) Hennebert syndrome (luetic otitic nystagmus syndrome)

        (3) Sarcoidosis syndrome (Schaumann syndrome)

        (4) Syphilis (acquired lues)

        (5) Tuberculosis

    B. Sclerocornea

    C. Brawny (gelatinous) scleritis

6. With chemical poisons

    A. Arsenic

    B. Gold

7. With corneal ring abscess

    A. Anterior segment necrosis

        (1) After circular diathermy

        (2) After a 'string' encircling procedure for retinal detachment

        (3) After multiple extraocular muscle surgery

    B. Bacillus subtilis

    C. Bacterium pyocyaneum

    D. Pneumococci

    E. Proteus

* = most important

8. With skin disease

    A. Herpes zoster

    B. Incontinentia pigmenti (Bloch Sulzberger syndrome)

    C. Lichen planus

    D. Molluscum contagiosum

    E. Palmoplantar keratosis

    F. Pityriasis rubra pilaris

    G. Psoriasis

Arffa, R.C.: Grayson's Diseases of the Cornea. 3rd Ed. St. Louis, Mosby–Year Book, 1991.

Pau, H.: Differential Diagnosis of Eye Diseases. 2nd Ed. New York, Thieme Med. Pub., 1988.

Roy, F.H.: Ocular Syndromes and Systemic Diseases. 2nd Ed. Philadelphia, W.B. Saunders, 1989.

Pannus (Superficial Vascular Invasion Confined to a Segment of the Cornea or Extending around the Entire Limbus)

*1. Acne rosacea

*2. Allergic marginal infiltration

*3. Anoxic contact lens overwear syndrome

4. Ariboflavinosis keratopathy

*5. Contact lens usage

6. Deerfly fever (tularemia)

7. Degenerative-blind degenerative eyes; often associated with bullous keratopathy

8. Dermatitis herpetiformis (Duhring-Brocq disease)

9. Drugs including:

benoxinate	F3T	phenylbutazone	trifluridine
benzalkonium	ibuprofen	piperocaine	urokinase(?)
butacaine	idoxuridine	proparacaine	vidarabine
cocaine	iodine solution	silicone	
dibucaine	oxyphenbutazone	tetracaine	
dyclonine	phenacaine	thimerosal	

10. Fuchs corneal dystrophy (degenerative pannus)

11. Glaucoma (degenerative pannus)

12. Hemophilus influenzae

13. Histiocytosis X (Hand-Schüller-Christian syndrome)

14. Hypoparathyroidism

15. Inclusion conjunctivitis in infants and adults (micropannus) (chlamydia)

16. Keratoconjunctivitis sicca

17. Leishmaniasis

18. Leprosy (Hansen disease)

19. Linear nevus sebaceous of Jadassohn

20. Lyell disease (toxic epidermal necrolysis or scalded skin syndrome)

21. Lymphopathia venereum

22. Molluscum contagiosum

23. Ocular cicatricial pemphigoid

24. Onchocerciasis (river blindness)

25. Papilloma (wart)

26. Pellagra (avitaminosis B_{12})

27. Pemphigus foliaceus (Cazenave disease)

28. Phlyctenular keratoconjunctivitis (see p. 247)

29. Siemen disease (keratosis follicularis spinulosa decalvans)

*30. Staphylococcal keratoconjunctivitis (micropannus)

31. Stevens-Johnson syndrome (mucocutaneous ocular syndrome)

*32. Superior limbic keratoconjunctivitis (micropannus)

33. Terrien disease (senile marginal atrophy)

34. Trachoma

35. Tuberculosis

36. Vaccinia

37. Vernal conjunctivitis (micropannus)

38. Vitamin B_{12} deficiency (Addison pernicious anemia syndrome)

Arffa, R.C.: Grayson's Diseases of the Cornea. 3rd Ed. St. Louis, Mosby–Year Book, 1991.

Dixon, W.S., and Bron, A.J.: Fluorescein angiographic demonstration of corneal vascularization in contact lens wearers. Am. J. Ophthalmol., 75:1010–1015, 1973.

Fraunfelder, F.T.: Drug-Induced Ocular Side Effects and Drug Interactions. 4th Ed. Philadelphia, Williams & Wilkins, 1996.

Pau, H.: Differential Diagnosis of Eye Diseases. 2nd Ed. New York, Thieme Med Pub., 1988.

Roy, F.H.: Ocular Syndromes and Systemic Diseases. 2nd Ed. Philadelphia, W.B. Saunders, 1989.

* = most important

Pannus (Superificial Invasion of Blood Vessels Confined to Segment of Cornea or Extending around Limbus)

	Trachoma	Leprosy	Phlyctenular Keratoconjunctivitis	Acne Rosacea	Molluscum Contagiosum	Vernal Conjunctivitis	Contact Lens Use	Inclusion Conjunctivitis	Superior Limbic Keratoconjunctivitis	Fuchs Dystrophy	Glaucoma	Staphylococcal Keratoconjunctivitis	Hypoparathyroidism	Keratoconjunctivitis Sicca
History														
1. All age groups									U			U	S	
2. Allergic ocular disease			U			U								
3. Bilateral	U	U		S	S	U		U	U	U	U	U		U
4. Chronic skin disorder		U		U										
5. Common in children/young adults			U		S	U								
6. Common in females			U	U						U				U
7. Common in newborns								U						
8. Congenital											S			
9. Familial										U	U			
10. Hereditary										U				
11. More than 30 to 50 years old						U				U				S
12. Ocular pain			U						U	S				
13. Photophobia			U			U							U	
14. Poor sanitation and medical care	U	S												
15. Pruritis			U									S		S
Physical Findings														
1. Anisocoria		S												
2. Blepharospasm		U	U						U				S	
3. Bullous keratopathy										U				
4. Cataract										S	S		S	
5. Chalazion				U								U		
6. Chronic blepharoconjunctivitis			U	U								U		S
7. Chronic keratoconjunctivitis	U					U								
8. Closed anterior chamber angle											U			
9. Conjunctival follicles/papillae		U				U		U						
10. Conjunctival nodules		U										U	U	
11. Conjunctival Tranta spots						U								
12. Conjunctival ulcers		U										S		
13. Conjunctival vegetations onto cornea						S								
14. Conjunctivitis, cicatricial	U													
15. Conjunctivitis, follicular								U						
16. Conjunctivitis, mucopurulent												U		
17. Conjunctivitis, mucous						U			U					U
18. Corneal abscess												S		
19. Corneal cicatrization				R						U				
20. Corneal edema							U			U	U			
21. Corneal endothelium degeneration										U				
22. Corneal filaments										S				U
23. Corneal hypesthesia											U			
24. Corneal infiltration							U							
25. Corneal nodules			S										U	
26. Corneal opacities	U	U	S					U	S					
27. Corneal perforation				R										R

Pannus (Superificial Invasion of Blood Vessels Confined to Segment of Cornea or Extending around Limbus) *Continued*

	Trachoma	Leprosy	Phlyctenular Keratoconjunctivitis	Acne Rosacea	Molluscum Contagiosum	Vernal Conjunctivitis	Contact Lens Use	Inclusion Conjunctivitis	Superior Limbic Keratoconjunctivitis	Fuchs Dystrophy	Glaucoma	Staphylococcal Keratoconjunctivitis	Hypoparathyroidism	Keratoconjunctivitis Sicca
Physical Findings														
28. Corneal phlyctenules			U									S		
29. Corneal plaques						U								
30. Corneal thinning				S										S
31. Corneal ulcer			S	S			S	R				S		S
32. Dacryocystitis		S												
33. Decreased intraocular pressure		S												
34. Decreased tear secretion									S					U
35. Entropion	U													
36. Epiphora	U		U			U	U	U	U					
37. Episcleritis		S		U										
38. Folds in Descemet membrane										U	U			
39. Forward displacement of the iris											U			
40. Glaucomatous disc cupping											U			
41. Increased intraocular pressure		S								S	U			
42. Iris atrophy											S			
43. Keratitis	U	U	S	S		S		S	S			U	U	U
44. Lagophthalmos		U							U					
45. Madarosis		U										S	U	
46. Multiple pupils		S												
47. Myopia													S	
48. Optic nerve atrophy											U			
49. Optic neuritis													S	
50. Papilledema													S	
51. Paralysis of seventh nerve		S												
52. Peripheral anterior synechiae											U			
53. Pigment on posterior corneal surface										U				
54. Ptosis	U								S			S		
55. Punctal occlusion						S								
56. Uveitis		U												
57. Visual field defects											U			
Laboratory Data														
1. Biopsy of skin (acid fast stain)		U												
2. Calcium diminished in plasma													U	
3. Chest roentgenogram			R											
4. Conjunctival fluorescent antibody staining	U							S						
5. Conjunctival smears														
Geimsa stain	U					U	U							
Gram stain			U									U		
Hematoxylin-eosin stain					U									
6. Phosphate elevated in plasma													U	
7. Purified protein derivative skin test			R											

R = rarely; S = sometimes; and U = usually.

Corneal Opacity, Diffuse

1. Acromesomelic dysplasia
*2. Birth trauma
3. Cockayne syndrome
*4. Congenital hereditary endothelial dystrophy
5. Congenital hereditary stromal dystrophy
6. Cystinosis
7. Fabry syndrome
8. Fetal rubella effects
9. GM gangliosidosis type 1
10. Hurler syndrome
11. Infection
12. Maroteaux-Lamy syndrome
13. Morquio syndrome
14. Mucolipidosis III
15. Mucolipidosis IV
16. Multiple sulfatase deficiency
17. MPS VII
18. Pachyonychia congenita syndrome
19. Pena-Shokeir type II syndrome (COFS syndrome)
20. Rutherford syndrome
21. Scheie syndrome
*22. Sclerocornea
23. Seip syndrome
24. Sialidosis, Goldberg type
25. Trisomy syndrome
26. 18q syndrome

Isenberg, S.J.: The Eye in Infancy. Chicago, Year Book Medical Publishers, 1989.
Roy, F.H.: Ocular Syndromes and Systemic Diseases. 2nd Ed. Philadelphia, W.B. Saunders, 1989.

Corneal Opacity, Localized, Congenital

1. Acromegaloid changes, cutis verticis gyrata and corneal leukoma
2. Aniridia
3. Autosomal dominant colomba
4. Cataract microcornea syndrome
*5. Dermoid limbal, central and ring
6. Fetal alcohol syndrome
7. Fetal rubella effects
8. Fetal transfusion syndrome
9. Fucosidosis
10. Group 13-trisomy phenotype

11. Keratoconus posticus circumscriptus

12. Meesman syndrome

13. Peters anomaly and short stature

14. Pillay syndrome (ophthalmomandibulomelic dysplasia)

15. Radial aplasia, anterior chamber cleavage syndrome

16. Richner-Hanhart syndrome

17. Rieger syndrome

18. Trisomy syndrome

19. Waarburg syndrome

20. Wedge shaped stromal opacity

21. 4p- syndrome

22. 11q syndrome

23. 18q- syndrome

Isenberg, S.J.: The Eye in Infancy. Chicago, Year Book Medical Publishers, 1989.

Roy, F.H.: Ocular Syndromes and Systemic Diseases. 2nd Ed. Philadelphia, W.B. Saunders, 1989.

Deep Corneal Stromal Deposits

*1. Cornea farinata

2. Deep filiform dystrophy

3. Deep punctiform dystrophy associated with ichthyosis

4. Fleck corneal dystrophy

5. Gold (chrysiasis)

6. Lattice corneal dystrophy

7. Macular corneal dystrophy

8. Polymorphic amyloid degeneration

Kincaid, M.C., et al.: Ocular chrysiasis. Arch. Ophthalmol., 100:1791, 1982.

Mannis, M.J., et al.: Polymorphic amyloid degeneration of the cornea. Arch. Ophthalmol., 99:1217–1219, 1981.

Intracorneal Hemorrhage

1. Associated with intraocular surgery

2. Diseases of cornea, such as corneal ulcers and chemical burns

3. Microbial keratitis

4. Migration from subconjunctival hemorrhage

5. Ocular trauma

6. Spontaneous in contact lens wearers

Hurwitz, B.S.: Spontaneous intracorneal hemorrhage caused by aphakic contact lens wear. Ann. Ophthalmol., 13:57, 1981.

Ormerod, L.D., and Egan, K.M.: Spontaneous hyphaema and corneal haemorrhage as complications of microbial keratitis. Brit. J. Ophthal., 71:933, 1988.

* = most important

Central Posterior Stromal Corneal Deposits

1. Bence Jones proteinuria
2. Dysproteinemia
3. Filiform corneal dystrophy
4. Immunoglobulin deposition
    A. Abnormal γ-globulin
    B. Benign monoclonal gammopathy
5. Multiple myeloma

Barr, C.C., et al.: Corneal crystalline deposits associated with dysproteinemia. Arch. Ophthalmol., 98:884–889, 1980.

Yassa, N.H., et al.: Corneal immunoglobulin deposition in the posterior stroma. Arch. Ophthalmol., 105:99–103, 1987.

Dellen (Shallow Corneal Excavation Near the Limbus, Usually on Temporal Side, with the Base of the Lesion Hazy and Dry)

1. Following the wearing of contact lens
2. In elderly persons—limbal vasosclerosis
3. Lagophthalmos
4. Lengthy administration of cocaine
5. Postcataract section
*6. Swelling of perilimbal tissues
    A. Allergic conjunctival edema
    B. Episcleritis
    *C. Filtering bleb
    D. Limbal tumor
    *E. Postoperative advancement of rectus muscle
    F. Postoperative retinal detachment
    G. Pinguecula
    H. Subconjunctival effusion or injection
7. With hemeralopia

Soong, H.K., and Quigley, H.A.: Dellen associated with filtering blebs. Arch. Ophthalmol., 101:385–387, 1983.

Phlyctenular Keratoconjunctivitis (Localized Conjunctival, Limbal, or Corneal Nodule about One to Three Millimeters in Size)

*1. Delayed hypersensitivity to bacterial protein, particularly tuberculoprotein and staphylococci; lymphopathia venereum and coccidioidomycosis may also be allergens
2. Malnutrition
3. Secondary infection of the conjunctiva, especially from Staphylococcus aureus, pneumococcus, Koch-Weeks bacillus, chlamydia, coccidioidomycosis, and gonorrhea
4. Systemic infection
    A. Bang disease (Brucellosis)

   B. Candidiasis

   C. Neurodermatitis

   D. Mikulicz-Radecki syndrome (dacryosialoadenopathy)

   E. Trachoma

   F. Sjögren syndrome (secretoinhibitor syndrome)

Newell, F.W.: Ophthalmology, Principles and Concepts. 7th Ed. St. Louis, C.V. Mosby, 1991.

Corneal Ring Lesion

1. Acanthamoebic keratitis

2. Associated with rheumatoid arthritis—inferior

3. Associated with Sjögren syndrome (secretoinhibitor syndrome)

4. Capnocytophaga ochracea

5. Double-ring formation—allergic keratitis

6. Marginal dystrophy—degenerative chronic corneal lesion with stromal thinning and intact epithelium; occurs in individuals younger than years of age

7. Marginal ulceration—secondary to massive granuloma of sclera or necrotizing nodular scleritis (see p. 272)

8. Mooren ulcer—deeply undermined central edges and chronic course with inflammation, painful

9. Ring abscess—rapidly destructive purulent lesion in the deepest parts of the cornea

10. Ring ulcer—see marginal corneal ulcers (p. 321)

11. Steroid use in furrow dystrophy

12. Terrien marginal degeneration-usually begins superiorly

13. Wegener granulomatosis (Wegener syndrome)

Ferry, A.P., and Leopold, I.H.: Marginal (ring) corneal ulcer as presenting manifestation of Wegener's granuloma. Trans. Am. Acad. Ophthalmol. Otolaryngol., 74:1276–1282, 1970.

Heidemann, D.G., et al.: Necrotizing keratitis caused by capnocytophaga ochracea. Am. J. Ophthalmol., 105:655–660, 1988.

Theodore, F.H., et al.: The diagnostic value of a ring infiltrate in acanthamoebic keratitis. Ophthalmology, 92:1471–1480, 1985.

Corneoscleral Keratitis

1. Boeck sarcoid (Schaumann syndrome)

2. Gout (hyperuricemia)

3. Leprosy (Hansen disease)

4. Infectious, e.g. pseudomonas

5. Malformations, such as in sclerocornea (see p. 342)

6. Sarcoma

7. Syphilis (acquired lues)

8. Trisomy 13 (trisomy D)

9. Tuberculosis

*10. Wegener granulomatosis

Arffa, R.C.: Grayson's Diseases of the Cornea. 3rd Ed. St. Louis, Mosby–Year Book, 1991.

* = most important

Central Corneal Ulcer

1. Of bacterial origin
   *A. Diplococcus pneumoniae (pneumococcus)—infiltrated gray-white or yellow disc-shaped central ulcer typically associated with diffuse keratitis, severe iridocyclitis, and hypopyon; follows corneal abrasion, occurs especially in the presence of chronic dacryocystitis, and is enhanced by general debility
   *B. Beta-hemolytic streptococcus and other streptococcus species
   *C. Pseudomonas aeruginosa but may also have pseudomonas acidovorans, pseudomonas stutzeri, pseudomonas mullei, and pseudomonas pseudomallei—primary corneal involvement, rapid spread often to panophthalmitis, large hypopyon, thick greenish pus; may be contaminant of eserine and fluorescein often associated with contact use.
   D. Escherichia coli
   E. Moraxella liquefaciens (diplococcus of Petit)—morphologically resembles diplobacillus of Morax-Axenfeld, which is never seen in central corneal ulcers
   F. Klebsiella pneumoniae
   G. Proteus vulgaris
   H. Actinomyces
   I. Tuberculous—secondary to conjunctival or uveal infections
   J. Serratia marcescens—gram-negative coccobacillus
   *K. Staphylococcus aureus, staphepidermitis and other staph species
   L. Mima polymorpha
   M. Dysgonic fermenter-2
   N. Others
2. Of viral origin
   *A. Herpes simplex virus
   B. Herpes zoster
   C. Vaccinia virus
   D. Variola
   E. Others
3. Of mycotic origin—follows corneal trauma, such as foreign bodies in the cornea or corneal abrasions caused by vegetable matter, or diseases, such as radiation keratitis, exposure keratitis, herpes zoster, and ocular pemphigus; chronic course; shallow crater; absent corneal vascularization; may follow treatment with antibiotics or, more likely, treatment with steroid-antibiotic combinations
   *A. Aspergillus
   B. Blastomyces dermatitidis
   *C. Candida albicans
   D. Cephalosporium
   *E. Fusarium solani
   F. Nocardia
   G. Others
4. Acquired immune deficiency syndrome (AIDS) related

5. Brittle cornea syndrome

6. Chemical—latex keratitis

*7. Dry eyes including Sjögren syndrome

8. Soluble tyrosine aminotransferase (STAT) deficiency

9. Extrusion of anterior chamber intraocular lens

Gelender, H.: Descemetocele after intraocular lens implantation. Arch Ophthalmol., 100:72–76, 1982.

Kiel, R.J., et al.: Corneal perforation caused by dysgonic fermenter-2. JAMA, 257:3269–3270, 1987.

McKnight, G.T., et al.: Transcorneal extrusion of anterior chamber intraocular lenses. Arch Ophthalmol., 105:1656–1664, 1987.

Pfister, R.R., and Murphy, G.E.: Corneal ulceration and perforation associated with Sjögren's syndrome. Arch Ophthalmol., 98:89, 1980.

Raber, I.M., et al.: Pseudomonas corneoscleral ulcers. Am J Ophthalmol., 92:353–362, 1981.

Roy, F.H.: Ocular Syndromes and Systemic Diseases. 2nd Ed. Philadelphia, W.B. Saunders, 1989.

Santos, C., et al.: Bilateral fungal corneal ulcers in a patient with AIDS-related complex. Am J Ophthalmol., 102:108–109, 1986.

Wilson, L.A., et al.: Pseudomonas corneal ulcers associated with soft contact-lens wear. Am J Ophthalmol., 92:546–554, 1981.

Marginal Corneal Ulcers

1. Ring ulcers—often bilateral, circumcorneal injection, and continuous ring or confluent multiple lesions

    A. Acute leukemia

    B. Bacillary dysentery

    C. Brucellosis (Bang disease)

    *D. Coalescence of several marginal ulcers

    E. Dengue fever

    F. Gold poisoning

    G. Gonococcal arthritis

    H. Following penetrating keratoplasty

    I. Hookworm infestation

    J. Influenza

    K. Last stages of trachoma, secondary to small circumferential pannus

    *L. Mooren's ulcer

    M. Polyarteritis nodosa (Kussmaul disease)

    N. Porphyria

    *O. Rheumatoid arthritis—Sjögren syndrome (secretion inhibitor syndrome)

    P. Scleroderma (progressive systemic sclerosis)

    Q. Systemic lupus erythematosus (Kaposi-Libman-Sacks syndrome)

    R. Tuberculosis

    R. Wegener granulomatosis (Wegener syndrome)

2. Simple marginal ulcers—superficial crescentic gray-colored ulcer

    A. Infection—due to staphylococcus, Koch-Weeks bacillus, pseudomonas, diplobacillus of Morax-Axenfeld—usually chronic

B. Toxic or allergic

C. Systemic disturbances, such as:

    (1) Acute upper respiratory infection

    (2) Bacillary dysentery

    (3) Barre-Lieou syndrome (posterior cervical sympathetic syndrome)

    (4) Brucellosis (Bang disease)

    (5) Crohn disease (granulomatous ileocolitis)

    (6) Gout (hyperuricemia)

    (7) Influenza

    (8) Lupus erythematosus (Kaposi-Libman-Sacks syndrome)

    (9) Polyarteritis nodosa (Kussmaul disease)

  (10) Postvaccinial ocular syndrome

 *(11) Rheumatoid arthritis—inferior cornea

Austin, P., and Brown, S.I.: Inflammatory Terrien's marginal corneal disease. Am J Ophthalmol., 92:189–192, 1981.

Mondino, B.J., et al.: Mooren's ulcer after penetrating keratoplasty. Am J Ophthalmol., 103:53–56, 1987.

Parker, A.V., et al.: Pseudomonas corneal ulcers after artificial fingernail injuries. Am J Ophthalmol., 107:548–560, 1989.

Roy, F.H.: Ocular Syndromes and Systemic Diseases. 2nd Ed. Philadelphia, W.B. Saunders, 1989.

Marginal Corneal Ulcers

	Staphylococcus Infection	Gout	Lupus Erythematosus	Rheumatoid Arthritis	Polyarteritis Nodosa	Acute Leukemia	Mooren Ulcer
History							
1. All ages	U						
2. Associated with diabetes	S						
3. Hereditary		U	R				
4. Malignant blood disorder							
5. More in females			U	U			
6. More in males					U		
7. Occurs in children						S	
8. Occurs during second to third decades					U		
9. Occurs during third to fourth decades			U				
10. Occurs during fourth to fifth decades					U		
Physical Findings							
1. Anterior uveitis	S	R	S	S	S		S
2. Band keratopathy				S			
3. Blepharitis	U			S			
4. Cataract				S	R		S
5. Chemosis of conjunctiva	S				S		
6. Conjunctival phlyctenules	U		S				
7. Conjunctivitis	U	U	S	U	S		U
8. Corneal epithelial keratitis	U		S	U	S		U
9. Corneal opacity				S			U
10. Corneal perforation	U				S		S
11. Corneal vascularization	S		S				S
12. Cotton-wool spots			U	R	S	S	
13. Dacryocystitis	S						
14. Ectropion	S						
15. Endophthalmitis	S						
16. Entropion	S						
17. Episcleritis		S	S				
18. Exophthalmos					R		
19. Hordeolum	U						
20. Hypopyon	S			S		S	
21. Keratoconjunctivitis sicca			S	U	S		
22. Lid edema	S				S		S
23. Macular edema						S	S
24. Madarosis	S						
25. Noncalcific band keratopathy		S					
26. Nystagmus			R				
27. Ocular motor disturbances		R	R	S	S	S	
28. Optic nerve atrophy			S		R	S	
29. Optic neuritis			S			S	
30. Papilledema			U		R	S	
31. Ptosis	R		R		R		
32. Retinal detachment						S	
33. Retinal hemorrhage			U		U	U	

* = most important

Marginal Corneal Ulcers *Continued*

	Staphylococcus Infection	Gout	Lupus Erythematosus	Rheumatoid Arthritis	Polyarteritis Nodosa	Acute Leukemia	Mooren Ulcer
Physical Findings							
34. Retinal vein occlusion			S		S		
35. Scleritis		S	S	S	S	S	S
36. Scleromalacia perforans				S			
37. Subconjunctivial nodules					S		
38. Tenonitis		S		S	S		
39. Visual field defects			S		R		
40. Vitreous opacities						S	
Laboratory Data							
1. Angiography—retinal					U		
2. Autoantibodies to nuclear and cytoplasmic constituents			U				
3. Blood tests							
Eosinophilia					S		
Sedimentation rate elevated					U	U	S
Leukocytic count elevated					U	U	
Neutropenia					U		
Normocytic hypochromic anemia					U	U	U
Thrombocytopenia					S	U	
4. Conjunctival/corneal exudates for culture/gram stain	U						
5. Diminished serum complement levels			S				
6. Electroretinogram abnormalities			U				
7. High uric acid urine/blood		U					
8. Joint changes—roentgenogram				U			
9. Latex agglutination test—rheumatoid factor				U			
10. Lupus erythematosus cell phenomenon			S				
11. Skeletal changes—roentgenogram						U	

R = rarely; S = sometimes; and U = usually.

Descemet Membrane Folds (Usually Follow Hypotony; see p. 367)

*1. Trauma, such as that due to cataract or corneal surgery

2. Mechanical cause, such as firm prolonged ocular bandaging or phthisis bulbi

3. Inflammatory condition, such as that following interstitial or herpes simplex keratitis

4. Diabetes (8% to 33%)

5. Ochronosis

6. Toxic

   A. Quinone and hydroquinone—vertical folds

   B. Formaldehyde 26%

   C. Experimental cold injury to cornea

   D. Digitoxin

7. Idiopathic

Angell, L.K., et al.: Visual prognosis in patients with ruptures in Descemet's membrane due to forceps injuries. Arch. Ophthalmol., 99:2137, 1981.

Descemet Membrane Tears (Haab Striae)

*1. Acute hydrops of the cornea, such as that due to keratoconus (see p. 328)

*2. Buphthalmos, e.g. from congenital glaucoma

3. Conical cornea

4. Myopia with marked anteroposterior diameter

*5. Trauma, such as birth injury or contusion

Angell, L.K., et al.: Visual prognosis in patients with ruptures in Descemet's membrane due to forceps injuries. Arch. Ophthalmol., 99:2137, 1981.

Cibis, G.W., and Tripathi, R.C.: The differential diagnosis of Descemet's tears (Haab's Striae) and posterior polymorphous dystrophy bands. Ophthalmology, 89:614, 1982.

Descemet Membrane Thickening

*1. Central cornea guttata

   A. Primary

   B. Secondary cornea guttata

      *(1) Congenital luetic interstitial keratitis

      (2) Endothelial cell insult

         a. Breaks in Descemet membrane, including scrolls of Descemet membrane in healed syphilitic interstitial keratitis

         b. Chandler syndrome (iridocorneal endothelial syndrome)

         c. Cogan-Reese syndrome (iris-nevus syndrome)

         *d. Corneal dystrophy, including Fuchs' syndrome

         e. Posterior keratoconus syndrome

   C. Transient cornea guttata associated with short-term episodes of iritis and corneal inflammation

2. Peripheral Hassall Henle warts

Alvarado, J.A., et al.: Pathogenesis of Chandler's syndrome, essential iris atrophy, and the Cogan-Reese syndrome. Invest. Ophthalmol. Vis. Sci., 27:873–882, 1986.

* = most important

Rodrigues, M.M., et al.: Fuchs' corneal dystrophy: A clinicopathologic study of the variation in corneal edema. Ophthalmology, 98:789–796, 1986.

Scattergood, K.D., et al.: Scrolls of Descemet's membrane in healed syphilitic interstitial keratitis. Ophthalmology, 90:1518–1523, 1983.

Retrocorneal Pigmentation

1. Endothelial phagocytosis of free melanin pigment as Krukenberg spindle

2. Iris melanocytes, iris pigment epithelial cells or pigment containing macrophages in the posterior corneal surface can follow operative or accidental ocular trauma

3. Status post hyphema

Snip, R.C., et al.: Posterior corneal pigmentation and fibrous proliferation by iris melanocytes. Arch Ophthalmol., 99:1232, 1981.

Low Endothelial Cell Count (Diminished Number of Corneal Endothelial Cells)

1. Acute and chronic uveitis

*2. Corneal endothelial dystrophy

3. Following cataract or other intraocular surgery

4. Cornea guttata, endothelial dystrophy and Fuch dystrophy

Olsen, T.: Changes in the corneal endothelium after acute anterior uveitis as seen with the specular microscope. Acta Ophthalmol., 58:250, 1980.

Murrell, W.J., et al.: The corneal endothelium and central corneal thickness in pigmentary dispersion syndrome. Arch Ophthalmol., 104:845–846, 1986.

Snail Tracks of Cornea (Irregular, Discontinuous Greyish-White Streaks or Patches, Usually Orientated Horizontally and Obliquely on the Corneal Endothelium)

1. Corneal buttons preserved in corneal storage medium

2. Following ocular surgery

3. Ocular trauma

Alfonso, E., et al.: Snail tracks of the corneal endothelium. Ophthalmology, 99:344–349, 1986.

Keratoconus (Conical Cornea) (Noninflammatory Ectasia of Cornea in its Axial Part with Considerable Visual Impairment Because of Development of a High Degree of Irregular Myopic Astigmatism). Keratoconus may be associated with:

1. Acute hydrops of the cornea

2. Aniridia

3. Apert syndrome (acrodysplasia)

4. Asthma, hay fever

*5. Atopic dermatitis, keratosis plantaris, and palmaris

6. Blue sclerotics, including van der Hoeve's syndrome (osteogenesis imperfecta) (see blue sclera, p. 263)

7. Chandler syndrome (iridocorneal endothelial syndrome)

8. Contact lens wear

9. Crouzon syndrome

10. Ehlers-Danlos syndrome (fibrodysplasia elastica generalisata, cutis hyperelastica)

11. Facial hemiatrophy

*12. Familial

13. Focal dermal hypoplasia (Goltz syndrome)

14. Fuchs corneal endothelial dystrophy

15. Gronblad-Strandberg syndrome (pseudoxanthoma elasticum)

16. Hereditary history

17. Hyperextensible joints and mitral valve prolapse

18. Infantile tapetoretinal degeneration of Leber

19. Iridoschisis

20. Laurence-Moon-Biedl syndrome (retinitis-polydactyly-adiposogenital syndrome)

21. Little syndrome (nail-patella syndrome)

22. Lymphogranuloma venereum

23. Marfan syndrome (arachnodactyly dystrophia mesodermalis congenita)

24. Mongolism (Down syndrome)

25. Neurocutaneous angiomatosis

26. Neurodermatitis

27. Neurofibromatosis (von Recklinghausen syndrome)

28. Noonan syndrome (male Turner syndrome)

29. Pellucid marginal corneal degeneration

30. Retinal disinsertion syndrome

31. Retinitis pigmentosa

32. Retinopathy of prematurity

33. Rieger syndrome

*34. Trauma, such as rubbing of eyes, birth injury or contusion

35. Vernal catarrh

36. 18q syndrome

Forstot, S.L., et al.: Familial keratoconus. Am J Ophthalmol., 105:92–93, 1988.

Isenberg, S.J.: The Eye in Infancy. Chicago, Year Book Medical Publishers, 1989.

Krachner, J.H., et al.: Keratoconus and related noninflammatory corneal thinning disorders. Surv Ophthalmol., 28:293–322, 1984.

Lipman, R.M., et al.: Keratoconus and Fuchs' corneal endothelial dystrophy in a patient and her family. Arch Ophthalmol., 108:993–994, 1990.

Pau, H.: Differential Diagnosis of Eye Diseases. 2nd Ed. Philadelphia, W.B. Saunders, 1989.

Roy, F.H.: Ocular Syndromes and Systemic Diseases. 2nd Ed. Philadelphia, W.B. Saunders, 1989.

Vinokur, E.T., et al.: The association of keratoconus, hyperextensible joints, and mitral valve prolapse. Ophthalmology, 93:95, 1986.

Cornea Plana (Decreased Corneal Curvature)

1. Isolated

2. Marfan syndrome

*3. Sclerocornea

Isenberg, S.J.: The Eye in Infancy. Chicago, Year Book Medical Publishers, 1989.

Staphyloma of Cornea (Corneal Stretching with Incarceration of Uveal Tissue)

1. Advanced keratoconus (see p. 328)

2. Avitaminosis A with keratomalacia

* = most important

3. Congenital

*4. Following corneal ulcer (see p. 322), neuroparalytic keratitis, corneal leprosy, and severe corneal injury

5. Mucoviscidosis (cystic fibrosis of the pancreas)

Arffa, R.C.: Grayson's Diseases of the Cornea. 3rd Ed. St. Louis, Mosby–Year Book, 1991.

Whorl-like Corneal Lesions

*1. Amiodarone toxicity

2. Amodiaquine hydrochloride administration

3. Atabrine administration

*4. Chloroquine and hydroxychloroquine toxicity

5. Chlorpromazine administration

*6. Fabry disease (diffuse angiokeratosis)

7. Indomethacin administration

8. Meperidine hydrochloride

9. Quinacrine administration

10. Urethan administration

Arffa, R.C.: Grayson's Diseases of the Cornea. 3rd Ed. St. Louis, Mosby–Year Book, 1991.

Fraunfelder, F.T.: Interim report. National registry of possible drug-induced ocular side effects. Ophthalmology, 87:88, 1982.

Kaplan, L.J., and Cappaert, W.E.: Amiodarone keratopathy. Arch Ophthalmol., 100:601, 1982.

Corneal Dermoids (Congenital Corneal Limbal Lesions That Grow Slowly). Tumors are yellowish, elevated, and variable in size; they consist of fibrofatty tissue covered by epidermal rather than by conjunctival epithelium and may contain ectodermal derivatives such as hair follicles, sebaceous glands, and sweat glands; trauma, irritation, and puberty hasten their growth

1. Bloch-Sulzberger syndrome (incontinentia pigmenti)

2. Cri du chat syndrome (cry of the cat syndrome)

3. Duane retraction syndrome

4. Multiple dermoids of the cornea associated with miliary aneurysms of the retina

5. Neurocutaneous syndrome (ectomesodermal dysgenesis)

6. Nevus sebaceous of Jadassohn (linear nevus sebaceous of Jadassohn)

*7. Oculoauriculovertebral dysplasia (Goldenhar syndrome)

8. Ring dermoid syndrome—autosomal dominant

9. Sporadic

10. Thalidomide teratogenicities

Arffa, R.C.: Grayson's Diseases of the Cornea. 3rd Ed. St. Louis, Mosby–Year Book, 1991.

Benjamin, S.N., and Allen, H.F.: Classification for limbal dermoid choristomas and brachial arch anomalies. Arch Ophthalmol., 87:305–314, 1972.

Henkind, P., et al.: Bilateral corneal dermoids. Am J Ophthalmol., 76:972–977, 1973.

Roy, F.H.: Ocular Syndromes and Systemic Diseases. 2nd Ed. Philadelphia, W.B. Saunders, 1989.

Corneal Dermoids

	Goldenhar Syndrome	Cri-du-chat Syndrome	Duane Retraction Syndrome	Block-Sulzberger Syndrome	Miliary Aneurysms of Retina	Thalidomide Teratogenicities	Neurocutaneous Syndrome	Nevus Sebaceous of Jadassohn Syndrome
History								
1. Drug ingestion during gestation						U		
2. Greater in females			U	U				
3. Greater left eye			U					
4. Hereditary	R	U	R	U	S		U	
5. Low birth weight		U						
6. Present at birth	U					U		U
7. Unilateral	S		U					
Physical Findings								
1. Absence/restricted adduction	S		U					
2. Antimongoloid palpebral fissures (temporal canthus lower)		U						S
3. Bulbar dermoid	U		S					S
4. Cataract	S	R		S			S	
5. Coloboma of lids	U							U
6. Corneal vascularization								S
7. Dacryocystitis	S							
8. Deficiency of tears		U						
9. Epicanthal folds		U						
10. Glaucoma						S		
11. Hypertelorism		U						
12. Iris and choroid coloboma	S		R			U		U
13. Microcornea	S							
14. Microphthalmos	S	R						
15. Nystagmus					S			S
16. Optic atrophy		R			S			
17. Papillary conjunctivitis							S	
18. Papillitis					S			
19. Paralysis of extraocular muscles	S					S		S
20. Persistent pupillary membrane	S							
21. Pigmented retinopathy						U	S	U
22. Retinal detachment					S	S		
23. Retinal microaneurysm					S	U		
24. Retinal vessel tortuosity		U						
25. Retraction of adducted globe	S		U					
26. Retrolenticular mass					S	S	U	
27. Strabismus	S	S	R	S				
28. Vitreous hemorrhage						S		
29. Widening of palpebral fissures on abduction	S		S					
Laboratory Data								
1. Chromosomal study reveals deletion of short-arm chromosome 5		U						
2. Electromyography shows disorder of paradoxic innervation			U					
3. Roentgenogram of cervical bones	U							

R = rarely; S = sometimes; and U = usually.

* = most important

Corneal Problems Associated with Keratotic Skin Lesions

1. Ectodermal dysplasia (anhidrotic)
*2. Ichthyosis
3. Keratosis follicularis
4. Keratosis follicularis spinulosa decalvans
5. Keratosis plantaris and palmaris
6. Pityriasis rubra pilaris

Arffa, R.C.: Grayson's Diseases of the Cornea. 3rd Ed. St. Louis, Mosby–Year Book, 1991.
Wilson, L.A.: External Diseases of the Eye. Philadelphia, Harper and Row, 1979.

Corneal Problems Associated with Lid Excrescences

1. Keratosis folliculosis
2. Lipid proteinosis
*3. Molluscum contagiosum
4. Verruca vulgaris

Arffa, R.C.: Grayson's Diseases of the Cornea. 3rd Ed. St. Louis, Mosby–Year Book, 1991.
Wilson, L.A.: External Diseases of the Eye. Philadelphia, Harper and Row, 1979.

Corneal Disease Associated with Lenticular Problems

1. Aberfeld syndrome (ocular and facial abnormalities syndrome)—cataracts, microcornea
2. Acrodermatitis chronica atrophicans—keratomalacia, corneal opacification, cataracts
3. Addison syndrome (idiopathic hypoparathyroidism)—keratoconjunctivitis, corneal ulcers, keratitic moniliasis, cataracts
4. Amiodarone—corneal deposits, anterior subcapsular cataracts
5. Amyloidosis—amyloid deposits of cornea, corneal dystrophy, pseudopodia lentis
6. Anderson-Warburg syndrome (oligophrenia-microphthalmos syndrome)—corneal opacification and lenticular destruction with a mass visible behind the lens
7. Andosky syndrome (atopic cataract syndrome)—atopic keratoconjunctivitis, keratoconus, uveitis, subcapsular cataract
8. Aniridia—microcornea and subluxated lenses
9. Anterior chamber cleavage syndrome (Reese-Ellsworth syndrome)—corneal opacities, anterior pole cataract
10. Anterior segment ischemia syndrome—corneal edema, corneal ulceration, cataract
11. Apert syndrome (absent digits cranial defects syndrome)—exposure keratitis, cataracts, ectopia lentis
12. Arteriovenous fistula (arteriovenous aneurysm)—bullous keratopathy, cataract
13. Aspergillosis—corneal ulcer, keratitis, cataract
* 14. Atopic disease (atopic eczema, Besnier prurigo)—keratoconjunctivitis, keratoconus, cataract
15. Autosomal dominant—cataracts and microcornea

16. Avitaminosis C (scurvy)—keratitis, corneal ulcer, cataract

17. Chickenpox (varicella)—corneal ulcer, corneal opacity, keratitis, cataract

18. Chlorpromazine—corneal and lens opacities

19. Cholera—keratomalacia, cataract

20. Chromosome partial deletion (short-arm) syndrome—cataracts, corneal opacities

21. Cockayne syndrome (Mickey Mouse syndrome)—cataracts, band keratopathy, corneal dystrophy

22. Congenital spherocytic anemia (congenital hemolytic jaundice)—congenital cataract, ring-shaped pigmentary corneal deposits

23. Crouzon syndrome (Parrot-Head syndrome)—exposure keratitis, cataract, corneal dystrophy

24. Cryptophthalmia syndrome (cryptophthalmos-syndactyly syndrome)—cornea differentiated from sclera, lens absence to hypoplasia, dislocation, and calcification

25. Cytomegalic inclusion disease (cytomegalovirus)—cataract, corneal opacities

26. Darier-White syndrome (keratosis follicularis)—keratosis, corneal subepithelial infiltrations, corneal ulceration, cataract

27. Dermatitis herpetiformis (Duhring-Broca disease)—corneal vascularization, cataract

28. Diphtheria-keratitis, corneal ulcer, cataract

29. Ehler-Danlos syndrome (fibrodysplasia elastica generalisata)—microcornea, keratoconus, lens subluxation

30. Electrical injury—corneal perforation, necrosis of cornea, anterior or posterior subcapsular cataracts

31. Exfoliation syndrome (capsular exfoliation syndrome)—cataract, dislocated lens, corneal dystrophy, lens capsule exfoliation

32. Folling syndrome (phenylketonuria)—corneal opacities, cataracts

* 33. Fuchs syndrome (I) (heterochromic cyclitis syndrome)—secondary cataract, edematous corneal epithelium

34. Goldscheider syndrome (epidermolysis bullosa)—bullous keratitis, corneal subepithelial blisters to corneal perforation, cataract

35. Gorlin-Goltz syndrome (multiple basal cell nevi syndrome)—cataract, corneal leukoma

36. Gronblad-Strandberg syndrome (elastorrhexis)—keratoconus, cataract, subluxation of lens

37. Hallermann-Streiff syndrome (oculomandibulofacial dyscephaly)—cataracts, microcornea

38. Hanhart syndrome (recessive keratosis palmoplantaris)—dendritic corneal lesions, keratitis, corneal haze, corneal neovascularization, cataract

39. Heerfordt syndrome (uveoparotid fever)—band keratopathy, keratoconjunctivitis, cataract

40. Hereditary ectodermal dysplasia syndrome (Siemens syndrome)—keratosis, corneal erosions, corneal dystrophy, cataract, lens luxation

*41. Herpes simplex—keratitis, corneal ulcer, cataract

*42. Herpes zoster—keratitis, corneal ulcer, cataract

* = most important

43. Histiocytosis X (Hand-Schüller-Christian syndrome)—pannus, bullous keratopathy, corneal ulcer, cataract

44. Hodgkin disease—keratitis, cataract

45. Homocystinuria syndrome—dislocated lens, cataract, keratitis

46. Hutchinson-Gilford syndrome (progeria)—cataract, microcornea

47. Hydatid cyst (echinococcosis)—keratitis, corneal abscess, cataract

48. Hypervitaminosis D—band keratopathy, cataract

49. Hypoparathyroidism—keratitis, cataract

50. Hypophosphatasia (phosphoethanolaminuria)—cataract, corneal subepithelial calcifications

51. Influenza—keratitis, cataract

52. Jadassohn-type anetodermal—keratoconus, cataract

53. Jadassohn-Lewandowsky syndrome (pachyonychia congenita)—corneal dyskeratosis, cataract

*54. Juvenile rheumatoid arthritis (Still disease)—band keratopathy, cataract

55. Kussmaul disease (periarteritis nodosa)—corneal ulcer, cataract

56. Kyrle disease (hyperkeratosis penetrans)—subcapsular cataracts, subepithelial corneal opacities

57. Leri syndrome (carpal tunnel syndrome)—corneal clouding, cataract

58. Listerellosis (listeriosis)—keratitis, corneal abscess and ulcer, cataract

59. Little syndrome (nail-patella syndrome)—microcornea, keratoconus, cataract

60. Lowe syndrome (oculocerebrorenal syndrome)—cloudy cornea, cataracts, megalocornea, corneal dystrophy

61. Malaria—keratitis, cataract

62. Marchesani syndrome (brachymorphia with spherophakia)—lentic ular myopia, ectopia lentis, megalocornea, corneal opacity

63. Marfan syndrome (arachnodactyly-dystrophia-mesodermalis congenita)—lens dislocation, cataract, megalocornea, lenticular myopia

64. Matsoukas syndrome (oculo-cerebro-articulo-skeletal syndromes)—cataract, corneal sclerosis

65. Meckel syndrome (dysencephalia splanchnocystica syndrome)—sclerocornea, microcornea, cataract

66. Morbilli (rubeola, measles)—corneal ulcer, cataract

67. Mucolipidosis IV (ML IV)—corneal clouding, cataract

68. Nematode ophthalmia syndrome (toxocariasis)—cataract, larvae present in the cornea

69. Neurodermatitis (lichen simplex chronicus)—keratoconjunctivitis, atopic cataracts, keratoconus

70. Ocular toxoplasmosis (toxoplasmosis)—keratitis, cataract

71. Oculodental syndrome (Peter syndrome)—macrocornea, opacities of the corneal margin, ectopic lentis, corneoscleral staphyloma

72. O'Donnell-Pappas syndrome—presenile cataract, peripheral corneal pannus

73. Paget syndrome (osteitis deformans)—corneal ring opacities, cataract

74. Passow syndrome (status dysraphicus syndrome)—neuroparalytic keratitis, zonular cataract

75. Pemphigus foliaceus (Cazenave disease)—pannus, corneal infiltration, cataract

76. Pigmentary ocular dispersion syndrome (pigmentary glaucoma)—Krukenberg's spindle, equatorial pigmentation of lens capsule

77. Pseudohypoparathyroidism (Seabright-Bantan syndrome)—punctate cataracts, keratitis

78. Radiation—corneal ulcer, punctate keratitis, cataracts, exfoliation of lens capsule

79. Refsum syndrome (phytanic acid oxidase deficiency)—corneal opacities, cataracts

80. Relapsing polychondritis—corneal ulcer, cataracts, keratoconjunctivitis sicca

81. Retinal disinsertion syndrome—lens subluxation, keratoconus

82. Retinopathy of prematurity—cataracts, corneal opacification

83. Rieger syndrome (dysgenesis mesodermalis corneae et irides)—microcornea, corneal opacities in Descemet membrane, dislocated lens

84. Romberg syndrome (facial hemiatrophy)—neuroparalytic keratitis, cataracts

85. Rubella syndrome (German measles)—corneal haziness, cataracts, microcornea

86. Sabin-Feldman syndrome—posterior lenticonus, microcornea

87. Sanfilippo-Good syndrome (mucopolysaccharidosis III)—deposits in cornea and lens

88. Schafer syndrome (keratosis palmoplantaris syndrome)—lesions in the lower portion of the cornea, cataract

89. Schaumann syndrome (sarcoidosis syndrome)—keratitis sicca, band-shaped keratitis, complicated cataract

90. Scheie syndrome (mucopolysaccharidosis IS)—diffuse haze to marked corneal clouding, cataracts

91. Stannus cerebellar syndrome—corneal vascularization, corneal opacities, cataracts

92. Stevens-Johnson syndrome (erythema multiforme exudativum)—keratitis, corneal ulcers, cataracts, pannus

93. Stickler syndrome (hereditary progressive arthro-ophthalmopathy)—keratopathy, cataracts

94. Thioridazine—corneal and lens opacities

95. Toxic lens syndrome—pigment precipitation on the surface of an intraocular lens, chronic uveitis

96. Trisomy syndrome—corneal and lens opacities

97. Turner's syndrome (gonadal dysgenesis)—corneal nebulae, cataracts

98. Ultraviolet radiation—band keratopathy, keratitis, discoloring of lens

99. van Bogaert-Scherer-Epstein syndrome (familial hypercholesterolemia syndrome)—lipid keratopathy, cataract, juvenile corneal arcus

100. von Recklinghausen syndrome (neurofibromatosis)—nodular swelling of corneal nerves, cataracts

101. Waardenburg syndrome (interoculoiridodermatoauditive dysplasia)—microcornea, cornea plana, lenticonus

* = most important

102. ~~Wagner syndrome (hereditary hyaloideoretinal degeneration and palatoschisis)~~—corneal degeneration, including band-shaped keratopathy, cataracts

103. Ward syndrome (nevus jaw cyst syndrome)—congenital cataracts, congenital corneal opacities

104. Wegener syndrome (Wegener granulomatosis)—corneal ulcer, corneal abscess, cataract

105. Weil disease (leptospirosis)—keratitis, cataract

106. Werner syndrome (progeria of adults)—juvenile cataracts, bullous keratitis, trophic corneal defects

107. Yersiniosis—corneal ulcer, cataract

108. Zellweger syndrome (cerebrohepatorenal syndrome of Zellweger)—corneal opacities, cataract

Bilgami, N.L., et al.: Marfan syndrome with microcornea, aphakia, and ventricular systolic defect. Indian Heart J., 33:78–80, 1981.

Dolan, B.J., et al.: Amiodarone keratopathy and lens opacities. J Am Optom. Assoc., 56:468–470, 1985.

Gualtieri, C.T., et al.: Corneal and lenticular opacities in mentally retarded young adults treated with thioridazine and chlorpromazine. Am J Psychiatry, 139:1178–1180, 1982.

Polomeno, R.C., and Cummings, C.: Autosomal dominant cataracts and microcornea. Can J Ophthalmol., 14:227–229, 1979.

Roy, F.H.: Ocular Syndromes and Systemic Diseases. 2nd Ed. Philadelphia, W.B. Saunders, 1989.

Corneal Disease Associated with Retinal Problems

1. Abdominal typhus (enteric fever)—corneal ulcer, retinal detachment, central retinal artery emboli

2. Acanthamoebae—keratitis, pannus, corneal ring abscess, retinal perivasculitis

3. African eyeworm disease—keratitis, central retinal artery occlusion, macular hemorrhages

4. Amyloidosis—amyloid corneal deposits, corneal dystrophy, retinal hemorrhages

5. Anderson-Warburg syndrome (oligophrenia-microphthalmos syndrome)—corneal opacification, malformed retina with retina pseudotumors

6. Angioedema (hives)—central serous retinopathy, corneal edema

7. Anterior segment ischemia syndrome—corneal edema midperiphery retinal hemorrhages

8. Apert syndrome (acrodysplasia)—exposure keratitis, retinal detachment

9. Arteriovenous fistula—bullous keratopathy, retinal hemorrhages

10. Aspergillosis—corneal ulcer, keratitis, retinal hemorrhages, retinal detachment

11. Atopic dermatitis—keratoconus and retinal detachment

12. Avitaminosis C—retinal hemorrhages, keratitis, corneal ulcer

13. Bacillus cereus-ring abscess of cornea, necrosis of retina

14. Bang disease (brucellosis)—keratitis, chorioretinitis, macular edema

15. Behçet syndrome (dermatostomata-ophthalmic syndrome)—keratitis, posterior corneal abscess, retinal vascular changes

16. Bietti disease (Bietti marginal crystalline dystrophy)—marginal corneal dystrophy, retinitis punctate albescens

17. Candidiasis-keratitis, corneal ulcer, retinal atrophy, retinal detachment

18. Carotid artery syndrome—corneal ulcer, loss of corneal sensation, retinal edema, engorgement of retinal veins

19. Chickenpox (varicella)—corneal ulcer, corneal opacity, retinitis, hemorrhagic retinopathy

*20. Chloroquine-corneal epithelial pigmentation, macular lesions

21. Chronic granulomatous disease of childhood-keratitis, destructive chorioretinal lesions

22. Cockayne syndrome (dwarfism with retinal atrophy and deafness)—pigmentary degeneration, band keratopathy, corneal dystrophy

23. Crohn disease (granulomatous ileocolitis)—marginal corneal ulcers, keratitis, macular edema, macular hemorrhages

24. Cryoglobulinemia—deep corneal opacities, venous stasis

25. Cystinosis (aminoaciduria)—crystals in cornea and pigment in retina

26. Dengue fever—keratitis, corneal ulcer, retinal hemorrhages

27. Diffuse keratoses syndrome—corneal nodular thickening in the stroma worse in fall, retinal phlebitis

28. Diphtheria—keratitis, corneal ulcer, central artery occlusion

29. Disseminated lupus erythematosus (Kaposi-Libman-Sacks syndrome)—keratitis, keratoconjunctivitis sicca, corneal ulcer, central retinal vein occlusion, retinal detachment

30. Ehlers-Danlos syndrome (cutis hyperelastica)—keratoconus, and retinitis pigmentosa

31. Electrical injury—corneal perforation, retinal edema, retinal hemorrhages, pigmentary degeneration, retinal holes, dilatation of retinal veins

32. Fabry disease (diffuse angiokeratosis)—whorl-like changes in cornea, central retinal artery occlusion, tortuosity of retinal vessels

33. Goldscheider syndrome (epidermolysis bullosa)—bullous keratitis with opacities, retinal detachment

34. Gronblad-Strandberg syndrome (systemic elastodystrophy)—angioid streaks of the retina, macular hemorrhages, retinal detachment, keratoconus

35. Hamman-Rich syndrome (alveolar capillary block syndrome)—keratomalacia ischemic retinopathy, cystic macular changes

36. Heerfordt syndrome (uveoparotid fever)—band keratopathy, retinal vasculitis

37. Hennebert syndrome (luetic otitic nystagmus syndrome)—interstitial keratitis, disseminated syphilitic chorioretinitis

38. Histiocytosis X (Hand-Schüller-Christian syndrome)—retinal hemorrhage, retinal detachment, bullous keratopathy, corneal ulcer, pannus

39. Hodgkin disease—keratitis, retinal hemorrhages

40. Hollenhorst syndrome (chorioretinal infarction syndrome)—hazy cornea, serous retinal detachment, pigmentary retinopathy

41. Hunter syndrome (mucopolysaccharidoses [MPS] II)—splitting or absence of pe-

ripheral Bowman membrane, stromal haze, pigmentary retinal degeneration, narrowed retinal vessels

42. Hurler-Scheie syndrome (MPS IH-S)—corneal clouding, pigmentary retinopathy

43. Hurler syndrome (gargoylism)—diffuse corneal haziness, retinal pigmentary changes, megalocornea, retinal detachment

44. Hydatid cyst (echinococcosis)—keratitis, abscess of cornea, retinal detachment, retinal hemorrhages

45. Hyperlipoproteinemia—arcus juvenilis, lipemia retinalis, xanthomata of retina

46. Hyperparathyroidism—band keratopathy, vascular engorgement of retina

47. Hypovitaminosis A—keratomalacia with perforation, corneal opacity, retinal degeneration

48. Idiopathic hypercalcemia (blue diaper syndrome)—band keratopathy, optic atrophy, papilledema

49. Indomethacin—corneal deposits, reduced retinal sensitivity

50. Influenza—keratitis, retinal hemorrhage

51. Japanese River fever (typhus)—keratitis, retinal hemorrhages

52. Juvenile rheumatoid arthritis (Still disease)—band keratopathy, macular edema

53. Kahler disease (multiple myeloma)—crystalline deposits of cornea, central retinal artery occlusion, retinal microaneurysms

54. Kussmaul disease (periarteritis nodosa)—retinal detachment, pseudoretinitis pigmentosa, corneal ulcer

55. Leber tapetoretinal dystrophy syndrome (retinal aplasia)—keratoconus, salt-and-pepper or "bone corpuscle" pigmentation, yellowish-brown or gray macular lesions

56. Lubarsch-Pick syndrome (primary amyloidosis)—amyloid corneal deposits, retinal hemorrhages

57. Lymphogranuloma venereum disease (Nicolas-Favre disease)—keratitis, pannus, corneal ulcer, keratoconus, tortuosity of retinal vessels, retinal hemorrhages

58. Marfan syndrome (arachnodactyly dystrophia mesodermalis congenita)—keratoconus, retinitis pigmentosa

59. Meckel syndrome (dysencephalia splanchnocystica syndrome)—sclerocornea, microcornea, retinal dysplasia

60. Meningococcemia—keratitis, retinal endophlebitis

61. Mikulicz-Radeski syndrome (dacryosialoadenopathy)—keratoconjunctivitis, retinal candlewax spots

62. ML IV (mucolipidosis IV)—corneal clouding, corneal opacities, retinal atrophy

63. Morbilli (measles-rubeola)—keratitis, corneal ulcer, pigmentary retinopathy, central retinal artery occlusion

64. Mucormycosis (phycomycosis)—corneal ulcer, striate keratopathy, retinitis, central retinal artery thrombosis

65. Mycosis fungoides syndrome (malignant cutaneous reticulosis syndrome)—keratoconjunctivitis, retinal edema, retinal hemorrhage

66. Myotonic dystrophy syndrome—corneal epithelial dystrophy, loss of corneal sensitivity, tapetoretinal degeneration, macular red spot, macular degeneration, chorioretinitis

67. Neurofibromatosis (von Recklinghausen syndrome)—nodular swelling nerves, hamartoma of retina

68. Norrie disease (atrophia oculi congenita)—malformation of sensory cells of retina, corneal nebulae

69. Oculodental syndrome (Peter's syndrome)—corneoscleral staphyloma, megalocornea, corneal marginal opacities, macular pigmentation

70. Onchocerciasis syndrome—punctate keratitis, sclerosing keratitis, chorioretinitis, retinal degeneration

71. Paget syndrome (osteitis deformans)—corneal ring opacities, retinal hemorrhages, pigmentary retinopathy, macular changes resembling Kuhnt-Junius degeneration

72. Phenothiazine—epithelial and endothelial pigment, retinal pigmentation

73. Pierre-Robin syndrome (micrognathia-glossoptosis)—retinal disinsertion, megalocornea

74. Plasma lecithin (cholesterol acyltransferase deficiency)—corneal stromal opacities, retinal hemorrhages

75. Porphyria cutanea tarda—keratitis, retinal hemorrhages, cotton-wool spots, macular edema

76. Postvaccinial ocular syndrome—corneal vesicles, and marginal ulcers, chorioretinitis, central serous retinopathy, central retinal vein thrombosis

77. Progressive systemic sclerosis—marginal corneal ulcers with cicatrization, cotton-wool spots, retinal hemorrhages

78. Radiation—corneal ulcer, punctate keratitis, keratoconjuctivitis sicca, retinal hemorrhage, macular degeneration, macular holes with vascularization

79. Refsum syndrome (phytanic acid oxidase deficiency)—band keratopathy, retinitis pigmentosa

80. Relapsing fever—interstitial keratitis, retinal hemorrhage

81. Relapsing polychondritis—corneal ulcer, retinal detachment, retinal artery thrombosis, keratoconjunctivitis sicca

82. Renal failure—cotton-wool spots, band keratopathy

83. Rendu-Osler syndrome (hereditary hemorrhagic telangiectasis)—intermittent filamentary keratitis, small retinal angiomas, retinal hemorrhages

84. Retinal disinsertion syndrome—bilateral keratoconus, retinal detachment

85. Retinoblastoma—corneal tumor, retinal neovascularization

86. Rothmund syndrome (telangiectasia-pigmentation cataract syndrome)—corneal lesions, retinal hyperpigmentation

87. Rubella syndrome (Gregg syndrome)—microcornea, pigmentary retinal changes

88. Sabin-Feldman syndrome—microcornea, chorioretinitis or atrophic degenerative chorioretinal changes

89. Sanfilippo-Good syndrome (mucopolysaccharidosis III)—slight narrowing of retinal vessels, acid mucopolysaccharide deposits in cornea.

90. Schaumann syndrome (sarcoidosis syndrome)—mutton fat keratitic precipitates, keratitis sicca, band-shaped keratitis, inflammatory retinal exudates

91. Scheie syndrome (mucopolysaccharidoses I-S)—diffuse to marked corneal clouding, tapetoretinal degeneration

92. Schwartz syndrome (glaucoma associated with retinal detachment)—retinal detachment, microcornea

93. Shy-Gonatas syndrome (orthostatic hypotension syndrome)—keratopathy, corneal ulcer, lattice-like white opacities in the area of Bowman membrane, retinal pigmentary degeneration

94. Smallpox—keratitis, congenital corneal clouding, chorioretinitis

95. Stannus cerebellar syndrome (riboflavin deficiency)—corneal vascularization, superficial diffuse keratitis, corneal opacities, brownish retinal patches

96. Stickler syndrome (hereditary progressive arthroophthalmopathy)—keratopathy, chorioretinal degeneration, total retinal detachment

97. Sturge-Weber syndrome (neuro-oculocutaneous angiomatosis)—retinal detachment, increased corneal diameter with cloudiness

98. Syphilis (acquired lues)—keratitis, retinal hemorrhages, retinal proliferation

99. Temporal arteritis syndrome (Hutchinson-Horton-Magath-Brown syndrome)—retinal detachments, narrowing of retinal vessels, central retinal artery occlusion, corneal hypesthesia

100. Trisomy 13 (Patau syndrome)—malformed cornea, retinal dysplasia

101. Tuberculosis—keratitis, pannus, corneal ulcer, retinitis

102. Ullrich syndrome (dyscraniopygophalangy)—cloudy cornea, corneal ulcers, chorioretinal coloboma

103. Ultraviolet radiation—photokeratitis, band keratopathy, herpes simplex keratitis, recurrent corneal erosions, retinal degeneration

104. Vaccinia—keratitis, pannus, corneal perforation, central serous retinopathy, pseudoretinitis pigmentosa

105. van Bogaert-Scherer-Epstein (primary hyperlipidemia)—arcus juvenilis of the cornea, lipid keratopathy, retinopathy with yellowish deposits

106. Vitreous tug syndrome—vitreous strands attached to corneal wound or scar, circumscribed retinal edema, posterior retinal detachment

107. von Gierke disease (glycogen storage disease type I)—corneal clouding, discrete nonelevated, yellow flecks in macula

108. Waardenburg syndrome (embryonic fixation syndrome)—microcornea, cornea plana, hypopigmentation and hypoplasia of retina

109. Wagner syndrome (hyaloideoretinal degeneration)—corneal degeneration, band-shaped keratopathy, hyaloideoretinal degeneration, narrowing of retinal vessels, retinal detachment, avascular preretinal membranes

110. Waldenstrom syndrome (macroglobulinemia syndrome)—crystalline corneal deposits, keratoconjunctivitis sicca, retinal venous thrombosis, retinal microaneurysms, cotton-wool spots

111. Weil disease (leptospirosis)—keratitis, retinitis

112. Werner syndrome (progeria of adults)—bullous keratitis, paramacular retinal degeneration

113. Wiskott-Aldrich syndrome (sex-linked draining ears, eczematoid dermatitis, bloody diarrhea)—corneal ulcers, retinal hemorrhages

114. Yersinosis—corneal ulcer, retinal hemorrhages

115. Zellweger syndrome (cerebrohepatorenal syndrome)—corneal opacities, narrowing of retinal vessels, retinal holes without detachment, tapetoretinal degeneration

116. Zieve syndrome (hyperlipemia hemolytic anemia-icterus syndrome)—cloudy cornea, corneal ulcers, retinal lipemia

Arffa, R.C.: Grayson's Disease of the Cornea. 3rd Ed. St. Louis, Mosby–Year Book, 1991.

Roy, F.H.: Ocular Syndromes and Systemic Diseases. 2nd Ed. Philadelphia, W.B. Saunders, 1989.

Corneal Diseases Associated with Deafness

1. Atopic dermatitis—limbal keratitis, conjunctivitis
*2. Cogan syndrome (nonsyphilitic interstitial keratitis)—interstitial keratitis
3. Meniere disease—iritis, glaucoma
*4. Polyarteritis nodosa (Kussmaul disease)—paralimbal keratitis, corneoscleral ulceration
5. Sarcoidosis syndrome (Schaumann syndrome)—primary stromal keratitis, keratoconjunctivitis sicca
*6. Syphilis (lues)—interstitial keratitis
7. 3-methyl-pentyn-3-yl acid phthalate (Whipcide, trichuricidal agent)—keratitis, uveitis, stromal keratitis
8. Tuberculosis—interstitial keratitis
9. Vogt-Koyonagi-Harada syndrome (uveitis-vitiligo-alopecia poliosis syndrome)—uveitis
10. Wegener granulomatosis—necrotizing sclerokeratitis

Heinemann, M.H., et al.: Cogan's syndrome. Ann. Ophthalmol., 12:667, 1980.

Trigger Mechanisms for Recurrent Herpes Simplex Keratitis

*1. Corticosteroids (topical)
*2. Emotional disturbances
*3. Exposure to sunlight (ultraviolet)
*4. Fever (most common)
5. Gastrointestinal upsets
6. Ingestion of food to which patient is allergic
7. Mechanical trauma
8. Menses

Kimura, S.J.: Infectious Diseases of the Conjunctiva and Cornea. Symposium of the New Orleans Academy of Ophthalmology. St. Louis, C.V. Mosby, 1963.

Predisposing Factors in Keratomycosis

1. Antibiotics
2. Steroids
3. Trauma

Francois, J., and Ryssdlaere, M.: Oculomycoses. Springfield, Ill., Charles C Thomas, 1972.

Gingrich, W.D.: Infectious Diseases of the Conjunctiva and Cornea. Symposium of the New Orleans Academy of Ophthalmology. St. Louis, C.V. Mosby, 1963, p. 154.

* = most important

Sclerocornea (Developmental Corneal Abnormality with Ill Defined Limbus Due to Extension of Opaque Scleral Tissue Into Cornea. Vision Varies with Involvement. Somatic Abnormalities Include Craniofacial, Digital, Skin and Testes Abnormalities, Deafness and Mental Retardation)

1. Associated ocular abnormalities including:
   A. Abnormalities of Descemet membrane, endothelium and corneal stroma
   B. Aniridia
   C. Cataract
   D. Coloboma
   E. Cornea plana—occurrence
   F. Dysgenesis of angle and iris
   G. Esotropia
   H. Glaucoma
   I. Iridocorneal synechiae
   J. Microphthalmia
   K. Nystagmus
   L. Persistent pupillary membrane
   M. Posterior embryotoxon
2. Associated syndromes including:
   A. Axenfeld syndrome
   B. Cross syndrome
   C. Dandy-Walker syndrome
   D. Hallermann-Streiff syndrome
   E. Hurler syndrome
   F. Hypomelanosis of Ito
   G. Lobstein syndrome
   H. Melnick-Needles syndrome
   I. Mieten syndrome
   J. Nail-Patella syndrome
   K. Rieger syndrome
   L. Robert syndrome
   M. Smith-Lemli-Opitz syndrome
   N. Unbalanced 17p-10q translocation
   O. Wolf syndrome (4p- syndrome)

Isenberg, S.J.: The Eye in Infancy. Chicago, Year Book Medical Publishers, 1989.

Tasman, W., and Jaeger, E., eds.: Duane's Clinical Ophthalmology. Philadelphia, J.B. Lippincott, 1990.

Intraocular Pressure

JAMES SAVAGE, M.D.

Contents

Glaucoma Suspect, Infant

1. Amblyopia ex anopsia
*2. Corneal edema (see p. 285)
3. Corneal enlargement
4. Cupping and atrophy of optic disc
5. Deep anterior chamber
*6. Epiphora, photophobia, and blepharospasm (see p. 73)
7. Iridodonesis and subluxation of lens (see p. 449)
8. Iris processes
*9. Tears in Descemet membrane (see p. 325)

Duane, T.D., and Jaeger, E.A.: Clinical Ophthalmology. Philadelphia, Harper & Row, 1994.

Harley, R.D.: Pediatric Ophthalmology. Philadelphia, W.B. Saunders, 1975.

Hoskins, H.D., and Kass, M.A.: Becker-Shaffer's Diagnosis and Therapy of Glaucoma. 6th Ed. St. Louis, C.V. Mosby, 1989.

Pollack, A., and Oliver, M.: Congenital glaucoma in two siblings. Acta. Ophthalmol., 62:359–363, 1984.

Shields, M.B.: Textbook of Glaucoma. 3rd ed. Baltimore, Williams & Wilkins. 1992.

Conditions Simulating Congenital Glaucoma

1. Blue sclera

    A. Albright's hereditary osteodystrophy (pseudohypoparathyroidism)

    B. Craniofacial dysostosis (Crouzon's disease)

    C. de Lange syndrome

    D. Ehlers-Danlos syndrome

    E. Fölling syndrome.

    F. Hallermann-Streiff syndrome (oculomandibulodyscephaly)

    G. Incontinentia pigmenti (Bloch-Sulzberger syndrome)

    H. Juvenile Paget's disease (hyperphosphatasia, hereditary)

    I. Lowe's (oculocerebrorenal syndrome)

    J. Marfan's syndrome

    K. Turner's (XO, gonadal dysgenesis) syndrome

    L. van der Hoeve's syndrome (osteogenesis imperfecta)

    M. Werner's syndrome

2. Corneal opacity

    A. Congenital malformations

        (1) Anterior corneal staphyloma

        (2) Cornea plana

        (3) Incontinentia pigmenti (Bloch-Sulzberger syndrome)

        (4) Norrie's disease

        *(5) Peters' anomaly

        (6) Riley-Day syndrome (congenital familial dysautonomia)

        *(7) Sclerocornea

        (8) Trisomy 13-15 syndrome (Patau syndrome)

    B. Edema

        *(1) Birth injury such as breaks in Descemet's membrane

        (2) Congenital hereditary corneal edema

        (3) Fetal uveitis

        *(4) Infectious keratitis (congenital syphilis, interstitial keratitis, rubella, variola, varicella, gonorrhea, mumps, others)

        (5) Keratitis (chemical)

        *(6) Keratoconus

    C. Metabolic disorders/dystrophies

        (1) Congenital hereditary stromal dystrophy

     (2) Corneal amyloidosis (Lubarsch-Pick syndrome)

     (3) Corneal lipidosis

     (4) Cystinosis (Lignac-Fanconi syndrome)

     (5) Fabry's disease

     (6) Hyperlipidemia

     (7) Mucopolysaccharidoses

        a. Hunter syndrome (MPS IIB)

        b. Hurler syndrome (MPS IH)

        c. Maroteaux-Lamy syndrome (MPS VI)

        d. Morquio syndrome (MPS IV)

        e. Sanfilippo syndrome (MPS IIIC)

        f. Scheie syndrome (MPS IS)

     (8) Porphyria (congenital)

     (9) von Gierke's glycogen storage disease

3. Epiphora (excessive tearing)

   *A. Lacrimal duct obstruction

   *B. Viral, chemical or allergic conjunctivitis

4. Large corneas

   A. Apert's syndrome

   B. High myopia

   C. Keratoglobus

   D. Marfan's syndrome

   E. Megalocornea

   F. van der Hoeve's syndrome (osteogenesis imperfecta)

*5. Photophobia- anterior uveitis (many causes)

Duane, T.D., and Jaeger, E.A.: Clinical Ophthalmology. Philadelphia, Harper & Row, 1994.

Geeraets, M.J.: Ocular Syndromes, 3rd Ed. Philadelphia, Lea & Febiger, 1976.

Harley, R.D.: Pediatric Ophthalmology. Philadelphia, W. B. Saunders, 1975.

Hoskins, H.D., and Kass, M.A.: Becker-Shaffer's Diagnosis and Therapy of Glaucoma. 6th Ed. St. Louis, C.V. Mosby, 1989.

Roy, F.H.: Ocular Syndromes and Systemic Diseases. 2nd Ed. Philadelphia, W.B. Saunders, 1989.

Shields, M. B.: Textbook of Glaucoma. 3rd Ed. Baltimore, Williams & Wilkins, 1992.

Syndromes and Diseases Associated with Glaucoma

1. Ocular Disease

   A. Corneal endothelial disorders

     (1) Fuchs' endothelial dystrophy

     (2) Iridocorneal endothelial (ICE) syndrome

        a. Chandler's syndrome

        b. Cogan-Reese (iris-nevus) syndrome

        c. Progressive iris atrophy

     (3) Posterior polymorphous dystrophy

* = most important

B. Developmental glaucomas with associated ocular anomalies

    (1). Aniridia (see p. 410)

    (2) Axenfeld-Rieger syndrome

    (3) Congenital ectropion uveae

    (4) Congenital iris hypoplasia

    (5) Megalocornea

    (6) Microcornea

    (7) Peters' anomaly

    (8) Sclerocornea

C. Elevated episcleral venous pressure (see p. 358)

D. Iris disorders

    (1) Iridoschisis

    *(2) Pigmentary glaucoma

E. Lens disorders

    (1) Cataract

        a. Lens particle glaucoma

        b. Phacoanaphylaxis

        c. Phacolytic (lens protein) glaucoma

        d. Phacomorphic (intumescent lens) glaucoma

    (2) Dislocation of the lens (see p. 449)

    *(3) Exfoliation syndrome

F. Medications/chemicals

    (1) Corticosteroids

    (2) Others (see p. 361)

G. Myopia

H. Ocular hemorrhage

    (1) Degenerated ocular blood

        a. Ghost cell glaucoma

        b. Hemolytic glaucoma

        c. Hemosideric glaucoma

    *(2) Hyphema

        a. Blunt trauma

        b. Intraocular surgery

          1. intraoperative

          2. postoperative

        c. Penetrating trauma

        d. Spontaneous

          1. anterior segment neovascularization

          2. intraocular tumor

          3. pupillary vascular tufts

(3) Orbital hemorrhage (massive)

(4) Vitreous hemorrhage (massive)

I. Ocular inflammation

   (1) Choroiditis and retinitis

      a. Cytomegalic inclusion retinitis

      b. Sympathetic ophthalmia

      c. Toxocariasis

      d. Vogt-Koyanagi-Harada syndrome

   (2) Episcleritis

*(3) Iridocyclitis

      a. Acute anterior iridocyclitis

      b. Ankylosing spondylitis

      c. Behçet's disease

      d. Fuchs' heterochromic cyclitis

      e. Glaucomatocyclitic crisis (Posner-Schlossman syndrome)

      f. Infectious diseases

         1. acquired immunodeficiency syndrome (AIDS)

         2. congenital rubella

         3. disseminated meningococcemia

         4. Hansen's disease (leprosy)

         5. hemorrhagic fever with renal syndrome

         6. onchocerciasis (also keratitis)

         7. syphilis

      g. Juvenile rheumatoid arthritis (JRA)

      h. Pars planitis

      i. Precipitates on the trabecular meshwork (Grant's syndrome)

      j. Reiter's syndrome

      k. Sarcoid

      l. Trauma

   (4) Keratitis

      a. Adenovirus Type 10

      b. Herpes simplex

      c. Herpes zoster

      d. Interstitial keratitis

   (5) Scleritis

*J. Ocular surgery

   (1) Aphakia or pseudophakia (see p. 453)

   (2) Corticosteroid induced

   (3) Cyclodialysis cleft (sudden closure)

   (4) Epithelial downgrowth

   (5) Malignant (ciliary block) glaucoma

* = most important

(6) ~~Penetrating keratoplasty~~

    a. Distortion of angle structures

    b. Graft rejection

(7) Vitreoretinal procedures

    a. Intravitreal gas

    b. Pars plana vitrectomy

    c. Retinal photocoagulation

    d. Scleral buckling surgery

    e. Silicone oil

K. Ocular trauma

  (1) Chemical burns (acid, alkali, other)

  (2) Contusion injuries

    a. Angle recession

    b. Hyphema

    c. Iritis

    d. Lens damage and/or dislocation

    e. Trabecular damage

  (3) Penetrating injuries

    a. Epithelial downgrowth

    b. Hyphema

    c. Lens damage and/or dislocation

    d. Peripheral anterior synechiae

  (4) Radiation damage

  (5) Retained intraocular foreign body (iron, copper)

  (6) Retrobulbar hemorrhage (massive)

L. Ocular tumors

  (1) Benign tumors of the anterior uvea

    a. Adenomas

    b. Cysts (primary vs. secondary)

    c. Iris nevi

    d. Leiomyomas

    e. Melanocytomas

    f. Melanoses

  (2) Histiocytosis X

  (3) Leukemias

  (4) Lymphomas

  (5) Metastatic tumors

    a. Carcinomas (most commonly breast in females and lung in males)

    b. Melanomas

  (6) Multiple myeloma

(7) Ocular tumors of childhood

   a. Juvenile xanthogranuloma

   b. Medulloepithelioma (diktyoma)

   c. Retinoblastoma

(8) Orbital tumors

(9) Primary uveal melanomas

(10) Retrobulbar tumors

M. Retinal, vitreous, and choroidal disorders

   (1) Angle closure

      a. Acute choroidal hemorrhage

      b. Central retinal vein occlusion (CRVO)

      c. Ciliochoroidal effusion

         1. Acquired immunodeficiency syndrome (AIDS)

         2. Arteriovenous malformations

         3. Inflammatory conditions

         4. Nanophthalmos

         5. Surgery

         6. Trauma

         7. Tumors

         8. Uveal effusion syndrome

      d. Hemorrhagic retinal and choroidal detachment

      e. Iris retraction syndrome with retinal detachment (Campbell)

      f. Persistent hyperplastic primary vitreous (PHPV)

      g. Postoperative panretinal photocoagulation

      h. Postoperative scleral buckle

      i. Retinal dysplasia

      j. Retinopathy of prematurity (retrolental fibroplasia)

  *(2) Neovascular glaucoma (see p. 366)

   (3) Retinitis pigmentosa

   (4) Rhegmatogenous retinal detachment (Schwartz syndrome)

2. Systemic disorders

  A. Acquired immunodeficiency syndrome (AIDS)

  B. Angioneurotic edema (giant urticaria)

  C. Ankylosing spondylitis (Marie-Strümpell disease)

  D. Aortic arch syndrome

  E. Behçet's disease

  F. Carotid artery occlusive disease

  G. Carotid-cavernous fistula

  H. Cavernous sinus thrombosis

  I. Crouzon's disease (craniofacial dysostosis)

* = most important

J. Cushing's disease

K. Developmental glaucoma as part of a syndrome

   (1) Bing-Neel (macroglobulinemia and CNS) syndrome

   (2) Chondrodystrophy, joint dislocation, glaucoma and mental retardation

   (3) Chromosomal abnormalities

      a. Chromosome partial deletion (long-arm) syndrome

      b. Pericentric inversion of chromosome II

      c. Trisomy 21(Down syndrome)

      d. Trisomy 16-18(Edward syndrome)

      e. Trisomy F (17–18)

      f. Trisomy 13-15 (Patau syndrome)

      g. Turner syndrome (XO, gonadal dysgenesis)

   (4) Cockayne's syndrome

   (5) Congenital rubella syndrome

   (6) Cretinism (juvenile hypothyroidism)

   (7) Cystinosis

   (8) Dental-ocular-cutaneous syndrome

   (9) Ehlers-Danlos syndrome

   (10) Familial histiocytic dermatoarthritis syndrome

   (11) Fetal alcohol syndrome

   (12) Gorlin-Goltz (multiple basal cell nevi) syndrome

   (13) Hallermann-Streiff syndrome (oculomandibulofacial dyscephaly)

   (14) Homocystinuria

   (15) Kartagener syndrome (sinusitis-bronchiectasis-situs inversus)

   (16) Kimmelstiel-Wilson syndrome

   (17) Kleinfelter's syndrome

   (18) Klippel-Trenaunay-Weber syndrome

   (19) Krabbe syndrome

   (20) Krause syndrome (congenital encephalo-ophthalmic dysplasia)

   (21) Lowe (oculocerebrorenal) syndrome

   (22) Marfan syndrome (arachnodactyly dystrophia mesodermalis congenita)

   (23) Meyer-Schwickerath-Weyers syndrome (oculodentodigital dysplasia)

   (24) Miller (Wilms aniridia) syndrome

   (25) Mucopolysaccharidoses

      a. Hurler syndrome (MPS IH)

      b. Maroteaux-Lamy syndrome (MPS VI)

      c. Morquio syndrome (MPS IV)

   (26) Nieden (telangiectasia-cataract) syndrome

   (27) Pierre-Robin syndrome (micrognathia-glossoptosis) syndrome

   (28) Prader-Willi syndrome (hypotonia, hypogonadism, obesity, and mental retardation)

    (29) Rubella syndrome

    (30) Rubenstein-Taybi (broad thumb) syndrome

    (31) Silverman (battered-child) syndrome

    (32) Stickler syndrome (hereditary progressive arthro-ophthalmopathy)

    (33) Treacher-Collins syndrome

    (34) Ullrich syndrome (dyscraniopygophalangy)

    (35) Waardenburg's syndrome

    (36) Wagner syndrome

    (37) Weber-Christian disease

    (38) Weil-Marchesani syndrome

    (39) Zellweger (cerebrohepatorenal) syndrome

*L. Diabetes

M. Epidemic dropsy (argemone oil poisoning)

N. Giant cell arteritis

*O. Graves disease

P. Hemorrhagic fever with renal syndrome (nephropathia epidemica)

*Q. Herpes simplex

*R. Herpes zoster

S. Histiocytosis X

T. Juvenile rheumatoid arthritis (JRA)

U. Juvenile xanthogranuloma

V. Leukemia

W. Lymphoma

X. Medications/Chemicals (see p. 361)

Y. Metastatic carcinoma

Z. Metastatic melanoma

AA. Multiple myeloma

BB. Phakomatoses

    (1) Nevus of Ota (oculodermal melanocytosis)

    (2) Sturge-Weber syndrome (encephalotrigeminal angiomatosis)

    (3) von Hippel-Lindau disease

    (4) von Recklinghausen's neurofibromatosis

CC. Reiter's syndrome

DD. Retinoblastoma

EE. Retrobulbar tumors

FF. Sarcoidosis

GG. Sickling disorders

HH. Superior vena cava (superior mediastinal) syndrome

II. Syphilis

JJ. Systemic corticosteroids

KK. Vogt-Koyanagi-Harada syndrome

* = most important

Duane, T.D. and Jaeger, E.A.: Clinical Ophthalmology. Philadelphia, Harper & Row, 1994.

Epstein, D.L.: Chandler and Grant's Glaucoma. 3rd Ed. Philadelphia, Lea & Febiger, 1986.

Evans, L.S.: Increased intraocular pressure in severely burned patients. Am. J. Ophthalmol., 111:56–58, 1991.

Geeraets, M.J.: Ocular Syndromes, 3rd Ed. Philadelphia, Lea & Febiger, 1976.

Grant, W.M. Toxicology of the Eye. 4th Ed. Springfield, Charles C. Thomas, 1993.

Harley, R.D.: Pediatric Ophthalmology. Philadelphia, W.B. Saunders, 1975.

Hoskins, H.D., et al.: Anatomical Classification of the Developmental Glaucomas. Arch. Ophthalmol., 102:1331–1336, 1984.

Isenberg, S.J.: The Eye in Infancy. Chicago, Year Book Medical Publishers, 1989.

Kushner, B.J., and Sondheimer, S.: Medical treatment of glaucoma associated with cicatricial retinopathy of prematurity. Am. J. Ophthalmol., 94:313–317, 1982.

McKusick, V.A.: Mendelian Inheritance in Man. 11th Ed. Baltimore, The Johns Hopkins University Press, 1994.

Ritch, R., and Shields, M.B.: The Secondary Glaucomas. St. Louis, C.V. Mosby, 1982.

Roy, F.H.: Ocular Syndromes and Systemic Diseases. 2nd Ed. Philadelphia, W.B. Saunders, 1989.

Shields, M.B.: Textbook of Glaucoma. 3rd ed. Baltimore, Williams & Wilkins, 1992.

Glaucoma Suspect, Adult

   1. Advanced age
   *2. Applanation reading 21mm Hg or higher
   3. Asymmetric intraocular pressures
   4. Black race
   5. Contusion angle deformity glaucoma in the fellow eye
   *6. Diabetes mellitus
   7. Diurnal fluctuation in intraocular pressure of 10mm Hg or greater
   8. Endothelial dystrophy of the cornea
   *9. Exfoliative syndrome (see p. 354)
   10. Family history of glaucoma
   *11. Hemorrhage at optic disc margin
   12. High myopia
   13. Intraocular pressure elevation following use of corticosteroids
   14. Krukenberg spindle and/or dense trabecular pigment band (see p. 284)
   *15. Prominent cupping of optic disc
   　　A. Asymmetry of cup/disc ratio
   　　B. Cup/disc ratio > 0.4
   　　C. Cupping to disc margin
   　　D. Vertical elongation of cup
   16. Retinal detachment (see p. 541)
   *17. Retinal vein occlusion (see p. 525)
   18. Schiotz scale reading 4.0/5.5 or 6.25/7.5 or less
   19. Thyrotropic exophthalmos
   *20. Visual field changes suggestive of glaucoma

Duane, T.D., and Jaeger, E.A.: Clinical Ophthalmology. Philadelphia, Harper & Row, 1994.

Epstein, D.L.: Chandler and Grant's Glaucoma. 3rd Ed. Philadelphia, Lea & Febiger, 1986.

Kimuna, R., and Levene, R.Z.: Gonioscopic difference between primary open angle glaucoma and normal subjects over 40 years of age. Am. J. Ophthalmol., 80:56–61, 1975.

Shields, M.B.: Textbook of Glaucoma. 3rd Ed. Baltimore, Williams & Wilkins, 1992.

Elevated Intraocular Pressure Measurement with Normal Appearing Optic Disc

1. Acromegaly
2. Anesthesia
   - A. Ketamine
   - B. Nitrous oxide with intravitreal gas
   - C. Succinylcholine
*3. Blepharospasm
4. Caffeine intake
5. Cardiopulmonary bypass surgery
*6. Dysthyroid ophthalmopathy
7. Elevation in hemoglobin concentration
8. Excessive water intake
9. High scleral rigidity and indentation (e.g. Schiotz) tonometry
10. Horizontal gaze position
11. Hyperthermia
12. Hyperthyroid
13. Marked emotional stress
14. Mechanical factors in checking intraocular pressure (e.g. by patient's hair interfering with applanation tonometer arm)
15. Medications/chemicals
    - *A. Corticosteroids
    - B. Cycloplegics
    - C. Others (see p. 361)
*16. Normal variation (ocular hypertension)
*17. Preglaucoma (intraocular pressure sufficiently elevated to cause damage to the optic nerve, but damage not yet visible ophthalmoscopically)
18. Reduced gravity
19. Tight collar, short neck, obesity
20. Tobacco smoking
*21. Tonometer in need of calibration
22. Valsalva's maneuver
23. Voluntary widening of palpebral fissure

Grant, W.M.: Toxicology of the Eye. 4th Ed. Springfield, Charles C. Thomas, 1993.

Munoz, M., and Capo, H.: Differential intraocular pressure in restrictive strabismus. Am. J. Ophthalmol., 112:352–353, 1991.

Ritch, R., and Reyes, A.: Moustache glaucoma. Arch. Ophthalmol., 106:1503, 1988.

Shields, M.B.: Textbook of Glaucoma. Baltimore, Williams & Wilkins, 1992.

* = most important

Secondary Open-Angle Glaucoma

1. Corneal endothelial disorders
    A. Fuchs' endothelial dystrophy
    B. Posterior polymorphous dystrophy
2. Elevated episcleral venous pressure (see p. 358)
3. Iris disorders
    A. Iridoschisis
    *B. Pigmentary glaucoma
4. Lens disorders
    A. Cataract
        (1) Lens particle glaucoma
        (2) Phacoanaphylaxis
        (3) Phacolytic (lens protein) glaucoma
    B. Displaced lens (see p. 449)
    *C. Exfoliation syndrome
5. Medications/chemicals
    *A. Corticosteroids
    B. Cycloplegic effect
    C. Others (p. 361)
6. Ocular hemorrhage (see p. 374)
7. Ocular inflammation (see p. 426)
8. Ocular surgery
    A. Alpha-chymotrypsin (enzyme glaucoma)
    *B. Corticosteroid induced
    C. Distortion of anterior chamber angle from limbal or keratoplasty sutures
    D. Early postoperative elevation of IOP following cataract surgery (especially in eyes with preexisting glaucoma)
    E. Hemorrhage
        (1) Degenerated ocular blood
            a. Ghost cell glaucoma
            b. Hemolytic glaucoma
            c. Hemosideric glaucoma
        *(2) Hyphema
        (3) Internal wound neovascularization (late postoperative hyphema)
        (4) Pseudophakia
            a. Anterior chamber IOL (including UGH syndrome)
            b. Iris-fixated IOL
            c. Posterior chamber IOL (usually sulcus fixation)
        (5) Retrobulbar hemorrhage (massive)
    F. Inflammation
    G. Intravitreal gas

      H. Neodymium: YAG laser capsulotomy

      I. Pseudophakic pigmentary dispersion (e.g. with posterior chamber implant)

      J. Retained lens cortex

    *K. Retained viscoelastic

      L. Silicone oil

      M. Sudden closure of cyclodialysis cleft

      N. Vitreous filling anterior chamber

9. Ocular trauma

      A. Chemical burns (acid, alkali, other)

      B. Contusion

          (1) Angle recession

        *(2) Hyphema

          (3) Iritis

          (4) Trabecular damage

      C. Radiation damage

      D. Retained intraocular foreign body (iron, copper)

      E. Retrobulbar hemorrhage (massive)

10. Ocular tumors (see p. 560 and 563)

11. Retinal, vitreous and choroidal disorders

    *A. Neovascular glaucoma-open angle stage (see p. 366)

      B. Retinitis pigmentosa

      C. Rhegmatogenous retinal detachment (Schwartz syndrome)

Duane, T.D., and Jaeger, E.A.: Clinical Ophthalmology. Philadelphia, Harper & Row, 1994.

Epstein, D.L.: Chandler and Grant's Glaucoma. 3rd Ed. Philadephia, Lea & Febiger, 1986.

Grant, W.M.: Toxicology of the Eye. 4th Ed. Springfield, Charles C. Thomas, 1993.

Ritch, R., and Shields, M.B.: The Secondary Glaucomas. St. Louis, C.V. Mosby, 1982.

Roy, F.H.: Ocular Syndromes and Systemic Diseases. 2nd Ed. Philadelphia, W.B. Saunders, 1989.

Steinert, R.F., et al.: Cystoid macular edema, retinal detachment, and glaucoma after Nd: YAG laser posterior capsulotomy. Am. J. Ophthalmol., 112:373–380, 1991.

Unilateral Glaucoma

1. Corneal endothelial disorders

      A. Fuchs' endothelial dystrophy with angle closure due to thickened peripheral cornea

      B. Iridocorneal endothelial (ICE) syndrome

          (1) Chandler's syndrome

          (2) Iris-nevus (Cogan-Reese) syndrome

          (3) Progressive iris atrophy

2. Elevated episcleral venous pressure (see p. 358)

3. Lens disorders

      A. Cataract

* = most important

      (1) Lens particle glaucoma

      (2) Phacoanaphylaxis

      (3) Phacolytic (lens protein) glaucoma

      (4) Phacomorphic (intumescent lens) glaucoma

  B. Displacement of the lens

      (1) Buphthalmos

      (2) Cataract (mature or hypermature)

      (3) Exfoliation syndrome

      (4) Intraocular tumor

      (5) Persistent hyperplastic primary vitreous (PHPV)

      (6) Sturge-Weber syndrome (encephalotrigeminal angiomatosis)

      (7) Trauma

      (8) Uveitis

 *C. Exfoliation syndrome (see p. 354)

4. Medications/chemicals

  A. Alpha chymotrypsin (enzyme glaucoma)

  B. Chemical burns (see p. 361)

 *C. Corticosteroids (topical or periocular)

  D. Cycloplegics (angle closure or open angle)

  E. Nitrous oxide inhalation with intraocular gas

  F. Urokinase (intraocular)

  G. Others (see p. 361)

5. Ocular hemorrhage (see p. 374)

6. Ocular inflammation (see p. 426)

*7. Ocular surgery (see p. 354)

8. Ocular trauma (see p. 355)

9. Ocular tumors (see p. 560 and 563)

10. Retinal, vitreous, and choroidal disorders

  A. Angle closure

      (1) Acute choroidal hemorrhage

    *(2) Central retinal vein occlusion (CRVO)

      (3) Ciliochoroidal effusion

        a. Arteriovenous malformations

        b. Inflammatory conditions

        c. Nanophthalmos

        d. Surgery

        e. Trauma

        f. Tumors

        g. Uveal effusion syndrome

      (4) Hemorrhagic retinal and choroidal detachment

      (5) Persistent hyperplastic primary vitreous (PHPV)

    *(6) Postoperative panretinal photocoagulation

    (7) Postoperative scleral buckle

    (8) Retinal dysplasia

    (9) Retinopathy of prematurity (Retrolental fibroplasia)

*B. Neovascular glaucoma (see p. 366)

    *(1) Diabetic retinopathy

    (2) Extraocular vascular disorders

        a. Carotid-cavernous fistula

        b. Carotid occlusive disease

        c. Giant cell arteritis

    (3) Ocular disorders-miscellaneous

        *a. Chronic glaucoma

        b. Endophthalmitis

        c. Intraocular malignancy

        d. Iris melanoma

        e. Persistent hyperplastic primary vitreous (PHPV)

        f. Photoradiation or helium ion irradiation for uveal melanoma

        g. Pseudophakia

        h. Sympathetic ophthalmia

        *i. Uveitis (chronic)

    (4) Retinal disorders-miscellaneous

        a. Coats' disease

        b. Eales' disease

        c. Optic nerve glioma with venous stasis

        d. Retinal detachment (usually chronic)

        e. Retinal vascular occlusive disorders

          1. retinal artery occlusion central or branch

         *2. retinal vein occlusion central or branch

        f. Retinoblastoma

        g. Retinopathy of prematurity (Retrolental fibroplasia)

        h. Retinoschisis

        i. Sickle cell retinopathy

C. Open angle glaucoma associated with rhegmatogenous retinal detachment (Schwartz syndrome)

Duane,T.D., and Jaeger, E.A.: Clinical Ophthalmology. Philadelphia, Harper & Row, 1994.

Epstein, D.L.: Chandler and Grant's Glaucoma. 3rd Ed. Philadelphia, Lea & Febiger, 1986.

Hoskins, H.D., and Kass, M.A.: Becker-Shaffer's Diagnosis and Therapy of Glaucoma. 5th Ed. St. Louis, C.V. Mosby, 1983.

Ritch, R., and Shields, M.B.: The Secondary Glaucomas. St. Louis, C.V. Mosby, 1982.

Roy, F.H.: Ocular Syndromes and Systemic Diseases. 2nd Ed. Philadelphia, W.B. Saunders, 1989.

Shields, M.B.: Textbook of Glaucoma. 3rd Ed. Baltimore, Williams & Wilkins, 1992.

* = most important

Glaucoma Associated with Displaced Lens

1. Alport's syndrome
2. Aniridia
3. Axenfeld-Rieger syndrome
4. Buphthalmos
*5. Cataract (mature or hypermature)
6. Cornea plana
7. Crouzon's disease (craniofacial dysostosis)
8. Ectopia lentis et pupillae
9. Ehlers-Danlos syndrome
*10. Exfoliation syndrome (see p. 354)
11. High myopia
12. Homocystinuria
13. Hyperlysinemia
14. Intraocular tumor
15. Isolated microspherophakia
16. Klinefelter's syndrome
17. Lowe's (oculocerebrorenal) syndrome
*18. Marfan's syndrome
19. Megalocornea
20. Oculo-dental syndrome
21. Refsum's syndrome
22. Retinitis pigmentosa
23. Scleroderma
24. Simple ectopia lentis
25. Stickler's syndrome
26. Sturge-Weber syndrome (encephalotrigeminal angiomatosis)
27. Sulfite oxidase deficiency
28. Syphilis
*29. Trauma
30. Treacher-Collins syndrome(mandibulofacial dysostosis)
31. Uveitis
32. Weill-Marchesani syndrome

Duane, T.D. and Jaeger, E.A.: Clinical Ophthalmology. Philadelphia, Harper & Row, 1994.

Epstein, D.L.: Chandler and Grant's Glaucoma. 3rd Ed. Philadelphia, Lea & Febiger, 1986.

Geeraets, M.J.: Ocular Syndromes. 3rd Ed. Philadelphia, Lea & Febiger, 1976.

Harley, R.D.: Pediatric Ophthalmology. Philadelphia, W.B. Saunders, 1975.

Portney, G.: Glaucoma Guidebook. Philadelphia, Lea & Febiger, 1977.

Shields, M.B.: Texbook of Glaucoma. 3rd Ed. Baltimore, Williams & Wilkins, 1992.

Glaucoma and Elevated Episcleral Venous Pressure

1. Arteriovenous fistulas
   A. Carotid-cavernous sinus fistulas

         (1) Spontaneous

         (2) Traumatic

     B. Orbital-meningeal shunts

     C. Orbital varices

   *D. Sturge-Weber syndrome (encephalotrigeminal angiomatosis)

2. Idiopathic elevation of episcleral venous pressure

   *A. Familial

    B. Sporadic

3. Venous obstruction

    A. Cavernous sinus thrombosis

   *B. Congestive heart failure

    C. Episcleral

         (1) Chemical burns (acid, alkali, others)

         (2) Radiation

    D. Jugular venous obstruction

    E. Orbital

       *(1) Dysthyroid

        (2) Orbital vein thrombosis

        (3) Phlebitis

        (4) Pseudotumor

        (5) Retrobulbar tumor

    F. Pulmonary venous obstruction

    G. Superior vena cava (superior mediastinal) syndrome

Duane, T.D., and Jaeger, E.A.: Clinical Ophthalmology. Philadelphia, Harper & Row, 1994.

Shields, M.B.: Textbook of Glaucoma. 3rd Ed. Baltimore, Williams & Wilkins, 1992.

Weinreb, R.N., et. al.: Glaucoma Secondary to Elevated Episcleral Venous Pressure. In: Ritch, R., et al.: The Glaucomas. St. Louis, C.V. Mosby, 1989.

Glaucoma Associated with Shallow Anterior Chamber

  *1. Primary angle closure

    A. Plateau iris syndrome

   *B. Relative pupillary block (most common)

2. Secondary angle closure

   *A. Central retinal vein occlusion (CRVO)

    B. Choroidal hemorrhage (acute)

    C. Ciliochoroidal effusion

        (1) Acquired immunodeficiency syndrome (AIDS)

        (2) Arteriovenous malformations

      *(3) Inflammation

        (4) Nanophthalmos

        (5) Trauma

* = most important

      (6) Tumor

      (7) Uveal effusion syndrome

  D. Cystinosis

  E. Drug-induced acute transitory myopia (diuretics, sulfonamides, others)

  F. Elevated episcleral venous pressure associated with arteriovenous fistula

  G. Fuchs' endothelial dystrophy- with peripheral corneal thickening

  H. Hemorrhagic retinal and choroidal detachment

   I. Hyperglycemia (acute)

  J. Inflammation

      (1) Episcleritis

      (2) Iridocyclitis with posterior synechiae and iris bombe

      (3) Posterior scleritis

  K. Intraocular tumor (posterior segment melanoma, metastatic carcinoma, retinoblastoma, medulloepithelioma, etc)

  L. Lens dislocation (see p. 449)

  M. Luetic interstitial keratitis

  N. Malignant (ciliary block) glaucoma

  O. Marotoux-Lamy syndrome (MPS VI)

  P. Multiple cysts of the iris and ciliary body

  Q. Nanophthalmos

  R. Persistent hyperplastic primary vitreous (PHPV)

*S. Phakic or aphakic pupillary block

  T. Phakomorphic (intumescent lens) glaucoma

  U. Postoperative panretinal photocoagulation

  V. Postoperative scleral buckle

  W. Retinal dysplasia

  X. Retinopathy of prematurity (Retrolental fibroplasia)

Duane, T.D., and Jaeger, E.A.: Clinical Ophthalmology. Philadelphia, Harper & Row, 1994.

Epstein, D.L.: Chandler and Grant's Glaucoma. 3rd Ed. Philadelphia, Lea & Febiger, 1986.

Fraunfelder, F.T., and Roy, F.H.: Current Ocular Therapy. 4th Ed. Philadelphia, W.B. Saunders. 1995.

Grant, W.M.: Toxicology of the Eye. 4th Ed. Springfield, Charles C. Thomas, 1993.

Shields, M.B.: Textbook of Glaucoma. 3rd Ed. Baltimore, Williams & Wilkins, 1992.

Glaucoma in Aphakia or Pseudophakia

  1. Alpha-chymotrypsin (enzyme glaucoma)

  2. Ciliary block (malignant) glaucoma

*3. Corticosteroid induced

  4. Degenerated intraocular blood

    A. Ghost cell glaucoma

    B. Hemolytic glaucoma

    C. Hemosideric glaucoma

5. Distortion of the anterior chamber angle by limbal sutures

*6. Early postoperative pressure elevation (especially in eyes with pre-existing glaucoma)

7. Epithelial downgrowth

8. Fibrous proliferation

*9. Following Neodymium: YAG capsulotomy

10. Hyphema

    A. Internal wound neovascularization (late postoperative hyphema)

    B. Pseudophakia

        (1) Anterior chamber IOL (including the UGH syndrome)

        (2) Iris-fixated IOL

        (3) Posterior chamber IOL (usually sulcus fixation)

11. Inflammation

12. Peripheral anterior synechiae

13. Primary open angle glaucoma

14. Pseudophakic pigmentary dispersion

*15. Pupillary block

*16. Retained lens cortex

*17. Retained viscoelastic

18. Vitreous filling the anterior chamber

19. Vitreous hemorrhage (massive)

Duane, T.D., and Jaeger, E.A.: Clinical Ophthalmology. Philadelphia, Harper & Row, 1994.

Epstein, D.L.: Chandler and Grant's Glaucoma. 3rd Ed. Philadelphia, Lea & Febiger, 1986.

Hoskins, H.D., and Kass, M.A.: Becker-Shaffer's Diagnosis and Therapy of Glaucoma. 6th Ed. St. Louis, C.V. Mosby, 1989.

Shields, M.B.: Textbook of Glaucoma. 3rd Ed. Baltimore, Williams & Wilkins, 1992.

Tessler, D.R., et al.: Persistently raised intraocular pressure following extracapsular cataract extraction. Brit. J. Ophthal. 74: 272–274, 1990.

Medications and Chemicals that May Cause Elevated Intraocular Pressure

1. Anesthetic agents

    A. Ketamine

    B. Nitrous oxide (inhalation, especially in eyes with retinovitreal surgery and intraocular gas)

2. Anticholinergics/Parasympatholytics

    A. Antidepressants[†]

        (1) Amitriptyline (Elavil)

        (2) Imipramine (Tofranil)

        (3) Nortriptyline (Pamelor)

        (4) Protriptyline (Vivactil)

        (5) Trimipramine (Surmontil)

* = most important

B. Antihistamines
  (1) Anazoline (Vasocon-A)
  (2) Bromphenirimine (Dimetane)
  (3) Cyclizine (Marezine)
  (4) Cyproheptadine (Periactin)
  (5) Diphenhydramine (Benadryl)
  (6) Orphenadrine (Norgesic)
  (7) Tripelennamine (Pyribenzamine)

C. Antiparkinson medications[†]
  (1) Biperiden (Akineton)
  (2) Cycrimine (Pagitane)
  (3) Trihexyphenidyl hydrochloride (Artane)

D. Antispasmolytic agents
  (1) Dicyclomine (Bentyl)
  (2) Diphemanil methylsulfate (Prantal)
  (3) Hexocyclium methylsulfate (Tral)
  (4) Hyoscyamine (Donnatal, Donnagel)
  (5) Mepenzolate (Cantil)
  (6) Methscopolomine bromide (Pamine)
  (7) Oxyphenonium bromide (Antrenyl)
  (8) Propantheline bromide (Pro-banthine)
  (9) Tridihexethyl chloride (Pathilon)

*E. Cycloplegics
  (1) Atropine
  (2) Cyclopentolate (Cyclogyl)
  (3) Homatropine
  (4) Tropicamide (Mydriacil)
  (5) Scopolamine (Hyoscine)

F. Miscellaneous
  (1) Atropine (systemic)
  (2) Glycopyrrolate (Robinul)

G. Phenothiazines[†]
  (1) Doxepin (Sinequan)
  (2) Haloperidol (Haldol)
  (3) Prochlorperazine (Compazine)
  (4) Promethazine (Phenergan)
  (5) Triflupromazine (Vesprin)

H. Poisoning
  (1) Belladonna
  (2) Jimson weed

3. Argemone oil (epidemic dropsy)

4. Caffeine

5. Carbon dioxide inhalation

6. Carmustine injection

7. Chemical burns

    A. Acid

        (1) Chromic acid

        (2) Hydrochloric (muriatic) acid

        (3) Sulfuric (battery) acid

    B. Alkali

        (1) Ammonium hydroxide (ammonia)

        (2) Calcium hydroxide (lime)

        (3) Sodium hydroxide (lye)

    C. Dibenz [b.f][1,4] oxazepine (CR tear gas)

    D. Formaldehyde gas (in aqueous solution = formalin)

8. CSN Stimulants/anorexics

    A. Dextroamphetamine

    B. Methamphetamine

    C. Phenmetrazine (Preludin)

    D. Phenteramine (Ionamin)

*9. Corticosteroids

    *A. Ocular (topical)

        (1) Dexamethasone (Decadron, Maxidex)

        (2) Fluorometholone (FML, Flarex)

        (3) Prednisolone acetate (Pred Forte)

        (4) Prednisolone sodium phosphate (Inflamase)

    *B. Subconjuctival depot injection

        (1) Methylprednisolone acetate

        (2) Triamcinolone

    C. Systemic

        (1) Betamethasone (Celestone)

        (2) Cortisone acetate

        (3) Dexamethasone (Decadron)

        (4) Hydrocortisone (Cortef, Solu-Cortef)

        (5) Methylprednisolone (Medrol)

        (6) Paramethasone (Haldrone)

        (7) Prednisolone

        (8) Prednisone (Deltasone)

        (9) Triamcinolone (Aristocort)

10. Idiopathic lens swelling

* = most important

    A. Acetylisalicylic acid (Aspirin)

    B. Sulfanilamide

    C. Others

11. Intraocular injection

    A. Alpha-chymotrypsin (enzyme glaucoma)

    B. Urokinase

    *C. Viscoelastic (Healon, others)

12. Methylphenidate (Ritalin)

13. Miotics

    A. Carbachol

    B. Demecarium (Humorsol)

    C. Echothiophate (Phospholine iodide)

    D. Pilocarpine

14. Succinylcholine (Anectine)

15. Sympathomimetics

    A. Ephedrine

    B. Mydriatics

        (1) Dipivalyl epinephrine (Propine)

        (2) Epinephrine (many products)

        (3) Hydroxyamphetamine (Paredrine)

        (4) Phenylephrine (Neosynephrine)

    C. Naphazoline (Naphcon)

    D. Pheniramine maleate (Naphcon-A)

    E. Phenylephrine (Neosynephrine)

    F. Tetrahydrozoline (Visine)

16. Testosterone

17. Vasodilators

    A. Elevation of IOP following subconjunctival injection

        (1) Bamethan (Bupatol)

        (2) Isoxsuprine (Vasodilan)

        (3) Tolazoline (Priscoline)

        (4) Triaziquone (Trenimon)

    B. Amyl nitrite (Vaporole)

18. Water (excessive intake)

† = May be potentiated by monoamine oxidase inhibitors such as phenelzine, pargyline, or tranyl-
    cypromine.

Duane, T.D., and Jaeger, E.A.: *Clinical Ophthalmology*. Philadelphia, Harper & Row, 1994.

Grant, W.M.: *Toxicology of the Eye*. 4th Ed. Springfield, Charles C. Thomas, 1993.

Shields, M.B.: *Textbook of Glaucoma*. 3rd Ed. Baltimore, Williams & Wilkins, 1992.

Primary Low Tension Glaucoma

1. Non-glaucomatous optic nerve disorders resembling glaucomatous damage
    - A. Developmental abnormalities
        - (1) Colobomas of the optic nerve head including optic pits
        - *(2) Large physiologic cups
        - (3) Tilted discs
    - B. Non-glaucomatous causes of acquired cupping
        - (1) Compressive lesions
            - a. Aneurysm
            - b. Chiasmic arachnoiditis
            - c. Cyst
            - d. Tumor
        - *(2) Ischemic optic neuropathy (especially arteritic)
    - *C. Non-glaucomatous causes of nerve fiber bundle defects on visual field testing
        - (1) Chorioretinal lesions
            - a. Chorioretinitis
            - b. Retinal vascular occlusions
            - c. Tumors
        - (2) Optic nerve head lesions
            - a. Colobomas
            - b. Drusen
            - c. Other
        - (3) Posterior lesion of the visual pathway
            - a. Meningioma
            - b. Pituitary tumor
            - c. Pseudotumor
            - d. Other
2. Undetected high-pressure glaucoma
    - A. Corneal edema giving false low measurement of IOP with applanation (e.g. Goldman or Perkins) tonometry
    - B. Intermittent elevation of IOP causing damage (IOP normal at time of exam)
        - (1) Glaucomatocyclitic crisis (Posner-Schlossman syndrome)
        - (2) Intermittent angle closure
        - (3) Other
    - C. Low scleral rigidity giving false low measurement of IOP with indentation (e.g. Schiotz) tonometry
    - *D. Prior elevation in pressure resulting in optic nerve damage
        - (1) 'Burned out' open angle glaucoma
        - (2) Corticosteroids
        - (3) Pigmentary glaucoma

* = most important

        (4) Trauma

        (5) Uveitis

    E. Wide diurnal variation (multiple measurements at different times of day required to rule-out high-pressure glaucoma)

Duane, T.D., and Jaeger, E.A.: Clinical Ophthalmology. Philadelphia, Harper & Row, 1994.

Shields, M.B.: Textbook of Glaucoma. 3rd Ed. Baltimore, Williams & Wilkins, 1992.

Werner, E.B.: Low-tension Glaucoma. In Ritch, R.,et. al.: The Glaucomas. St. Louis, C.V.Mosby, 1989.

Neovascular Glaucoma

*1. Diabetic retinopathy

  2. Extraocular vascular disorders

    A. Aortic arch syndrome

    *B. Carotid artery occlusive disease

    C. Carotid-cavernous fistula

    D. Giant cell arteritis

  3. Ocular disorders-miscellaneous

    A. Chronic glaucoma

    B. Endophthalmitis

    C. Iris melanoma

    D. Persistent hyperplastic primary vitreous (PHPV)

    E. Pseudophakia

    F. Sympathetic ophthalmia

    *G. Uveitis

  4. Retinal disorders-miscellaneous

    A. Choroidal melanoma

    B. Coats' exudative retinopathy

    C. Eales'disease

    D. Metastatic carcinoma

    E. Norrie's disease

    F. Optic nerve glioma with subsequent venous stasis retinopathy

    G. Photoradiation or helium ion irradiation for uveal melanoma

    *H. Retinal detachment (usually chronic)

    I. Retinal vascular occlusive disorders

        (1) Branch retinal artery occlusion.

        *(2) Branch retinal vein occlusion

        *(3) Central retinal artery occlusion

        *(4) Central retinal vein occlusion

    J. Retinoblastoma

    K. Retinopathy of prematurity (Retrolental fibroplasia)

    L. Retinoschisis

    M. Sickle cell retinopathy

N. Stickler's syndrome (inherited vitreoretinal degeneration)

O. Syphilitic retinal vasculitis

Duane, T.D., and Jaeger, E.A.: Clinical Ophthalmology. Philadelphia, Harper & Row, 1994.

Shields, M.B.: Textbook of Glaucoma. 3rd Ed. Baltimore, Williams & Wilkins, 1992.

Hypotony

*1. Essential hypotension

2. Secondary hypotony

   A. Cartilaginous -arthritic-ophthalmic deafness

   B. Ciliochoroidal detachment

      (1) Chorioretinal inflammation

      (2) Ocular neoplasm

      *(3) Trauma including ocular surgery

   *C. Cyclitis

   *D. Cyclodialysis

   E. Decreased intraocular pressure from medications and chemicals

      (1) Alcuronium

      (2) Aminophylline (intravenous)

      *(3) Carbonic anhydrase inhibitors (e.g. acetazolamide, methazolamide, ethoxzo-lamide)

      (4) Cardiac glycosides (digitoxin, digoxin, lanatoside-C, ouabain)

      (5) Dibenamine

      (6) Dihydroergotoxine (Hydergine)

      *(7) Hyperosmotics (urea, glycerin, mannitol, ascorbic acid, glycerol, ethanol, trometa-mol)

      (8) Isosorbide

      (9) Pargyline (Eutonyl)

      (10) Phentolamine (Regitine)

      (11) Propranolol (Inderal)

      (12) Thiopental (Pentothal)

   *F. Deep anesthesia

   G. Deep coma and severe cerebral disease

   *H. Dehydration-severe (e.g., cholera, dysentery, diabetic coma, etc)

   *I. Diabetic coma

   *J. Glaucoma medications (beta blockers, sympathomimetics, miotics, carbonic anhydrase inhibitors)

   K. Hilding syndrome

   L. Horner syndrome

   M. Hyperosmolarity

   N. Intestinal perforation or obstruction

* = most important

   O. Irradiation

   P. Morquio-Brailsford syndrome (MPS IV)

   Q. Myotonic dystrophy

*R. Ocular trauma with or without visible ciliary body injury

*S. Perforating ocular trauma

*T. Phthisis

   U. Post-encephalitic syndrome

*V. Postoperative surgical procedures especially for glaucoma

   W. Raeder syndrome

*X. Retinal detachment

*Y. Systemic hypotension-severe (circulatory collapse, medications)

   Z. Uremic coma

*AA. Wound leak

Fraunfelder, F.T.: Drug-Induced Ocular Side Effects and Drug Interactions. Philadelphia, Williams & Wilkins, 1996.

Grant, W.M.: Toxicology of the Eye 4th Ed. Springfield, Charles C. Thomas, 1993.

Roy, F.H.: Ocular Syndromes and Systemic Diseases. 2nd Ed. Philadelphia. W. B. Saunders, 1989.

Shields, M.B.: Textbook of Glaucoma. 3rd Ed. Baltimore, Williams & Wilkins, 1992.

Anterior Chamber

CHRISTOPHER J RAPUANO, M.D.

Contents

Hypopyon (Pus in Anterior Chamber)

1. Hypopyon ulcer— corneal ulcer with pus in the anterior chamber
   A. Acanthamoeba
   B. Acquired Immunodeficiency Syndrome (AIDS)
   C. Aspergillus
   D. Candida albicans

E. Chemical injury
F. Diplococcus pneumoniae
G. Escherichia coli
H. Fusariam
I. Herpes simplex
J. Herpes zoster
K. Measles
L. Moraxella
M. Neisseria gonorrhoeae
N. Proteus vulgaris
*O. Pseudomonas aeruginosa
P. Serratia
Q. Smallpox
R. Spitting cobra venom
S. Staphyloccus
*T. Streptococcus

2. Severe acute iridocyclitis
3. Necrosis of intraocular tumors or metastasis
4. Retained intraocular foreign bodies, including toxic lens syndrome
5. Endophthalmitis—at time of surgical treatment, accidental trauma, drug users or spontaneous (see p. 257)

A. Acanthamoebae
B. Actinomycosis
C. Amebiasis
D. Aspergillosis
E. Bacterial including bacillus cereus
F. Behçet syndrome
G. Candida albicans
H. Coccidioidomycosis
I. Coenurosis
J. Cysticercosis
K. Fusavium
L. Hydatid cyst
M. Influenza
N. Listeria monocytogenes
O. Lockjaw (Clostridium tetani)
P. Metastatic bacterial endophthalmitis
Q. Moraxella
R. Mucor species
S. Mycobacterium avium

*T. Pseudomonas

U. Relapsing fever

V. Serratia marcescens

W. Saprophytic fungi

*X. Staphylococcus

*Y. Streptoccus

Z. Sterile hypopyon

    (1) Behçet syndrome (oculobuccogenital syndrome)

    (2) Endotoxin contamination of ultrasonic bath

    (3) Following cyanoacrylate sealing of a corneal perforation

    (4) Following refractive surgery

    (5) Histiocytosis X (Hand-Schüller-Christian syndrome)

    (6) Intraocular lens or instrument polishing compounds or sterilization techniques

    *(7) Juvenile rheumatoid arthritis

    (8) Laser iridotomy

    (9) Leukemia

    *(10) Reaction to lens protein

    (11) Rough intraocular lens edges

    (12) von Bechterev-Strumpel syndrome (rheumatoid spondylitis)

AA. Stevens-Johnson syndrome (dermatostomatitis)

BB. Tight contact lens or contact lens overwear syndrome

CC. Tuberculosis

DD. Weil disease (leptospirosis)

EE. Yersiniosis

6. Drugs, including:

benoxinate	ferrous sulfate
butacaine	iodide and iodine solutions and compounds
cocaine	iron dextran
colchicine(?)	iron sorbitex
dibucaine	phenacaine
dyclonine	piperocaine
ferrocholinate	polysaccharide-iron complex
ferrous fumarate	proparacaine
ferrous gluconate	radioactive iodides
ferrous succinate	tetracaine urokinase

Spontaneous Hyphema

	Systemic Hypertension	Intraocular Neoplasm Melanos	Diseases of Blood Leukemia	Severe Iritis Herpes Zoster	Rubeosis Iridis	Fibrovascular Membrane in Areas Retinopathy of Prematurity	Juvenile Xanthogranuloma
History							
1. Acute or chronic blood disorder			S				
2. Premature Infants						U	
3. History varicella-zoster virus				U			
4. Carotid artery insufficiency					S		
5. Central retinal artery or vein occlusion					S		
6. Childhood disease							U
7. Diabetic retinopathy					S		
8. Elevated blood pressure	U						
9. Oxygen in excess in closed incubators						U	
10. Rare in children		U					
11. Rare in non-caucasians		U					
Physical Findings							
1. Anterior chamber depth variations		S					
2. Arteriosclerosis	U						
3. Cataract				S		S	
4. Conjunctivitis				U			
5. Corneal, lid and epibulbar tumor							S
6. Cotton wool spots	U		U				
7. Chronic uveitis		S		S	R		S
8. Decreased visual acuity		S				S	
9. "Dragged disc" appearance						U	
10. Ectropion uvea							
11. Engorgement of conjunctival vessels				U			
12. Fatty exudates	U						
13. Fibrovascular membrane on anterior iris and chamber angle						U	
14. Freckles on iris		U					
15. Glaucoma	R	S	S	S	S	S	S
16. Heterochromia of iris		S		R	R	S	
17. Hyptony		S	S				
18. Hypopyon				S	R		
19. Iris atrophy				S			
20. Keratitis				U			
21. Macular edema				S			
22. Neuralgia				U			
23. Orbital apex syndrome				S			
24. Optic atrophy				S		S	
25. Optic disc edema	S			S			
26. Optic neuritis				S	U		
27. Papillary conjunctival hypertrophy				S			
28. Paralysis of intraocular muscles	S			S	S		
29. Pigmentary retinal changes						S	
30. Pigmented mass on iris							
31. Peripheral anterior synechiae				R	U		
32. Prominent episcleral vessels		U					

Spontaneous Hyphema *Continued*

	Systemic Hypertension	Intraocular Neoplasm Melanos	Diseases of Blood Leukemia	Severe Iritis Herpes Zoster	Rubeosis Iridis	Fibrovascular Membrane in Areas Retinopathy of Prematurity	Juvenile Xanthogranuloma
Physical Findings							
33. Proptosis							R
34. Pupillary distortion		U		R			S
35. Recurrent corneal ulcer							
36. Retinal artery narrowing	U					U	
37. Retinal detachment			S				
38. Retinal edema	S						
39. Retinal hemorrhages	U		U			S	
40. Retinal neovascularization						U	
41. Retinal venous engorgement and tortuosity			U			S	
42. Retrolental mass						U	
43. Scleritis				S			
44. Uveal tract tumor		S					S
45. Vitreous hemorrhage	S		S		S	S	
46. Vitreous traction						U	
49. Zoster rash of eyelids				S			

R = rarely; S = sometimes; U = usually

7. Vitreous "fluff-ball"

8. Following refractive surgery

9. Pseudo-hypopyon

    A. Ghost-cell glaucoma with khaki-colored cells

    B. Accidental intraocular steroid injection

10. Acute angle-closure glaucoma

11. Non-Hodgkin lymphoma

12. Pars plana vitrectomy and silicone oil injection

Au Eong, K.G., et al.: Hypopyon-an unusual sign in acute angle-closure glaucoma. International Ophthal. 17:127–129, 1991.

Fraunfelder, F.T.: Drug-Induced Ocular Side Effects and Drug Interactions. 4th Ed. Philadelphia, Williams & Wilkins, 1996.

Elliott, D., et al.: Elevated intraocular pressure, pigment dispersion and dark hypopyon in endogenous endophthalmitis from Listeria monocytogenes. Survey of Ophthalmol. 37: 117–124, 1992.

Hansen, E.A., et al.: Spitting Cobra Ophthalmia in United Nations Forces in Somalia. Amer J Ophthal 117: 671–672, 1994.

Johnson, R.N., et al.: Transient hypopyon with marked anterior chamber fibrin following pars plana vitrectomy and silicone oil injection. Arch Ophthalmol., 107:683–686, 1989.

Pau, H.: Differential Diagnosis of Eye Diseases. 2nd Ed. New York, Thieme Med. Pub., 1988.

Roy, F.H.: Ocular Syndromes and Systemic Diseases. 2nd Ed. Philadelphia, W.B. Saunders, 1989.

Saran, B.R. et al.: Hypopyon Uveitis in Patients with Acquired Immunodeficiency Syndrome treated for Systemic Mycobacterium avium Complex Infection with Rifabutin. Arch Ophthalmol. 112;1159–1161, 1994.

Hyphema (Bleeding into the Anterior Chamber)

1. Trauma

    A. Following laser iridectomy or strabismus surgery in aphakia

    B. Honan balloon use in Fuchs' heterochromic iridocyclitis

    *C. Tear of ciliary body—post contusion deformity of anterior chamber

    *D. To ciliary body, such as cyclodialysis

    E. To iris, such as iridodialysis or intraocular lens irritation

    F. After air bag inflation

2. Overdistention of vessels

    A. Obstruction of central retinal vein

    B. Sudden lowering of high intraocular pressure

3. Fragility of vessel walls

    A. Acute gonorrheal iridocyclitis

    B. Acute herpes iridocyclitis

    C. Acute rheumatoid iridocyclitis

    D. Ankylosing spondylitis

4. Blood abnormality

    A. Anemias

    B. Association with use of aspirin

C. Hemophilia

D. Leukemia

E. Purpura

5. Metabolic disease

A. Diabetes mellitus (Willis disease)

B. Scurvy (avitaminosis C)

6. Neovascularization of iris (see rubeosis iridis, p. 412)

7. Vascularized tumors of iris (see pigmented and nonpigmented iris lesions, pp. and 419)

A. Angioma

*B. Juvenile xanthogranuloma (JXG)

C. Lymphosarcoma

D. Retinoblastoma

8. Wound vascularization following cataract extraction

9. Persistent pupillary membrane hemorrhage

Feldman, S.T., and Deutsch, T.A.: Hyphema following Honan balloon use in Fuchs' heterochromic iridocyclitis. Arch. Ophthalmol., 104:967, 1986.

Geisse, L.J.: Nd:YAG laser treatment for recurrent hyphemas in pseudophakia. Am J Ophthalmol., 111:513, 1991.

Gottsch, J.D.: Hyphema: diagnosis and management. Retina. 10: 65–72, 1990.

Keszel, V.A., and Helveston, E.M.: Hyphema as a complication of strabismus surgery in an aphakic eye. Arch Ophthalmol., 104:637–638, 1986.

Klemperer, I., et al.: Spontaneous hyphema; an unusual complication of uveitis associated with ankylosing spondylitis. Annals of Ophthal. 24:177–179, 1992.

Moster, M.R., et al.: Laser iridectomy. Ophthalmology, 93:20–24, 1986.

Lesher, M.P., et al.: Corneal edema, hyphema, and angle recession after air bag inflation. Arch Ophthal. 111: 1320–1322, 1993.

Roy, F.H.: Ocular Syndromes and Systemic Diseases. 2nd Ed. Philadelphia, W.B. Saunders, 1989.

Spontaneous Hyphema

1. Delayed following glaucoma surgery

2. Diseases of blood or blood vessels

A. Hemophilia

B. Leukemia

C. Malignant lymphoma

D. Purpura

E. Scurvy

3. Fibrovascular membranes in retrolenticular or zonular area

A. Persistent primary vitreous

B. Retinoschisis

C. Retinopathy of prematurity

4. Systemic hypertension

* = most important

　　5. Hydrophthalmos

　　6. Iatrogenic

　　7. Intraocular neoplasms

　*8. Juvenile xanthogranuloma—yellow nodules of skin & iris

　　9. Malignant exophthalmos

　10. Microbial keratitis, especially Moraxella

　11. Occult trauma or trauma with late effect

　*12. Rubeosis iridis

　13. Severe iritis with or without

　　　　A. Behçet disease (dermatostomato-ophthalmic syndrome)

　　　　B. Diabetes mellitus (Willis disease)

　　　　C. Gonococcal infection

　　　　D. Herpes zoster or Herpes simplex

　14. Use of warfarin, heparin, aspirin, and alcohol

　15. Vascular anomalies of iris

　16. Wound vascularization following cataract extraction

Koehler, M.P., and Shelton, D.B.: Spontaneous hyphema resulting from warfarin. Ann Ophthalmol., 15:858–859, 1983.

Mason, G.I., et al.: Bilateral spontaneous hyphema arising from iridic microhemangiomas. Ann Ophthalmol., 11:87, 1979.

Ormerod, L.D., and Egan, K.M.: Spontaneous hyphaema and corneal haemorrhages as complications of microbial keratitis. Brit J Ophthalmol., 71:933, 1987.

Pandolfi, M.: Hemorrhages in Ophthalmology. New York, Thieme-Stratton, 1979.

Ritch, R., et al.: The Glaucomas. St. Louis, C.V. Mosby, 1989.

Spontaneous Hyphema in Infants

　　1. Acute rheumatoid iridocyclitis

　　2. Blood dyscrasias, such as anemia, leukemia, and disseminated intravascular coagulation

　　3. Iritis (see p. 422)

　*4. Juvenile xanthogranuloma

　　5. Perinatal asphyxia

　　6. Persistent hyperplastic primary vitreous

　　7. Retinoblastoma

　　8. Retinoschisis

　　9. Retinopathy of prematurity

　*10. Trauma without history (consider child abuse)

Appelboom, T., and Durso, F.: Retinoblastoma presenting as a total hyphema. Ann. Ophthalmol., 17:508–510, 1985.

Harley, R.D., et. al.: Juvenile xanthogranuloma. J. Pediatr. Ophthalmol. Strabismus, 19:33–39, 1982.

Ortiz, J.M., et. al.: Disseminated intravascular coagulation in infancy and in the neonate. Arch. Ophthalmol., 100:1413–1415, 1982.

Wu, G., and Behrens, M.M.: Hyphema in the newborn: Report of a case. J. Pediatr. Ophthalmol. Strabismus, 19:56–57, 1982.

Spontaneous Hyphema in Infants

	Juvenile Xanthogranuloma	Retinoblastoma*	Blood Dyscrasias as Anemia/Leukemia*	Acute Rheumatoid Iridocylytis	Trauma without History*	Retrolental Fibroplasia	Persistent Hyperplastic Primary Vitreous	Retinoschisis	Iritis as Behçet Syndrome
History									
1. Bilateral		R	S	U		U		U	S
2. Child abuse					U				
3. Common in males					U			U	
4. Congenital							U	U	
5. Familial		U	S	S					
6. Hereditary		U	S						
7. Japanese/Italian extraction									S
8. Oxygen therapy						U			
9. Prematurity						U	S		
10. Virus infection									U
Physical Findings									
1. Anterior/posterior synechiae					S				S
2. Band keratopathy					U				
3. Blood stained cornea	U								
4. Cataract					U	S			S
5. Cherry red spot of macula									S
6. Conjunctival/subconjunctival mass	R								S
7. Corneal abrasions					S				
8. Corneal edema	S								
9. Corneal opacity									S
10. Cotton-wool spots			U						
11. Endophthalmitis		S							
12. Endothelial corneal damage					S				
13. Extraocular muscle paralysis			S						S
14. Eyelids, yellow/brown papules/nodules	U								
15. Galucoma	S	S		S	S	R	S		S
16. Heterchromic iris	U	U							
17. Hypopyon		U			U				R
18. Hypotony					S				
19. Iridodialysis					S				
20. Iris neovascularization		U							
21. Leukokoria		U					U		
22. Lid edema		U			S				
23. Macular edema					S				S
24. Microphthalmia						S	S		
25. Mydriasis		U							
26. Nystagmus								S	
27. Ocular pain		S			U	S			S
28. Optic atrophy									S
29. Optic neuritis					U				S
30. Oval/eccentric pupil	S								
31. Panophthalmitis		S							
32. Papilledema		S	S						
33. Phthisis bulbi						S	S		

* = most important

Spontaneous Hyphema in Infants *Continued*

	Juvenile Xanthogranuloma	Retinoblastoma*	Blood Dyscrasias as Anemia/Leukemia*	Acute Rheumatoid Iridocyclytis	Trauma without History*	Retrolental Fibroplasia	Persistent Hyperplastic Primary Vitreous	Retinoschisis	Iritis as Behçet Syndrome
Physical Findings									
34. Proptosis	R								
35. Recessed chamber angle					S				
36. Retinal detachment		S	S		S	U	S	S	
37. Retinal edema			U		S				S
38. Retinal mass						S	S		
39. Retinal tractional tear					S				
40. Salmon colored iris lesion	U								
41. Scleral rupture					S				
42. Scleritis									S
43. Subluxed lens					S				
44. Strabismus		U						S	S
45. Thread-like arterioles			S						
46. Uveitis	U			U		S			
47. Vitreous cells				U					
48. Vitreous detachment					S				
49. Vitreous hemorrhage		S	S			R		S	S
50. Vitreous veils								U	
Laboratory Data									
1. Antinuclear antibody titers				U					
2. Biopsy of lid lesion	U								
3. Biopsy of tumor		S							
4. Bone marrow puncture			U						
5. Computed tomographic scan		U			S				
6. Cytology of anterior chamber	S	S	S						
7. Complete blood study (white blood cell count, hemoglobin, hematocrit)			U	S					
8. Electroretinogram abnormal								U	
9. Fluorescein angiography			S	S	S	S	S	U	
10. Homologous leucocytic antibody determination				S					U
11. Lumbosacral-spine roentgenogram									U
12. Macroglobulins negative									U
13. Orbital roentgenogram (globe calcium)		S			S				
14. Ultrasonography, ocular	U	U			U	U	S		
15. Visual fields								U	

R = rarely; S = sometimes; and U = usually.

Plasmoid Aqueous (Aqueous with a High Protein Content)

1. Rheumatoid arthritis

2. Serum sickness

3. Infection with gonococcus

4. Following paracentesis or intraocular operation, such as cataract extraction

5. Severe corneal ulceration

6. Trauma

Newell, F.W.: Ophthalmology, Principles and Concepts. 7th Ed. St. Louis, C.V. Mosby, 1991.

Cholesterolosis of the Anterior Chamber (Cholesterol Crystals in the Anterior Chamber; Usually in a Blind Eye following Trauma, but May Be Associated with Hyphema or Secondary Glaucoma). Associated with:

*1. Chronic uveitis

2. Eales disease (periphlebitis)

3. Lens subluxation (see p. 449)

4. Mature or hypermature cataract

5. Microphthalmia

*6. Phthisis bulbi

7. Retinal detachment (see p. 541)

8. Traumatic cataract

9. Vascular disorders

10. Vitreous hemorrhage (see p. 474)

Mishra, R.K., et al.: Cholesterol crystals in Eales disease. Indian J Ophthalmol., 28:67–68, 1980.

Wand, M., and Garn, R.A.: Cholesterolosis of the anterior chamber Am J Ophthalmol., 78:143–144, 1974.

Gas Bubbles in the Anterior Chamber

1. Clostridium perfringens

2. E. coli

3. Yag laser treatment to the anterior segment

4. Post-operative intraocular surgery

Frantz, J.F., et al.: Acute endogenous panophthalmitis caused by clostridium perfringens. Am J Ophthalmol., 78:295–303, 1974.

Obertymski, H., and Dyson, C.: Clostridium perfringens panophthalmitis. Can J Ophthalmol., 9:258–259, 1974.

Pigmentation of Trabecular Meshwork

1. In elderly individuals—inferior nasal or faint band circumferential

*2. Pseudo-exfoliation of lens with or without glaucoma—unilateral or bilateral

*3. Pigmentary glaucoma

*4. Krukenberg spindle without glaucoma

* = most important

*5. Malignant melanoma—one eye

6. Cyst of pigment layer of iris—unilateral

7. Previous intraocular operation, inflammation, or hyphema—scattered, mostly in lower angle

8. Nevus—dense, isolated patch

9. Open-angle glaucoma—patchy band, whole circumference

10. Following gamma irradiation for malignancy of nasal sinus

Epstein, D.L.: Chandler and Grant's Glaucoma. 3rd Ed. Philadelphia, Lea & Febiger, 1986.

Roth, M., and Simmons, R.J.: Glaucoma associated with precipitates on the trabecular meshwork. Ophthalmology, 86:1614, 1982.

Pigment Liberation into Anterior Chamber with Dilatation of Pupil

1. Diabetes mellitus (Willis disease)

2. Exercise

3. Hurler disease (mucopolysaccharidoses IH)

4. Low tension glaucoma with pigment dispersion

Epstein, D.L.: Chandler and Grant's Glaucoma. 3rd Ed. Philadelphia, Lea & Febiger, 1986.

Ritch, R.: Nonprogressive low tension glaucoma with pigmentary dispersion. Am J Ophthalmol., 94:190–196, 1982.

Grading of Anterior Chamber Angle Width (Usually Determined by Gonioscopy)

1. Grade 0: No angle structures visible—narrow angle, complete or partial closure (angle closure)

2. Grade 1: Unable to see posterior one half of trabecular meshwork—extremely narrow angle (probably capable of angle closure)

3. Grade 2: Part of Schlemm's canal is visible—moderately narrow angle (may be capable of angle closure)

4. Grade 3: Posterior portion of Schlemm canal is visible—moderately open angle (incapable of angle closure)

5. Grade 4: Ciliary body is visible—open angle (incapable of angle closure)

Epstein, D. L.: Chandler and Grant's Glaucoma. 3rd Ed. Philadelphia, Lea & Febiger, 1986.

Shields, M.B.: Textbook of Glaucoma. 2nd Ed. Baltimore, Williams & Wilkins, 1986.

Blood in Schlemm Canal (Reversal of Normal Pressure Gradient)

*1. Artifact of goniolens flange occluding the episcleral veins in one or more quadrants

2. High episcleral venous pressure

    *A. Carotid-cavernous sinus fistula (Red-eyed shunt syndrome)

    *B. Dural-cavernous fistula

    C. Mediastinal tumors

    D. Orbital arteriovenous fistula

    E. Sturge-Weber syndrome (meningocutaneous syndrome)

F. Superior vena cava obstruction (superior vena cava syndrome)

G. Tetralogy of Fallot

3. Low intraocular pressure

A. Following trabeculectomy

B. Hypotony (see p. 367)

C. Intraocular inflammation

4. Normal eye

Namba, H.: Blood reflux into anterior chamber after trabeculectomy. Jpn. J. Ophthalmol., 27:616–625, 1983.

Phelps, C.D., et. al.: Arterial anastomosis with Schlemm's canal. Trans. Am. Ophthalmol. Soc., 83:304–315, 1985.

Phelps, C.D., et. al.: The diagnosis and prognosis of atypical carotid cavernous fistula. Am. J. Ophthalmol., 93:423–436, 1982.

Deep Anterior Chamber Angle

1. Normal variation

2. Aphakia

3. Myopia

4. Megalocornea or conical cornea including keratoconus (see p. 295)

5. Congenital glaucoma

6. Posterior dislocation of the lens (see p. 449)

7. Recession of anterior chamber angle

Newell, F.W.: Ophthalmology, Principles and Concepts. 7th Ed. St. Louis, C.V. Mosby, 1991.

Shields, M.B.: Textbook of Glaucoma. 2nd Ed. Baltimore, Williams & Wilkins, 1986.

Narrow Anterior Chamber Angle (May Be Capable of Angle Closure Glaucoma)

1. Normal variation

*2. Predisposition to angle closure

3. Anterior dislocation of the lens

4. Hyperopia

5. Spherophakia and microcornea (see p. 448)

6. Postoperative intraocular operation with leaking wound (see hypotony, p. 367)

7. Choroidal detachment (see p. 591)

*8. Pupillary block

9. Loss of aqueous from perforating ulcer, corneal wound, or staphyloma (see hypotony, p. 367)

10. Intumescent senile cataract

11. Traumatic cataract that fluffs up

12. Primary hyperplastic primary vitreous (PHPV)

13. Peripheral anterior synechiae (see p. 382)

* = most important

*14. Posterior entrapment of aqueous humor (malignant glaucoma or ciliary-block glaucoma)

15. Drugs, including:

acetazolamide	neostigmine	sulfamethizole
acetylcholine	physostigmine	sulfamethoxazole
alpha-chymotrypsin	pilocarpine	sulfamethoxypyridazine
demecarium	sulfacetamide	sulfanilamide
dichlorphenamide	sulfachlorpyridazine	sulfaphenazole
echothiophate	sulfadiazine	sulfapyridine
edrophonium	sulfamethazine	sulfasalazine
ethoxzolamide	sulfadimethoxine	sulfathiazole
isoflurophate	sulfamerazine	sulfisoxazole
methazolamide	sulfameter	

*16. Plateau iris

17. Diffuse ciliary body or iris tumor

Fraunfelder, F.T.: Drug-Induced Ocular Side Effects and Drug Interactions. 4th Ed. Philadelphia, Williams & Wilkins, 1996.

Newell, F.W.: Ophthalmology, Principles and Concepts. 7th Ed. St. Louis, C.V. Mosby, 1991.

Scheie, H.G., and Morse, P.H.: Shallow anterior chamber as a sign of non-surgical choroidal detachment. Ann. Ophthalmol., 6:317–322, 1974.

Taylor, B.C., and Winslow R.L.: Pseudophakic flat anterior chamber following retinal detachment repair. Ophthalmology, 88:935, 1981.

Irregular Depth of the Anterior Chamber

1. Partial dislocation of lens
2. Tumor of iris or ciliary body
3. Peripheral anterior synechiae on one side of the chamber (see p. 382)
4. Iris bombe or pupillary block
5. Ruptured lens capsule with swelling on one side
6. Anatomic narrowing superiorly
7. Subacute angle closure glaucoma
8. Cyclodialysis and traumatic recession of chamber angle

Epstein, D.L.: Chandler and Grant's Glaucoma. 3rd Ed. Philadelphia, Lea & Febiger, 1986.

Newell, F.W.: Ophthalmology, Principles and Concepts. 7th Ed. St. Louis, C.V. Mosby, 1991.

Peripheral Anterior Synechiae (Adhesion of Iris Tissue across Anterior Chamber Structures in Variable Amounts Noted with Gonioscopy)

1. Bridge corneoscleral trabecular meshwork to Schwalbe's line or anterior to Schwalbe's line (uncommon)
   A. Anterior chamber cleavage syndrome
      (1) Axenfeld syndrome (posterior embryotoxon)
      (2) Congenital central anterior synechiae

      (3) Following intraocular lens implantation

      (4) Reiger syndrome (dysgenesis mesostromalis)

    B. Essential iris atrophy (see p. 418)

    C. Iris bombe from occlusion of pupil

    D. Iris or ciliary body tumor pushing iris into contact with cornea

    E. Local adhesion with of epithelium or fibrous ingrowth

    F. Penetrating injury of the cornea

    G. Postoperative flat anterior chamber

2. Synechiae of iris limited to ciliary band, scleral spur, and trabecular meshwork (common)

    *A. Following cataract surgery, intraocular implantation, refractive surgery, or laser trabeculoplasty

    *B. Intraocular inflammation

    *C. Neovascular glaucoma from fibrovascular membrane (see p. 366)

    *D. Sequelae to angle closure glaucoma

Deg, J.K., et al.: Delayed corneal wound healing following radial keratotomy. Ophthalmology, 92.734–740, 1985.

Epstein, D.L.: Chandler and Grant's Glaucoma. 3rd Ed. Philadelphia, Lea & Febiger, 1986.

Kolker, A.E., and Hetherington, J.: Becker-Shaffer's Diagnosis and Therapy of the Glaucomas. 6th Ed. St. Louis, C.V. Mosby, 1989.

Newell, F.W.: Ophthalmology, Principles and Concepts. 7th Ed. St. Louis, C.V. Mosby, 1991.

Rouhiainen, H.J., et al.: Peripheral anterior synechiae formation after trabeculoplasty. Arch Ophthalmol., 106:189–191, 1988.

Schwartz, A.L., et al.: Argon laser trabecular surgery in uncontrolled phakic open angle glaucoma. Ophthalmology, 88:203, 1981.

Neovascularization of Anterior Chamber Angle (Newly Formed Vessels Extend Into the Trabecular Meshwork)

1. Anterior chamber angle

    A. Congenital pupillary iris lens membrane with goniodysgenesis

    B. Traumatic chamber angle

2. Iris tumors

    A. Hemangioma

    B. Melanoma

    C. Metastatic carcinoma

3. Ocular vascular disease

    *A. Central retinal artery thrombosis (see p. 512)

    *B. Central retinal vein thrombosis (see p. 525)

    C. Hemiretinal branch vein occlusion (HBVO)

4. Postinflammatory

    A. Anterior chamber implants

    B. Fungal endophthalmitis

* = most important

C. Radiation

D. Retinal detachment operation

E. Uveitis, chronic

5. Proximal vascular disease

    A. Aortic arch syndrome (Takayasu syndrome)

    B. Carotid cavernous fistula

    C. Carotid ligation

    D. Carotid occlusive disease

    E. Cranial arteritis (temporal arteritis syndrome)

6. Retinal disease

    A. Coats disease (Leber miliary aneurysms)

    *B. Diabetic retinopathy

    C. Eales disease (periphlebitis)

    D. Glaucoma, chronic

    E. Melanoma of choroid

    F. Norrie disease (fetal iritis syndrome)

    G. Persistent hyperplastic primary vitreous

    H. Retinal detachment

    I. Retinal hemangioma

    J. Retinal vessel occlusion

    K. Retinoblastoma

    L. Retrolental flbroplasia

    M. Sickle cell retinopathy (Herrick syndrome)

Cibis, G.W., et. al.: Congenital pupillary iris-lens membrane with goniodysgenesis. Ophthalmology, 93:847–852, 1986.

Kimura, R.: Fluorescein gonioangiography of newly formed vessels in the anterior chamber angle. Tohoku J. Exp. Med., 140:193–196, 1983.

Moses, L.: Complications of rigid anterior chamber implants. Ophthalmology, 91:819–825, 1984.

Roy, F.H.: Ocular Syndromes and Systemic Diseases. 2nd Ed. Philadelphia, W.B. Saunders, 1989.

Shihab, Z.M., and Lee, P.F.: The significance of normal angle vessels. Ophthalmic. Surg., 16:382–385, 1985.

Iris Processes (Pectinate Ligaments in Anterior Chamber Angle)

1. Achondroplasia, diastrophic dwarfism, cartilage-hair hypoplasia, and spondyloepiphyseal dysplasia, anterior chamber clevage syndrome, Axenfeld syndrome, Reiger syndrome, Peter's anomaly.

2. Congenital glaucoma—may be associated with congenital microcoria and goniodysgenesis

3. Congenital scoliosis

4. Legg-Perthes disease (coxa plana)

5. Marfan syndrome (hypoplastic form of dystrophia mesodermalis congenita)

6. Mucopolysaccharidoses (including Hunter syndrome, Hurler syndrome, Scheie syndrome, and Sanfilippo-Good syndrome)

7. Myopic patients

*8. Normal especially brown-eyed persons

9. Pigmentary ocular dispersion syndrome

Dunn, S.P., et. al.: New findings in posterior amorphous corneal dystrophy. Arch. Ophthalmol., 102: 236–239, 1984.

Pollock, A., and Oliver, M.: Congenital glaucoma and incomplete congenital glaucoma in two siblings. Acta. Ophthalmol. (Copenh.), 62:359–363, 1984.

Roy, F.H.: Ocular Syndromes and Systemic Diseases. 2nd Ed. Philadelphia, W.B. Saunders, 1989.

Tawara, A., and Inomato, H.: Familial cases of congenital microcoria associated with late onset congenital glaucoma and goniodysgenesis. Jpn. J. Ophthalmol., 27:63–72, 1983.

White Mass in Anterior Chamber

*1. Endophthalmitis

2. Ocular aspergillosis

3. Sterile inflammation following surgery or trauma

*4. Tumor

Katz, G., et al.: Ocular Aspergillosis Isolated in the Anterior Chamber. Ophthalmology. 100:1815–1818, 1993.

* = most important

Pupil

EDWARD G. BUCKLEY

Contents

Mydriasis (Dilated Pupil) (Usually Greater than Five Millimeters)

1. Physiologic

   A. Larger pupils in women than in men

   B. Larger pupils in myopes than in hypermetropes

   C. Larger pupils in blue irides than in brown irides

   D. Larger pupils in adolescents and middle-aged persons than in very young or old persons

   E. Surprise, fear, pain, strong emotion, or vestibular stimulation

   F. General anesthesia of stages I, II, and IV

G. Autosensory pupillary reflex—stimulation of middle ear

H. Auditory pupillary reflex—tuning fork adjacent to ear

I. Vestibular pupillary reflex—stimulation of labyrinth by heat, cold, or rotation

J. Vagotonic pupillary reflex—stimulation on deep inspiration

2. Drugs, including:

acetaminophen	betamethasone
acetanilid	biperiden
acetophenazine	bromide
acetylcholine	bromisovalum
adiphenine	brompheniramine
albuterol	butabarbital
alcohol	butalbital
aldosterone	butallylonal
alkavervir	butaperazine
allobarbital	butethal
alprazolam	caramiphen
alseroxylon	carbamazepine
amantadine	carbinoxamine
ambutonium	carbon dioxide
amitriptyline	carbromal
amobarbital	carisoprodol
amoxapine	carphenazine
amphetamine	chloral hydrate
amyl nitrite	chloramphenicol
anisotropine	chlorcyclizine
antazoline	chlordiazepoxide
antimony lithium thiomalate	chlorisondamine
antimony potassium tartrate	chloroform
antimony sodium tartrate	chlorpheniramine
antimony sodium thioglycollate	chlorphenoxamine
aprobarbital	chlorphentermine
aspirin	chlorpromazine
atropine	chlorprothixene
atropine methylnitrate	cimetidine
azatadine	clemastine
baclofen	clidinium
barbital	clomiphene
belladonna	clomipramine
benzathine	clonazepam
penicillin G	clonidine
benzphetamine	clorazepate
benztropine	cocaine

codeine
colistimethate
colistin
cortisone
cryptenamine
cyclizine
cyclobarbital
cyclopentobarbital
cyclopentolate
cycrimine
cyproheptadine
deserpidine
desipramine
desoxycorticosterone
dexamethasone
dexbrompheniramine
dexchlorpheniramine
dextroamphetamine
diazepam
diacetylmorphine
dicyclomine
diethazine
diethylpropion
digitalis
digoxin
dimethindene
diphemanil
diphenhydramine
diphenylhydantoin
diphenylpyraline
diphtheria toxoid (adsorbed)
dipivefrin
disopyramide
disulfiram
doxepin
doxylamine
droperidol
emetine
ephedrine
epinephrine
ergot
erythromycin
ether

ethopropazine
fenfluramine
fludrocortisone
fluorometholone
fluphenazine
fluprednisolone
flurazepam
gentamicin(?)
glutethimide
glycopyrrolate
guanethidine
halazepam
haloperidol
hashish
heptabarbital
hexachlorophene
hexamethonium
hexethal
hexobarbital
hexocyclium
homatropine
hydrabamine penicillin V
hydrabamine phenoxymethyl penicillin
hydrocortisone
hydromorphone
hydroxyamphetamine
imipramine
indomethacin(?)
insulin
iodide and iodine solutions and compounds
isocarboxazid
isoniazid
isopropamide
levallorphan
levarterenol
levodopa
lidocaine
lorazepam
loxapine
LSD
lysergide
maprotiline
marijuana

measles and rubella virus vaccine (live)

measles, mumps and rubella virus vaccine (live)

measles virus vaccine (live)

mecamylamine

meclizine

medrysone

mepenzolate

meperidine

mephentermine

mephobarbital

meprednisone

meprobamate

mescaline

mesoridazine

metaraminol

methadone

methamphetamine

methantheline

methaqualone

metharbital

methdilazine

methitural

methixene

methohexital

methotrimeprazine

methoxamine

methscopolamine

methyl alcohol

methylatropine nitrate

methylene blue

methylpentynol

methylphenidate

methylprednisolone

methyprylon

metoclopramide

midazolam

morphine

mumps virus vaccine (live)

nalidixic acid

nalorphine

naloxone

naltrexone

naphazoline

nialamide

nitrazepam

nitroglycerin(?)

nitrous oxide

norepinephrine

nortriptyline

opium

oral contraceptives

orphenadrine

oxazepam

oxygen

oxymorphone

oxyphencyclimine

oxyphenonium

paraldehyde

paramethasone

pargyline

pentobarbital

pentolinium

pentylenetetrazol

perazine

pericyazine

perphenazine

phenacetin

phendimetrazine

phenelzine

pheniramine

phenmetrazine

phenobarbital

phenoxymethyl penicillin

phentermine

phenylephrine

phenylpropanolamine

phenytoin

pilocarpine

pipenzolate

piperacetazine

piperidolate

poldine

polymyxin B

potassium penicillin G

potassium penicillin V

~~potassium phenethicillin~~	~~stibophen~~
potassium phenoxymethyl penicillin	syrosingopine
prazepam	talbutal
prednisolone	temazepam
prednisone	tetraethylammonium
primidone	tetrahydrocannabinol
probarbital	tetrahydrozoline
procaine penicillin G	THC(?)
prochlorperazine	thiamylal
procyclidine	thiethylperazine
promazine	thiopental
promethazine	thiopropazate
propantheline	thioproperazine thioridazine
propiomazine	thiothixene
propoxyphene	tranylcypromine
protoveratrines A and B	trazodone
protriptyline	triamcinolone
psilocybin	triazolam
pyrilamine	tridihexethyl
quinidine	trifluoperazine
quinine	trifluperidol
radioactive iodides	triflupromazine
rauwolfia serpentina	trihexyphenidyl
rescinnamine	trimeprazine
reserpine	trimethaphan
rubella and mumps virus vaccine (live)	trimethidinium
rubella virus vaccine (live)	trimipramine
scopolamine	tripelennamine
secobarbital	tropicamide
sodium antimonylgluconate	urethan
sodium salicylate	veratrum viride alkaloids
stibocaptate	vinbarbital
stibogluconate	

3. Toxins, including: after-shave lotion, arsenic, clostridium botulinum (gas gangrene), tetanus (lockjaw), cannabis, adrenergic agents, such as nasal sprays, or asthma therapy in newborns, para-aminosalicylic acid, lead, carbon monoxide, organic phosphorus, bovine milk protein in infants with allergic malabsorption, Datura stramonium (Jimson weed), Datura Wrightii (Moonflower), and Solanacease (Nightshade), nitro and aminocompounds of benzene, carbon disulfide, papaverine.

4. Ocular causes (Mydriasis) (see fixed pupil section p. 386)

   A. Glaucoma, usually acute

   B. Glaucomocylitic crisis (Posner-Schlossman syndrome)

   C. Hollenhorst syndrome (chorioretinal infarction syndrome)

*D. Iritis; uveitis

  E. Intraocular foreign body (iron mydriasis)

  F. Iris atrophy

  G. Iris sphincter rupture

*H. Paralytic mydriasis, following trauma

  I. Photocoagulation complications

  J. Retinoblastoma

5. Lesions of ciliary ganglion causing internal ophthalmoplegia (e.g., dilated pupil and absent accommodation)

  A. Adie's tonic pupil

  B. Congenital lesion

  C. Herpes zoster

  C. Orbital floor fracture repair

  D. Systemic lupus erythematosus (disseminated lupus erythematosus)

  E. Varicella (chickenpox)

  F. Yellow fever

6. Acute or chronic ophthalmoplegias (see p. 193)

7. Third-nerve lesion—also ptosis and ophthalmoplegia on affected side (see p. 75)

8. Coma because of alcohol ingestion, eclampsia, diabetes, uremia, epilepsy, apoplexy, or meningitis—the pupils are equally dilated and do not constrict with stimulation

9. Midbrain tumors, in which dilated pupils, paralysis of vertical gaze (especially upward gaze), and retraction nystagmus are manifest

  A. Craniopharyngioma

  B. Parinaud syndrome (paralysis of upgaze movements)

10. Epidural or subdural hematoma

11. Paralytic parasympathetic lesions

12. Irritative sympathetic lesion—pupillary dilatation widening of palpebral aperture, and slight exophthalmos

  A. Irritative lesion, such as tumor, encephalitis, or syringomyelia of the hypothalamus, midbrain, medulla, or cervical cord

  B. Thoracic lesions, such as cervical rib, aneurysms of the thoracic vessels, mediastinal tumors, or tubercular pleurisy

*C. Cervical lesions, including nasopharyngeal tumors, thyroid swelling, or cervical nodes

  D. Rabies (hydrophobia)

*E. Trauma

  F. Visceral disease

  G. Aortic dilatation or exudative endocarditis (Roque sign)

  H. Acute abdominal conditions, such as appendicitis, cholecystitis, or colitis (Moskowskij sign)

  I. Psychiatric patients with pressure over McBurney point (Meyer phenomenon)

* = most important

13. Tumors, injury, or hemorrhage of frontoparietal, parietal, temporal, or temporo-occipital area—contralateral mydriasis and ipsilateral defect in the visual field

14. Fractured skull

15. Acute autonomic neuropathy

16. Acute pandysautonomia

17. Avitaminosis B$_z$ (pellagra)

18. Chorea

19. Clivus edge syndrome

20. Craniocervical syndrome (whiplash injury)

21. Foramen lacerum syndrome (aneurysm of internal carotid artery syndrome)

22. Hemiacrosomia syndrome (hemifacial or unilateral hypertrophy)

23. Iron deficiency anemia

24. Lockjaw (tetanus)

25. Mycosis fungoides syndrome (Sezary syndrome)

26. Optic canal syndrome

27. Parkinson syndrome (shaking palsy)

28. Prematurity

29. Pulseless disease

30. Reye syndrome (acute encephalopathy syndrome)

31. Rollet syndrome (orbital apex-sphenoidal syndrome)

32. Suprarenal-sympathetic syndrome (adrenal medulla tumor syndrome)

33. Temporal arteritis

34. Weber syndrome (cerebellar peduncle syndrome)

35. Wernicke syndrome (I) (avitaminosis B$_1$ thiamine deficiency)

36. Zellweger syndrome (cerebrohepatorenal syndrome)

Bodker, F.S., et al.: Postoperative mydriasis after repair of orbital floor fracture. Am J Ophthalmol. 115:372–375, 1993.

Cuppeto, J.R., and Greco, T.: Mydriasis in giant cell arteritis. J Clin Neuroophthalmol. 9: 267, 1985.

Fraunfelder, F.T.: Drug-Induced Ocular Side Effects and Drug Interactions. 4th Ed. Philadelphia, Williams & Wilkins, 1996.

Hendrix, L.E., et al.: Papaverine-induced mydriasis. Am J Neuroradiology. 15: 716–718, 1994.

Isenberg, S.J., et al.: The fixed and dilated pupils of premature neonates. Am J Ophthalmol. 110: 168, 1990.

Pau, H.: Differential Diagnosis of Eye Diseases. 2nd Ed. New York, Thieme Med. Pub., 1988.

Richardson, P., and Schulenburg, W.E.: Bilateral congenital mydriasis. Brit J Ophthalmol. 76:632–633, 1992.

Roy, F.H.: Ocular Syndromes and Systemic Diseases. 2nd Ed. Philadelphia, W.B. Saunders, 1989.

Relative Fixed, Dilated Pupil

1. Midbrain damage—vascular accidents, tumors, degenerative and infectious diseases

    A. Dorsal (Edinger-Westphal nucleus and its connections)—rare, involves both pupils, pupillary near reaction often retained, and often associated with supranuclear vertical gaze palsy (upgaze)

*B. Ventral (fascicular part of third nerve)—associated with other neurologic deficits, such as Nothnagel syndrome, Benedikt syndrome, Weber syndrome involves other extraocular components of the third nerve

*2. Damage to the third nerve (from interpeduncular fossa to ciliary ganglion)

    A. Basal aneurysms

    B. Supratentorial space—occupying masses, causing displacement of the brain stem or transtentorial herniation of the uncus—patient is stuporous or comatose

    C. Basal meningitis—often bilateral internal ophthalmoplegia

    *D. Ischemic oculomotor palsy

    E. Parasellar tumor (e.g., pituitary adenoma, meningioma, craniopharyngioma, nasopharyngeal carcinoma, or distant metastases)

    F. Parasellar inflammation (e.g., Tolosa-Hunt syndrome, temporal arteritis, herpes zoster)

*3. Damage to the ciliary ganglion

    A. Viral ciliary ganglionitis or involvement of the ciliary nerves, such as from herpes zoster

    B. Orbital trauma or tumor

    C. Trauma from inferior oblique surgery

    D. Trauma from retrobulbar injections

4. Damage to short ciliary nerves

    A. Blunt trauma to the globe may injure the ciliary plexus at the iris root (traumatic iridoplegia)

    B. Choroidal trauma or tumor

*5. Damage to the iris

    A. Degenerative or inflammatory diseases of the iris

    B. Posterior synechiae

    C. Acute rise of intraocular pressure (hypoxia or sphincter damage)

    D. Blunt injury to the globe with sphincter damage (traumatic iridoplegia)

    E. Pharmacologic blockade by atropinic substances

    F. Post cataract surgery

5. Total blindness, including cortical blindness (see p. 704)

    A. Bilateral optic nerve

        (1) Anterior ischemic optic neuropathy

        (2) Avulsion (traumatic)

        (3) Optic neuritis

    B. Bilateral retina

        (1) Acute retinal necrosis

        (2) Central retinal artery occlusion

        (3) Central retinal vein occlusion

        (4) Retina detachment

* = most important

Isenberg, S.J., et al.: The fixed and dilated pupils of premature neonates. Am. J. Ophthalmol., 110:168–171, 1990.

Lam, S., et al.: Atonic pupil after cataract surgery. Ophthalmol., 96:589–590, 1989.

Newell, F.W.: Ophthalmology, Principles and Concepts. 7th Ed. St. Louis, C.V. Mosby, 1991.

Thompson, H.S., et al.: The fixed dilated pupil. Arch. Ophthalmol., 86:21–27, 1971.

Miosis (Small Pupil) (Usually Less than Two Millimeters)

1. Physiologic

   A. Smaller pupil in men than in women

   B. Smaller pupil in hypermetropes than in myopes

   C. Smaller pupil in brown irides than in blue irides

   D. Smaller pupil in very young or old than in adolescents and middle-aged

   E. Sleep, fatigue, coma

   F. Stage III anesthesia

   G. Near vision (synkinesis with convergence and accommodation)

   H. Vestibular stimulation

2. Drugs including:

aceclidine	chloroprocaine
acetophenazine	chlorpromazine
acetylcholine	chlorprothixene
alcohol	clonidine
allobarbital	codeine
ambenonium	cyclobarbital
amobarbital	cyclopentobarbital
aprobarbital	demecarium
baclofen	diacetylmorphine
barbital	dibucaine
bethanechol	diethazine
bromide	digitalis(?)
bromisovalum	dronabinol
bupivacaine	droperidol
butabarbital	echothiophate
butalbital	edrophonium
butallylonal	ephedrine(?)
butaperazine	ergot
butethal	ergotamine
carbachol	ether
carbromal	ethopropazine
carisoprodol	fluphenazine
carphenazine	haloperidol
chloral hydrate	hashish
chloroform	heptabarbital

hexachlorophene

hexethal

hexobarbital

hydromorphone

iodide and iodine solutions and compounds(?)

isocarboxazid

isoflurophate

isosorbide dinitrate(?)

levallorphan

levodopa

lidocaine

marijuana

meperidine

mephobarbital

mepivacaine

meprobamate

mesoridazine

methacholine

methadone

methaqualone(?)

metharbital

methdilazine

methitural

methohexital

methotrimeprazine

methyprylon

midazolam

morphine

nalorphine

naltrexone

naloxone

neostigmine

nialamide

nitrous oxide

opium

oxprenolol

oxymorphone

paraldehyde

pentazocine

pentobarbital

perazine

pericyazine

perphenazine

phencyclidine

phenelzine

phenobarbital

phenoxybenzamine

phenylephrine

physostigmine

pilocarpine

piperacetazine

piperazine

piperocaine

prilocaine

primidone

probarbital

procaine

prochlorperazine

promazine

promethazine

propiomazine

propoxycaine

propoxyphene

propranolol

pyridostigmine

radioactive iodides(?)

secobarbital

sulindac

talbutal

tetracaine

tetrahydrocannabinol

thiamylal

thiethylperazine

thiopental

thiopropazate

thioproperazine

thioridazine

thiothixene

tolazoline

tranylcypromine

trifluoperazine

trifluperidol

triflupromazine

trimeprazine

vinbarbital

vitamin A

3. Ocular causes

   *A. Accommodative spasm (Hysteria)

   B. Corneal irritation, such as keratitis or corneal injury

   C. Conjunctival irritation

   D. Congenital miosis (absent dilator muscle)

   E. Dislocated lenses

   F. Iritis

   *G. Posterior iris synechiae, usually irregular

   H. Retinitis pigmentosa

4. Central nervous system defects

   A. Acute pontine angle lesion, such as hemorrhage or tumor associated with disturbed conjugate gaze

   B. Arteriosclerotic and degenerative disease of the cerebrum

   C. Encephalitis

   D. Facial tetanus

   E. Infections/tumors of the cavernous sinus or superior orbital fissure

   F. Purulent meningitis

   G. Severe hypoxia

5. "Cluster headache" or histamine cephalgia-ptosis; miosis; red, watering eye on side of headache

6. Raeder paratrigeminal syndrome—ipsilateral miosis and pain—may be associated with third-nerve paralysis or corneal anesthesia

   A. Extracranial aneurysm of internal carotid

   B. Idiopathic

   C. Meningioma

   D. Migraine

   E. Post-trauma

7. Argyll Robertson pupil—small and irregular; reacts better to accommodation than to light

   A. Aberrant regeneration of the third nerve

   B. Carbon disulfide poisoning

   C. Cerebral aneurysm

   D. Chronic alcoholism

   *E. Diabetes mellitus (Willis disease)

   F. Encephalitis

   G. Friedreich ataxia

   H. Malaria

   I. Midbrain tumors, such as pinealomas and craniopharyngioma

   J. Multiple sclerosis (disseminated sclerosis)

   K. Senile and degenerative diseases of the central nervous system

   L. Syphilis (acquired lues)

      M. Syringomyelia

      N. Trauma to skull or orbit

  8. Ataxia, spastic with congenital miosis—dominant

  9. Babinski-Nageotte syndrome (medulla tegmental paralysis)

10. Coenurosis

11. Craniocervical syndrome (whiplash injury)

12. Dejerine-Klumpke syndrome (lower radicular syndrome)

13. Devic syndrome (neuromyelitis optica)

*14. Diabetes mellitus

15. Eaton-Lambert syndrome (myasthenic syndrome)

16. Elevated intracranial pressure

*17. Horner syndrome (cervical sympathetic paralysis syndrome)

18. Jugular foramen syndrome (Vernet syndrome)

19. Lowe syndrome (oculocerebrorenal syndrome)

20. Marfan syndrome (arachnodactyly dystrophia mesodermalis congenita)

21. Morquio syndrome (mucopolysaccharidosis IV)

22. Myotonic dystrophy (Curschmann-Stewart syndrome)

23. Naffziger syndrome (scalenus anticus syndrome)

24. Pancoast syndrome (superior pulmonary sulcus syndrome)

25. Parkinsonism (shaking palsy)

26. Psychogenic diseases, such as schizophrenia, dementia precox, or hysteria

27. Refsum syndrome (phytanic acid storage disease)

28. Retroparotid space syndrome (Villaret syndrome)

29. Romberg syndrome (facial hemiatrophy)

30. Spider bites

31. Stormorken's syndrome (thrombocytopathia bleeding tendency)

32. Tetanus (lockjaw)

33. von Herrenschwand syndrome (sympathetic heterochromia)

34. Wallenberg syndrome (dorsolateral medullary syndrome)

35. Wernicke syndrome (avitaminosis B_1, thiamine deficiency)

Fraunfelder, F.T.: Drug-Induced Ocular Side Effects and Drug Interactions. 4th Ed. Philadelphia, Williams & Wilkins, 1996.

Roy, F.H.: Ocular Syndromes and Systemic Diseases. 2nd Ed. Philadelphia, W.B. Saunders, 1989.

Sjaastad, O.: The hereditary syndrome of thrombocytopathia, bleeding tendency extreme miosis, muscular fatigue, asplenia, headache, etc. (Stormorken's syndrome). Headache. 34:221–225, 1994.

Paradoxical Pupillary Reaction (Constricts when Light is Withdrawn)

  1. Best's disease

*2. Congenital achromatopsia

*3. Congenital stationary night blindness

* = most important

4. Leber's congenital amaurosis

5. Optic nerve hypoplasia

6. Retinitis pigmentosa

Barricks, M.E., et al.: Paradoxical pupillary responses in congenital stationary night blindness. Arch. Ophthalmol. 95:1800–1804, 1977.

Flynn, J.T., et al.: Paradoxical pupil in congenital achromatopsia. Int Ophthalmol. 2:91–96, 1981.

Frank, J.W., et al.: Paradoxic pupillary phenomena. Arch Ophthalmol. 106:1564, 1988.

Absence or Decrease of Pupillary Reaction to Light

Absence or decreased pupillary reaction to light caused by drugs, including:

acetaminophen	carbenicillin(?)
acetanilid	carbinoxamine
acetophenazine	carbon dioxide
alcohol	carbromal
allobarbital	carisoprodol
alprazolam	carmustine
amitriptyline	carphenazine
amobarbital	chloramphenicol
amoxapine	chlorcyclizine
amoxicillin	chlordiazepoxide
amphetamine	chlorpheniramine
ampicillin	chlorphenoxamine
antazoline	chlorpromazine
antimony lithium thiomalate	chlorprothixene
antimony potassium tartrate	cholecalciferol
antimony sodium tartrate	cimetidine
antimony sodium thioglycollate	clemastine
aprobarbital	clomipramine
aspirin	clonazepam
atropine	clonidine
baclofen	clorazepate
barbital	cloxacillin(?)
belladonna	cocaine
benztropine	cyclizine
biperiden	cyclobarbital
bromide	cyclopentobarbital
bromisovalum	cycrimine
brompheniramine	desipramine
butabarbital	dexbrompheniramine
butalbital	dexchlorpheniramine
butallylonal	dextroamphetamine
butethal	diacetylmorphine
calcitriol	diazepam

dicloxacillin(?)

diethazine

dimethindene

diphtheria toxoid adsorbed

doxepin

doxylamine

diphenhydramine

diphenylpyraline

emetine

ergocalciferol

ergot

ethopropazine

fenfluramine

fluphenazine

flurazepam

glutethimide

halazepam

heptabarbital

hetacillin(?)

hexachlorophene

hexethal

hexobarbital

homatropine

imipramine

insulin

isocarboxazid

isoniazid

lidocaine

lorazepam

meclizine

meperidine

mephobarbital

meprobamate

mesoridazine

mescaline

methamphetamine

methaqualone

metharbital

methdilazine

methicillin(?)

methitural

methohexital

methotrimeprazine

methyl alcohol

methyprylon

midazolam

nafcillin(?)

neomycin

nialamide

nitrazepam

nortriptyline

orphenadrine

oxacillin(?)

oxazepam

pargyline

pentylenetetrazol

pentobarbital

perazine

periciazine

perphenazine

phenacetin

phencyclidine

phenelzine

pheniramine

phenmetrazine

phenobarbital

phenylpropanolamine

phenytoin

piperacetazine

prazepam

primidone

probarbital

prochlorperazine

procyclidine

promazine

promethazine

propantheline

propiomazine

protriptyline

psilocybin

pyrilamine

quinine

scopolamine

secobarbital

sodium antimonylgluconate

sodium salicylate

stibocaptate	triazolam
stibogluconate	trichloroethylene
stibophen	trifluoperazine
talbutal	triflupromazine
temazepam	trihexyphenidyl
tetanus immune globulin	trimeprazine
tetanus toxoid	trimipramine
thiamylal	tripelennamine
thiethylperazine	triprolidine
thiopental	urethan
thiopropazate	vinbarbital
thioproperazine	vitamin D
thioridazine	vitamin D_2
thiothixene	vitamin D_3
tranylcypromine	

Fraunfelder, F.T.: Drug-Induced Ocular Side Effects and Drug Interactions. 4th Ed. Philadelphia, Williams & Wilkins, 1996.

Anisocoria (An Inequality of Pupils of One Millimeter or Greater)

1. Central nervous system

    *A. Adie (tonic) pupil

    B. Aneurysm of the aorta or carotid artery

    C. Cerebrovascular accidents

    D. Cervical rib (ipsilateral constricted pupil)

    E. Encephalitis (mild cases)

    *F. Horner syndrome (cervical sympathetic paralysis syndrome)

    G. Pontine lesions

    H. Tabes dorsalis

    I. Third-nerve paresis

    J. Trigeminal neuralgia (tic douloureux)

    K. Wernicke hemianopic pupil

2. Drugs, including:

alcohol	clemastine	ethchlorvynol	methaqualone
antazoline	dexbrompheniramine	etidocaine	nialamide
bromide	dexchlorpheniramine	jimsonweed	oral contraceptives
bromisovalum	diacetylmorphine	hashish	phenelzine
brompheniramine	dimethindene	isocarboxazid	pheniramine
bupivacaine	diphenhydramine	lidocaine	phenylpropanolamine
carbinoxamine	diphenylpyraline	lysergide	prilocaine
carbromal	disulfiram	marijuana	procaine
chloroprocaine	doxylamine	mepivacaine	propoxycaine
chlorpheniramine	dronabinol	mescaline	psilocybin

pyrilamine   tetrahydrocannabinol   trichloroethylene   triprolidine
scopolamine   tranylcypromine   tripelennamine

3. Ocular conditions

    A. Artificial eye (pseudoanisocoria)

    B. Cornea such as keratitis or abrasion

    C. Glaucoma including pigmentary dispersion

  *D. Iris, such as iritis, synechiae, iris atrophy, or iris sphincter rupture

    E. Ocular trauma

    F. Spastic miosis

4. Physiologic

    A. Anisometropia—larger pupil with the more myopic eye

    B. Familial

    C. Lateral illumination of one eye gives more miosis in that eye than in the other

    D. Nonfamilial—normal variation (small percentage of the population)

    E. Tournay reaction—with the eyes turned sharply to the side, dilatation of the pupil of the abducting eye and miosis of pupil of the adducting eye

6. Unilateral miosis (see p. 394)

7. Unilateral mydriasis (see p. 386)

Cheng, M.M. and Catalano, R.A.: Fatigue-induced familial anisocoria. Am J Ophthalmol. 109:480–481, 1990.

Feibel, R.M., and Perlmutter, J.C.: Anisocoria in the pigmentary dispersion syndrome. Am J Ophthalmol. 111:384, 1991.

Fraunfelder, F.T.: Drug-Induced Ocular Side Effects and Drug Interactions. 4th Ed. Philadelphia, Williams & Wilkins, 1996.

Nakagawa, T.A., et al.: Aerosolized atropine as an unusual cause of anisocoria in a child with asthma. Pediatric Emergency Care. 9:153–154, 1993.

Slamovits, T.I., et al.: Intracranial oculomotor nerve paresis with anisocoria and pupillary parasympathetic hypersensitivity. Am J Ophthalmol., 104:401–406, 1987.

Irregularity of Pupil (Including Oval or Peaked Pupil)

1. Adherent leukoma as one part of iris is pulled up to corneal scar, peripheral anterior synechiae, or corneal laceration with prolapse of iris

2. Anterior chamber intraocular lens that is too long or erodes into uveal tissue

3. Argyll-Robertson pupil—small and irregular; reacts better to accommodation than to light; same type as seen in diabetic patients (pseudodiabetic pupil)

4. Congenital coloboma of the iris, usually below

5. Following laser iridectomy

6. Glaucoma—oval, dilated pupil

*7. Injury of the iris

8. Iris tuck of anterior chamber intraocular lens

*9. Iritis—usually small but pupil may be any shape with anterior or posterior synechiae

*10. Long-term intraocular inflammation

* = most important

11. Medication, with faster reaction of one sector of iris than of another—miosis or mydriasis

12. Operation—as sector iridectomy or peripheral iridectomy

13. Optic atrophy due to causes such as syphilis, quinine poisoning and internal ophthalmoplegia of vascular or traumatic origin

14. Piece of anterior capsule into anterior chamber

15. Posterior chamber intraocular lens with loop of intraocular lens holding the midportion of iris peripherally

16. Posterior chamber lens with two haptics having the lens either behind the pupil with the haptics in front or having the lens anterior to the pupil with the haptics behind the iris

17. Segmental iris atrophy

18. Tumors of iris or ciliary body

19. Vitreous or zonules into corneal laceration

20. Vitreous strand from behind pupil to wound

21. Wound leak with or without iris prolapse

Moster, M.R., et al.: Laser iridectomy. Ophthalmology, 93:20–24, 1986.

Newell, F.W.: Ophthalmology, Principles and Concepts. 7th Ed. St. Louis, C.V. Mosby, 1991.

Reidy, J.J., et al.: An analysis of semiflexible, closed-loop anterior chamber intraocular lenses. Am. Intraocular Implant Soc. J., 11:344–352, 1985.

Hippus (Visible, Rhythmic but Irregular Pupillary Oscillations, Deliberate in Time, and Two Millimeters or More Excursions; No Localizing Significance)

1. Normal

2. Incipient cataracts

3. Central nervous system diseases, including: presence of total third cranial nerve palsy, hemiplegia, meningitis (acute), cerebral syphilis, tabes and general paralysis, myasthenia gravis, tumors of corpora quadrigemina, epileptics, Cheyne-Strokes breathing, multiple sclerosis (disseminated sclerosis) and cerebral tumors

4. Neurasthenia (nervous exhaustion, Beard disease)

5. Drugs, including:

allobarbital	butethal	metharbital	probarbital
amobarbital	cyclobarbital	methitural	secobarbital
aprobarbital	cyclopentobarbital	methohexital	talbutal
barbital	heptabarbital	pentobarbital	thiamylal
butabarbital	hexethal	pentylenetetrazol	thiopental
butalbital	hexobarbital	phenobarbital	vinbarbital
butallylonal	mephobarbital	primidone	

Fraunfelder, F.T.: Drug-Induced Ocular Side Effects and Drug Interactions. 4th Ed. Philadelphia, Williams & Wilkins, 1996.

Zinn, K.M.: The Pupil. Springfield, Ill., Charles C Thomas, 1972.

Tonohaptic Pupil (Long Latent Period Preceding Both Contraction to Light and Redilatation Followed in Each Instance by a Short but Prompt Movement)

1. Catatonic state
2. Diabetes mellitus (Willis disease)
3. Diabetes insipidus
4. Dystrophia adiposogenitalis (Frohlich syndrome) or pituitary cachexia (Simmond disease)
5. Introverted persons of the schizophrenic group
6. Parkinsonism (shaking palsy)
7. Pigmentary retinal dystrophy
8. Postencephalitic condition
9. Schizoid state

Duke-Elder, S., and Scott, G.I.: System of Ophthalmology, Vol. 12. St. Louis, C.V. Mosby, 1971.

Leukokoria (White Pupil) (See Lesions Confused with Retinoblastoma, p. 556)

1. Angiomatosis of retina (cercbelloretinal hemangioblastomatosis)
2. Astrocytoma
*3. Cataract (congenital)
4. Choroidal hemangioma
*5. Coats disease (retinal telangiectasia)
6. Coloboma of choroid and optic disc
7. Congenital cytomegalovirus retinitis
8. Congenital retinal detachment
9. Exudative retinitis, chorioretinitis, or both
10. Falciform fold of retina
11. Herpes simplex retinitis
12. High myopia with advanced chorioretinal degeneration
*13. Medullation of nerve fiber layer
14. Metastatic endophthalmitis
15. Morning glory syndrome (hereditary central glial anomaly of the optic disc)
16. Nematode endophthalmitis (Toxocara canis)
17. Norrie disease (atrophia oculi congenita)
*18. Ocular toxocariasis
19. Organized vitreous hemorrhage
20. Persistent hyperplastic primary vitreous
21. Retinal dysplasia (massive retinal fibrosis)
*22. Retinoblastoma
23. Retinopathy of prematurity (ROP)
24. Retrolental membrane associated with Bloch-Sulzberger syndrome (incontinentia pigmenti)

* = most important

Leukokoria (White Pupil)

	Cataract	Nematode Endophthalmitis	Coats Disease*	Persistent Hyperplastic Primary Vitreous*	Retrolental Fibroplasia	Retinal Dysplasia	Organized Vitreous Hemorrhage	Falciform Fold of Retina	Angiomatosis of Retina	Bloch-Sulzberger Syndrome	Exudative Retinitis	Diktyoma	Congenital Retinal Detachment	Norrie Disease	Juvenile Retinoschisis	Metastatic Endophthalmitis	Retinoblastoma*	Coloboma of Choroid	Medullation Nerve Layer	Traumatic Chorioretinitis	High Myopia with Retinal Degeneration
History																					
1. Bilateral	S	R	R	S	S	S	R	S	S	S		R		U	U	S	S	S	R		U
2. Congenital	U		S	U		U		U	R	U			U	U	U		U	U	U		U
3. More in females										U											
4. More in males			S											U	U		R				
5. Occurs during first decade			U																		
6. Occurs from birth to 2 years of age	U	U		U	U	U		U		U		U	U	U	U	U	S	U	U	U	
7. Occurs during second and third decades									U												
8. Occurs during third to fifth decades																			U		U
9. Ocular trauma	S							S												U	
10. Oxygen therapy					S																
11. Prematurity				S	U																
Physical Findings																					
1. Angiomatosis of iris									S												
2. Chorioretinitis							S				U					U				U	
3. Ciliary body tumor												U									
4. Dark macular spot																					U
5. Endophthalmitis		U														U					
6. Myopic crescent																					U
7. Foveal retinoschisis															U						
8. Glaucoma	S	S	S	S	R			S									S				
9. Iris tumor												U									
10. Lid ecchymosis																R					
11. Microphthalmia			U	U			S	S								U			S		
12. Nystagmus	S		S		U						S			S		S	R	S			
13. Optic atrophy											S										
14. Optic neuritis											S										
15. Orbital mass												S				R					
16. Papilledema																					S
17. Persistent hyaloid vessel				S			S	U													
18. Phthisis bulbi			S	S				S		S	S				U		S				
19. Pigmented retinopathy											U										
20. Retinal detachment	S	U	S	U	S	S	S	S			S		U	U	S		S			S	S
21. Retinal folds						U							S								
22. Retinal hemorrhage	S	U					S	U	S	U											
23. Retrolental mass			U	U			U	U	U		U	U		U		U	S				
24. Ruptures in Bruch membrane																				U	U
25. Soft retinal exudates		R	S								S										

Leukokoria (White Pupil) *Continued*

	Cataract	Nematode Endophthalmitis	Coats Disease*	Persistent Hyperplastic Primary Vitreous*	Retrolental Fibroplasia	Retinal Dysplasia	Organized Vitreous Hemorrhage	Falciform Fold of Retina	Angiomatosis of Retina	Bloch-Sulzberger Syndrome	Exudative Retinitis	Diktyoma	Congenital Retinal Detachment	Norrie Disease	Juvenile Retinoschisis	Metastatic Endophthalmitis	Retinoblastoma*	Coloboma of Choroid	Medullation Nerve Layer	Traumatic Chorioretinitis	High Myopia with Retinal Degeneration
Physical Findings																					
26. Solitary, elevated, and rounded macular lesions		U															R				
27. Strabismus	U	U		S	U		U		S	S			S		S		S	R			
28. Telangiectatic retinal vessels			U				R		S												
29. Uveitis		U	S	S			S	S	S		S					U					
30. Vitreous hemorrhage		S	S		R		U								S		U				
31. Vitreous veils															U						
Laboratory Data																					
1. Blood eosinophilia		U																			
2. Electroretinogram abnormal					S	S									U						
3. Fluorescein angiography		U	U		R	S	S	U	U		U				U		R	U	U	U	U
4. Ocular ultrasonography	U	U	U	U	U		U		S	U		U	U	U		U	U				S
5. Orbital roentgenogram							U										U				

R = rarely; S = sometimes; and U = usually.

* = most important

*25. Toxoplasmosis (congenital)

26. Traumatic chorioretinitis

27. Tumors other than retinoblastoma

    A. Choroidal hemangioma

    B. Combined retinal hamartoma

    C. Diktyoma

    D. Glioneuroma

    E. Leukemia

    F. Medulloepithelioma

    G. Retinal astrocytic hamartoma

    H. Retinal capillary hemangioma

28. Uveitis (peripheral)

29. Vitreous organization following unsuspected penetrating wounds

Abramson, D.H., et al.: The management of unilateral retinoblastoma without primary enucleation. Arch. Ophthalmol., 100:1249, 1982.

Enyedi, L.B., et al.: Ultrastructural study of Norrie's disease. Am. J. Ophthalmol., 111:439–445, 1991.

Federman, J.L., et al.: The surgical and nonsurgical management of persistent hyperplastic primary vitreous. Ophthalmology. 89:20, 1982.

Roy, F.H.: Ocular Syndromes and Systemic Diseases. 2nd Ed. Philadelphia, W.B. Saunders, 1989.

Shapiro, D.R., and Stone, R.D.: Ultrasonic characteristics of retinopathy of prematurity presenting with leukokoria. Arch Ophthalmol., 103:1690–1694, 1985.

Shields, J.A., et al.: Malignant teratoid medulloepithelioma of the ciliary body simulating persistent hyperplastic primary vitreous. Am J Ophthalmol. 107:296–300, 1989.

Long Ciliary Processes Extending into Dilated Pupillary Space

1. Aniridia

2. Anterior rotation of ciliary processes

    A. After scleral buckling operation

    B. Angle closure

    C. Anterior choroidal separation

    D. Cyst or tumor behind iris

    E. Dislocated lens

    F. From adherence to limbal scar

    G. Plateau iris

3. Extreme mydriasis

4. Falciform detachment of the retina

5. Incontinentia pigmenti (Bloch-Sulzberger syndrome)

6. Norrie disease (atrophia oculi congenita)

7. Persistent hyperplastic primary vitreous (PHPV)

8. Retinal dysplasia of Reese

9. Retrolental fibroplasia (RLF)

10. Surgical coloboma

11. Trisomy 13 (trisomy D)

Epstein, D.L.: Chandler & Grant's Glaucoma. 3rd Ed. Philadelphia, Lea & Febiger, 1986.

Hansen, A.C.: Norrie's disease. Am. J. Ophthalmol., 66:320–332, 1963.

Persistent Pupillary Membrane

1. Fetal iritis

2. Hereditary

3. Physiologic

*4. Use of oxygen therapy in premature nursery

Hornblass, A.: Persistent pupillary membrane and oxygen therapy in premature infants. Ann. Ophthalmol., 3:95–99, 1971.

Decentered Pupillary Light Reflex

1. Positive angle kappa—pseudoexotropia

2. Negative angle kappa—pseudoesotropia

*3. Eccentric fixation—deep unilateral amblyopia

*4. Ectopic macula—macular displacement by retinal scarring or strands, such as retrolental fibroplasia

5. Ectopic pupil

Beyer-Machule, C., and Noorden, G.K., von: Atlas of Ophthalmic Surgery: Vol 1: Lids, Orbits, Extraocular Muscles. New York, Thieme Med Pub., 1984.

Pupillary Block Following Cataract Extraction

1. Air pupillary block

2. Dense, impermeable anterior hyaloid membrane

3. Free vitreous block

4. Intraocular lens effectively closing off pupil and iridectomies

5. Leaky wound

6. Nonperforating iridectomy

7. Posterior vitreous detachment associated with pooling or retrovitreal aqueous

8. Postoperative iridocyclitis

9. Subchoroidal hemorrhage

10. Swollen lens material behind the iris

Tomey, K.F., and Traverso, C.E.: Neodymium-YAG laser posterior capsulotomy for the treatment of aphakic and pseudophakic pupillary block. Am. J. Ophthalmol., 104:502–507, 1987.

Afferent Pupillary Defect (Pupil of Eye with Diminished Vision from Disease of Retina or Optic Nerve Will Fail to React Directly to Light but Will Constrict Consensually when the Healthy Eye Is Stimulated)

1. Amblyopia (rare)

2. Branch retinal artery/vein occlusion

* = most important

3. Central retinal artery/vein occlusion

4. Diabetic retinopathy (severe)

5. Hyphema

6. Macular degeneration (rarely)

7. Neovascular glaucoma

*8. Optic neuritis

*9. Optic nerve lesion

10. Radiation

11. Reticulum cell sarcoma

12. Retinal detachment

13. Toxoplasma retinochoroiditis

14. Traumatic optic neuropathy and retinopathy

15. Unilateral optic nerve hypoplasia

Browning, D.J., and Tiedeman, J.S.: The test light affects quantitation of the afferent pupillary defect. Ophthalmology, 94:53–55, 1987.

Burde, R.M., et al.: Clinical Decisions in Neuro-ophthalmology. 2nd Ed. St. Louis, C.V. Mosby, 1991.

Striph, G.G., et al.: Afferent pupillary defect caused by hyphema. Am. J. Ophthalmol., 106:352–353, 1988.

* = most important

Iris

KENNETH GOINS

Contents

Aniridia (Absence of Iris, Partial or Complete)

1. AGR triad-sporadic (bilateral or unilateral) aniridia, genitourinary abnormalities, and mental retardation
2. Associated ocular findings
   A. Cataracts
   B. Corneal dystrophy
   C. Ectopia lentis
   D. Glaucoma
   *E. Macular aplasia—autosomal dominant
   F. Microcornea and subluxated lenses
   G. Nystagmus
   H. Optic nerve hypoplasia
   I. Photophobia
   J. Poor foveal reflex
   *K. Strabismus
3. Associated with autosomal recessive inheritance with fully developed macula
4. Associated with unilateral renal agenesis and psychomotor retardation
5. Beckwith-Wiedemann syndrome
6. Deletion of short arm of eleventh chromosome
7. Gillespie syndrome (incomplete aniridia, cerebellar ataxia and oligophrenia)
8. Homocystinuria syndrome
9. Marinesco-Sjögren syndrome (congenital spinocerebellar ataxia)
10. Miller syndrome (Wilms aniridia syndrome)
11. Partial trisomy 2q
12. Peters syndrome (oculodental syndrome)
13. Rieger syndrome (dysgenesis mesostromalis)
14. Ring chromosome 6
15. Scaphocephaly syndrome
16. Siemens syndrome (anhidrotic ectodermal dysplasia)
*17. Traumatic
18. Ullrich syndrome (dyscraniopygophalangy)

Green, D.M., et al.: Screening of children with hemihypertrophy, aniridia and Beckwith-Wiedemann syndrome in patients with Wilms tumor: a report from the National Wilms Tumor Study. Medical & Pediatric Oncology. 21: 188–192, 1993.

Nelson, I.B., et al.: Aniridia: A review. Surv Ophthalmol., 28:621–642, 1984.

Pearce, W.G.: Variability of iris defects in autosomal dominant aniridia. Canadian J Ophthalmol., 29: 25–29, 1994.

Roy, F.H.: Ocular Syndromes and Systemic Diseases. 2nd Ed. Philadelphia, W.B. Saunders, 1989.

Coloboma of Iris (Failure of Fusions of Fetal Fissure in Optic Vesicle, Usually Inferior or Inferonasal)

1. Acroreno-ocular syndrome
2. Aicardi syndrome

3. Aniridia

4. Biemond syndrome

5. Cat eye syndrome (partial G-trisomy syndrome)

6. CHARGE association (coloboma, heart anomaly, choanal atresia, retardation, genital and ear anomalies)

7. Chromosome partial short-arm deletion syndrome

8. Ellis-van Crefeld syndrome (chondroectodermal dysplasia)

9. Epidermal nevus syndrome (ichthyosis hystrix)

10. Focal dermal hypoplasia syndrome (Goltz syndrome)

11. Hallermann-Streiff-François syndrome (dyscephalic mandibulooculo facial syndrome)

12. Hemifacial microsoma syndrome (otomandibular dysostosis)

*13. Hereditary usually dominant may be recessive

14. Hurler syndrome (mucopolysaccharidoses I)

15. Hyperchromic heterochromia

16. Jeune disease (asphyxiating thoracic dystrophy)

17. Joubert syndrome

18. Kartagener syndrome

19. Klinefelter syndrome

20. Klippel-Trenaunay-Weber syndrome (angio-osteohypertrophy syndrome)

21. Langer-Giedion syndrome

22. Lanzieri syndrome

23. Laurence-Moon-Bardet-Biedl syndrome (retinitis pigmentosapolydactyly-adiposogenital syndrome)

*24. Marfan syndrome (dolichostenomelia-arachnodactyly-hyperchondroplasia-dystrophia mesodermalis congenita)

25. Maternal use of thalidomide

26. Maternal vitamin A deficiency

27. Meckel syndrome

28. Median facial cleft syndrome

29. Microphthalmos syndrome (Meyer-Schwickerath and Weyers syndrome)

30. Nevoid basal cell carcinoma syndrome

31. Nevus sebaceous of Jadassohn (linear sebaceous nevus syndrome of Jadassohn)

32. Obesity-cerebral-ocular-skeletal anomalies syndrome

33. Oculoauriculovertebral dysplasia syndrome

34. Otomandibular dysostosis (hemifacial microsomia syndrome)

35. Partial deletion of group D chromosome

36. Rieger syndrome (dysgenesis mesodermalis corneae et irides)

37. Retinal dysplasia

38. Rubinstein-Taybi syndrome (broad thumbs syndrome)

*39. Sporadic

* = most important

40. Treacher Collins syndrome (Franceschetti syndrome)
41. Trisomy *13* (D trisomy) (Patau syndrome)
42. Trisomy 17-syndrome (Edward syndrome)
43. Turner syndrome
44. Warburg syndrome
45. White Spone naevus
46. Wolf syndrome (monosomy partial syndrome)
47. 11q syndrome
48. 13q syndrome
49. 13r syndrome
50. 18q syndrome
51. 18r syndrome

Bard, L.A.: Genetic counseling of families with Marfan syndrome and other disorders showing a marfanoid body habitus. Ophthalmology, 86:1764, 1980.

Isenberg, S.J.: The Eye in Infancy. Chicago, Year Book Medical Publishers, 1989.

Roy, F.H.: Ocular Syndromes and Systemic Diseases. 2nd Ed. Philadelphia, W.B. Saunders, 1989.

Rubeosis Iridis (Neovascularization [Newly Formed Blood Vessels] on Iris)

1. Proximal vascular disease
   A. Aortic arch syndrome (pulseless disease; Takayasu syndrome)
   B. Carotid-cavernous fistula (carotid artery syndrome)
   C. Carotid ligation
   D. Carotid occlusive disease
   E. Cranial arteritis syndrome (giant-cell arteritis)

2. Ocular vascular disease
   *A. Central retinal artery thrombosis (see p. 512)
   *B. Central retinal vein thrombosis (see p. 525)
   C. Long posterior ciliary artery occlusion
   D. Reversed flow through the ophthalmic artery

3. Retinal diseases
   A. Coats disease (retinal telangiectasia)
   *B. Diabetes mellitus
   C. Eales disease (periphlebitis)
   D. Glaucoma, chronic
   E. Melanoma of choroid
   F. Norrie disease (oligophrenia-microphthalmos syndrome)
   G. Persistent hyperplastic primary vitreous
   H. Retinal detachment
   I. Retinal hemangioma
   J. Retinoblastoma

    K. Retrolental fibroplasia

    L. Sickle cell disease (Herrick syndrome)

4. Iris tumors

    A. Hemangioma

    B. Melanoma

    C. Metastatic carcinoma

5. Postinflammatory

    A. Argon laser coreoplasty

    B. Exfoliation syndrome

    C. Fibrinoid syndrome

    D. Fungal endophthalmitis (see p. 255)

    E. Iris neovascularization with pseudoexfoliation

    F. Radiation

    G. Retinal detachment operation

    H. Uveitis, chronic

6. Vascular tufts at the pupillary margin

    A. Cataract

    B. Diabetes mellitus

    C. Myotonic dystrophy syndrome (myotonia atrophica syndrome)

    D. Ocular hypotony

    E. Respiratory failure

Ringvold, A., and Davanger, M.: Iris neovascularization in eyes with pseudoexfoliation syndrome. Br J Ophthalmol., 65:138–141, 1981.

Roy, F.H.: Ocular Syndromes and Systemic Diseases. 2nd Ed. Philadelphia, W.B. Saunders, 1989.

Sassani, J.W., et al.: Massively invasive diffuse choroidal melanoma. Arch Ophthalmol., 103:945–948, 1956.

Ulbig, M.R., et al.: Anterior Hyaloidal Fibrovascular Proliferation after Extracapsular cataract Extraction in Diabetic Eye. Am J Ophthalmol., 115; 321–326, 1993.

Hyperemia of Iris (Dilatation of Pre-existing Vessels of Iris)

    1. Corneal ulcer

    2. Foreign body on the cornea

    3. Injury, intraocular

 *4. Iridocyclitis

 *5. Iritis

    6. Scleritis

 *7. Uveitis

O'Brien, C.S.: Ophthalmology: Notes for Students. Iowa City, Athens Press, 1930.

* = most important

Hyperchromic Heterochromia (Abnormal eye with iris of darker color than fellow eye)

	Siderosis	Malignant Melanoma of Iris	Neurofibromatosis	Klein-Wardenburg Syndrome	Bremer's Status Dysraphicus	Rubeosis Iridis
History						
1. Activated at puberty, during pregnancy or menopause			U			
2. Carotid artery insufficiency						S
3. Central retinal vein or artery occlusion						S
4. Diabetic retinopathy						S
5. Family or sporadic occurrence		R			U	
6. Hereditary			U	U		
7. Intraocular iron or steel foreign body	U					
8. Pigmented mass on iris		U	S			
Physical Findings						
1. Anterior chamber depth variations			U			R
2. Blepharophimosis				U		
3. Blue irides				U		
4. "Cafe au lait" spots in fundus			S			
5. Cataract	S		U		S	
6. Cells and flare	U	S				
7. Corneal edema	S					S
8. Corneal neovascularization	S					
9. Decreased visual acuity	S	S		S		S
10. Dyschromatopsia	S					
11. Ectropion uvea		S				U
12. Elephantiasis of the lids			U			
13. Enophthalmos					U	
14. Fibrovascular membrane on anterior iris and chamber angle						U
15. Fleischer's ring	U					
16. Glaucoma	R	S	R	U		U
17. Hamartoma of retina			R			
18. Hypertelorism				U		
19. Hypertrichosis				U		
20. Hyphema		S				S
21. Hypopyon	U					S
22. Hudson-Stalhi line on cornea	U					
23. Interstitial keratitis	S					
24. Iridoplegia	S					S
25. Keratitis					S	
26. Lens luxation or subluxation	S					
27. Macular edema	S					
28. Miosis					S	
29. Narrowing of palpebral fissure					S	
30. Neurofibroma of the choroid, iris, lids and ciliary body			U			
31. Night blindness	S					
32. Nodular swelling of corneal nerves			U			
33. Nystagmus						
34. Ocular hypotony					S	
35. Optic atrophy			S		S	

Hyperchromic Heterochromia (Abnormal eye with iris of darker color than fellow eye) *Continued*

	Siderosis	Malignant Melanoma of Iris	Neurofibromatosis	Klein-Wardenburg Syndrome	Bremer's Status Dysraphicus	Rubeosis Iridis
Physical Findings						
36. Optic nerve glioma			S			
37. Papilledema					S	
38. Paresis of ocular muscles					S	
39. Phthisis bulbi	S					
40. Prominent episcleral vessels		S				
41. Proptosis			U			
42. Pulsation of the globe			U			
43. Pupillary distortion	R	S				
44. Ptosis			U		U	
45. Retinal detachment	S					
46. Rusty discoloration of conjunctiva	U					
47. Subconjunctival hemorrhage	S					
48. Synechiae	S	R				U
49. Uveitis	U	S				S
Lab Data						
1. B scan	S	U	U			
2. CT scan	S		U			
3. X ray	U					

R = Rarely; U = Usually; S = Sometimes

Hypochromic Heterochromia (Abnormal eye with iris of lighter color than the fellow eye)

	Horner's Syndrome	Fuch's Heterochromia	Posner-Schlossman Syndrome	Parry-Romberg's Syndrome	Chediak-Higashi Syndrome	Klein-Waardenberg's Syndrome	Bremer's Status Dysraphicus
History							
1. Familial							U
2. Greater in children	U						
3. Greater 20 to 50 years old			U	U			
4. Hereditary				U	U	U	
5. Lesion in the pons, cervical cord or hypothalmus							
6. Mild infective cyclitis		S	S				
7. Occurs in albinoid siblings born of consanguineous parents					U		
8. Paralysis of cervical sympathetic	S						
9. Photophobia					U		
Physical Findings							
1. Absence of nasal portion of eyebrows					S		
2. Blephanophimosis						U	
3. Blue iris						U	
4. Cataracts					S		S
5. Cells and flare in anterior chamber							
6. Corneal anesthesia							
7. Choroiditis		R					
8. Decreased pigmentation in choroid					S		
9. Elevated disc					S		
10. Enophthalmos	U			U			U
11. Epithelial corneal edema		S	U				
12. Glaucoma			U				
13. Glaucomatous cupping			R				
14. Hypertelorism						U	
15. Hypertrichosis							S
16. Hypotony							
17. Keratic precipitates			U				U
18. Keratitis					U		U
19. Miosis							
20. Mydriasis							
21. Narrowness and decreased number of retinal vessels					U		
22. Nystagmus					S		S
23. Oculocutaneous albinism							
24. Optic atrophy							S
25. Outer canthus lower than inner					S		
26. Papilledema					S		
27. Paresis of ocular muscles					S		
28. Ptosis	U			U			U
29. Vitreous opacities		S					

R = rarely; S = sometimes; and U = usually.

Heterochromia (Difference of Color between Two Irides)

1. Hypochromic heterochromia—abnormal eye with iris of lighter color than that of the fellow eye
    - A. Anemia with unilateral iritis
    - B. Chediak-Higashi syndrome (anomalous leukocytic inclusions with constitutional stigmata)
    - *C. Congenital, sporadic, and/or familial
    - D. Conradi syndrome (epiphyseal congenital dysplasia)
    - E. Fuchs syndrome (I) (heterochromic cyclitis syndrome)
    - F. Gansslen syndrome (familial hemolytic icterus)
    - G. Glaucomatocyclitic crisis (Posner-Schlossman syndrome)
    - *H. Horner syndrome (cervical sympathetic paralysis syndrome)
    - I. Hypomelanosis of Ito syndrome (incontinentia pigmenti achromiens)
    - J. Infiltration of nonpigmented tumor into iris
    - *K. Iris atrophy (diffuse and unilateral), including that because of trauma, inflammation, or senility
    - L. Parry-Romberg syndrome (facial hemiatrophy)
    - M. Status dysraphicus syndrome (Bremer syndrome)
    - N. Tuberous sclerosis hypopigmented iris spot (Bourneville syndrome)
    - O. Waardenburg-Klein syndrome (embryonic fixation syndrome)
2. Hyperchromic heterochromia—abnormal eye with iris of darker color than that of the fellow eye
    - A. Anterior or posterior chamber hemorrhage, prolonged
    - B. Coloboma
    - *C. Congenital, sporadic, and/or familial
    - D. Embryonic fixation syndrome (Waardenburg-Klein syndrome)
    - E. Incontinenta pigmenti (Bloch-Sulzberger syndrome)
    - F. Iris abscess
    - G. Malignant melanoma of the iris or other pigmented tumors of the iris
    - H. Microcornea (see p. 291)
    - I. Monocular melanosis in which there are excess chromatophores in the stroma of the iris (melanosis bulbi)
    - *J. Neovascular, such as rubeosis iridis or hyperemia of iris, unilateral (see p. 412 or p. 413)
    - K. Neurofibromatosis (von Recklinghausen syndrome)
    - *L. Nevi of iris
    - M. Perforating injuries or contusion of the globe occurring before the subject is years of age
    - N. Retention of intraocular iron foreign body-siderosis
    - O. Severe contusion with hypertrophy of the superficial layers of the stroma of the iris
    - P. Status dysraphicus (Bremer syndrome)

* = most important

3. Dark central pupillary margin, pale pigment around its circumference
    A. Hereditary osteo-onychodysplasia
    B. Normal iris

Diesenhouse, M.C., et al: Acquired Heterochromia with Horner Syndrome in Two Adults. Ophthalmology. 99:1815–1817, 1992.

Gutman, I., et al.: Hypopigmented iris spot. Ophthalmology, 89:1155, 1982.

Isenberg, S.J.: The Eye in Infancy. Chicago, Year Book Medical Publishers, 1989.

Monteiro, M.L.R., et al.: Iron mydriasis. Am J Ophthalmol., 97:794–795, 1984.

Newell, F.W.: Ophthalmology, Principles and Concepts. 7th Ed. St. Louis, C.V. Mosby, 1991.

Roy, F.H.: Ocular Syndromes and Systemic Diseases. 2nd Ed. Philadelphia, W.B. Saunders, 1989.

Iris Atrophy

1. Anterior segment ischemia syndrome
2. Arteriovenous fistula
3. Chandler syndrome (iridocorneal endothelial syndrome)
4. Complication of light coagulation and beta radiation
5. Complication of retinal detachment operation
*6. Congenital—autosomal dominant
7. Crohn disease (granulomatous ileocolitis)
*8. Essential (progressive) atrophy
9. Glaucomatous atrophy
    A. Acute—atrophy and/or iridoschisis
    *B. Chronic—stromal and epithelial
10. Hallermann-Streiff-François syndrome (dyscephalic mandibulooculo facial syndrome)
11. Hilding syndrome (destructive iridocyclitis and multiple joint dislocations)
12. Homocystinuria syndrome
13. Hypothermal injury
14. Iris-nevus syndrome (Cogan-Reese syndrome)
15. Ischemia
    A. Acute angle closure glaucoma
    B. Carotid-cavernous fistula
    C. Hemoglobin sickle cell C disease
    D. Occlusive artery disease
    E. Orbital irritation
    F. Surgery angle closure glaucoma
    *G. Trauma
16. Krause syndrome (congenital encephalo-ophthalmic dysplasia)
17. Neurogenic-tabes with stromal atrophy
18. Norrie disease (fetal iritis syndrome)
*19. Old age
20. Pierre-Robin syndrome (micrognathia-glossoptosis syndrome)

21. Posterior pigment layer is swollen and degenerated

    A. Diabetes mellitus (Willis disease)

    B. Hurler syndrome (mucopolysaccharidoses I-H)

22. Postinflammatory—iritis because of such disease as tuberculosis, syphilis, (acquired lues) herpes zoster, herpes simplex, smallpox, leprosy (Hansen disease), onchocerciasis syndrome (River blindness), sporotrichosis

23. Shy-Magee-Drager syndrome (orthostatic hypotension syndrome)

24. Spontaneous progressive

    A. Congenital hypoplasia iris stroma

    B. Reiger syndrome (dysgenesis mesostromalis)

25. Takayasu syndrome (aortic arch syndrome, pulseless disease)

26. Use of quinine, chloramine, mustard gas

27. Wagner syndrome (hyaloideoretinal degeneration)

28. Xeroderma pigmentosa, including skin lesions

Rodrigues, M.M., et al.: Clinical electron microscopic, and immunohistochemical study of the corneal endothelium and Descemet's membrane in the iridocorneal endothelial syndrome. Am J Ophthalmol., 101:16–27, 1986.

Roy, T.H.: Ocular Syndromes and Systemic Diseases. 2nd Ed. Philadelphia, W.B. Saunders, 1989.

Shields, M.B., et al.: The essential iris atrophies. Am J Ophthalmol., 85:749–769, 1978.

Iridodonesis (Tremulous Iris)

   *1. Aphakia following cataract extraction

   *2. Dislocation of the lens (see p. 449)

    3. Hydrophthalmos or buphthalmos (see p. 256)

    4. Hypermature senile cataract

Filatov, V., et al.: Dislocation of the crystalline lens in a patient with Sturge Weber syndrome. Amer J Ophthal., 24:260–262, 1992.

Huggon, I.C., et al.: Contractural arachnodactyly with mitral regurgitation and iridodonesis. Arch Disease in Childhood. 65: 317–319, 1990.

Tumors Arising from Pigment Epithelium of Iris

1. Hyperplasia

    A. Primary (congenital)

      (1) At pupillary margin

      (2) At margins of colobomas

    B. Acquired

      (1) Region of sphincter—migrating epithelial cells appear in stroma as clump cells (equivocal origin)

      (2) Cells can reach anterior surface of iris and proliferate (velvety black in appearance)

    C. Secondary

      (1) Intraocular inflammation—pigmented cells proliferate around the pupillary margin onto anterior iris surface

      (2) Long-standing glaucoma

        a. Proliferation around the pupillary margin onto anterior iris surface

        b. Migration through stroma to anterior surface at collarette

* = most important

*(3) Trauma (including operation—proliferation of pigment epithelium on anterior surface of iris, across pupil, or on posterior surface of cornea

  *(4) Drugs, including: demecarium, echothiophate, edrophonium, isoflurophate, neostigmine, physostigmine, pilocarpine often associated with cystic formation

2. Neoplasia

  *A. Benign—well-differentiated epithelial cells, usually pigmented, often with pseudoacinar arrangement and cysts; may have limited locally invasive properties

  B. Malignant

    (1) Carcinoma

    (2) Local invasion, intraocular metastases

    (3) Medulloepithelioma, embryonal type (diktyoma)

    (4) Papillary cystadenoma

Fraunfelder, F.T.: Drug-Induced Ocular Side Effects and Drug Interactions. 4th Ed. Philadelphia, Williams & Wilkins, 1996.

Morris, P.A., and Henkind, P.: Neoplasms of the iris pigment epithelium. Am. J. Ophthalmol., 66:31, 1968.

Pigmented Lesions of Iris

1. Adenoma of iris

2. Anterior chamber intraocular lens and segmental uveal ectropion

3. Anterior staphyloma

4. Corneal or scleral perforation

*5. Cyst—congenital, spontaneous, or traumatic, including pigmentation

6. Ectopic lacrimal gland tissue

*7. Ectropion uvea

8. Epithelioma of the ciliary body

9. Exudative mass in the anterior chamber

10. Foreign body of iris, including iron with siderosis

11. Fuchs syndrome of heterochromic cyclitis with the darker normal iris considered to contain a diffuse melanoma

12. Hemangioma of the iris with pigmentation because of hemorrhage

13. Hemosiderosis because of contusions with hyphema or injuries and disease in the posterior portion of the eye with recurrent bleeding

14. Juvenile xanthogranuloma (nevoxanthoendothelioma)

15. Leiomyoma or leiomyosarcoma of the iris

16. Leukemic infiltrates and malignant lymphomas

17. Malignant melanoma of the iris

18. Metastatic carcinomas arising in the lung, breast, gastrointestinal tract, thyroid gland, prostate gland, kidney, or testicle

19. Neurofibromatosis with increased pigmentation of the iris

*20. Nevi of the iris

21. Nodular thickening and scarring of the iris

22. Pigmentary glaucoma

23. Pigment epithelial tumors of the iris

24. Segmental melanosis oculi, including congenital melanosis

25. Stromal mass in the anterior chamber

26. Uveitis, such as that because of conglomerate tuberculous lesions of the stroma or sarcoid involvement of the iris

Chang, M., et al.: Adenoma of the pigment epithelium of the ciliary body simulating a malignant melanoma. Am J Ophthalmol., 88:40–48, 1979.

Richburg, F.A.: Anterior chamber lenses and severe segmental uveal ectropion. Am Intra-Ocular Implant Soc J, 7:328, 1981.

Shields, C.L., et al.: Differentiation of adenoma of the iris pigment epithelium from iris cyst and melanoma. Am J Ophthalmol, 100:678–681, 1986.

Nonpigmented Lesions of Iris

1. Amelanotic melanoma

2. Endothelioma

3. Exudative mass in the anterior chamber

4. Fibrosarcoma

*5. Foreign body

6. Forward extension of diktyoma

7. Hemangioma of the iris

*8. Iris cyst

9. Iris nodules

   A. Ectodermal (Koeppe nodules)—pupillary margin and gray with ocular inflammation

   B. Mesodermal (Busacca nodules)—anterior surface of iris in collarette region

10. Juvenile xanthogranuloma—may be associated with diffuse infiltration of the iris

11. Leiomyoma or leiomyosarcoma of the iris

12. Leprosy (Hansen disease)

   A. Lepromas of the iris

   B. Leprotic pearl—minute white spots on surface of iris

13. Metastatic carcinoma of the iris arising from the lungs, breast, gastrointestinal tract, thyroid gland, prostate gland, kidney, or testicle

14. Neurofibroma and neuroglioma

15. Sarcoid nodules—multiple, discrete, irregularly distributed over the iris

16. Seeding of tumor, such as retinoblastoma, from the posterior segment

17. Syphilis (acquired lues)

   A. Gummas—solitary, large, avascular, white lesions

   B. Papules (condylomas)—multiple, small, vascular, yellowish lesions

18. Teratoma

19. Tuberculosis

   A. Acute miliary—small grayish-yellow or reddish nodules

   B. Hyalinized or fibrotic scar (Michel flecks)

   C. Tuberculoma—white-gray lesion

*= most important

Rummelt, V, et al.: Congenital Nonpigmented Epithelial Iris Cyst after Amniocentesis. Ophthalmology. 100:776–781, 1993.

Shields, J.A., et al.: Metastatic tumors to the iris in patients. Amer J Ophthal., 119:422–430, 1995.

Wyzinski, P., et al.: Simultaneous bilateral iris metastases from renal cell carcinoma. Am J Ophthalmol., 92:206–209, 1981.

Conditions Simulating Anterior Uveitis or Iritis

1. Brushfield spots
2. Fuchs syndrome (II) (Stevens-Johnson syndrome)
3. Hereditary deep dystrophy of cornea
4. Hyalinized keratitic precipitate
5. Iridoschisis—splitting of iris
6. Juvenile xanthogranuloma of the iris (nevoxanthoendothelioma)
7. Malignant lymphomas or leukemia
8. Malignant melanoma
9. Metastatic tumor arising from the lungs, breast, gastrointestinal tract, thyroid gland, prostate gland, kidney, or testicle
10. Neurofibromas of the iris
11. Pigment floaters in the anterior chamber, especially after mydriasis
*12. Pseudoexfoliation of the lens capsule (glaucoma capsulare)
13. Reticulum cell sarcoma
14. Retinoblastoma
15. Scleroderma (progressive systemic sclerosis)
*16. Siderosis bulbi

Denslow, G.T., and Kielar, R.A.: Metastatic adenocarcinoma to the anterior uvea and increased carcinoembryonic antigen levels. Am. J. Ophthalmol., 85:378–382, 1978.

Schlaegel, T.F.: Essentials of Uveitis. Boston, Little, Brown & Company, 1969.

Syndromes and Diseases Associated with Iritis

1. Actinomycosis
2. Amebiasis (entamoeba histolytica)
3. Amendola syndrome (Brasilian pemphigus)
4. Anderson-Warburg syndrome (congenital progressive oculoacousticocerebral dysplasia)
5. Ankylosing spondylitis (von Beckterev-Strumpell syndrome)
6. Ascariasis
7. Aspergillosis
8. Bee sting of the cornea
9. Behçet syndrome (oculobuccogenital syndrome)
10. Blastomycosis
11. Brucellosis (Bang disease)
12. Candidiasis

13. Charlin syndrome (nasociliary nerve syndrome)

14. Chlamydia pneumoniae

15. Coccidioidomycosis

16. Cryptococcosis

17. Cysticercosis

18. Cytomegalic inclusion disease (cytomegalovirus)

19. Dengue fever

20. Endophthalmitis phacoanaphylactica

*21. Following laser iridectomy

22. Fuchs syndrome

   (1) (heterochromic cyclitis syndrome)

23. Henoch-Schönlein purpura (anaphylactoid purpura)

24. Herbicide exposure—2,4-dichlorophenoxyacetic acid

*25. Herpes simplex

*26. Herpes zoster

27. Histoplasmosis

28. Histiocytosis X (xanthomatous granuloma syndrome)

29. Hypervitaminosis D

30. Leptospirosis (Weil disease)

31. Mucormycosis (phycomycosis)

32. Mycoplasma pneumoniae

33. Nocardiosis

34. Onchocerciasis syndrome (onchocerca volvulus)

35. Reiter syndrome (conjunctivourethrosynovial syndrome)

36. Romberg syndrome (facial hemiatrophy)

37. Rubella syndrome (Gregg syndrome)

*38. Sarcoidosis syndrome (Schaumann syndrome)

39. Sporotrichosis

*40. Still disease (juvenile rheumatoid arthritis)

41. Syphilis (acquired lues)

42. Toxoplasmosis (ocular toxoplasmosis)

43. Tuberculosis

44. Vaccinia

45. Vogt-Koyanagi-Harada syndrome (uveitis, vitiligo-alopecia-poliosis syndrome)

Makley, T.A., and Orlando, R.G.: Uveitis in older patients. Ann Ophthalmol., 14:942, 1982.

Millin, R.B., and Samples, J.R.: Iritis after herbicide exposure. Am J Ophthalmol., 99:726, 1985.

Roy, F.H.: Ocular Syndromes Systemic Diseases. 2nd Ed. Philadelphia, W.B. Saunders, 1989.

Salzman, M.B., et al.: Ocular manifestations of mycoplasma pneumoniae infection. Clinical Infectious Diseases. 1465:1137–1139, 1992.

Yamada, I., et al.: A child with iritis due to chlamydia pneumoniae infection. J Japanese Assoc for Infectious Diseases. 68:1543–1547, 1994.

* = most important

Iritis (Anterior Uveitis) in Children

	Still Syndrome	Ankylosing Spondylitis	Behçet Syndrome	Sarcoidosis	Chronic Cyclitis (Para Planitis)	Fuchs Heterochromic Cyclitis	Herpes Simplex	Herpes Zoster	Vogt-Koyanagi-Harada Syndrome	Sympathetic Ophthalmia
History										
1. Before puberty	U	U								
2. Bilateral					S					
3. Familial	S									
4. Following trauma/surgery										U
5. Greater in females	S				U					
6. Greater in males		U				S				
7. Hereditary		U								
8. Occurs in young adults									U	R
9. Prominent in whites						U				
10. Prominent in blacks				U						
11. Seen in Japanese			S						U	
12. Virus infection			S				U	U	S	
Physical Fitness										
1. Anterior and posterior synechiae	S	U	S				S			
2. Band keratopathy	S	S		R						
3. Cataract	S	S	S	R	S	S		S	S	S
4. Conjunctivitis			S	R			S	S		
5. Corneal opacity			S			S				
6. Corneal ulcer							S			
7. Corneal edema						S	S	U		
8. Cyclitic membrane					U					
9. Cystoid macular edema					U					
10. Choroiditis						S			S	S
11. Dacryoadenitis				U						
12. Dacryocystitis				S						
13. Decreased corneal sensitivity							U	U		
14. Dendritic corneal figure							U	S		
15. Entropion								S		
16. Exophthalmos				S						
17. Extraocular muscle paralysis			U	S			R	S		
18. Glaucoma	S	S	S	S		S	S	S	S	S
19. Hyphema	S									
20. Hypopyon	S	S	R				R	R		
21. Iris bombé	S									
22. Iris hypoheterchromia						U	R	R		

R = rarely; S = sometimes; and U = usually.

Iritis (Anterior Uveitis) in Children *Continued*

	Still Syndrome	Ankylosing Spondylitis	Behçet Syndrome	Sarcoidosis	Chronic Cyclitis (Pars Planitis)	Fuchs Heterochromic Cyclitis	Herpes Simplex	Herpes Zoster	Vogt-Koyanagi-Harada Syndrome	Sympathetic Ophthalmia
Physical Fitness										
23. Keratitis				S			U	U		S
24. Keratitic precipitates	U	U								
25. Macular edema	S		S							
26. Macular hemorrhage				R						
27. Optic atrophy			S	S						
28. Optic neuritis	S		S	S				S		U
29. Retinal detachment					S				S	
30. Retinal hemorrhages			S	S					R	
31. Retinal vasculitis			S							
32. Scleritis		S	S							
33. Sheathing of peripheral retinal veins					U					
34. Snowballs of peripheral inferior retina					U					
35. Strabismus			S							
36. Subconjunctival nodules			U			S				
37. Vitreous hemorrhages			S		S					
38. Vitreous opacity						S			S	S
39. White lashes									S	
40. Zoster rash of lid								S		
Laboratory Data										
1. Antinuclear antibody test (+)	U									
2. Biopsy of inferior forniceal follicles				U						
3. Cerebrospinal fluid protein level high				S						
4. Chest roentgenogram				U						
5. Elevated sed rate		U								
6. Fluorescein angiography		U			U				U	
7. Homologous leucocytic antibody determination	U	U	S							
8. Lumbosacral spine roentgenogram		U	U							
9. Macroglobulins (−)				U						
10. Rheumatoid factor and lupus erythematosis cell test (+)	U	U								
11. Serum angiotensin-converting enzyme				U						
12. Tuberculosis skin test				U						U
13. Ultrasonography				S						
14. Viral culture serial antibody titer							U	U		

R = rarely; S = sometimes; and U = usually.

Iritis (Anterior Uveitis) in Children

1. Anterior and posterior uveitis
    A. Retinoblastoma
    *B. Sarcoidosis syndrome (Schaumann syndrome)
    C. Sympathetic ophthalmia
    D. Vogt-Koyanagi-Harada syndrome (uveitis-vitiligo-alopecia-poliosis syndrome)
*2. Chronic cyclitis (peripheral uveitis)
3. Fuchs heterochromic cyclitis
4. Iridocyclitis
    A. Ankylosing spondylitis (von Beckterev-Strumpell syndrome)
    B. Behçet syndrome (oculobuccogenital syndrome)
    *C. Sarcoidosis syndrome (Schaumann syndrome)
    D. Still syndrome (juvenile rheumatoid arthritis)
    *E. Trauma
    F. Unknown
5. Keratouveitis
    *A. Herpes simplex
    *B. Herpes zoster

Kimura, S.J., and Hogan, M.J.: Uveitis in children: Analysis of cases. Trans. Am. Ophthalmol. Soc., 62:173, 1964.

Powell, C.J., et al.: Diffuse infiltrating retinoblastoma masquerading as a panuveitis. Ophthalmology, 92:119, 1986.

Nongranulomatous Uveitis

1. Physical insult
    A. Endogenous
    B. Exogenous
*2. Toxic insults
    A. Autointoxication—ptomaines, protein split products, and so forth from food poisoning
    B. Bacterial endotoxins
    C. Reticulum cell sarcoma of brain
    D. Toxins from disintegrating helminths
    *E. Viral toxins
3. Immediate hypersensitive reaction
    *A. Airborne allergens
    B. Drugs, including:

acetazolamide   aurothioglucose
amphotericin B   aurothioglycanide
auranofin   benoxinate

butacaine

chymotrypsin

cocaine

cytarabine

demecarium

dibucaine

dichlorphenamide

diethylcarbamazine

dyclonine

echothiophate

edrophonium

emetine

epinephrine

ethoxzolamide

fluorouracil

gold Au 198

gold sodium thiomalate

gold sodium thiosulfate

iodide and iodine solutions and compounds

isoflurophate

methazolamide

metipranolal

neostigmine

phenacaine

physostigmine

piperocaine

pralidoxime

proparacaine

radioactive iodides

streptokinase

tetracaine

    C. Foods

    D. Protein antigens (anaphylaxia)

4. Delayed hypersensitive reaction

    A. Bacterial antigens

    B. Viral antigens

5. Doubtful entities—nongranulomatous uveitis

    A. Amebiasis

    B. Diabetic iritis

    C. Gouty iritis

    D. Heterochromic iridocyclitis

    *E. Sarcoidosis syndrome (Schaumann syndrome)

    F. Secondary to metabolic disease, such as biliary cirrhosis and systemic xanthomatosis

    G. Uveitis associated with collagen diseases

6. Mixed granulomatous and nongranulomatous

    A. Lens-induced uvealis

    *B. Peripheral uveitis

Fraunfelder, F.T.: Drug-Induced Ocular Side Effects and Drug Interactions. 4th Ed. Philadelphia, Williams & Wilkins, 1996.

Gray, M.Y., and Lazarus, J.H.: Iritis after treatment with streptokinase. Brit Med J. 97: 309, 1994.

Martins, J.C.: Corticosteroid-induced uveitis. Am J Ophthalmol., 77:433–437, 1974.

Miller, R.B., and Wong, I.G.: Metipranolol associated granulomatous iritis. Amer J Ophthalmol., 118: 805–806, 1994.

Minckler, D.S., et al.: Uveitis and reticulum cell sarcoma of brain with bilateral neoplastic seeding of vitreous without retinal or uveal involvement. Am J Ophthalmol., 80:433–439, 1975.

Mohan, et al.: Acute granulomatosis iritis following fluorouracil therapy for failed trabeculectomy. Indian J Ophthal 39: 125–126, 1991.

* = most important

Granulomatous Uveitis

1. Proven or probable etiology

  A. Associated with nonpyogenic systemic infections

    (1) Brucellosis (Brucella melitensis, B. abortus, B. suis)

    (2) Leprosy (Mycobacterium leprae)

    (3) Leptospirosis (Leptospira canicola, L. icterohaemorrhagiae, L. pomona)

    *(4) Syphilis (Treponema pallidum)

    *(5) Tuberculosis (Mycobacterium tuberculosis)

  B. Protozoan infections

    (1) Amebiasis (Entamoeba coli, E. histolytica, Endolimax nana, Acanthamoeba hartmannella)

    (2) Toxoplasmosis (Toxoplasma gondii)

    (3) Trypanosomiasis (Trypanosoma cruzi, T. gambiense)

  C. Fungal infections

    (1) Actinomycosis

    (2) Aspergillosis

    (3) Blastomycosis

    (4) Candidiasis (moniliasis)

    (5) Coccidioidomycosis

    (6) Cryptococcosis (Cryptococcus neoformans or Torula histolytica)

    *(7) Histoplasmosis (Histoplasma capsulatum)

    (8) Mycomycosis (phycomycosis)

    (9) Nocardiosis

    (10) Sporotrichosis (Sporotrichum schenckii)

  D. Helminth infestations

    (1) Ascaridiosis (Ascaris lumbricoides)

    (2) Cestodes

      a. Cysticercosis (Cysticercus cellulosae)

      b. Taeniasis (Taenia echinococcus)

    (3) Diptera larvae (exogenous)

    (4) Nematodes

      a. Ancylostomiasis (Toxocara canis, Ancylostoma duodenale, Ancylostoma caninum, Necator americanus)

      b. Onchocerciasis (Onchocerca volvulus)

2. Recognized clinical and histopathologic entity, of unknown cause

Characteristics of Granulomatous and Nongranulomatous Inflammation in Anterior Uvea

Symptomatology	Granulomatous Uveitis	Nongranulomatous Uveitis	
		Acute, Self-limited Insult	Chronic or Often-repeated Insult
Clinical onset	Slow and insidious, chronic and protracted; often remissions and exacerbations	Acute, usually self-limited (1–6 weeks)	Acute or insidious, usually protracted or chronic over months
Inflammation	Low-grade ciliary inflammation; acute only when there is a secondary allergic reaction	Acute, intense ciliary inflammation	Usually low-grade or intermittent inflammation
Keratitic deposits	Heavy, often "mutton-fat" epitheloioid cell deposits	Pinpoint lymphoid cell deposits	Pinpoint lymphocytic cell deposits
Aqueous	Few cells; fibrin only if there is a superimposed allergic reaction; usually weak aqueous flare	Many cells; often fibrin; intense flare in active stages	Moderate number of cells; rarely fibrin; low-grade or absent flare
Nodules	Frequent—Koeppe, Busacca, stromal	None	None
Iris changes	Slight edema; organic thickening from cellular infiltration	Edema; blurring of iris pattern; acute capillary dilatation frequent	Slight blurring of iris pattern; slight capillary dilatation; pigmentary degeneration
Posterior synechiae	Heavy, organized adhesions form slowly, usually difficult or impossible to break	None, or easily broken fibrinous adhesions in early attacks; become organized only after repeated attacks	Slowly forming but may become organized
Organic damage	If disease is unchecked usually progressive damage from onset of first attack, fibrosis, posterior synechiae, occlusio pupillae, secondary glaucoma, capsular clouding and phthisis bulbi	Usually none in early attacks; band keratitis, posterior synechiae, secondary glaucoma, cataracts, and phthisis bulbi may occur after repeated attacks	Gradually increasing irreversible changes, such as in recurrent acute attacks

* = most important

    *A. Multiple sclerosis

    *B. Sarcoidosis syndrome (Schaumann syndrome)

    C. Sympathetic ophthalmia

3. Nonspecific granulomatous uveitis of unknown cause, including granulomatous ileocolitis

4. Mixed granulomatous and nongranulomatous

    A. Lens-induced uveitis

    B. Peripheral uveitis

5. Viral uveitis

    A. Proven or probable

        (1) Cytomegalic inclusion disease

        (2) Herpes simplex

        (3) Herpes zoster

        (4) Vaccinia

    B. Suspected

        (1) Behçet syndrome (oculobuccogenital syndrome)

        (2) Vogt-Koyanagi-Harada syndrome (uveitis-vitiligo-alopecia-poliosis syndrome)

6. Histiocytosis X (includes eosinophilic granuloma, Hand-Schüller-Christian disease and Letterer-Siwe disease)

7. Following treatment of a choroidal melanoma with proton-beam irradiation

Cartwright, M.J., et al.: Sporothrix schenckii endophthalmitis presenting as granulomatous uveitis. Brit J Ophthalmol., 77:61–62, 1993.

Lim, J.I., et al.: Anterior granulomatous uveitis in patients with multiple sclerosis. Ophthalmol., 98: 142–145, 1991.

Margo, C.E, and Pautler, S.E.: Granulomatous uveitis after treatment of a choroidal melanoma with proton-beam irradiation. Retina. 10: 140–143, 1990.

Pigmented Ciliary Body Lesions

    *1. Ciliary body cyst

    *2. Drugs including:

adrenal cortex injection	edrophonium	neostigmine
aldosterone	epinephrine	paramethasone
betamethasone	fludrocortisone	physostigmine
cortisone	fluprednisolone	pilocarpine
demecarium	hydrocortisone	prednisolone
desoxycorticosterone	isoflurophate	prednisone
dexamethasone	meprednisone	triamcinolone
echothiophate	methylprednisolone	

3. Malignant melanoma

4. Melanocytoma of ciliary body

5. Peripheral uveal detachment

6. Post-traumatic pigmentary migration

Fraunfelder, F.T.: Drug-Induced Ocular Side Effects and Drug Interactions. 4th Ed. Philadelphia, Williams & Wilkins, 1996.

Shields, J.A., et al.: Uveal pseudomelanoma due to post-traumatic pigmentary migration. Arch Ophthalmol., 89:519–522, 1973.

Neuroepithelial Tumors of Ciliary Body

1. Congenital
    A. Glioneuroma
    B. Medulloepithelioma
        *(1) Benign
        (2) Malignant
    C. Teratoid medulloepithelioma
        (1) Benign
        (2) Malignant
2. Acquired
    A. Adenocarcinoma
        *(1) Papillary
        (2) Pleomorphic
        (3) Solid
    B. Adenoma
        *(1) Papillary
        (2) Pleomorphic
        (3) Solid
    C. Mesectodermal leiomyoma
    D. Pseudoadenomatous hyperplasia

Croxatto, J.O., and Malbran, E.S.: Unusual ciliary body tumor. Ophthalmology, 89:1208, 1982.

Spencer, W.H., and Jesberg, D.O.: Glioneuroma (choristomatous malfunctions of the optic cup margin). Arch Ophthalmol., 89:387–391, 1973.

Shields J.A., et al.: Observations on seven cases of intraocular leiomyoma. Arch Ophthalmol., 112: 521–528, 1994.

Shields, J.A., et al.: Natural causes and histopathologic findings of lacrimal gland chorestoma of the iris and ciliary body. Amer J Ophthalmol., 119: 219–224, 1995.

Internal Ophthalmoplegia (Paresis of Ciliary Body with Loss of Power of Accommodation and Pupil Dilatation Because of Lesions of Ciliary Ganglion)

1. Acute porphyria—frequently bilateral
*2. Adie syndrome (myotonic pupil)
3. Aneurysm of the posterior communicating artery at its junction with the internal carotid—unilateral
4. Congenital—rare
*5. Cycloplegic ocular medication—most common
6. During acute illness—transient
7. During blepharoplasty—transient

* = most important

8. Fisher syndrome (ophthalmoplegia-ataxia-areflexia syndrome)

9. Foramen lacerum syndrome (aneurysm of internal carotid artery)

10. Histiocytosis X (Hand-Schüller-Christian syndrome)

11. Hollenhorst syndrome (chorioretinal infarction syndrome)

*12. Increased intracranial pressure

13. Infections, including chickenpox, measles, diphtheria, syphilis, scarlet fever, pertussis, smallpox, influenza, herpes zoster, botulism, sinusitis, and viral hepatitis

14. Lubarsch-Pick syndrome (amyloidosis)

15. May be early lesion of acute or chronic ophthalmoplegia

16. Metastatic tumors of choroid

17. Nasopharyngeal carcinoma—early

18. Nothnagel syndrome (ophthalmoplegia-cerebellar ataxia syndrome)

19. Partial seizures

20. Retrobulbar injections of alcohol

21. Transcleral diathermy

22. Trauma to eye or orbit

23. Vogt-Koyanagi-Harada syndrome (uveitis-vitiligo-alopecia-poliosis syndrome)

Perlman, J.P., and Conn, H.: Transient internal ophthalmoplegia during blepharoplasty. A report of three cases. Ophthalmic Plastic & Reconstructive Surgery, 7:141–143, 1991.

Rosenberg, M.L., and Jabbari, B.: Miosis and internal ophthalmoplegia as a manifestation of partial seizures. Neurology, 41:737–739, 1991.

Roy, F.H.: Ocular Syndromes and Systemic Diseases. 2nd Ed. Philadelphia, W.B. Saunders, 1989.

Lens

RICHARD WARD ALLINSON, M.D.

Contents

Anterior Subcapsular Cataract

	Atopic Eczema*	Electric Injury	Diabetes Mellitus*	Werner Syndrome	Myotonic Dystrophy	Intraocular Copper and Iron	Trauma (Blunt)*	Wilson Disease
History								
1. Consanguinity				S				
2. Diplopia			S		S			
3. Familial			U		U			U
4. Hereditary				U	U			
5. Intraocular foreign body history						U		
6. More than 200 volts injury		U						
7. Night blindness		S				S		U
8. Often occurs in childhood	U			S				
9. Occurs in first decade								U
10. Occurs during second to third decade					U	S		
11. Onset, usually fourth decade			U					
12. Trauma history							U	
Physical Findings								
1. Absent eyelashes/eyebrows				U				
2. Angle recession							S	
3. Astigmatism					S			
4. Blepharospasm		S						
5. Blue sclera					S			
6. Bullous keratopathy					S			
7. Chemosis conjunctiva	U						S	
8. Chorioretinitis					S	S		
9. Choroidal atrophy		S						
10. Choroidal rupture		S						
11. Conjunctival giant papillary hypertrophy	S							
12. Conjunctival necrosis							S	
13. Conjunctival scarring	S						S	
14. Copper colored macular sheen						U		
15. Corneal epithelial dystrophy					S			
16. Corneal necrosis		S						
17. Corneal opacity					S	S		
18. Corneal perforation		S						
19. Corneal scarring	S	S						
20. Corneal vascularization	S							
21. Cotton-wool spots			U					
22. Dyschromatopsia						S		
23. Ectropion uvea			S					
24. Endophthalmitis						U		
25. Exophthalmos				S			S	
26. Filamentary conjunctival discharge	S							
27. Fixed and dilated pupil			S				S	
28. Hudson-Stahli line in cornea						S		
29. Hyphema		S				S	S	
30. Hypopyon						S		
31. Interstitial keratitis						S		

Anterior Subcapsular Cataract *Continued*

	Atopic Eczema*	Electric Injury	Diabetes Mellitus*	Werner Syndrome	Myotonic Dystrophy	Intraocular Copper and Iron	Trauma (Blunt)*	Wilson Disease
Physical Findings								
32. Iris greenish/rusty tinge						S		
33. Ischemic optic neuropathy			S			S		
34. Kayser-Fleischer ring						S		U
35. Keratoconus	S							
36. Laceration of lid							S	
37. Lid exudates/erythema	S							
38. Lid hemorrhage							S	
39. Lid necrosis/burn		U						
40. Lid telangiectasia			U					
41. Loss corneal sensitivity					U			
42. Low intraocular pressure							S	
43. Macular degeneration				S	S			
44. Macular edema			S			S		
45. Macular red spot					S			
46. Microaneurysms of retina			U					
47. Nystagmus		S		S				S
48. Optic nerve atrophy		S	S		S		S	
49. Optic neuritis		S	S					
50. Papilledema			S					
51. Paralysis of extraocular muscles		S	U	U				S
52. Phthisis bulbi						S		U
53. Presbyopia, early			S	S				
54. Ptosis			S		S			
55. Punctate keratitis	S							
56. Retinal cysts		S						
57. Retinal degeneration		S			S	S		
58. Retinal detachment	S		S			S	S	
59. Retinal exudate/edema			S	U				
60. Retinal gliosis						S		
61. Retinal hemorrhage			S	U		S	S	
62. Retinal holes		S						
63. Retinal neovascularization			S					
64. Retinal rusty discoloration						S		
65. Retrobulbar hemorrhage							S	
66. Rubeosis iridis			S					
67. Staphylococcal blepharitis	S							
68. Synechiae of iris						S		
69. Tranta dot	S							
70. Uveitis		S				S		
71. Vitreous hemorrhage			S				S	
72. Vitreous opacity/degeneration						S		
Laboratory Data								
1. Allergy testing	U							
2. Blood sugar elevated			S					

* = most important

Anterior Subcapsular Cataract *Continued*

Physical Findings	Atopic Eczema*	Electric Injury	Diabetes Mellitus*	Werner Syndrome	Myotonic Dystrophy	Intraocular Copper and Iron	Trauma (Blunt)*	Wilson Disease
3. Computed tomography scan of head		R						S
4. Genetic studies				U	U			
5. Hepatic tests								U
6. Orbital roentgenogram						U	S	
7. Serum gamma globulin concentration reduced					U			
8. Serum immunoglobulin E concentration elevated	U							
9. Ultrasonography		S				U	U	
10. Urine copper elevated								S
11. Visual field defects		S	R		S			

R = rarely; S = sometimes; and U = usually.

Anterior Subcapsular Cataract

1. Acrodermatitis chronica atrophicans
2. Addison syndrome (adrenal cortical insufficiency)
3. Albinism
4. Allopurinol therapy
5. Alport syndrome (hereditary nephritis)
6. Amiodarone usage
7. Andogsky syndrome (dermatogenous cataract)
8. Aniridia
9. Anterior chamber air
10. Atopic (eczema cataract)
11. Bee sting of cornea
12. Cerebrohepatorenal syndrome (Smith-Lemti-Opitz syndrome)
13. Chlorpromazine therapy
14. Chromosomal 3; 18 translocation
15. Comedo cataract
16. Coughing
17. Cryotherapy
18. Electric cataract
*19. Diabetes mellitus (Willis disease)
20. Facial paralysis (partial)
21. Frenkel syndrome (ocular contusion syndrome)
22. Goldscheider syndrome (epidermolysis bullosa)
23. Gyrate atrophy (ornithine ketoacid aminotransferase deficiency)
24. Head-banging (chronic)
25. Hemifacial microsomia syndrome (François-Haustrate syndrome)
26. Hypermature cataract with other changes
27. Hypoparathyroidism
28. Idiopathic—10% normal population
29. Intraocular copper and iron
30. Isotretinoin
31. Jadassohn-Lewandowsky syndrome (epidermolysis bullosa)
32. Leber's congenital amaurosis
33. Marinesco-Sjögren syndrome (oligophrenia syndrome)
34. Myotonic dystrophy (Curschmann-Steinert syndrome)
35. Naphthalene ingestion
36. Neurodermatitis
37. Pemphigus foliaceous (Cazenave disease)
38. Phenothiazine therapy
39. Phospholine iodide usage
40. Pseudohypoparathyroidism

* = most important

41. Reese-Ellsworth syndrome (anterior chamber cleavage syndrome)

42. Rothmund syndrome (telangiectasia-pigmentation-cataract syndrome)

43. Scaphocephaly

44. Thorazine ingestion

*45. Trauma, such as contusion

46. Tyrosinosis

47. Vitrectomy for diabetic retinopathy

48. Werner syndrome (progeria of adults)

49. Wilson disease (hepatolenticular degeneration)

50. Zinc chloride (concentrated)

Asamoto, A., and Yablonski, M.E.: Posttrabeculectomy anterior subcapsular cataract formation induced by anterior chamber air. Ophthalmic Surgery, 24:314–319, 1993.

Flack, A.J., et al.: Anterior subcapsular cataracts: A review of potential etiologies. Ann. Ophthalmol., 17:78–80, 1985.

Herman, D.C., and Dyer, J.A.: Anterior subcapsular cataracts as a possible adverse ocular reaction. Am. J. Ophthalmol., 103:236, 1987.

McKusick, V.A.: Mendelian Inheritance In Man. 9th Ed. Baltimore, Johns Hopkins University Press, 1994.

Roy, F.H.: Ocular Syndromes and Systemic Disease. 2nd Ed. Philadelphia, W.B. Saunders, 1989.

Steel, D., et al.: Anterior subcapsular plaque cataract in hyperornithinemia gyrate atrophy a case report. Brit. J. Ophthal., 76:762–763, 1992.

Weidle, E.C.: Lenticular chrysiasis in oral chrysotherapy. Am. J. Ophthalmol., 103:240–241, 1987.

Nuclear Cataracts

1. Alcohol

2. Arteriovenous fistula

3. Associated with photocoagulation such as argon laser use

4. Capsular exfoliation syndrome

5. Congenital dysplasia

6. Conradi syndrome (multiple epiphyseal congenital dysplasia)

7. Coppock cataract, discoid cataract, zonular cataract—autosomal dominant

8. Hyperbaric oxygen therapy

9. Maple syrup urine disease (branched chain ketoaciduria)

10. Matsouka syndrome (oculo-cerebro-articulo-skeletal syndrome)

11. Nuclear diffuse nonprogressive cataract—autosomal dominant, rarely recessive

*12. Nuclear sclerosis

      *a. Pars plana vitrectomy for macular pucker

      b. smoking

13. Nuclear total cataract—autosomal dominant, rarely recessive

14. Paradichlorobenzene (mothballs)

15. Perforating injuries

*16. Rubella syndrome (German measles)

17. Siemen syndrome (hereditary ectodermal dysplasia syndrome)

18. von Gierke disease (glucose-phosphate deficiency)

Cherfan, G.M., et al.: Nuclear sclerotic cataract after vitrectomy for idiopathic epiretinal membranes causing macular pucker. Am. J. Ophthalmol., 111:434–438, 1991.

Heiba, I.M., et al.: Genetic etiology of nuclear cataract: evidence for a major gene. Amer. J. Medical Genetics, 47:1208–1214, 1993.

Klein, R.E., et al.: Cigarette smoking and lens opacities–the Beaver Dam Eye Study. Amer. J. of Preventive Medicine., 9:27–30, 1993.

Meloni, T., et al.: Glucose 6-phosphate dehydrogenase deficiency and cataract of patients in Northern Sardinia. Am. J. Ophthalmol., 110:661–664, 1990.

Palmquist, B.M., et al.: Hyperbaric oxygen therapy. Br. J. Ophthalmol., 68:113–117, 1984.

Pogrebniak, A.E., et al.: Argon Laser-induced Cataract in an Infant with Retinopathy of Prematurity. Amer. J. Ophthal., 117:261–263, 1994.

Ritter, L.L., et al.: Alcohol and lens opacities in the Beaver Dam Eye Study. Arch. Ophthal., 111:113–117, 1993.

Roy, F.H.: Ocular Syndromes & Systemic Diseases. 2nd Ed. Philadelphia, W.B. Saunders, 1989.

Lamellar (Stellate, Zonular, Cortical, Coronary) Cataracts

1. Alcohol

2. Aniridia

3. Argon laser

4. Autosomal dominant congenital cataract

5. Congenital zonular cataract

6. Cortical cataract and congenital ichthyosis

7. Dermochonoral corneal dystrophy

8. Diabetes mellitus (Willis disease)

9. Females

10. Galactokinase deficiency (von Reuss syndrome)

11. Hagberg-Santavuori (neuronal ceroid-lipofuscinoses)

12. Hypoglycemia

13. Hypophosphatasia (phosphoethanolaminuria)

14. Iritis

15. Leiomyoma

16. Mannosidosis

17. Marfan syndrome (dolichostenomelia-arachnodactyly-hyperchondroplasia-dystrophia mesodermalis congenita)

18. Marshall syndrome (atypical ectodermal dysplasia)

19. Myotonic dystrophy syndrome (Curschmann-Steinert syndrome)

20. Neurofibromatosis 2 (central neurofibromatosis)

21. Nieden syndrome (telangiectasia cataract syndrome)

22. Nonwhites

23. Passow syndrome (status dysraphicus syndrome)

24. Riboflavin deficiency (Stannus cerebellar syndrome)

25. Roy syndrome (cataract associated with smoking)

*26. Sunlight

27. Tetany cataract (hypoparathyroidism)

*28. Ultraviolet-B light

29. Van Bogaert-Scherer-Epstein syndrome (primary hyperlipidemia)

30. Van der Hoeve syndrome (osteogenesis imperfecta)

31. Wagner syndrome (hyaloideoretinal degeneration)

32. Zonular cataract and nystagmus—X-linked

Bateman, J.B., et al.: Genetic linkage analysis of autosomal dominant congenital cataracts. Am. J. Ophthalmol., 101:218–225, 1986.

Bateman, J.B., and Philipport, M.: Ocular features of the Hagberg-Santavuori syndrome. Am. J. Ophthalmol., 102:262–271, 1986.

Isenberg, S.J.: The Eye in Infancy. Chicago, Year Book Medical Publishers, 1989.

McKusick, V.A.: Mendelian Inheritance In Man. 11th Ed. Baltimore, Johns Hopkins University Press, 1994.

Roy, F.H.: Ocular Syndromes and Systemic Diseases. 2nd Ed. Philadelphia, W.B. Saunders, 1989.

Roy, F.H.: Cigarette smoking and the risk of cataract (letter). JAMA, 269:748, 1993.

Schein, O.D., et al.: Cortical lenticular opacification: distribution and location in a longitudinal study. Invest. Ophthal. and Visual Science, 35:363–366, 1994.

Punctate Cataracts (Small Numerous Opacities)

1. Albright hereditary osteodystrophy (pseudohypoparathyroidism)

2. Argon laser

3. Autosomal dominant vitreoretinochoroidopathy (ADVIRC)

4. Cockayne syndrome (dwarfism with retinal atrophy and deafness)

5. Cretinism (hypothyroidism)

6. Galactokinase deficiency (von Reuss syndrome)

7. Hypercalcemia (adult)

8. Hyperprolactinemia

9. Incontinentia pigmenti achromians

10. Lowe syndrome (oculocerebrorenal syndrome)

11. Rothmund syndrome (telangiectasia-pigmentation-cataract syndrome)

12. Supravalvular aortic stenosis (Williams-Beuren syndrome)

Blair, N.P., et al.: Autosomal dominant vitreoretinochorodopathy. Br. J. Ophthalmol., 68:2–9, 1984.

Costagliola, C.: Hyperprolactinemia and lens opacities. Annals of Ophthal., 24:418–419, 1992.

Drack, A.V., et al.: Transient punctate lenticular opacities as a complication of Argon laser photocoagulation in an infant with retinopathy of prematurity. Amer. J. Ophthal., 113:583, 1992.

Goldberg, M.F., et al.: Inherited snowflake cataracts. Ophthalmic Paediatr. Genet., 4:123–139, 1984.

McKusick, V.A.: Mendelian Inheritance In Man. 8th Ed. Baltimore, Johns Hopkins University Press, 1988.

Roy, F.H.: Ocular Syndromes and Systemic Diseases. 2nd Ed. Philadelphia, W.B. Saunders, 1989.

Posterior Subcapsular Cataract

1. Complicated cataract

    A. Anterior segment involvement, such as that because of:

        (1) Acute and chronic corneal ulcer

       *(2) Iridocyclitis

       *(3) Chronic anterior uveitis

        (4) Acute or chronic glaucoma

    B. Posterior segment involvement such as that because of:

       *(1) Chronic posterior uveal inflammation

        (2) Long-standing retinal detachment

        (3) High myopia

        (4) Hereditary retinal lesions, including retinitis pigmentosa

        (5) Persistent hyperplastic primary vitreous

2. Congenital posterior polar lens changes

    A. Spurious posterior capsular cataract (Mittendorf dot)

    B. Posterior polar cataract—persistent fibrovascular sheath of lens with or without secondary cataract

    C. Posterior lenticonus

3. Abefeld syndrome (ocular and facial abnormalities syndrome)

4. Acrodermatitis chronica atrophicans

5. Alcoholism

6. Aniridia

7. Anterior segment ischemia syndrome

8. Aspergillosis

9. Bassen-Kornzweig syndrome (familial hypolipoproteinemia)

10. Bloch-Sulzberger syndrome (incontinentia pigmenti)

11. Buerger disease (thromboangiitis obliterans)

12. Capsular exfoliation syndrome

13. Carotid artery syndrome

14. Chromosome partial deletion (short-arm) syndrome

15. Congenital amaurosis of Leber (Leber's congenital amaurosis)

16. Cushing syndrome

*17. Diabetes mellitus (Willis disease)

18. Drugs, including: dinitrophenol busulfan (Myleran), triparanol (MER-29), PUVA, allopurinol, indapamide, megestrol acetate and phenothiazine usage

19. Electrical injury

20. Engelmann syndrome (diaphyseal dysplasia)

21. Fabry disease (glycosphingolipid lipidosis)

22. Familial hypogonadism syndrome

23. Frenkel syndrome (ocular contusion syndrome)

24. Fuchs syndrome
    (1) (heterochromic cyclitis syndrome)
25. Glassblowers (heat) cataract
26. Gyrate atrophy (ornithine ketoacid aminotransferase deficiency)
27. Hagberg-Santavuori syndrome (neuronal ceroid-lipofuscinoses)
28. Hair dye
29. Hand-Schüller-Christian syndrome (xanthomatous granuloma syndrome)
30. Harada syndrome (uveitis-vitiligo-alopecia-poliosis syndrome)
31. Heerfordt syndrome (uveoparotitis)
32. Hemochromatosis
33. Herpes simplex
34. Hodgkin disease
35. Hypertension
36. Hypoparathyroidism
37. Ionizing radiation, such as that encountered in x-ray, radium, or neutron therapy
38. Jacobsen-Brodwall syndrome
39. Kussmaul disease (necrotizing angiitis)
40. Kyrle disease (hyperkeratosis follicularis et parafollicularis in cutem penetrans)
41. Laurence-Moon-Bardet-Biedl syndrome (retinitis pigmentosa-polydactyly-adiposogenital)
42. Leprosy (Hansen disease)
43. Leri syndrome (carpal tunnel syndrome)
44. Leukemia
45. Lightning induced
46. Malaria
47. Meckel syndrome (dysencephalia splanchnocystic syndrome)
48. Myotonic dystrophy (Curschmann-Steinert syndrome)
49. Neurodermatitis (lichen simplex chronicus)
50. Neurofibromatosis 1 (von Recklinghausen syndrome)
51. Neurofibromatosis 2 (central neurofibromatosis)
52. Ocular trauma (blunt)
53. Oculo-oto-ororenoerythropoietic disease
54. O'Donnell-Pappas syndrome (foveal hypoplasia and presenile cataract—autosomal dominant)
55. Paget syndrome (osteitis deformans)
56. Pemphigus foliaceus (Cazenave disease)
57. Pernicious anemia syndrome
58. Pierre-Robin syndrome (micrognathia-glossoptosis syndrome)
59. Posterior polar cataract—autosomal dominant
60. Pseudohypoparathyroidism

61. Refsum syndrome (phytanic acid storage disease)

62. Renal transplantation

63. Retinitis pigmentosa-deafness-ataxia syndrome

64. Roy syndrome (unilateral cataract associated with smoking)

*65. Senile posterior cortical cataract

66. Sjögren syndrome (secretoinhibitor syndrome)

67. Silicone oil (intraocular)

*68. Steroid usage (topical or systemic)

69. Stickler syndrome (hereditary progressive arthro-ophthalmopathy)

70. Still disease (juvenile rheumatoid arthritis)

71. Toxocariasis (Nematode ophthalmia syndrome)

72. Trisomy (Patau syndrome)

73. Tuomaala-Haapanen syndrome (similar to pseudohypoparathyroidism)

74. Turner syndrome (gonadal dysgenesis)

75. Ultraviolet-B light

76. Uric acid (increased serum levels)

77. Vitrectomy for diabetic retinopathy

78. Weil disease (leptospirosis)

79. Werner syndrome (progeria of adults)

80. Yersiniosis

Aronson, N.E., et al.: Posterior Subcapsular Cataracts Associated with Megestrol Acetate Therapy. J. Cataract Refract. Surg., 19:90–92, 1993.

Bateman, J.B., et al.: Genetic linkage analysis of autosomal dominant congenital cataracts. Am. J. Ophthalmol., 101:218–225, 1986.

Bouzas, E.A., et al.: Posterior subcapsular cataract in endogenous Cushing syndrome—an uncommon manifestation. Invest. Ophthal. and Visual Science, 34:3497–3500, 1993.

Bouzas, E.A., et al.: Lens opacities in neurofibromatosis 2: further significant correlations. Brit. J. Ophthal., 77:354–357, 1993.

Haik, B.G., et al.: Radiation and chemotherapy of parameningeal rhabdomyosarcoma involving the orbit. Ophthalmology, 98:1001–1009, 1986.

Jahn, C.E., et al.: Identification of metabolic risk factors for posterior subcapsular cataract. Ophthalmic Res., 18:112–116, 1986.

Kaiser-Kupfer, M.I., et al.: The association of posterior capsular lens opacities with bilateral acoustic neuromas in patients with Neurofibromatosis Type2. Arch. Ophthalmol., 107:541–544, 1989.

McKusick, V.A.: Mendelian Inheritance In Man. 9th Ed. Baltimore, Johns Hopkins University Press, 1994.

Minotty, P.V., and Gordan, J.K.: Posterior subcapsular cataracts in a patient with hemochromatosis. Ann. Ophthalmol., 15:266–267, 1983.

Roy, F.H. Cigarette smoking and the risk of cataract (letter). JAMA, 269:748, 1993.

Roy, F.H.: Ocular Syndromes and Systemic Diseases. 2nd Ed. Philadelphia, W.B. Saunders, 1989.

Sponsel, W.E., and Rapoza, P.A.: Posterior subcapsular cataract associated with indapamide therapy (letter). Arch. of Ophthal., 110:454, 1992.

* = most important

Posterior Subcapsular Cataract

	Corneal Ulcer	Glaucoma	Chronic Uveitis*	High Myopia	Retinitis Pigmentosa	Ionizing Radiation*	Diabetes Mellitus	Blunt Ocular Trauma	Steroid Use*	Fabry Disease	Kyrle Disease	Werner Syndrome	Myotonic Dystrophy
History													
1. Acute onset	U						U						
2. Associated diabetes mellitus											U		
3. Bilateral				U	U		S		U	U	S	S	U
4. Caused by microbes, parasites, or noninfectious systemic diseases			U										
5. Common during second to third decades					S							U	U
6. Common during third to fifth decades				S			U			U			
7. Common after fourth decade		U											
8. Congenital				S									
9. Consanguinity												U	
10. Exposure to roentgenograms, gamma and infrared rays, or microwaves						U							
11. Familial		S			U		U			U		U	U
12. Hereditary					U		U			U		U	U
13. Most common in blacks		S											
14. More common in males					S								
15. Preceded by mild trauma to corneal epithelium	U												
16. Prolonged topical or systemic steroids									U				
17. Trauma	S							U					
Physical Findings													
1. Absent eyelashes/scanty eyebrows									S			U	
2. Angle recession								S					
3. Anterior/posterior synechiae	S	S	U										
4. Anterior uveitis			U				S						
5. Astigmatism							S					S	
6. Blue sclera												U	
7. Bullous keratopathy												U	
8. Chorioretinitis			U					S				S	S
9. Choroidal exudative areas			U										
10. Chronic blepharitis						U							
11. Closed anterior chamber angle		U											
12. Conjunctival keratinization									S				
13. Conjunctival necrosis									S				
14. Cornea verticillata										S			
15. Corneal dystrophy										U			U
16. Corneal hypesthesia						S	S						U
17. Corneal necrosis						S							
18. Corneal opacities						S				U	U		
19. Corneal perforation	S												
20. Cystoid macular edema					S	S							
21. Dark macular spot				U									
22. Disc hamartomas/drusens					S								
23. Ectropion						U							
24. Endophthalmitis	S												
25. Enlarging myopic crescent				U									

Posterior Subcapsular Cataract *Continued*

Physical Findings	Corneal Ulcer	Glaucoma	Chronic Uveitis*	High Myopia	Retinitis Pigmentosa	Ionizing Radiation*	Diabetes Mellitus	Blunt Ocular Trauma	Steroid Use*	Fabry Disease	Kyrle Disease	Werner Syndrome	Myotonic Dystrophy
26. Entropion						U							
27. Epithelial corneal edema		U											
28. Exophthalmos								S		S			
29. Extraocular muscle palsy						S	S						
30. Folds Bowman/Descemet membranes		U											
31. Hard retinal exudates							U						
32. Hyphema								S					
33. Hypopyon	U												
34. Increased intraocular pressure		U		S		S	S		S				
35. Internuclear ophthalmoplegia											S		
36. Iridocyclitis	U												
37. Iris atrophy						S	S						
38. Keratoconus					R								
39. Lid hemorrhage								S					
40. Lid laceration								S					
41. Lid telangiectasia												S	
42. Low intraocular pressure			S					S					
43. Macular degeneration						S							S
44. Macular holes						S		S					
45. Macular red spot													U
46. Madarosis						U							
47. Microphthalmos					R								
48. Mutton fat keratic precipitates			U										
49. Myopia					U		S						
50. Nystagmus					R	S						S	
51. Optic nerve atrophy		U			S	S	R	S				S	
52. Papilledema			S					S			S		
53. Paramacular retinal degeneration												S	
54. Pigmentary changes in retina (Bone corpuscles or spiderlike figures)					U	S		S				S	
55. Pigmentary degeneration of iris		U					S						
56. Presbyopia, early							S					S	
57. Progressive external ophthalmoplegia					R							U	
58. Ptosis													R
59. Punctate keratitis						U							
60. Pupil dilated and fixed		U					S	S					
61. Retinal detachment			S	S				S					
62. Retinal exudates						S	U						
63. Retinal hemorrhage						S	U	S					
64. Retinal microaneurysms							U				U		
65. Retinal neovascularization						S	U						
66. Retinal vascular occlusion		U				S					S		
67. Retrobulbar hemorrhage								S					
68. Rupture in Bruch membrane								S					
69. Rupture of pupillary sphincter								S					
70. Strabismus					R								

* = most important

Posterior Subcapsular Cataract *Continued*

	Corneal Ulcer	Glaucoma	Chronic Uveitis*	High Myopia	Retinitis Pigmentosa	Ionizing Radiation*	Diabetes Mellitus	Blunt Ocular Trauma	Steroid Use*	Fabry Disease	Kyrle Disease	Werner Syndrome	Myotonic Dystrophy
Physical Findings													
71. Stromal abscess formation	U												
72. Symblepharon						S							
73. Trophic corneal defects												U	
74. Uveitis			U									S	
75. Visual field defects		U		S	U	S			U				S
76. Vitreous opacities			U										
Laboratory Data													
1. Albuminuria											S		
2. Angiotensin—converting enzyme/ lysozyme tests for sarcoid			U										
3. Blood sugar elevated							U					S	
4. Color vision abnormal					U								
5. Complement fixation test for histoplasmosis			U										
6. Chest roentgenogram			U										
7. Dark adaptation abnormal					U								
8. Electrooculogram abnormal					U								
9. Electroretinogram consistently abnormal					U								
10. Fluorescein angiograaphy			S	U	U	S	S						
11. Genetic studies										U		U	U
12. Giemsa strain smear	U												
13. Gram stain smear	U												
14. Homologous leucocytic antibody B2F testing			U										
15. Leukocyte/eosinophilic count and sedimentation rate elevated			S										S
16. Lipid storage testing										U			
17. Lumbosacral roentgenogram			U										
18. Ocular ultrasonography			S					U					
19. Purified protein derivative skin test			U										
20. Profile for immunologic abnormalities			U										
21. Venereal disease reaction level or fluorescent treponemal antibody-absorption test			U										
22. Visual field test		U		S	U	S			U				S

R = rarely; S = sometimes; and U = usually.

Iridescent Crystalline Deposits in Lens

1. Idiopathic
2. Hypothyroid (cretinism)
3. Hypocalcemia
   A. Postoperative—removal of thyroid and accidental parathyroid removal
   B. Idiopathic hypoparathyroidism
   C. Pseudohypoparathyroidism (hypoparathyroid cretinism) or with hyperphosphatemia (Albright disease)
   D. Pseudopseudohypoparathyroidism (brachymetacarpal dwarfism)
4. Myotonic dystrophy (Curschmann-Steinert syndrome)
5. Drugs, including:

acetophenazine	gold Au 198	prochlorperazine
amiodarone	gold sodium thiomalate	promazine
auranofin	gold sodium thiosulfate	promethazine
aurothioglucose	mercuric oxide	propiomazine
aurothioglycanide	mesoridazine	silver nitrate
butaperazine	methdilazine	silver protein
carphenazine	methotrimeprazine	thiethylperazine
chlorpromazine	mild silver protein	thiopropazate
chlorprothixene	perazine	thioridazine
colloidal silver	pericyazine	thiothixene
diazepam(?)	perphenazine	trifluoperazine
diethazine	phenylmercuric acetate	triflupromazine
ethopropazine	phenylmercuric nitrate	trimeprazine
fluphenazine	piperacetazine	

6. Cataract (coralliform and aculeiform) usually autosomal dominant; sometimes recessive

Fraunfelder, F.T.: Drug-Induced Ocular Side Effects and Drug Interactions. 4th Ed. Philadelphia, Williams & Wilkins, 1996.

McKusick, V.A.: Mendelian Inheritance In Man. 9th Ed. Baltimore, Johns Hopkins University Press, 1994.

Roy, F.H.: Ocular Syndromes and Systemic Diseases. 2nd Ed. Philadelphia, W.B. Saunders, 1989.

Oil Droplet in Lens

1. Anterior displacement of lens
*2. Galactosemia-transferase deficiency (von Reuss syndrome)
3. Lenticonus

Bellows, J.G., and Bellows, R.T.: Displacement of the lens. In Bellows, J.G. (ed.): Cataract and Abnormalities of the Lens. New York, Grune & Stratton, 1975, p. 277.

Beutler, E., et al.: Galactokinase deficiency as cause of cataract. N. Engl. J. Med., 288:1203–1206, 1973.

Lenticonus (Conical Lens Surface Protuberance) and Lentiglobus (Globular Lens Surface Protuberance)

1. Anterior—rare and usually bilateral
   *A. Alport syndrome (hereditary nephritis)

* = most important

~~B. Spina bifida~~

    C. Waardenburg syndrome (embryonic fixation syndrome)

  2. Posterior—more common and often unilateral

    A. Associated with persistent hyperplastic primary vitreous

    B. Associated with remnants of hyaloid artery

    C. Familial posterior lenticonus and microcornea

    *D. Lowe syndrome (oculocerebrorenal syndrome)

    E. Trauma

Bleik, J.H., et al.: Familial posterior lenticonus and microcornea. Arch. of Ophthal., 110:1208, 1992.

Crounch, E.R., and Parks, M.M.: Management of posterior lenticonus complicated by unilateral cataract. Am. J. Ophthalmol., 85:503–508, 1978.

Tripathi, R.C., et al.: Pathogenesis of cataracts in patients with Lowe's syndrome. Ophthalmology, 93:1046–1051, 1986.

Lens Absorption

  1. Congenital rubella syndrome (German measles)

  2. Hallerman-Streiff syndrome (dyscephalic mandibulo-oculo facial syndrome)

  3. Surgical trauma as discission

  4. Trauma, blunt or penetrating

Roy, F.H.: Ocular Syndromes and Systemic Diseases. 2nd Ed. Philadelphia, W.B. Saunders, 1989.

Exfoliation of Lens Capsule (Superficial Layers of Lens Capsule Split Off and Float in Aqueous as a Fine Membrane)

  *1. Senile exfoliation

  2. Toxic exfoliation

    A. Atrophic eyes

    B. Prolonged iridocyclitis

    C. Lodgment of metallic foreign body, such as iron or copper

  3. Traumatic

    A. Perforating injury

    B. Contusions with suspensory ligament separated from a dislocated lens

  4. Heat exposure, such as that experienced by glass-blowers

Duke-Elder, S.: System of Ophthalmology. Vol. XI. St. Louis, C.V. Mosby, 1969.

Meades, K., and Versace, P.: True exfoliation of the lens capsule. Australian & New Zealand Journal of Ophthal., 20:347–348, 1992.

Microphakia or Spherophakia or Microspherophakia (Small Lens or Highly Spherical Lens)

  1. Achard syndrome (Marfan syndrome with dysostosis mandibulofacialis)

  2. Alport syndrome (hereditary nephritis)

  3. Familial anomaly

  4. Homocystinuria syndrome

5. Hyperlysinemia

6. Lenticular myopia as recessive inheritance trait

7. Little syndrome (hereditary osteo-orcychodysplasia)

8. Lowe syndrome (renal rickets)

*9. Marchesani syndrome (brachymorphy with spherophakia) (Weill-Marchesani syndrome)

10. Marfan syndrome (dolichostenomelia-arachnodactyly hyperchondroplasia dystrophica mesodermalis congenita)

11. Peter's anomaly (anterior chamber clevage syndrome)

12. Reticular dystrophy of the retinal pigment epithelium

13. Rubella syndrome (Gregg syndrome)

14. Waardenburg syndrome (embryonic fixation syndrome)

Roy, F.H.: Ocular Syndromes and Systemic Diseases. 2nd Ed. Philadelphia, W.B. Saunders, 1989.
Sorsby, A.: Ophthalmic Genetics. 2nd Ed. New York, Appleton-Century-Crofts, 1970.

Dislocated Lens

1. Achard syndrome (Marfan with dysostosis)

2. Adenoma of the nonpigmented epithelium of the ciliary body

3. Apert syndrome (sphenoacrocraniosyndactyly)

4. Ascariasis

5. Associated ocular findings

   *A. Aniridia

   B. Coloboma of iris and choroid

   *C. Congenital glaucoma

   D. Ectopia lentis et pupillae

   E. Focal hermal hypoplasia (Goltz syndrome)

   F. High myopia

   G. Isolated lens dislocation (up)

   H. Megalocornea

   I. Microcornea

   J. Microspherophakia with hernia

   K. Pseudoxanthoma

6. Autosomal recessive or dominant abnormality without other defects, except usually ectopic pupils

7. Capsular exfoliation syndrome

8. Cryptophthalmia syndrome (cryptophthalmos-syndactyly syndrome)

9. Dwarfism, genetic type

10. Ehlers-Danlos syndrome (cutis hyperelastica)

11. Gillum-Anderson syndrome (blepharoptosis, myopia, ectopia lentis)

12. Gorlin-Goltz syndrome

13. Grönblad-Strandberg syndrome (pseudoxanthoma elasticum)

* = most important

14. Hereditary ectodermal dysplasia syndrome

*15. Homocystinuria—usually downward displacement of lens

16. Hyperlysinemia

17. Late-onset localized junctional epidermolysis bullosa and mental retardation

18. Mandibulofacial dysostosis (Franceschetti syndrome)

19. Marchesani syndrome (brachymorphy with spherophakia)(Weill-Marchesani syndrome)

*20. Marfan syndrome (dolichostenomelia-arachnodactyly-hyperchondroplasia dystrophia mesodermalis congenita)—usually superior displacement of lens

21. Molybdenum cofactor deficiency (combined deficiency of sulfite oxidase and xanthine dehydrogenase)

22. Oculodental syndrome (Peters syndrome)

23. Pseudoexfoliation (exfoliation syndrome)

24. Recession of anterior chamber angle

25. Retinal disinsertion syndrome

26. Retinoblastoma

27. Rieger syndrome (dysgenesis mesostromalis)

28. Spherophakia (see p. 448)

29. Spontaneous (degenerative)

30. Sulfite oxidase deficiency

31. Surgical accidents (iatrogenic)

*32. Syphilis (lues)

*33. Trauma as in Frenkel syndrome (ocular contusion syndrome), bee sting, and following YAG laser

34. Treacher-Collins syndrome (mandibulofacial dysostosis)

35. Uveitis

36. Wildervanck syndrome (cervico-oculoacoustic syndrome)

Byrnes, B.A., et al.: Retinoblastoma presenting with spontaneous hyphema and dislocated lens. J. Pediatr. Ophthal. Strabismus, 30:334–336, 1993.

Chen, C.J., and Richardson, C.D.: Bee sting-induced ocular changes. Ann. Ophthalmol., 18:285–286, 1986.

Isenberg, S.J.: The Eye in Infancy. Chicago, Year Book Medical Publishers, 1989.

Johnson, J.L., et al.: Inborn error of molybdenum metabolism: Combined deficiencies of sulfite oxidase and xanthaline dehydrogenase in a patient lacking the molybdenum cofactor. Proc. Nat. Acad. Sci. U.S.A., 77:3719–3751, 1980.

Melamed, S., et al.: Neodymium: YAG laser iridotomy as a possible contribution to lens dislocation. Ann. Ophthalmol., 18:281–282, 1986.

Roy, F.H.: Ocular Syndromes and Systemic Diseases. 2nd Ed. Philadelphia. W.B. Saunders, 1989.

Strisciuglio, P., et al.: Wildervanck's syndrome with bilateral subluxation of lens and facial paralysis. J. Med. Genet., 20:72–73, 1983.

Dislocated Lens

	Marfan Syndrome*	Weill-Marchesani Syndrome	Dwarfism as Cockayne Disease	Trauma*	Homocystinuria*	Syphilis*	Ehlers-Danlos Syndrome	Rieger Syndrome	Hyperlysinemia	Sulfite Oxidase Deficiency	Treacher-Collins Syndrome
History											
1. Autosomal dominant	U						U	U			S
2. Autosomal recessive		S	U		U						
3. Blunt ocular trauma				U							
4. Congenital	U	S				S					
5. Hereditary	U	U	U		U		U	S	S	S	U
Physical Findings											
1. Angioid streaks							U				
2. Angle recession				S							
3. Aniridia					R			S			
4. Antimongoloid obliquity (temporal canthus lower)		U									
5. Bialteral interstitial keratitis						U					
6. Blue sclera							U				
7. Cataract	U		U	S	R						
8. Central retinal artery occlusion					R						
9. Coloboma of iris	R				R						U
10. Corneal opacity		S						U			
11. Choroidal hemorrhage							S				
12. Choroiditis						U					
13. Decreased tearing			S								
14. Disciform macular degeneration							S	U			
15. Epicanthal folds							U				
16. Glaucoma		R		S	U			U			
17. Hyphema				U							
18. Iridodialysis				S							
19. Iris hypoplasia								U			
20. Iritis				U							
21. Keratoconus							U				
22. Macular edema				U							
23. Megalocornea	S	U									
24. Microcornea					R			U			
25. Microphthalmos					R			U			U
26. Myopia	U	U			U						
27. Nystagmus	U		U							U	
28. Optic atrophy		S	S		U	U		S			
29. Optic disc hypoplasia											U
30. Optic neuritis						U					
31. Papilledema					R						
32. Peripheral cystoid retinal degeneration					U						
33. Peripheral anterior synechiae				S				U			
34. Pigmented retinal appearance	S		U		U				U		
35. Retina detachment	S										
36. Spherophakia	U	U							U		
37. Strabismus	U										
38. Underdeveloped orbicularis oculi muscle											U
39. Vitreous hemorrhage								S			

* = most important

Dislocated Lens *Continued*

	Marfan Syndrome*	Weill-Marchesani Syndrome	Dwarfism as Cockayne Disease	Trauma*	Homocystinuria*	Syphilis*	Ehlers-Danlos Syndrome	Rieger Syndrome	Hyperlysinemia	Sulfite Oxidase Deficiency	Treacher-Collins Syndrome
Laboratory Data											
1. Cystathionine blood/urine										U	
2. Fluorescent treponemal antibody-absorption test						U					
3. Hemocystine/methionine in blood/urine					U						
4. Lysine/homoarginine in blood/urine									U		

R = rarely; S = sometimes; and U = usually.

Aphakia (Absence of Lens in Usual Position behind Iris)

1. Congenital absence of lens—rare
2. Dislocation of the lens into vitreous cavity, anterior chamber, or subconjunctival area
3. Following cataract extraction
4. Gradual absorption of the lens

Hanna, C., et al.: Extraocular traumatic luxation of the lens. J. Arkansas Med. Soc., 66:210, 1969.

O'Brien, C.S.: Ophthalmology: Notes for Students. Iowa City, Athens Press, 1930.

Equatorial Lens Pigmentation

1. Associated with myopia and retinal detachment
2. Congenital malformation
3. Pigmentary glaucoma
4. Uveitis

Delaney, W.V., Jr.: Equatorial lens pigmentation, myopia, and retinal detachment. Am. J. Ophthalmol., 79:194–205, 1975.

Unilateral Cataracts

1. Argon laser treatment
*2. Trauma
3. Complicated cataract
    A. Anterior segment involvement, such as that because of:
        (1) Acute and chronic corneal ulcer
        *(2) Iridocyclitis
        (3) Chronic anterior uveitis
        (4) Acute or chronic glaucoma
    B. Posterior segment involvement, such as that because of:
        (1) Chronic posterior uveal inflammation
        (2) Long-standing retinal detachment
        (3) High myopia
        (4) Hereditary retinal lesions
        (5) Persistent hyperplastic primary vitreous
4. Roy syndrome (unilateral cataract associated with smoking)
5. Congenital posterior polar lens changes
6. Glaucomatocyclitic crisis (Posner-Schlossman syndrome)
7. Conditions that give bilateral manifestations with earlier onset in one eye

Jarrett, W.H.: Dislocation of the lens. Arch. Ophthalmol., 78:289, 1967.

Roy, F.H.: Ocular Syndromes and Systemic Diseases. 2nd Ed. Philadelphia, W.B. Saunders, 1989.

Roy, F.H.: Cigarette smoking and the risk of cataract (letter). JAMA, 269:748, 1993.

* = most important

Lenticular Disease Associated with Corneal Problems

1. Aberfeld syndrome (ocular and facial abnormalities syndrome)—cataracts, microcornea
2. Acrodermatitis chronica atrophicans—keratomalacia, corneal opacification, cataracts
3. Addison syndrome (idiopathic hypoparathyroidism)—keratoconjunctivitis, corneal ulcers, keratitic moniliasis, cataracts
4. Alport syndrome (hereditary nephritis)—anterior lenticonus, posterior polymorphous corneal dystrophy
*5. Amiodarone—corneal deposits, anterior subcapsular cataracts
6. Amyloidosis—amyloid deposits of cornea, corneal dystrophy, pseudopodia lentis
7. Anderson-Warburg syndrome (oligophrenia-microphthalmos syndrome)—corneal opacification and lenticular destruction with a mass visible behind the lens
8. Andogsky syndrome (atopic cataract syndrome)—atopic keratoconjunctivitis, keratoconus, uveitis, subcapsular cataract
9. Aniridia—microcornea and subluxated lenses
10. Anterior chamber cleavage syndrome (Reese-Ellsworth syndrome)—corneal opacities, anterior pole cataract
11. Anterior segment ischemia syndrome—corneal edema, corneal ulceration, cataract
12. Apert syndrome (absent digits cranial defects syndrome)—exposure keratitis, cataracts, ectopia lentis
13. Arteriovenous fistula (arteriovenous aneurysm)—bullous keratopathy, cataract
14. Aspergillosis—corneal ulcer, keratitis, cataract
*15. Atopic dermatitis (atopic eczema, Besnier prurigo)—keratoconjunctivitis, keratoconus, cataract
16. Autosomal dominant—cataracts and microcornea
17. Avitaminosis C (scurvy)—keratitis, corneal ulcer, cataract
18. Chalcosis (intraocular copper containing foreign body) deposits in Descemet' membrane and anterior lens capsule
19. Chickenpox (varicella)—corneal ulcer, corneal opacity, keratitis, cataract
20. Chlorpromazine—corneal and lens opacities
21. Cholera—keratomalacia, cataract
22. Chromosome partial deletion (short-arm) syndrome—cataracts, corneal opacities
23. Chrysiasis (gold)—corneal and lens deposits
24. Cockayne syndrome (Mickey Mouse syndrome)—cataracts, band keratopathy, corneal dystrophy
25. Congenital spherocytic anemia (congenital hemolytic jaundice)—congenital cataract, ring-shaped pigmentary corneal deposits
26. Crouzon syndrome (Parrot-Head syndrome)—exposure keratitis, cataract, corneal dystrophy
27. Cryptophthalmia syndrome (cryptophthalmos-syndactyly syndrome)—cornea differentiated from sclera, lens absence to hypoplasia, dislocation, and calcification
28. Cytomegalic inclusion disease (cytomegalovirus)—cataract, corneal opacities

29. Darier-White syndrome (keratosis follicularis)—keratosis, corneal subepithelial infiltrations, corneal ulceration, cataract

30. Dermatitis herpetiformis (Duhring-Broca disease)—corneal vascularization, cataract

31. Dermochondral corneal dystrophy (of François)—cataract, corneal dystrophy

32. Diabetes mellitus—cataract, corneal edema secondary to rubeosis

33. Diphtheria—keratitis, corneal ulcer, cataract

34. Down syndrome (Trisomy 21)—lens opacities, keratoconus

35. Ehler-Danlos syndrome (fibrodysplasia elastica generalisata)—microcornea, keratoconus, lens subluxation

36. Electrical injury—corneal perforation, necrosis of cornea, anterior or posterior subcapsular cataracts

37. Endothelial dystrophy and anterior polar cataract (Dohlman)

38. Exfoliation syndrome (capsular exfoliation syndrome)—cataract, dislocated lens, corneal dystrophy, lens capsule exfoliation

39. Fabry disease (glycosphingolipid lipidosis)—cataract, corneal dystrophy

40. Folling syndrome (phenylketonuria)—corneal opacities, cataracts

41. Fuchs syndrome (I) (heterochromic cyclitis syndrome)—secondary cataract, edematous corneal epithelium

42. Goldscheider syndrome (epidermolysis bullosa)—bullous keratitis, corneal subepithelial blisters to corneal perforation, cataract

43. Gorlin-Goltz syndrome (multiple basal cell nevi syndrome)—cataract, corneal leukoma

44. Grönblad-Strandberg syndrome (elastorrhexis)—keratoconus, cataract, subluxation of lens

45. Hallermann-Streiff syndrome (oculomandibulofacial dyscephaly)—cataracts, microcornea

46. Hanhart syndrome (recessive keratosis palmoplantaris)—dendritic corneal lesions, keratitis, corneal haze, corneal neovascularization, cataract

47. Heerfordt syndrome (uveoparotid fever)—band keratopathy, keratoconjunctivitis, cataract

48. Hereditary ectodermal dysplasia syndrome (Siemens syndrome)—keratosis, corneal erosions, corneal dystrophy, cataract, lens luxation

49. Herpes simplex—keratitis, corneal ulcer, cataracts

50. Herpes zoster—keratitis, corneal ulcer, cataract

51. Histiocytosis X (Hand-Schüller-Christian syndrome)—pannus, bullous keratopathy, corneal ulcer, cataract

52. Hodgkin disease—keratitis, cataract

53. Homocystinuria syndrome—dislocated lens, cataract, keratitis

54. Hutchinson-Gilford syndrome (progeria)—cataract, microcornea

55. Hydatid cyst (echinococcosis)—keratitis, corneal abscess, cataract

56. Hypervitaminosis D—band keratopathy, cataract

57. Hypoparathyroidism—keratitis, cataract

58. Hypophosphatasia (phosphoethanolaminuria)—cataract, corneal subepithelial calcifications

* = most important

59. Influenza—keratitis, cataract

60. Jadassohn-type anetodermal—keratoconus, cataract

61. Jadassohn-Lewandowsky syndrome (pachyonychia congenita)—corneal dyskeratosis, cataract

*62. Juvenile rheumatoid arthritis (Still disease)—band keratopathy, cataract

63. Kussmaul disease (periarteritis nodosa)—corneal ulcer, cataract

64. Kyrle disease (hyperkeratosis penetrans)—subcapsular cataracts, subepithelial corneal opacities

65. Leber's congenital amaurosis—cataracts, keratoconus

66. Leri syndrome (carpal tunnel syndrome)—corneal clouding, cataract

67. Listerellosis (listeriosis)—keratitis, corneal abscess and ulcer, cataract

68. Little syndrome (nail-patella syndrome)—microcornea, keratoconus, cataract

*69. Lowe syndrome (oculocerebrorenal syndrome)—cloudy cornea, cataracts, megalocornea, corneal dystrophy

70. Malaria—keratitis, cataract

71. Marchesani syndrome (brachymorphy with spherophakia)—lenticular myopia, ectopia lentis, megalocornea, corneal opacity

72. Marfan syndrome (arachnodactyly-dystrophia-mesodermalis congenita)—lens dislocation, cataract, megalocornea, lenticular myopia

73. Matsoukas syndrome (oculo-cerebro-articulo-skeletal syndromes)—cataract, corneal sclerosis

74. Meckel syndrome (dysencephalia splanchnocystic syndrome)—sclerocornea, microcornea, cataract

75. Micro syndrome (autosomal recessive microcephaly, microcornea, congenital cataract, mental retardation, optic atrophy and hypogenitalism)

76. Morbilli (rubeola, measles)—corneal ulcer, cataract

77. Mucolipidosis IV (ML IV)—corneal clouding, cataract

78. Myotonic dystrophy (Curschmann-Steinert syndrome)—lens opacity, cornea-epithelial dystrophy

79. Nematode ophthalmia syndrome (toxocariasis)—cataract, larvae present in the cornea

80. Neurodermatitis (lichen simplex chronicus)—keratoconjunctivitis, atopic cataracts, keratoconus

81. Neurofibromatosis 1

82. Neurofibromatosis 2

83. Ocular toxoplasmosis (toxoplasmosis)—keratitis, cataract

84. Oculodental syndrome (Peter syndrome)—macrocornea, opacities of the corneal margin, ectopic lentis, corneoscleral staphyloma

85. O'Donnell-Pappas syndrome—presenile cataract, peripheral corneal pannus

86. Paget syndrome (osteitis deformans)—corneal ring opacities, cataract

87. Passow syndrome (status dysraphicus syndrome)—neuroparalytic keratitis, zonular cataract

88. Pemphigus foliaceus (Cazenave disease)—pannus, corneal infiltration, cataract

89. Peter's anomaly (anterior chamber cleavage syndrome—lens apposition to leukoma

90. Pigmentary ocular dispersion syndrome (pigmentary glaucoma)—Krukenberg's spindle, equatorial pigmentation of lens capsule

91. Pseudohypoparathyroidism (Seabright-Bantan syndrome)—punctate cataracts, keratitis

92. Radiation—corneal ulcer, punctate keratitis, cataracts, exfoliation of lens capsule

93. Refsum syndrome (phytanic acid oxidase deficiency)—corneal opacities, cataracts

94. Relapsing polychondritis—corneal ulcer, cataracts, keratoconjunctivitis sicca

95. Retinal disinsertion syndrome—lens subluxation, keratoconus

96. Retrolental fibroplasia (RLF)—cataracts, corneal opacification

97. Rieger syndrome (dysgenesis mesodermalis corneae et irides)—microcornea, corneal opacities in Descemet membrane, dislocated lens

98. Romberg syndrome (facial hemiatrophy)—neuroparalytic keratitis, cataracts

99. Rothmund syndrome (telangiectasia-pigmentation-cataract syndrome)—cataract, corneal lesions

*100. Rubella syndrome (German measles)—corneal haziness, cataracts, microcornea

101. Sabin-Feldman syndrome—posterior lenticonus, microcornea

102. Sanfilippo-Good syndrome (mucopolysaccharidosis III)—deposits in cornea and lens

103. Schafer syndrome (keratosis palmoplantaris syndrome)—lesions in the lower portion of the cornea, cataract

104. Schaumann syndrome (sarcoidosis syndrome)—keratitis sicca, band-shaped keratitis, complicated cataract

105. Scheie syndrome (mucopolysaccharidosis IS)—diffuse haze to marked corneal clouding, cataracts

106. Siderosis (intraocular iron foreign body)—iron deposition in lens and cornea

107. Stannus cerebellar syndrome—corneal vascularization, corneal opacities, cataracts

108. Steroids—cataract, may worsen certain types of corneal infections

109. Stevens-Johnson syndrome (erythema multiforme exudativum)—keratitis, corneal ulcers, cataracts, pannus

110. Stickler syndrome (hereditary progressive arthro-ophthalmopathy)—keratopathy, cataracts

111. Thioridazine—corneal and lens opacities

112. Toxic lens syndrome—pigment precipitation on the surface of an intraocular lens, chronic uveitis

113. Trisomy syndrome—corneal and lens opacities

114. Turner's syndrome (gonadal dysgenesis)—corneal nebulae, cataracts

115. Ultraviolet radiation—band keratopathy, keratitis, discoloring of lens

116. van Bogaert-Scherer-Epstein syndrome (familial hypercholesterolemia syndrome)—lipid keratopathy, cataract, juvenile corneal arcus

117. von Recklinghausen syndrome (neurofibromatosis)—nodular swelling of corneal nerves, cataracts

118. Waardenburg syndrome (interoculoiridodermatoauditive dysplasia)—microcornea, cornea plana, lenticonus

* = most important

119. Wagner syndrome (hereditary hyaloideoretinal degeneration and palatoschisis)—corneal degeneration, including band-shaped keratopathy, cataracts

120. Ward syndrome (nevus jaw cyst syndrome)—congenital cataracts, congenital corneal opacities

121. Wegener syndrome (Wegener granulomatosis)—corneal ulcer, corneal abscess, cataract

122. Weil disease (leptospirosis)—keratitis, cataract

123 Werner syndrome (progeria of adults)—juvenile cataracts, bullous keratitis, trophic corneal defects

*124. Wilson disease (hepatolenticular degeneration)—sunflower cataract, Kayser-Fleischer ring

125. Yersiniosis—corneal ulcer, cataract

126. Zellweger syndrome (cerebrohepatorenal syndrome of Zellweger)—corneal opacities, cataract

Bilgami, N.L., et al.: Marfan syndrome with microcornea, aphakia, and ventricular systolic defect. Indian Heart J., 33:78–80, 1981.

Dolan, B.J., et al.: Amiodarone keratopathy and lens opacities. J. Am. Optom. Assoc., 56:468–470, 1985.

Gualtieri, C.T., et al.: Corneal and lenticular opacities in mentally retarded young adults treated with thioridazine and chlorpromazine. Am. J. Psychiatry, 139:1178–1180, 1982.

Polomeno, R.C., and Cummings, C.: Autosomal dominant cataracts and microcornea. Can. J. Ophthalmol., 14:227–229, 1979.

Roy, F.H.: Ocular Syndromes and Systemic Diseases. 2nd Ed. Philadelphia, W.B. Saunders, 1989.

Warburg, M., et al.: Autosomal recessive microcephaly, microcornea, congenital cataract, mental retardation, optic atrophy, and hypogenitalism-Micro syndrome. Amer. J. Diseases of Children, 147:309–312, 1993.

Drugs Associated with Cataracts

Acetophenazine	carbamazepine(?)	demecarium
acetylcholine	carbromal(?)	desoxycorticosterone
adrenal cortex injection	carphenazine	dexamethasone
alcohol	chloroquine	dextrothyroxine(?)
aldosterone	chlorperazine	diazoxide
allopurinol	chlorpromazine	diethazine
amiodarone(?)	chlorphentermine(?)	diethylpropion(?)
amodiaquine	chlorpromazine	droperidol(?)
azathioprine(?)	(phenothiazine)	echothiophate
BCG vaccine(?)	chlorprothixene	ergocalciferol
benzodiazepine	cholecalciferol(?)	ergonovine(?)
benzphetamine(?)	clomiphene(?)	ergot(?)
betamethasone	cobalt	ergotamine(?)
betaxolol(?)	colchicine(?)	ethopropazine
busulfan	cortisone	ethotoin
butaperazine	danazol(?)	etretinate
calcitriol(?)	deferoxamine	fenfluramine(?)

fludrocortisone
fluorometholone
fluphenazine
fluprednisolone
gold
haloperidol(?)
hydrocortisone
hydroxychloroquine
ibuprofen(?)
indomethacin(?)
isofluorphate
isotretinoin(?)
levobunolol(?)
lithium carbonate(?)
medrysone
megestrol acetate
mephenytoin(?)
meprednisone
mesoridazine
methdilazine
methotrimeprazine
methoxsalen(?)
methylergonovine(?)
methylprednisolone
methysergide(?)

mitomycin C (topical) (?)
mitotane
naltrexone
naproxen(?)
neostigmine
nifedipine(?)
oral contraceptives(?)
oxygen
paramethasone
penicillamine(?)
perazine
pericyazine
perphenazine
phendimetrazine(?)
phentermine(?)
phenytoin
physostigmine
pilocarpine
piperacetazine
piperazine(?)
prazosin(?)
prednisolone
prednisone (steroid)
prochlorperazine
promazine

promethazine
propiomazine
puva (?)
silicone
sulfonamides (maternal ingestion)
sulindac(?)
thiethylperazine
thiopropazate
thioproperazine
thioridazine
thiothixene
timolol(?)
triamcinolone
trifluoperazine
trifluperidol(?)
triflupromazine
trimeprazine
trioxsalen(?)
troleandomycin (?)
urokinase(?)
verapamil(?)
vitamin D_2(?)
vitamin D_3(?)

Syndromes and Diseases Associated with Cataracts

1. Abefeld syndrome (blepharophimosis associated with generalized myopathy)
2. Acrodermatitis chronica atrophicans
3. Addison syndrome (adrenal cortical insufficiency)
4. Albinism
5. Albright hereditary osteodystrophy (pseudohypoparathyroidism)
6. Alopecia areata
*7. Alport syndrome (hereditary nephritis)
8. Alström disease (cataract and retinitis pigmentosa)
9. Andogsky syndrome (atopic cataract syndrome)
10. Anterior segment ischemia syndrome
11. Apert syndrome (acrocephalosyndactylism syndrome)
12. Apical malformations associated with cataracts
13. Arteriovenous fistula
14. Arthrogryposis multiplex congenita
15. Aspergillosis
*16. Atopic dermatitis syndrome

* = most important

17. Autosomal dominant foveal hypoplasia and presenile cataract syndrome (O'Donnell-Pappas syndrome)
18. Bassen-Kornzweig syndrome (abetalipoproteinemia)
19. Bloch-Sulzberger syndrome (incontinentia pigmenti)
20. Bonnevie-Ullrich syndrome (pterygolymphangiectasia)
21. Bourneville syndrome (tuberous sclerosis)
22. Buerger disease (thromboangiitis obliterans)
23. Caisson syndrome (bends)
24. Capsular exfoliation syndrome
25. Carotid artery syndrome
26. Cataract and hypertrophic neuropathy—autosomal recessive
27. Cataract with microcornea and coloboma of iris—autosomal dominant
28. Cataract, floriform—autosomal dominant
29. Cataract and cardiomyopathy—autosomal recessive
30. Cataract, congenital, or juvenile—autosomal recessive
31. Cataract, congenital total, with posterior sutural opacities in heterozygotes—X-linked
32. Cataract, congenital with absence deformity of leg—autosomal recessive
33. Cataract, congenital, with microcornea or slight microphthalmia—X-linked
34. Cataract, cortical and congenital ichthyosis—autosomal recessive
35. Cataract, mental retardation, hypogonadism (Martsolf syndrome)
36. Cataract, microcephaly, arthrogryposis kyphosis syndrome (CAMAK syndrome)—autosomal recessive
37. Cataract microcephaly, failure to thrive, kyphoscoliosis syndrome (CAMFAK syndrome)—autosomal recessive
38. Cataract, nuclear and total nuclear—usually autosomal dominant rarely recessive
39. Cataract, zonular, and nystagmus—X-linked
40. Cat-eye syndrome (Schachenmann syndrome)
41. Cerebral cholesterinosis (cerebrotendinous xanthomatosis)
42. Cerebellar ataxia, cataract, deafness, and dementia or psychosis
43. Cerebral palsy
44. Cerebrohepatorenal syndrome (Smith-Lemli-Opitz syndrome)
45. Cerebrotendinous xanthomatosis
46. Cholera
47. Chromosome 13q partial deletion (long-arm) syndrome
48. Chromosomal 3; 18 translocation
49. Chromosome deletion (short-arm) syndrome
50. Cockayne syndrome (dwarfism with retinal atrophy and deafness)
51. Cerebro-oculofascioskeletal syndrome (COFS syndrome)
52. Congenital cataract and hypertrophic cardiomyopathy syndrome
53. Congenital cataract with oxycephaly (tower skull)
54. Congenital hemolytic icterus

55. Congenital ichthyosiform erythroderma
56. Congenital rubella syndrome (German measles)
57. Conradi syndrome (stippled epiphyses syndrome)
58. Comedo-cataract
59. Craniofacial dysostosis (Crouzon disease)
60. Cretinism (hypothyroidism)
61. Crome syndrome (congenital cataracts, epileptic fits, mental retardation, small stature)
62. Cushing syndrome
63. Cytomegalovirus
64. Darier-White syndrome (keratosis follicularis)
65. Dermatitis herpetiformis
*66. Diabetes mellitus (Willis disease)
66. Diarrhea
67. Diphtheria
68. Ectodermal dysplasia
69. Electrical injury
70. Ellis-van Creveld syndrome (chondroectodermal dysplasia)
71. Engelmann syndrome (diaphyseal dysplasia)
72. Epidermal nevus syndrome (ichthyosis hystrix)
73. Fabry disease (diffuse angiokeratosis)
74. Familial congenital cataracts, microcornea, abnormal irides, nystagmus, and glaucoma syndrome
75. Familial congenital cataract, nonprogressive neurologic disorders, and mental deficiency syndrome
76. Familial histiocytic dermatoarthritis syndrome
77. Familial hypogonadism syndrome
78. Familial t (2;16) translocation
79. Fetal alcohol syndrome
80. Folling syndrome (phenylketonuria)
81. François dyscephalic syndrome (Hallerman-Streiff syndrome)
82. Frenkel syndrome (ocular contusion syndrome)
83. Fuchs syndrome (1) (heterochromic cyclitis syndrome)
84. Galactokinase deficiency—autosomal recessive
*85. Galactosemia-transferase deficiency
86. Goldenhar syndrome (oculoauriculovertebral dysplasia)
87. Goldscheider syndrome (epidermolysis bullosa)
88. Gorlin-Goltz syndrome (multiple basal cell nevi syndrome)
89. Grönblad-Strandberg syndrome (pseudoxanthoma elasticum)
90. Gyrate atrophy (ornithine ketoacid aminotransferase deficiency)
91. Hagberg-Santavuori syndrome (neuronal ceroid-lipofuscinosis)
92. Hallerman-Streiff syndrome (oculomandibulofacial dyscephaly)

* = most important

93. Hand-Schüller-Christian syndrome (histiocytosis X)

94. Harada disease (uveitis-vitiligo-alopecia-poliosis syndrome)

95. Heerfordt syndrome (uveoparotid fever)

96. Hemifacial microsomia syndrome (François-Haustrate syndrome)

97. Herpes simplex virus

98. Hilding syndrome (destructive iridocyclitis and multiple joint dislocations)

99. Hodgkin disease

100. Homocystinuria

101. Hookworm disease

102. Hruby-Irvine-Gass syndrome (cystoid maculopathy following cataract extraction with vitreous loss)

103. Hutchinson-Gilford syndrome (progeria)

104. Hydatid cyst

105. Hypercalcemia (adult)

106. Hypercalcemia (infantile) with mental retardation (supravalvular aortic stenosis syndrome)

107. Hyperprolactinemia

108. Hypertrophic cardiomyopathy

109. Hypervitaminosis A

110. Hypervitaminosis D

111. Hypocalcemia

112. Hypoglycemia

113. Hypoparathyroidism

114. Hypophosphatasia (phosphoethanolaminuria)

115. Incontinentia pigmenti achromians

116. Infantile hypoglycemia (male)

117. Influenza

118. Infrared radiation

119. Intrauterine infections
    A. herpes virus
    B. mumps
    C. rubella
    D. toxoplasmosis
    E. vaccinia

120. Jacobsen-Brodwall syndrome

121. Jadassohn-Lewandowsky syndrome (pachyonychia congenita)

122. Karsch-Neugebauer syndrome (nystagmus-split hand syndrome)

123. Klippel-Trenaunay-Weber syndrome (angio-osteohypertrophy syndrome)

124. Krause syndrome (congenital encephalo-ophthalmic dysplasia)

125. Kussmaul disease (periarteritis nodosa)

126. Kyrle disease (hyperkeratosis penetrans)
127. Lanzieri syndrome (craniofacial malformations)
128. Laser treatment for retinopathy of prematurity
129. Laurence-Moon-Biedl syndrome (retinitis pigmentosa-polydactyly-adiposogenital)
130. Leber syndrome (optic atrophy-amaurosis-pituitary syndrome)
131. Leiomyoma
132. Leri syndrome (carpal tunnel syndrome)
133. Lightning
134. Listerellosis
*135. Lowe syndrome (oculocerebrorenal syndrome)
136. Majewski syndrome (short rib polydactyly syndrome)
137. Malaria
138. Male Turner syndrome (Noonan syndrome)
139. Malignant hyperpyrexia syndrome
140. Mandibulofacial dysostosis (Franceschetti syndrome)
141. Mannosidosis
142. Maple syrup urine disease (branched chain ketoaciduria)
143. Marfan syndrome (arachnodactyly dystrophia mesodermaliscongenita)
144. Marinesco-Sjögren syndrome (congenital cataract-oligophrenia syndrome)
145. Marshall syndrome (atypical ectodermal dysplasia)
146. Martsolf syndrome
147. Matsoukas syndrome (oculo-cerebro-articulo-skeletal syndrome)
148. Meckel syndrome (dysencephalia splanchnocystic syndrome)
149. Microcephaly, microphthalmia, cataracts and joint contractures syndrome
150. Microphthalmia—congenital anterior polar cataract syndrome—autosomal dominant
151. Miller syndrome (Wilms aniridia syndrome)
152. Monilethrix
153. Morgan syndrome (intracranial exostosis)
154. Morquio-Brailsford syndrome (mucopolysaccharidoses IV)
155. Multiple sulfatase deficiency
156. Myopic (high)
157. Myotonic dystrophy (Curschmann-Steinert syndrome)
158. Nail-patella syndrome (Little syndrome)
159. Nance-Horan syndrome (cataract-dental syndrome)
160. Neurodermatitis
161. Neurofibromatosis 1 (von Recklinghausen syndrome)
162. Neurofibromatosis 2 (central neurofibromatosis)
163. Nieden syndrome (telangiectasia-cataract syndrome)
164. Norrie's disease
165. Oculo-oto-ororenoerythropoietic disease

* = most important

166. Optic atrophy, cataract, and neurologic disorder—autosomal dominant
166. Osteogenesis imperfecta congenita, microcephaly and cataracts—autosomal recessive
167. Osteopetrosis (Albers-Schönberg syndrome)
168. Oxycephaly
169. Pachyonychia congenita syndrome
170. Paget syndrome (idiopathic hyperphosphatasemia)
171. Partial trisomy 10q trisomy
172. Passow syndrome (syringomyelia)
173. Pellagra (avitaminosis B_2)
174. Pemphigus foliaceus (Cazenave disease)
175. Pernicious anemia syndrome (vitamin B_{12} deficiency)
176. Pierre-Robin syndrome (micrognathia-glossoptosis syndrome)
177. Prader-Labhart-Willi syndrome (hypogenital dystrophy with diabetic tendency)
178. Pseudoexfoliation syndrome
179. Pseudohypoparathyroidism
180. Radiation
181. Reese-Ellsworth syndrome (anterior chamber cleavage syndrome)
182. Refsum syndrome (phytanic acid storage disease)
183. Renal failure (chronic)
184. Renal transplantation
185. Retinal ischemic infarction syndrome
*186. Retinitis pigmentosa-deafness-ataxia syndrome
187. Rhizomelic chondrodysplasia punctata
188. Riboflavin deficiency syndrome (oculo-orogenital syndrome)
189. Ring chromosome in the D group
190. Robert syndrome
191. Romberg syndrome (facial hemiatrophy)
192. Rothmund syndrome (infantile poikiloderma)
*193. Roy syndrome (unilateral cataract associated with smoking)
194. Rubeola (measles)
195. Rubinstein-Taybi syndrome (broad thumbs syndrome)
196. Scaphocephaly syndrome (craniofacial dysostoses)
197. Schaefer syndrome (congenital dyskeratosis)
198. Schwartz syndrome
199. Scurvy (avitaminosis C)
200. Sickle-cell disease (Herrick syndrome)
201. Siemen syndrome (congenital atrophy of the skin)
203. Sjögren syndrome (secreto-inhibitor syndrome)
204. Sjögren Larsson syndrome (oligophrenia ichthyosis)
205. Smith-Lemli-Opitz syndrome
206. Split-hand with congenital nystagmus, fundal changes, cataracts—autosomal dominant

207. Spondyloepiphyseal dysplasia (SED) dwarfism

208. Stannus cerebellar syndrome (vitamin B_2 deficiency)

209. Stickler syndrome (hereditary progressive arthro-ophthalmopathy)

*210. Still disease (juvenile rheumatoid arthritis)

211. Toxocariasis (nematode ophthalmia syndrome)

212. Treacher-Collins syndrome (mandibulofacial dysostosis)

213. Trichomegaly, spherocytosis, and cataract—autosomal dominant

214. Trichorrhexis nodosa (argininosuccinicaciduria)

215. Trisomy 13-syndrome (Patau syndrome)

216. Trisomy 16-syndrome (Edward syndrome)

217. Trisomy 20p syndrome

218. Trisomy 21 (Down's syndrome)

219. Tuomaala-Haapanen syndrome

220. Turner syndrome (gonadal dysgenesis)

221. Tyrosinosis (Hanhart syndrome)

222. Usher syndrome (hereditary retinitis pigmentosa—deafness syndrome)

223. Uvea-touch syndrome

224. Van der Hoeve syndrome (brittle bone disease)

225. Van Bogaert-Scherer-Epstein syndrome (primary hyperlipidemia)

226. Varicella infection

227. von Recklinghausen syndrome (neurofibromatosis)

228. Wagner syndrome (hyaloideoretinal degeneration)

229. Warburg syndrome (hydrocephalus, agyria, and absent cortical laminar retinal dysplasia with or without encephalocele)

230. Ward syndrome (nevus-jaw cyst syndrome)

231. Wegener syndrome (Wegener granulomatosis)

232. Weil disease (leptospirosis)

233. Werner syndrome (scleropoililoderma)

234. Wilson disease (hepatolenticular degeneration)

235. Yersiniosis

236. Zellweger syndrome (cerebrohepatorenal syndrome)

237. 3+ syndrome

238. 4p syndrome

239. 18p syndrome

240. 18q syndrome

Bateman, J.B., and Philippart, M.: Ocular features of the Hagberg-Santavuori syndrome. Am. J. Ophthalmol., 102:262–271, 1986.

Christiansen, J.P., and Bradford, J.D.: Cataract in infants treatment with argon laser photocoagulation for threshold retinopathy of prematurity. Amer. J. Ophthal., 119:175–80, 1995.

Cruysberg, J.R.M., et al.: Features of a syndrome with congenital cataract and hypertrophic cardiomyopathy. Am. J. Ophthalmol., 102:740–749, 1986.

Isenberg, S.J.: The Eye in Infancy. Chicago, Year Book Medical Publishers, 1989.

* = most important

Pau, H.: Differential Diagnosis of Eye Diseases. 2nd Ed. New York, Thieme Med. Pub., 1988.

Roy, F.H.: Ocular Syndromes and Systemic Diseases. 2nd Ed. Philadelphia, W.B. Saunders, 1989.

Roy, F.H.: Cigarette smoking and the risk of cataract. (letter) JAMA, 269:748, 1993.

Lenticulocorneal Adherence (Lens Adjacent to Endothelium of Cornea)

1. Acquired anterior corneal disease as ulcer with perforation or trauma
2. Aniridia
3. Peters anomaly (oculodental syndrome)
4. Rieger anomaly (dysgenesis mesostromalis)

Kivlin, J.D., et al.: Peters' anomaly as a consequence of genetic and nongenetic syndromes. Arch. Ophthalmol., 104:61–64, 1986.

Waring, G., et al.: Ultrastructure and successful keratoplasty of sclerocornea in Mieten's syndrome. Am. J. Ophthalmol., 90:469–475, 1980.

Spasm of Accommodation (Increased Tone of Ciliary Body with Increased Convexity of Crystalline Lens) (see Acquired Myopia)

1. Alcoholism
2. Cerebrovascular accident
3. Contusion injury to the globe or head
4. Cyclic oculomotor palsy or spasm
5. Diabetes mellitus
6. Drugs, such as aceclidine, acetylcholine, carbachol, demecarium, DFP, digitalis, echothiophate, guanethidine, isoflurophate, methylene blue, morphine, neostigmine, opium, physostigmine, pilocarpine
7. Fatigue cramp of overworked ciliary muscle; most frequent with compound hyperopia and mixed astigmatism associated with anisometropia
8. Graves disease (hyperthyroidism, Basedow syndrome)
9. Infectious, such as diphtheria, helminthic infestations, or sinus disease
10. Irritative lesions of brain stem and oculomotor trunk, such as epidemic encephalitis, tabes, meningitis, influenza, scleritis, measles, or orbital inflammation
11. Middle cerebral artery occlusion
12. Ocular inflammation, such as ciliary muscle irritant
13. Pineal tumor
14. Reflex irritation, such as in trigeminal neuralgia
15. Sympathetic paralysis
16. Trauma

Fraunfelder, F.T.: Drug-Induced Ocular Side Effects and Drug Interactions. 4th Ed. Philadelphia, Williams & Wilkins, 1996.

Pau, H.: Differential Diagnosis of Eye Diseases. 2nd Ed. New York, Thieme Med. Pub, 1988.

Ohtsuka, K., et al.: Accommodation and convergence insufficiency with left middle cerebral artery occlusion. Am. J. Ophthalmol., 106:60–64, 1988.

Walsh, F.B., and Hoyt, W.F.: Clinical Neuro-ophthalmology. 4th Ed. Baltimore, Williams & Wilkins, 1988.

Paresis of Accommodation (Partial or Total Loss of Physiologic Ability to Change Shape of Lens and Thus Focus of Eye [see Mydriasis, p. 386]; This Ability is Related to Age [see Acquired Hyperopia])

 *1. Presbyopia—gradual decrease in amplitude of accommodation related to age

 2. Accommodative insufficiency

  A. Asthenic individuals

  B. Illness or debilitation, including intestinal toxemia, tuberculosis, influenza, whooping cough, measles, and tonsillar and dental infections

  C. Anemia

  D. Overwork

  E. Whiplash injury

 3. Ciliary body aplasia—with or without pupillary and iris abnormalities

 4. Iridocyclitis—acute and chronic

 5. Glaucoma with atrophy of ciliary body

 6. Choroidal metastasis with suprachoroidal extension

 7. Trauma, such as tears in iris sphincter, tears at root of iris, or recession of the anterior chamber angle with posterior displacement of the ciliary attachment and ocular hypotension

 8. Rupture of zonular fibers and partial subluxation of lens

 9. Myotonic dystrophy (Curschmann-Steinert syndrome)

 10. Drugs, including:

acetazolamide	benztropine
acetophenazine	betamethasone
adiphenine	bethanechol
alcohol	biperiden
alprazolam	bromide
ambutonium	butaperazine
aminosalicylate(?)	captopril(?)
aminosalicylic acid(?)	caramiphen
amitriptyline	carbachol
amodiaquine	carbamazepine
amoxapine	carbinoxamine
amphetamine	carbon dioxide
anisindione	carphenazine
anisotropine	chloramphenicol
antazoline	chlordiazepoxide
atropine	chlorisondamine
belladonna	chlorothiazide
bendroflumethiazide	chlorphenoxamine
benzathine penicillin G	chlorpromazine
benzphetamine	chlorthalidone
benzthiazide	cimetidine

*= most important

clemastine
clidinium
clomipramine
clonazepam
clorazepate
cocaine
cortisone
cyclopentolate
cyclothiazide
cycrimine
desipramine
dexamethasone
dextroamphetamine
diacetylmorphine
diazepam
dibucaine
dichlorphenamide
dicyclomine
diethazine
diphemanil
diphenadione
diphenhydramine
diphenylpyraline
emetine
ergot
ethopropazine
fluorometholone
fluphenazine
glycopyrrolate
hexamethonium
hexocyclium
homatropine
hydrochlorothiazide
hydrocortisone
hydroflumethiazide
hydromorphone
hydroxyamphetamine
imipramine
indapamide
iodide and iodine solutions and compounds
isoniazid
isopropamide
maprotiline

marijuana
mecamylamine
medrysone
mepenzolate
meprobamate
mescaline
mesoridazine
methacholine
methamphetamine
methantheline
methaqualone
methazolamide
methdilazine
methixene
methotrimeprazine
methscopolamine
methyclothiazide
methylatropine nitrate
methylene blue
methyprylon
methysergide metolazone
mianserin
midazolam
morphine
nalidixic acid
naproxen
nitrazepam
nortriptyline
opium
orphenadrine
oxazepam
oxymorphone
oxyphencyclimine
oxyphenonium
pargyline
pentazocine
pentolinium
perazine
periciazine
perphenazine
phendimetrazine
phenindione
phenmetrazine

phentermine

pilocarpine

pimozide

pipenzolate

piperacetazine

piperazine

piperidolate

piperocaine

piroxicam(?)

poldine

polythiazide

potassium penicillin G

potassium penicillin V

potassium phenethicillin

pralidoxime

prazepam

prednisolone

primidone

procaine penicillin G

procarbazine

prochlorperazine

procyclidine

promazine

promethazine

propantheline

propiomazine

propranolol

protriptyline

psilocybin

pyrilamine

quinethazone

radioactive iodides

rubella virus vaccine (live)

scopolamine

streptomycin

temazepam

tetanus immune globulin

tetanus toxoid

tetracaine

tetraethylammonium

tetrahydrocannabinol

thiethylperazine

thiopropazate

thioproperazine

thioridazine

thiothixene

triazolam

trichlormethiazide

trichloroethylene

tridihexethyl

trifluoperazine

trifluperidol

triflupromazine

trihexyphenidyl

trimeprazine

trimethaphan

trimethidinium

trimipramine

tripelennamine

tropicamide

vinblastine

vincristine

11. Neurogenic causes

    A. Infectious conditions

        (1) Epidemic encephalitis

        (2) Anterior poliomyelitis

        (3) Exanthemas and acute infections, such as scarlet fever, mumps, measles, influenza, typhoid fever, dengue fever, viral hepatitis, amebic dysentery, and malaria

        (4) Herpes zoster

        (5) Syphilis (lues)

        (6) Tuberculosis

        (7) Leprosy (Hansen disease)

        (8) Focal infections, such as from teeth or nasal sinuses

B. Toxic conditions

   (1) Alcohol

   (2) Lead

   (3) Arsenic

   (4) Carbon monoxide

   (5) Diphtheritic paralysis

   (6) Botulism

   (7) Extensive burn

   (8) Snake venom

C. Degenerative conditions

   (1) Congenital hereditary ophthalmoplegia

   (2) Progressive congenital ophthalmoplegia

   (3) Hereditary ataxia

   (4) Myotonic dystrophy (Curschmann-Steinert syndrome)

   (5) Myasthenia gravis

D. Metabolic conditions

   (1) Acute hemorrhagic anterior polioencephalitis of Wernicke

   (2) Diabetes mellitus

   (3) Lactation

   (4) Following pregnancy

E. Isolated internal ophthalmoplegia

F. Isolated failure of near reflex, such as with inverse Argyll-Robertson pupil

G. Lesions of parasympathetic nuclei in midbrain

   (1) Encephalitis

   (2) Pineal tumor

   (3) Other signs of mesencephalic disease, including multiple sclerosis, infectious polyneuropathy, and vascular lesions

   (4) Syphilis—bilateral

H. Trauma to head or neck

   (1) Cerebral concussion

   (2) Craniocervical extension injuries

Pau, F.H.: Differential Diagnosis of Eye Diseases. 2nd Ed. New York, Thieme Med. Pub., 1988.

Roy, F.H.: Ocular Syndromes and Systemic Diseases. 2nd Ed. Philadelphia, W.B. Saunders, 1989.

Walsh, F.B., and Hoyt, W.F.: Clinical Neuro-Ophthalmology. 4th Ed. Baltimore, Williams & Wilkins, 1985.

Vitreous

MANDI CONWAY, M.D.

Contents

Pseudodetachment of Vitreous (Conditions Simulating Detachment of Vitreous)

1. Enormous cavity in the vitreous body with a relatively thin posterior wall
2. Membranous formations within the vitreous associated with uveitis and hemorrhage
3. Outline of the ascending portion of Cloquet's canal just anterior to the disc

Tolentino, F.I., et al.: Vitreoretinal Disorders Diagnoses and Management. Philadelphia, W.B. Saunders, 1976.

Anterior Vitreous Detachment (Anterior Vitreous Cortex May Be Separated from Posterior Lens or Posterior Zonular Fibers)

1. Retrolenticular—usually caused by vitreous shrinkage

   *A. Trauma (most common)

    B. Hemorrhage—usually secondary to trauma

    C. Senescence (rare)

    D. Inflammation

    E. Retinal detachment (see p. 541)

  *F. Iatrogenic after injection of vitreous substitutes (gas)

2. Retro-ocular

    A. Vitreous shrinkage (see p. 471)

    B. Ciliary body tumor

    C. Blood

    D. Exudate

3. Retrolenticular and retro-ocular combined occurs with rupture of the hyaloideo-capsular ligament

Tolentino, F.I., et al.: Vitreoretinal Disorders Diagnosis and Management. Philadelphia, W.B. Saunders, 1976.

Posterior Vitreous Detachment

1. Complete posterior detachment

    A. Simple detachment—occurs in young persons

      (1) Exudate from chorioretinal focus

      (2) Hemorrhage between the vitreous and the retina

      (3) Retraction of the cortical vitreous caused by exudate within the vitreous

      (4) Vitreous hemorrhage in a young individual with vitreous shrinking due to thrombosis of central retinal vein, retinal neovascularization

    B. Complete posterior detachment with collapse

      (1) Senescent changes are primary cause

      (2) Uveitis

      (3) Trauma

      (4) Hemorrhage

      (5) Sodium hyaluronate

    C. Funnel-shaped posterior detachment

      (1) Perforating injuries of globe

      (2) Retinal neovascularization

      (3) Massive vitreous detachment

    D. Atypical complete posterior detachment—residual adherence of vitreous to a peripheral retinal area

      (1) Focus of chorioretinitis

      (2) Following cataract extraction with loss of vitreous

      (3) Following perforating wounds

      (4) Posterior uveitis with inflammatory cells

2. Partial posterior detachment (unusual)

    A. Superior detachment—primarily a senescent change; generally forerunner of posterior vitreous detachment with collapse

    B. Partial posterior detachment (not infrequent)

     (1) Preretinal hemorrhage

     (2) Retinal neovascularization

C. Partial lateral or partial inferior detachment

     (1) Focus of choroiditis

     (2) Circumscribed retinal periphlebitis

     (3) Intraocular foreign body

Foos, R.Y., et al.: Posterior vitreous detachment in diabetic subjects. Ophthalmology, 87:122, 1980.

Jaffe, N.S.: The Vitreous in Clinical Ophthalmology. St. Louis, C.V. Mosby, 1969.

Nirankari, V.S., et al.: Pseudo-vitreous hemorrhage: A new intraoperative complication of sodium hyaluronate. Ophthal. Surg., 12:503, 1981.

Rand, S., et al.: Visual outcome in moderate and severe proliferative diabetic retinopathy. Arch. Ophthalmol., 99:1551, 1981.

Posterior Vitreous Detachment

	Complete, Simple Posterior Vitreous Detachment	Compete Posterior Vitreous Detachment with Collapse
Age	Young	Old or myopes of any age
Etiology	Inflammation, hemorrhage, trauma	Senescence
Refractive error	Unimportant	Myopia in younger patients
Prior vitreous degeneration	None	Fibrillary degeneration and cavities
Vitreous cells	Cells and vitreous precipitates	None
Rocking movements of vitreous	Rare	Frequent
Retinal breaks	Rare (except trauma)	10–15%
Hemorrhages	Rare in inflammatory disorders	10–15%
Vitreoretinal traction	Rare	10–15%
Prepapillary opacity	Yes	Yes
Onset	Slowly progressive	
Shape of posterior vitreous border	Spherical	Collapsed

* = most important

Vitreous Hemorrhage

1. Acquired lues (syphilis)
2. Arsenic toxicity
3. Ascariasis
4. Avulsed retinal vessel syndrome
5. Battered baby syndrome (Silverman syndrome)
6. Behçet syndrome (dermatostomato-ophthalmic syndrome)
7. Blood disease—retinal hemorrhage breaking into vitreous
    A. Anemias
        (1) Aplastic anemia
        (2) Hemolytic anemia
        (3) Hypochromic anemia
        (4) Pernicious anemia
    B. Dysproteinemias—macroglobulins and cryoglobulins
    C. Hemophilia associated with trauma
    D. Leukemias
    E. Multiple myeloma (Kahler disease)
    F. Polycythemia vera (Vaquez disease)
    G. Thrombocytopenic purpura
8. Coats disease (retinal telangiectasia)
9. Collagen disease
    A. Dermatomyositis
    B. Disseminated lupus erythematosus (Kaposi-Libman-Sacks syndrome)
    C. Polyarteritis nodosa (Kussmaul disease)
    D. Scleroderma (progressive systemic sclerosis)
10. Complete posterior vitreous detachment with collapse (10–15% at time of event)
11. Cysticercosis
12. Dengue fever
13. Diabetes mellitus-proliferative retinopathy
14. Dislocation of intraocular lenses
15. Disseminated intravascular coagulation
16. Drusen of optic disc
17. Eales disease
18. Exudative age-related macular degeneration
19. Familial exudative vitreoretinopathy
20. Gronblad-Strandberg syndrome (systemic elastodystrophy)
21. Hemorrhages in the newborn
    A. Hemorrhagic disease of the newborn factor VII and prothrombin deficiency
    B. Persistent vessels of the hyaloid system
    C. Retinal hemorrhage of newborn breaking through to vitreous cavity

22. Iatrogenic globe perforation associated with strabismus surgery

23. Indomethacin reaction

24. Influenza

25. Intraocular foreign body

26. Intraocular tumor

27. Hypertension (venous occlusive disease)

28. Juvenile retinoschisis

*29. Macroaneurysm (retinal arterial)

30. Malaria

31. Malignant melanoma

32. Migration from anterior bleeding as from angle supported, iris supported or posterior chamber lenses

*33. Neovascularization following vascular occlusion (primarily venous occlusive disease)

34. Neovascularization of cataract wound

35. Ocular ischemic syndrome with neovascularization of disc

36. Pars planitis

37. Persistent hyaloid artery

38. Persistent hyperplastic primary vitreous (PHPV)

*39. Posterior vitreous detachment (PVD)

40. Purtscher disease (traumatic retinal angiopathy)

41. Retinal angiomatosis (von Hippel disease)

*42. Retinal break or tear with or without retinal detachment and avulsed retinal vessels

*43. Retinal hemorrhage, including vein occlusion and sickle retinopathy, arterial macroaneurysm

44. Retinal tacks (intrusion)

45. Retinoblastoma

46. Retinopathy of prematurity-proliferative stage

47. Scleral buckle (intrusion)

48. Sleep apnea

49. Sickle cell disease (Herrick syndrome)—SA, SS or SC

50. Surgical cataract complication with lenticular fragments dislocated into vitreous

51. Terson syndrome of associated vitreous and subarachnoid hemorrhage syndrome

52. Thalassemia (Cooley anemia)

53. Thromboangiitis obliterans (Buerger disease)

54. Tuberous sclerosis

55. von Hippel-Lindau disease (angiomatosis retinae)

56. von Willebrand's syndrome

57. Trauma

58. Traumatic asphyxia

* = most important

59. Tuberculosis

60. Uveitis (associated with)

Brown, G.C., et al.: Ophthalmic Manifestation of Carotid Artery Disease in Singerman, L.T., et al.: Retinal and Choroidal Manifestation of Systemic Disease. Philadelphia, Williams & Wilkins, 1991.

Chen, T.L., and Yarng, S.S.: Vitreous hemorrhage from a persistent hyaloid artery. Retina, 13:148–151, 1993.

Dana, M.R., et al.: Spontaneous and traumatic vitreous hemorrhage. Ophthal., 100:1377–1383, 1993.

Ferrone, P.J. and de Juan, E.: Vitreous hemorrhage in infants. Arch. Ophthal., 112:1185–1189, 1994.

Gass, J.D.: Hemorrhage into the vitreous; a presenting manifestation of malignant melanoma of the choroid. Arch. Ophthal., 69:778–779, 1963.

Phillips, W.B., et al.: Pars planitis presenting with vitreous hemorrhage. Ophthal. Surgery, 24:630–631, 1993.

Roy, F.H.: Ocular Syndromes and Systemic Diseases. 2nd Ed. Philadelphia, W.B. Saunders, 1989.

Vitreous Hemorrhage

	Retinal Break	Diabetes Mellitus	Blunt Ocular Trauma	Sickle Cell Disease	Blood Disease ie Anemia	Collagen Disease ie Lupus Erythematosus	Eales Disease	Coat's Disease	Von-Hippel-Lindau Disease	Malignant Melanoma	Retinopathy of Prematurity	Retinal Vein Occlusion
History												
1. Aphakic, myopic and traumatized eyes	U											
2. Bilateral		U		U	U	S	U		U		U	
3. Congenital				U				U	R			
4. Familial	S	U		U					U	R		
5. Greater in blacks				U								
6. Greater in females						U						
7. Greater in males			U				U	U				
8. Greater in whites										U		
9. Greater over 40 years of age												U
10. History of arteriosclerosis, hypertensive disease or hyperviscosity syndromes												U
11. Occurs birth to 2 years											U	
12. Occurs 1st decade								U				
13. Occurs 2nd to 3rd decade			S			S	S		U			
14. Occurs 3rd to 4th decade				S		S	S					R
15. Oxygen therapy											U	
16. Prematurity											U	
17. Wide age range	U		U									
Physical Findings												
1. Afferent pupillary reaction abnormal	S											
2. Angioid streaks				S								
3. Angiomatosis of iris									S			
4. Anterior ischemic optic neuropathy		S										S
5. Anterior uveitis						R						
6. Arteriovenous retinal shunts		S		U								S
7. Bright choroidal plaques				U								
8. Cataract		S								R		
9. Conjunctival comma signs				U								
10. Conjunctival icterus or pallor				S								
11. Conjunctival phlyctenules						S						
12. Corneal abrasions			U									
13. Corneal epithelial keratitis						S						
14. Corneal neovascularization						S						
15. Cotton wool spots		U		U		S						U
16. Choroidal nevus										S		
17. Choroidal rupture			S							S		
18. Degenerative changes in R.P.E.	R									S		
19. Disc neovascularization		S		S								S
20. Ectropion uvea		S										S
21. Endothelial corneal damage			S									
22. Episcleritis						S						

Vitreous Hemorrhage *Continued*

	Retinal Break	Diabetes Mellitus	Blunt Ocular Trauma	Sickle Cell Disease	Blood Disease ie Anemia	Collagen Disease ie Lupus Erythematosus	Eales Disease	Coat's Disease	Von-Hippel-Lindau Disease	Malignant Melanoma	Retinopathy of Prematurity	Retinal Vein Occlusion
Physical Findings												
23. Extraocular muscle paralysis		R				R				R		
24. Glaucoma		R	S					R	S	R	R	S
25. Hard Exudates		U					U	U	S			S
26. Hyphema			S									
27. Increased pigmentation of lids										R		
28. Iridodialysis			S									
29. Keratoconjunctivitis sicca						S						
30. Low intraocular pressure	S		S									
31. Macular edema	R	S					S			R		S
32. Macular hemorrhage		S	S	S	S							S
33. Macular holes	R		R	S								
34. Microphthalmia											R	
35. Optic atrophy		S	S	S		S				R		
36. Orbital myositis										S		
37. Panophthalmitis										R		
38. Papilledema		S			R	S						S
39. Peerivascular sheathing							U	S				S
40. Phthisis bulbi											S	
41. Pigmented or amelanotic choroidal mass										U		
42. Ptosis						R						
43. Retinal detachment	S			S			U	U	U	S	R	R
44. Retinal hemorrhages	S	U		S	S	S	U	U	S			U
45. Retinal microaneurysms		U		S	S							R
46. Retinal neovascularization		U		S	R							S
47. Retinal arterial venous anastomosis		S		U		S	R				S	S
48. Retinal vein occlusion		S		S	R	S						U
49. Retrolental mass											S	
50. Rubeosis iridis		S		S						R		S
51. Salmon patches in retina				S								
52. Scleritis						S						
53. Soft retinal exudates (cottonwool spots)		U					U	S	S			U
54. Telangiectatic retinal vessels		U						U	U			U
55. Uveitis						S						
56. Venous dilation		U		U		S	U		U		S	U
57. Visual field defects						R				R		
58. White wedge shaped infarcts in choroid				S								S
Lab Data												
1. Autoantibodies to nuclear and cytoplasmic constituents						U						
2. Biopsy										S		
3. Blood sugar elevated		U										
4. Cerebral angiography									U			

Vitreous Hemorrhage *Continued*

	Retinal Break	Diabetes Mellitus	Blunt Ocular Trauma	Sickle Cell Disease	Blood Disease ie Anemia	Collagen Disease ie Lupus Erythematosus	Eales Disease	Coat's Disease	Von-Hippel-Lindau Disease	Malignant Melanoma	Retinopathy of Prematurity	Retinal Vein Occlusion
Lab Data												
5. Chest X ray abnormal							S			S		
6. CT scan:												
—Orbital mass detectable										U		
—Traumatic ocular lesion detectable			U									
7. Diminished complement levels						S						
8. Electroretinogram abnormal	S	S				R						S
9. Fluorescein angiography	U	U	U	S		U	U	U	U	U	R	U
10. Hemoglobin eletrophoresis presence of Hb-S				U								
11. L.E. cell phenomenon						S						
12. Lipid profile elevated	S											S
13. Ocular ultrasonography			U				S	U	U	U	S	
14. Orbital X ray			R									
—Diffusely enlarged orbit										S		
—Erosion of optic canal										R		
15. Platelet count and Hb low					U							
16. P-32 uptake (rarely performed)										R		
17. Visual field test abnormal (rarely performed)										S		

R = rarely; S = sometimes; and U = usually.

Vitreous Opacities

1. Opaque sheets anterior to the vitreous
   A. Elschnig pearls after extracapsular cataract extraction or needling (posterior capsule opacification)
   B. Normal posterior capsule—often following extracapsular cataract extraction or needling
   C. Soemmerring ring following extracapsular cataract extraction or needling
   D. Vitreous adhesions to iris, capsule, or IOL after cataract extraction with vitreous loss

2. Pseudoglioma-leukokoria (see p. 403)

3. Scattered opacities
   A. Amyloid disease—rare (seen in older persons)
   B. Ankylosing spondylitis
   C. Coagula of the colloid basis of the gel
   D. Crystalline deposits
      (1) Asteroid hyalosis
      (2) Synchysis scintillans
   E. Heterochromic uveitis—20–50 years old; of all uveitis, iris atrophy, lens changes
   F. Myeloma, multiple—rare: in 50 to 70 years old, associated with bone pain, anemia
   G. Myopia, severe
   H. Pigment cells—post-traumatic (hemorrhage), senile, or melanotic, associated with rhegmatogenous retinal detachment.
   I. Protein coagulaplasmoid vitreous
      (1) Choroidal tumors (very rare—reported in metastatic breast cancer once)
      (2) Contusions
      (3) Intermediate uveitis (pars planitis)
      (4) Retinochoroiditis
   J. Red blood cells (see vitreous hemorrhage p. 474)
   K. Snowball opacities—rare, associated with pars planitis or sarcoidosis, endophthalmitis—indolent
   L. Tissue cells—epithelial, histiocytic, glial
   M. Toxoplasmosis—active
   N. Tumor cells—retinoblastoma in older child, reticulum cell sarcoma (older persons)
   O. Vitreous degeneration—Wagner's disease, Ehlers-Danlos and Marfan's syndrome, senescent aging changes, myopia
   P. Whipple's disease
   Q. White blood cells—inflammatory disease—vitreitis

4. Single opacities
   A. Anterior hyaloid remnant (Mittendorf dot)—25% normal eyes, dot on posterior lens surface

    B. Hyaloid remnants (uncommon)—persistent hyperplastic primary vitreous

    C. Foreign body—history of trauma or surgery

    D. Dislocated lens (see p. 449)

    E. Parasitic cysts

        (1) Hydatid disease (echinococcosis)—rare, children and young adults, tropical

        (2) Cysticercosis—rare

    F. Vitreous detachment—common in older or myopic persons

Belmont, J.B., and Michelson, J.B.: Vitrectomy in uveitis associated with ankylosing spondylitis. Am. J. Ophthalmol., 94:300, 1982.

Durant, W.J., et al.: Vitrectomy and Whipple's disease. Arch. Ophthalmol., 102:851, 1984.

Fitzgerald, C.R.: Pars plana vitrectomy for vitreous opacity secondary to presumed toxoplasmosis. Arch. Ophthalmol., 98:321, 1980.

Perkins, E.S., and Dobree, J.H.: The Differential Diagnosis of Fundus Conditions. St. Louis, C.V. Mosby, 1972, p. 23.

Sandgren, O., et al.: Vitreous amyloidosis associated with homozygosity for the transthyretin methionine gene. Arch. Ophthalmol., 108:1586, 1990.

Schwartz, M.F., et al.: An unusual case of ocular involvement in primary systemic nonfamilial amyloidosis. Ophthalmology, 89:394, 1982.

Beads in Vitreous (Snowballs in Vitreous)

    1. African eye-worm disease (loiasis)

    2. Amyloidosis (Lubarsch-Pick syndrome)

    3. Behçet syndrome (dermatostomato-ophthalmic syndrome)

    4. Birdshot retinochoroidopathy

    5. Brucellosis (Bang disease)

    6. Familial exudative vitreoretinopathy (Criswick-Schepens syndrome)

    7. Hemophilus influenzae

    8. Irvine syndrome

    9. Jacobsen-Brodwall syndrome

    10. Ocular toxocariasis

    11. Ocular toxoplasmosis

    12. Oculo-oto-ororenoerythropoietic disease

    13. Pars planitis

    14. Retinoblastoma

    15. Sarcoidosis

    16. Severe uveitis

    17. Sympathetic ophthalmia

    18. Toxic lens syndrome

    19. Typhus (Japanese river fever)

    20. Vogt-Koyanagi-Harada syndrome (uveitis-vitiligo-alopecia-poliosis syndrome)

Noda, S., et al.: Patients with asteroid hyalosis and visible floaters. Japanese J. Ophthal., 37:452–455, 1995.

Schlaegel, T.F.: The Uvea. Arch. Ophthalmol., 85:635, 1971.

Asteroid Hyalosis versus Synchysis Scintillans

	Asteroid Hyalosis	Synchysis Scintillans
Age of patient	Elderly	Usually young
Bilaterality	Usually unilateral (75%)	Usually bilateral
Incidence	Rare	Extremely rare
Appearance	Spherical white bodies	Flat, angular crystals
Motility	Moves with vitreous structures and returns to original positions	Moves freely and falls to floor of vitreous
Chemistry	Calcium soaps	Cholesterol crystal
Associated ocular disease	None; diabetes mellitus?	Secondary to other ocular disease or trauma

Complications Following Operative Vitreous Loss

1. Inflammatory complications
    A. Irritable eye (chronically)
    B. Recurrent or persistent uveitis
    C. Vitreitis with vitreous opacities
2. Wound complications
    A. Epithelial invasion or downgrowth
    B. Fibrous ingrowth
    C. Fistula or gaping of wound (with or without vitreous wick syndrome)
    *D. Infection and/or endophthalmitis
    E. Excessive astigmatism
3. Corneal complications
    A. Corneal edema (vitreocorneal touch)
    B. Bullous keratopathy
    C. Corneal opacification
4. Secondary glaucoma
    A. Vitreous obstruction of anterior chamber angle
    B. Pupillary block (iridohyaloid adhesions, anterior hyaloid displacement, uveitis)
    C. Iris and vitreous adherence to wound (peripheral anterior synechiae)
5. Fibroblastic and traction phenomena
    A. Pupillary membrane
    B. Pupillary distortion—"peaked" or updrawn synechiae
    C. Cystoid macular edema (CME)
    D. Retinal detachment
    E. Optic neuritis or papilledema
    F. Vitreous hemorrhage
    G. Posterior vitreous detachment

Krupin,T., and Kolker, A.G.: Atlas of Complications in Ophthalmic Surgery. St. Louis, Mosby, 1993.

Peyman, G.A., and Shulman, J.A.: Intravitreal Surgery, Principles and Practice. New York. Appleton-Lange, 1994.

Postoperative Vitreous Retraction (Usually Manifested by Circular Equatorial Retinal Fold or Star-Shaped Retinal Fold)

1. Accidental perforation of the sclera at operation, which may be associated with hemorrhage and loss of vitreous resulting in a pathologic formation of new epiretinal membrane or proliferative vitreoretinopathy
2. Giant retinal breaks allowing a large area of direct contact between the choroid and the vitreous
3. Perforating diathermy and excessively strong or repeated applications of superficial diathermy, which may cause vitreous hemorrhage or thermal injury to the vit-

* = most important

reous; impairment of chorioretinal blood circulation may result in exudation and hemorrhage into the vitreous

4. Venous stasis caused by the compression of vortex veins by the indentation resulting from a buckling procedure

Jaffe, N.S.: The Vitreous in Clinical Ophthalmology. St. Louis, C.V. Mosby, 1969.

Vitreous Cyst (Cystic Structure in Vitreous Body)

1. Congenital (developmental)—may be associated with hyaloid remnants
2. Acquired
   - A. Infectious cyst
     - (1) Coenurosis (coenurus cerebrah's larva of dog tapeworm)
     - (2) Luetic retinochoroiditis
     - (3) Toxoplasmosis
   - B. Myopia
   - C. Parasitic cysts
     - (1) Cysticercosis—rare
     - (2) Echinococcosis
     - (3) Hydatid disease (echinococcosis)—rare, children and young adults, tropical
     - (4) Nematode cyst (toxocariasis)
   - D. Pigmentary retinopathy
   - E. Retinal detachment
   - F. Trauma

Bullock, J.D.: Development vitreous cysts. Arch. Ophthalmol., 91:84, 1974.

Flynn, W.J., and Carlson, D.W.: Pigmented vitreous cyst. Archives of Ophthal., 112:1113, 1994.

Nussenblat, R.B., and Palestine, A.G.: Uveitis Fundamentals and Clinical Practice. Chicago, Yearbook Med. Publishers, 1989.

Wood, T.R., and Binder, P.S.: Intravitreal and intracameral cysticercosis. Ann. Ophthalmol., 11:1033, 1979.

Vitreous Liquefaction

1. Myopia
2. Peripheral uveitis
3. Retinitis pigmentosa
4. Spontaneous
5. Trauma
6. With aging
7. With vitreous traction such as Wagner disease

Nussenblatt, R.B., and Palestin, A.G.: Uveitis Fundamental and Clinical Practice. Chicago, Yearbook Med. Publishers, 1989.

Takhashi, M., et al.: Biomicroscopic evaluation and photography of liquefied vitreous in some vitreoretinal disorders. Arch. Ophthalmol., 99:1555, 1981.

Retina

LEONARD S. KIRSCH, M.D., F.R.C.S.(C)

Contents

Anatomic Classification of Macular Diseases

1. Vitreoretinal surface

    A. Preretinal hemorrhage and subinternal limiting membrane hemorrhage

    B. Vitreous traction on the macula

    C. Epiretinal membrane and macular pucker

2. Nerve fiber—ganglion cell layers

    A. Hereditary cerebromacular degeneration

        (1) Sphingolipidoses

            a. Tay-Sachs disease (GM_2—gangliosidosis type I)

            b. Sandhoff disease ($GM.MDSD_2$—gangliosidosis type II)

            c. Niemann-Pick disease type A (essential lipoid histiocytosis)

            d. Niemann-Pick disease type B (sea-blue histiocyte syndrome)

            e. Lactosyl ceramidosis

            f. Metachromatic leukodystrophy (arylsulfatase A deficiency)

        g. Gaucher disease (glucocerebroside storage disease)

        h. Farber lipogranulomatosis

        i. Generalized gangliosidosis (GM_1—gangliosidosis type I)

        j. Mucolipidosis I (lipomucopolysaccharidosis)

    (2) Goldberg disease (unclassified syndrome with features of mucopolysaccharidoses, sphingolipidoses; and mucolipidoses)

    (3) Ceroid lipfucinoses

        a. Hagberg-Santevuori (infantile)

        b. Jansky-Bielschowsky disease (late infantile)

        c. Spielmeyer-Vogt Batten

  B. Vitreoretinal dystrophies

    (1) Macular degeneration in congenital hereditary x-linked retinoschisis

    (2) Goldmann-Favre syndrome (vitreotapetoretinal degeneration)—recessive

3. Nerve fiber, ganglion cell, inner plexiform, inner nuclear, outer plexiform layers

  A. Ischemia secondary to inadequate perfusion of retinal vessels

    (1) Branch artery occlusion

    (2) Branch vein occlusion

    (3) Diabetes mellitus

4. Outer plexiform layer

  A. Cystoid macular degeneration (see p. 493)

    (1) With retinal vascular leakage

        a. Acute nongranulomatous iridocyclitis

        b. Acute cyclitis

        c. Hypertension

        d. Medication (epinephrine, nicotinic acid)

        e. Neoproleferative diabetic retinopathy

        f. Pars planitis

        g. Postoperative (Irvine-Gass syndrome)

        h. Radiation retinopathy

        i. Retinitis pigmentosa

        j. Sarcoidosis

        k. Vascular anomalies

    (2) Without obvious retinal vascular leakage

        a. Vitreous traction on the macula

        b. Serous detachment of sensory epithelium

        c. Serous detachment of pigment epithelium

        d. Hemorrhagic detachment of macula

        e. Choroidal tumors

  B. Lipid deposits in macula secondary to vascular disease in retina

    (1) Stellate retinopathy (see p. 500)

       a. Hypertensive retinopathy

       b. Diabetic retinopathy

       c. Coats disease (retinal telangiectasia)

       d. Trauma—ocular or cerebral

       e. Retinal artery or vein occlusion (see p. 653)

       f. Retinal periphlebitis

       g. Juxtapapillary choroiditis

       h. Papilledema (see p. 653)

       i. Angiomatosis retinae

       j. Papillitis (see p. 641)

       k. Acute, febrile illness, such as measles, influenza, meningitis, erysipelas, psittacosis, Behçet's disease

       l. Chronic infections, such as tuberculosis or syphilis

       m. Coccidioidomycosis

       n. Parasitic infection, such as that due to teniae, Giardia, Ancylostoma

       o. Idiopathic

    (2) Circinate retinopathy

       a. Senile vascular disease

       b. Venous obstruction

       c. Diabetic retinopathy

       d. Coats disease (retinal telangiectasia)

       e. Retinal detachment

       f. Anemia

       g. Leukemia

       h. Idiopathic (primary)

       i. Retinal arterial macroaneurysm

    (3) Diabetic retinopathy

5. Outer nuclear layer or photoreceptor elements

  A. Congenital hereditary vision defects

    (1) Trichromatism (anomalous)

    (2) Dichromatism

    (3) Monochromatism

  B. Hereditary macular dystrophies

    (1) Progressive cone dystrophy

    (2) Inverse (macular) retinitis pigmentosa

  C. Olivopontocerebellar degeneration

  D. Light toxicity

    (1) Operating microscope burn

    (2) Solar burn

6. Pigment epithelium

A. Hereditary macular dystrophies

  (1) Vitelliform dystrophy (Best's disease)

  (2) Adult onset foveomacular vitelliform dystrophy (Adult Best's)

  (3) Fundus flavimaculatus

  (4) Fundus flavimaculatus with macular involvement (Stargardt disease)

  (5) Dominant drusen (Doyne honeycomb dystrophy)

  (6) Reticular pigment dystrophy (Sjögren)

  (7) Butterfly-shaped pigment dystrophy (Deutman)

  (8) Central areolar choroidal and pigment epithelial dystrophy

  (9) Sorsby's fundus dystrophy

B. Inflammatory lesions

  (1) Rubella syndrome (German measles)

  (2) Acute posterior multifocal placoid pigment epitheliopathy

C. Toxic lesions

  (1) Chloroquine

  (2) Hydroxychloroquine

  (3) Phenothiazine

    a. chlorpromazine

    b. thioridazine

  (4) Sparsomycin

  (5) Ethambutol

  (6) Indomethacin

  (7) Quinine

  (8) Desferrioxamine

  (9) Penicillamine

D. Drusen (senile, degenerative)

E. Refsum syndrome (phytanic acid storage disease)

F. Myotonic dystrophy syndrome

7. Bruch's membrane

A. Angioid streaks associated with (see p. 584)

  (1) Pseudoxanthoma elasticum (Groenblad-Strandberg syndrome)

  (2) Senile elastosis of skin

  (3) Osteitis deformans (Paget disease)

  (4) Fibrodysplasia hyperelastica (Ehler-Danlos syndrome)

  (5) Sickle cell anemia

  (6) Acromegaly

  (7) Beta-thalassemia

  (8) Abetalipoproteinemia (Bassen-Kornzweig syndrome)

B. Lacquer cracks in pathologic myopia

C. Traumatic fracture of Bruch's membrane

8. Pigment epithelium-Bruch's membrane choriocapillaris

A. Degenerative lesions

   (1) Disciform macular degeneration (senile, juvenile)

   (2) Age-related macular degeneration

   (3) Adult hereditary cerebromacular degeneration (Kufs?)

B. Serous detachment of neuroepithelium or pigment epithelium associated with:

   (1) Central serous chorioretinopathy

   (2) Hemangioma of choroid

   (3) Malignant melanoma

   (4) Pit of optic disk

   (5) Hypotony (see p. 367)

   (6) Leukemic infiltrates of choroid

   (7) Terminal illness

   (8) Trauma

   (9) Uveitis

   (10) Optic neuritis (see p. 643)

   (11) Papilledema (see p. 653)

   (12) Acute hypertension

   (13) Vitreous traction

   (14) Angioid streaks (see p. 584)

   (15) Vogt-Koyangi-Harada syndrome

   (16) Toxocara canis

   (17) Myopic choroidal degeneration

   (18) Metastatic carcinoma

   (19) Choroidal nevus

   (20) Collagen vascular disease

   (21) Hemorrhagic or organized disciform detachment

9. Choroid

  A. Degenerative lesions

    (1) Central areolar choroidal atrophy

    (2) Myopic choroidal atrophy

    (3) Helicoid peripapillary chorioretinal atrophy (?)

  B. Inflammatory lesions

    (1) Histoplasmosis

  C. Vascular occlusive lesions

10. Miscellaneous

  A. Retinal inflammations (multilayer alterations that may involve the macula)

    (1) Toxoplasma gondii

    (2) Toxocara canis

    (3) Septic emboli

(4) Cytomegalovirus retinitis

(5) Candida

(6) Bacteria

B. Congenital anomalies of the macula

(1) Aplasia

(2) Hypoplasia

(3) Heterotopia

(4) Colobomas (see p. 615)

(5) Aberrant macular vessels

Maumenee, A.E., and Emery, J.M.: An anatomic classification of diseases of the macula. Am. J. Oph-thalmol., 74:594–599, 1972.

Yannuzzi, L.A., et al.: The Macula: A Comprehensive Text and Atlas. Baltimore, Williams & Wilkins, 1979.

Bilateral Macular Lesions

1. Development defects (colobomas)

2. Drugs, including:

allopurinol(?)	clonidine(?)	iodochlorhydroxyquin
amodiaquine	griseofulvin(?)	iodoquinol
broxyquinoline	hydroxychloroquine	quinine
chloroquine	ibuprofen(?)	thioridazine
chlorpromazine	indomethacin(?)	

3. Infectious entities

   A. Herpes simplex

   *B. Cytomegalic retinitis

   C. Candidiasis and nocardiosis

   D. Toxocara canis (visceral larva migrans syndrome)

   E. Congenital syphilis

   *F. Tuberculosis

   *G. Ocular histoplasmosis

   H. Congenital toxoplasmosis

4. Intrauterine inflammations

5. Noninfectious entities

   A. Best disease

   B. Stargardt disease

   *C. Exudative age-related macular degeneration

6. Presumed inflammatory origin

Bronstein, M.A., et al.: Bilateral macular lesions. Ann. Ophthalmol., 13:859–861, 1981.

Fraunfelder, F.T.: Drug-Induced Ocular Side Effects and Drug Interactions. 4th Ed. Philadelphia, Williams & Wilkins, 1996.

Pseudomacular Edema

1. Exudative senile maculopathy—serous and/or hemorrhagic detachment of the macular retina in individuals 50 years of age or older, including "giant cyst of macula"

2. Serous detachment of retinal pigment epithelium

3. Central serous retinopathy caused by drugs, including:

adrenal cortex injection	desoxycorticosterone	hydrocortisone	paramethasone
aldosterone	dexamethasone	indomethacin	prednisolone
betamethasone	fludrocortisone	methylprednisolone	prednisone
cortisone	fluprednisolone	oral contraceptives	triamcinolone(?)

Fraunfelder, F.T.: Drug induced Ocular Side Effects and Drug Interactions. Philadelphia, Williams & Wilkins, 1996.

Gass, J.D.M.: Pathogenesis of disciform detachment of neuroepithelium. Am. J. Ophthalmol., 63:573–711, 1967.

Macular Edema (Loss of Foveal Depression with Ophthalmoscope and Outline of Multiple Cystoid Spaces Retroilluminated with Slit Lamp; Often a Yellow Exudate Lies Deep within or beneath Retina in Foveal Area)

1. Acquired parafoveal telangiectasis

2. Amebiasis (amebic dysentery)

3. Bang disease (brucellosis)

4. Behçet syndrome (dermatostomato-ophthalmic syndrome)

*5. Carotid artery obstruction

6. Central angiospastic retinopathy

7. Coats disease

8. Choroidal tumors

9. Crohn's disease

*10. Cytomegalovirus retinitis

*11. Diabetic retinopathy

12. Dominant inheritance macular dystrophy

13. Drugs, including:

acetazolamide	benzthiazide
acetophenazine	betamethasone
adrenal cortex injection	betaxolol(?)
aldosterone	broxyquinoline
allopurinol(?)	butaperazine
aluminum nicotinate	carbromal
amithiozone	carphenazine
amodiaquine	chloramphenicol
aspirin	chloroquine
bendroflumethiazide	chlorothiazide

* = most important

chlorpromazine
chlorthalidone
chymotrypsin(?)
cobalt(?)
cortisone
cyclothiazide
desoxycorticosterone
dexamethasone
dichlorphenamide
diethazine
diiodohydroxyquin
dipivefrin
epinephrine
ergot
ethambutol
ethopropazine
ethoxzolamide
fludrocortisone
fluphenazine
fluprednisolone
griseofulvin
hexamethonium
hydrochlorothiazide
hydrocortisone
hydroflumethiazide
hydroxychloroquine
indapamide
indomethacin(?)
iodide and iodine solutions and compounds
iodochlorhydroxyquin
iodoquinol
iothalamate
meglumine and sodium
iothalamic acid
levobunolol(?)
meprednisone
mesoridazine
methazolamide
methdilazine

methotrimeprazine
methyclothiazide
methylprednisolone
metolazone
naproxen(?)
niacin
niacinamide
nicotinic acid
nicotinyl alcohol
paramethasone
perazine
periciazine
perphenazine
phenylephrine(?)
piperacetazine
polythiazide
prednisolone
prednisone
prochlorperazine
promazine
promethazine
propiomazine
quinethazone
quinine
radioactive iodides
sodium salicylate
tamoxifen
thiethylperazine
thiopropazate
thioproperazine
thioridazine
timolol
triamcinolone
trichlormethiazide
trichloroethylene
trifluoperazine
triflupromazine
trimeprazine(?)

14. Electrical injuries to the retina

15. Epikeratophakia complication

16. Fabry disease (ceramide trihexoside lipidosis)

17. Felty syndrome (rheumatoid arthritis with hypersplenism)
18. Following corneal-relaxing incisions
19. Goldmann-Favre disease (hyaloideoretinal degeneration)
20. Gyrate atrophy
21. Hallerman-Streiff syndrome (dyscephalic mandibulo-oculo-facial syndrome)
22. Hemangiomas of choroid
23. Hemangioma of choroid
24. Hunter syndrome (MPS II)
25. Hurler syndrome (MPS I-H)
26. Hypertensive retinopathy
27. Hypotony (postoperative)
*28. Irvine-Gass syndrome
29. Large central foveal cyst
30. Leukemia
31. Meningococcemia (Neisseria meningitidis)
32. Macular dystrophy—dominant
33. Nematode, intraretinal
34. Nylon suture toxicity
35. Optic nerve pit
36. Pars planitis (peripheral uveitis)
37. Photocoagulation
38. Porphyria cutanea tarda
39. Posterior capsule rupture
*40. Preretinal fibrosis (macular pucker)
41. Punctata albescens retinopathy
42. Radiation retinopathy
43. Retinitis pigmentosa
44. Retino-hypophysary syndrome (Lijo-Pavia-Lis syndrome)
45. Scheie syndrome
46. Scleral buckle
47. Silverman syndrome (battered baby syndrome)
48. Subacute sclerosing panencephalitis (Dawson disease)
49. Toxoplasmic chorioretinitis
50. Trauma to globe (commotio retinae)
51. Ultraviolet light from sun, operating microscope, or other bright light sources
52. Uveitis (anterior or posterior)
*53. Vein occlusion, including branch vein occlusion (see p. 525)
54. von Hippel-Lindau syndrome (retinocerebral angiomatosis)
55. YAG laser posterior capsulotomy

Balyeat, H.D., et al.: Nylon suture toxicity after cataract surgery. Ophthalmology, 95:1509–1514, 1988.

* = most important

Carter, J., et al.: Cystoid macular edema following corneal-relaxing incisions. Arch. Ophthalmol., 105:70–72, 1987.

Fraunfelder, F.T.: Drug-Induced Ocular Side Effects and Drug Interactions. 4th Ed. Philadelphia, Williams & Wilkins, 1996.

Loeffler, K.U., et al.: Dominantly inherited cystoid macular edema. A histopathologic study. Ophthal., 99:1385–1392, 1992.

Millay, R.H., et al.: Niacin maculopathy. Ophthalmology, 95:930–936, 1988.

Miyake,Y., et al.: Classification of aphakic cystoid macular edema with focal macular electroretinograms. Amer. J. Ophthal., 116:576–583, 1993.

Pinckers, A., et al.: Colour vision in retinitis pigmentosa. Influence of cystoid macular edema. International Ophthal., 17:143–146, 1993.

Rosen, S.I.: Cystoid macular edema following epikeratophakia. Am. J. Ophthalmol., 106:746, 1988.

Rumelt, S., et al.: Retinal Neovascularization and Cystoid Macular Edema in Punctata Albescens Retinopathy. Amer. J. Ophthal., 114:507–509, 1992.

Roy, F.H.: Ocular Syndromes and Systemic Diseases. 2nd Ed. Philadelphia, W.B. Saunders, 1989.

Smith, R.T., et al.: Quantification of diabetic macular edema. Arch. Ophthalmol., 105:218–222, 1987.

Steinert, R.F., et al.: Cystoid macular edema, retinal detachment, and glaucoma after Nd: YAG laser posterior capsulotomy. Am. J. Ophthalmol., 112:373–380, 1991.

Weene, L.E.: Cystoid macular edema after scleral buckling responsive to acetazolamide. Ann. Ophthal., 24:423–434, 1992.

Absence of Foveal Reflex

1. Absence of foveal reflex caused by drugs, including: amodiaquine, chloroquine, diiodohydroxyquin, hydroxychloroquine, iodochlorhydroxyquin, quinine

Fraunfelder, F.T.: Drug-Induced Ocular Side Effects and Drug Interactions. 4th Ed. Philadelphia, Williams & Wilkins, 1996.

Macular Pucker—Tiny Folds Often Arranged in a Stellate Manner around Macula and Usually Associated with a Preretinal Membrane (Preretinal Macular Fibrosis, Preretinal Vitreous Membrane, Surface Wrinkling Retinopathy, Cellophane Maculopathy)

1. Associated with proliferative retinopathy
    *A. Diabetes retinopathy
    B. Eales disease
    *C. Hypertension
    D. Sickle cell disease
    E. Vein occlusion
2. Congenital
3. Following photocoagulation or cryoretinopexy
4. Following traumatic posterior vitreous separation, such as blunt trauma to the eye and whiplash injury (craniocervical syndrome)
5. Loss of formed vitreous at operation
6. Idiopathic (probably related to spontaneous posterior vitreous detachment)
7. Macular detachment
8. Multiple retinal operations

9. Penetrating or blunt injuries

10. Posterior uveitis

*11. Proliferative vitreoretinopathy following vitreoretinal surgery

12. Retinal detachment

13. Trauma (blunt)

14. Vitreous hemorrhage

Appiah, A.P., and Hirose, T.: Secondary causes of premacular fibrosis. Ophthalmology, 96:389–392, 1989.

McDonald, H.R., et al.: Surgical management of idiopathic epiretinal membranes. Ophthalmology, 93:978–983, 1986.

Smiddy, W.E., et al.: Clinicopathologic study of idiopathic macular pucker in children and young adults. Retina, 12:232–236, 1992.

Uemura, A., et al.: Macular pucker after retinal detachment surgery. Ophthal. Surgery, 23:116–119, 1992.

Stellate Retinopathy (Exudates in a star formation radiating around the macula in the nerve fiber layer)

	Hypertension	Ocular Trauma	Retinal Periphlebitis	Papillitis	Papilledema	Acute Febrile Illness i.e. Behçet's Disease	Chronic Infections i.e. Tuberculosis	Coccidioidomycosis
History								
1. Communicable disease							U	
2. Elevated blood pressure	U							
3. Hereditary	S							
4. History of ocular trauma		U						
5. In young men			U					
6. Increased intracranial pressure					U			
7. Monocular loss of vision				S	U			
8. Occurs between 15 and 45 years of age					U			
9. Occurs in adults						U		
10. Occurs in people living in an endemic area								U
Physical Findings								
1. Absence of spontaneous venous pulse						S		
2. Arteriosclerosis	U							
3. Blepharitis							S	
4. Capillary nonperfusion			S					U
5. Cellulitis							S	
6. Conjunctivitis							S	
7. Corneal ulcer							S	
8. Cotton wool spots	S	S						
9. Choroidal rupture		S						
10. Choroiditis							S	
11. Dacryocystitis							S	
12. Diffuse gray-white appearance of the neurosensory retina	S							
13. Diplopia		S						
14. Disc hemorrhages						S		
15. Disc pallor (late)				U				
16. Enophthalmos		S						
17. Episcleritis	S							S
18. Fatty exudates						S		
19. Granulomatous lesion of optic nerve head								S
20. Hypopyon								S
21. Intravitreal hemorrhage		S	S					
22. Iritis		S						
23. Keratitis						S	S	
24. Keratoconjunctivitis sicca						U		
25. Lens subluxation or dislocation		S						
26. Macular edema								
27. Meibomianitis								
28. Miosis		S						
29. Mutton-fat keratic precipitates								S
30. Nystagmus						R		
31. Ocular pain		S						
32. Ocular pain on movements				U				

Stellate Retinopathy (Exudates in a star formation radiating around the macula in the nerve fiber layer) *Continued*

	Hypertension	Ocular Trauma	Retinal Periphlebitis	Papillitis	Papilledema	Acute Febrile Illness i.e. Behçet's Disease	Chronic Infections i.e. Tuberculosis	Coccidioidomycosis
Physical Findings								
33. Optic disc edema	S		U		S			
34. Optic nerve atrophy						S	S	
35. Optic nerve capillary hyperemia				U				
36. Optic neuritis						S	S	
37. Palsies of extraocular muscles								S
38. Pannus						S	S	
39. Panophthalmitis						S	S	
40. Paralysis of accommodation		S						
41. Paralysis of sixth cranial nerve								S
42. Perivascular exudates		S						
43. Perivascular sheathing		S				S		
44. Recurrent uveitis						U		
45. Relative afferent pupillary defect				U				
46. Retinal arterial narrowing	U							
47. Retinal detachment		S						
48. Retinal edema					S			
49. Retinal hemorrhages	S							
50. Retinal tears or disinsertion		S	S					
51. Retinal vasculitis		S				S		
52. Retinitis						U	S	
53. Scleral perforation							S	
54. Scleritis							S	
55. Secondary glaucoma						S		S
56. Subconjunctival nodules							S	
57. Subtle vertical striae on the temporal side of disc					S			
58. Uveitis							S	S
59. Venous dilation			S			S		
60. Venous obstruction			S					
61. Vision may be reduced		S						
62. Vitreal floaters								S
63. Vitreal opacity								S
64. Vitreous cells				S			S	S
65. Vitreous inflammation				S			S	S

R = Rarely; S = sometimes; and U = usually.

Macular Star or Stellate Retinopathy (Exudates in a Star Formation Radiating around Macula in the Nerve-fiber Layer)

1. Acute febrile illness, such as measles, influenza, meningitis, erysipelas, psittacosis, Behçet disease (dermatostomato-ophthalmic syndrome)

2. Chronic infections, such as tuberculosis or syphilis

3. Coccidioidomycosis

4. Gansslen syndrome (familial hemolytic icterus)

*5. Hypertension

6. Idiopathic

7. Juxtapapillary choroiditis (Jensen disease)

*8. Neuroretinitis

9. Obstruction of the artery or vein supplying the macular area (see p. 512 or 525)

10. Ocular or cerebral trauma

11. Parasitic infection, such as that due to teniae, Giardia, Ancylostoma

*12. Papilledema (see p. 653)

13. Papillitis (see p. 643)

14. Retinal periphlebitis

Roy, F.H.: Ocular Syndromes and Systemic Diseases. 2nd Ed. Philadelphia, W.B. Saunders, 1989.

Yannuzzi, L.A., et al.: The Macula: A Comprehensive Text and Atlas. Baltimore, Williams & Wilkins, 1979.

Retinociliary Vein—Disappears from Retina at Disc Margin without Connection to Central Retinal Vein

1. Acquired

    A. Arachnoid cyst of the optic nerve

    B. Central retinal vein occlusion (see p. 525)

    C. Chronic atrophic papilledema from causes including craniopharyngioma (see p. 653)

    D. Glioma of the optic disc

2. Congenital

Wolter, J.J.: Retinociliary vein associated with a craniopharyngioma. Ann. Ophthalmol., 11:751, 1979.

Cherry-red Spot in Macula (Rule Out Macular Hemorrhage)

1. Cardiac myxomas

2. Cryoglobulinemia

3. Dapsone poisoning

4. Hallervorden-Spatz disease (pigmentary degeneration of globus pallidus)

5. Hollenhorst syndrome (chorioretinal infarction syndrome)

6. Hurler syndrome (MPS I-H)

*7. Hypertension (severe)

8. Intralesional chalazion corticosteroid injection

9. Leber congenital amaurosis

10. Macular hemorrhage

*11. Macular hole with surrounding retinal detachment

12. ML I (lipomucopolysaccharidosis)

13. Myotonic dystrophy syndrome (Curschmann-Steinert syndrome)

14. Multiple sulfatase deficiency

*15. Occlusion of central retinal artery (see p. 512)

16. Quinine toxicity

17. Sphingolipidoses

   A. Cherry-red spot myoclonus

   B. Farber syndrome (Farber lipogranulomatosis)

   C. Gangliosidosis GM_1—type (juvenile gangliosidosis)

   D. Gaucher disease (glucocerebroside storage disease)

   E. Goldberg syndrome

   F. Infantile metachromatic leukodystrophy (van Bogaert-Nijssen disease)

   G. Niemann-Pick disease type A

   H. Niemann-Pick disease type B

   I. Sandoff disease (gangliosidosis GM_2—type 2)

   *J. Tay-Sachs disease (gangliosidosis GM—type I)

18. Steroid injection intranasally

*19. Temporal arteritis (giant cell arteritis)

20. Traumatic retinal edema (commotio retinae; Berlin edema)

21. Vogt-Spielmeyer cerebral degeneration (Batten-Mayou syndrome)

Abhayambika, K., et al.: Peripheral neuropathy and haemolytic anaemia with cherry red spot on macula in dapsone poisoning. J. Assoc. of Physician of India, 38:564–565, 1990.

Garland, P.E., et al.: Visual disturbance resulting from intranasal steroid injection. Arch. Ophthalmol., 107:22–23, 1989.

Isenberg, S.J.: The Eye in Infancy. Chicago, Year Book Medical Publishers, 1989.

Roy, F.H.: Ocular Syndromes and Systemic Diseases. 2nd Ed. Philadelphia, W.B. Saunders, 1989.

Sorcinelli, I., et al.: Cherry-red spot, optic atrophy and corneal cloudings in a patient suffering from GM.MDSD/gangliosidosis type I. Metabolic, Pediatric and Systemic Ophthalmol., 10:64, 1987.

Macular Hemorrhage

1. Choroidal neovascular membranes

   *A. Age-related macular degeneration

   B. Angioid streaks

   C. Histoplasmosis

   D. Idiopathic

   E. Pathologic myopic

   F. Posterior uveitis

* = most important

2. Infectious retinitis

    *A. cytomegalovirus retinitis

    B. Subacute bacterial endocarditis

3. Retinal vascular disease

    A. Radiation retinopathy

    B. Retinal arterial macroaneurysm

    *C. Vein occlusion

4. Systemic diseases

    A. Blood dyscrasias

      (1) anemia

      (2) leukemia

      (3) polycythemia vera

      (4) sickle-cell disease

      (5) thrombocytopenia

      (6) Waldenstrom's macroglobulinemia

    B. Cardiovascular shock (especially gastrointestinal hemorrhage)

    *C. Diabetes mellitus

    *D. HIV-related retinopathy

    *E. Hypertension

    F. Toxemia of pregnancy

5. Trauma

    A. Choroidal rupture

    B. Purtscher's retinopathy

    C. Shaken baby syndrome

    D. Terson syndrome

    E. Valsalva retinopathy

    F. Vitreous detachment

Ballantyne, A.J., and Michaelson, I.C.: Textbook of the Fundus of the Eye. 3rd Ed. Baltimore, Williams & Wilkins Co., 1981.

Paris, C.L., et al.: Neonatal macular hemorrhage. International Ophthal., 15:153–155, 1991.

Stevenson, A., et al.: Is Aspirin a Factor in Macular Hemorrhage. Ophthalmology Times, 18:32–34, 1993.

Schachat, A.P., and Sommer, A.: Macular hemorrhages associated with posterior vitreous detachment. Am. J. Ophthalmol., 102:647–649, 1986.

Yannuzzi, L.A., et al.: The Macula: A Comprehensive Text and Atlas. Baltimore, Williams & Wilkins, 1979.

Parafoveal Telangiectasia (Retinal Microvascular Anomaly Involving the Parafoveal Capillary Network as Well as Immediately Adjacent Vascular Bed, Best Demonstrated by Fluorescein Angiography)

    1. Carotid artery obstruction

    *2. Diabetes mellitus, usually bilateral

*3. Idiopathic

4. Localized form of Coats disease, usually unilateral

*5. Small branch vein occlusion

6. Small retinal capillary hemangioma, usually unilateral

7. Roentgenogram, irradiation

Gass, J.D., and Oyakawa, T.: Idiopathic juxtafoveal telangiectasia. Arch. Ophthalmol., 100:769, 1982.

Millay, R.H., et al.: Abnormal glucose metabolism and parafoveal telangiectasia. Am. J. Ophthalmol., 102:363–370, 1986.

Macular Hemorrhage

	High Myopia (Fuchs Spot)*	Disciform Macular Degeneration	Inflammation as Histoplasmosis*	Angioid Streaks	Familial
History					
1. Familial					U
2. Greater in whites than blacks			U		
3. In persons 30 to 50 years	U			U	
4. In persons 50 years and older		U			
5. Mainly central visual loss		U			
6. Metamorphopsia		U			
7. More often men			U		
8. Myopia more than 12 diopters	U				
Physical Findings					
1. Circumpapillary choroiditis			U		
2. Dark spot in macula	U	S			
3. Enlarging myopic crescent	U				
4. Macular lesion in active stage, pigment ring with sensory retinal detachment			U		
5. Mottled macular appearance	U				
6. Pigment epithelial retinal detachment	U	U			
7. Ruptures in Bruch membrane	U			U	
8. Scattered atrophic chorioretinal spots in mid and far periphery			U		
9. Serous retinal separation	S	U			
Laboratory Data					
1. Fluorescein angiography	U	U	U	U	U
2. Histoplasmin skin test			U		

R = rarely; S = sometimes; and U = usually.

Microhemorrhagic Maculopathy—Small Monocular Macular Hemorrhage that is Punctate, Round or Bilobed

1. Increased venous stasis (Valsalva stress)
2. Impaired blood platelet aggregation
3. Medications that impair platelet function including aspirin, ibuprofen (Motrin), pentazocine, propranolol hydrochloride and oral contraceptives.

Pruett, R.C., Carvalho, A.C.A., and Trempe, C. L.: Microhemorrhagic maculopathy. Arch. Ophthalmol., 99:425, 1980.

Macular Cyst (Must be Differentiated from Macular Hole with Hruby Lens or Contact Lens and Slit Lamp)

1. Amebiasis
2. Cysticercosis—subretinal cyst
*3. Cystic degeneration—common following trauma, uveitis, and vascular disease
4. Hamman-Rich syndrome (alveolar capillary block syndrome)
5. Histoplasmosis
6. Hydatid disease (echinococcosis)
7. Parasitic and mycotic cysts

McDonnell, P.J., et al.: Clinical features of idiopathic macular cysts and holes. Am. J. Ophthalmol., 93:777–786, 1982.

Roy, F.H.: Ocular Syndromes and Systemic Diseases. 2nd Ed. Philadelphia, W.B. Saunders, 1989.

Macular Hole (Must Be Differentiated from Macular Cyst with Hruby Lens or Contact Lens and Slit Lamp)

*1. Idiopathic (most common, may be bilateral)
2. From:
  A. Edema (see p. 493)
    (1) Inflammatory
    (2) Toxic
    (3) Vascular
    (4) Following papilledema
  B. High myopia
  C. Ischemic, such as with retinal detachment or choroidal tumor—the macula is separated from choriocapillaris
  D. Degenerative conditions of the retina and retinal dystrophy
  E. Trauma
  F. Radiation injury
  G. Glaucoma
  H. Posterior senile retinoschisis
  I. High tension electric shock
  J. Central serous chorioretinopathy
  K. Optic disc coloboma

L. Posterior retinal detachment associated with optic pits

M. Industrial laser burns

N. Lightening—induced

O. Posterior microphthalmos

P. Subhyaloid hemorrhage

Q. Topical pilocarpine use

R. YAG laser

3. Dawson disease (subacute sclerosing panencephalitis)

4. Foveomacular retinitis—usually young males

*5. Pseudohole due to epiretinal membrane (may differentiated from true hole by fluorescein angiography)

Benedict, W.L., and Shami, M.: Impending Macular Hole Associated with Topical Pilocarpine. Amer. J. Ophthal., 114:765–779, 1992.

Blacharski, P.A., and Newsome, D.A.: Bilateral macular holes after Nd: YAG laser posterior capsulotomy. Am. J. Ophthalmol., 105:451–459, 1988.

Brent, B.D.: Macular holes after pneumatic retinopexy. Arch. Ophthalmol., 106:724–725, 1988.

Brown, G.C.: Macular hole following rhegmatogenous retinal detachment repair. Arch. Ophthalmol., 106:765–772, 1988.

Gass, J.D.M.: Idiopathic senile macular hole. Arch. Ophthalmol., 106:629–639, 1988.

Lansing, M.B., et al.: The effect of pars plana vitrectomy and transforming growth factor-beta without epiretinal membrane peeling on full-thickness macular holes. Ophthal., 100:868–871, 1993.

Smiddy, W.E.: Atypical presentations of macular holes. Arch. Ophthal., 111:626–631,1993.

Macular Coloboma—Bilaterally Symmetric Circumscribed, Excavated Defects in Choroid and Retina in Region of Macula Associated with Reduced Vision

1. Autosomal dominant

2. Autosomal recessive inheritance with skeletal anomalies

3. Conditions that exhibit choroidal coloboma (see p. 615)

4. Down syndrome

5. Hypercalciuria, myopia, and macular coloboma

6. Isolated

7. Macular coloboma with brachydactyly

8. Sorsby syndrome I

Isenberg, S.J.: The Eye in Infancy. Chicago, Year Book Medical Publishers, 1989.

Yamaguchi K., and Tamai, M.: Congenital macular coloboma in Down syndrome. Ann. Ophthal., 22:222–223, 1990.

Elevated Macular Lesion

1. Angiospastic retinopathy

2. Central serous detachment of retina

3. Chorioretinitis especially histoplasmosis and toxoplasmosis

4. Choroidal hemangioma

5. Dawson disease (subacute sclerosing panencephalitis)

6. Malignant melanoma

7. Varix of the vortex ampulla

Newell, F.W.: Ophthalmology, Principles and Concepts. 7th Ed. St. Louis, C.V. Mosby, 1991.

Osher, R.H., et al.: Varix of the vortex ampulla. Am. J. Ophthalmol., 92:653–660, 1981.

Heterotopia of the Macula (Abnormal Location of Macula in Relation to Optic Disc; Eye with Ectopic Macula Tends to Deviate in Same Direction as Macular Displacement; Visual Fields Show Displacement of Blind Spot and Cover-Uncover Test Shows No Shift of Fixation)

1. Chorioretinitis

2. Congenital

*3. Retinopathy of prematurity

4. Inflammatory

*5. Proliferative diabetic retinopathy

Bresnick, G.H.: Visual function abnormalities in macular heterotopia caused by proliferative diabetic retinopathy. Am. J. Ophthalmol., 92:85–102, 1981.

Stem, S.D., and Arenberg, I.K.: Heterotopia of the macula with associated retinal detachment. J. Pediatr. Ophthalmol., 6:198–202, 1969.

White or Yellow Flat Macular Lesion and Pigmentary Change

1. Post-traumatic—pigmentary disturbance; cysts or hole at macula

2. Postinflammatory—chorioretinal atrophy with pigment clumping at center and periphery of lesion

3. Coloboma of macula—atrophic area at macula often associated with coloboma of disc; sclera may be ectatic (see p. 617)

4. Radiation injuries—common after solar eclipse; punched-out appearance

5. Fuchs dark spot—pigmented spot associated with other signs of degenerative myopia

6. Drugs, including:

adrenal cortex injection	dexamethasone(?)	iodochlorhydroxyquin
aldosterone	diiodohydroxyquin	methylprednisolone
allopurinol(?)	fludrocortisone	oral contraceptives
amodiaquine	fluprednisolone(?)	paramethasone(?)
betamethasone(?)	griseofulvin	prednisolone(?)
chloroquine	hydrocortisone(?)	prednisone(?)
cortisone(?)	hydroxychloroquine	quinine
desoxycorticosterone(?)	indomethacin(?)	triamcinolone

7. Stellate retinopathy—star-shaped exudates (see p. 500)

8. Hard exudates and circinate retinopathy (see p. 551)

9. Drusen—common, discrete yellow spots beneath retina

10. Doyne honeycomb choroiditis—rare; honeycomb pattern of yellow patches at posterior pole; degenerative changes at macula

11. Heredomacular dystrophies

   A. Best disease (vitelliruptive macular dystrophy) up to years of age; egg-yolk lesion at macula, later absorbed to leave atrophic scar

   B. Fundus flavimaculatus—yellow patches at posterior pole; degenerative changes at macula

   C. Stargardt disease (juvenile macular degeneration) to years of age; variable appearance in different families; bilateral lesions showing some degree of symmetry

   D. Behr disease (optic atrophy-ataxia syndrome)—adults, similar to Stargardt type

   E. Presenile and senile—pigmentary changes followed by atrophy, bilateral and symmetrical

13. Central choroidal sclerosis—rare, atrophic retina with sclerosed choroidal vessels showing clearly

14. Central areolar choroidal atrophy—rare, exudate and edema followed by sharply defined atrophic area with white strands of choroidal vessels

15. Pseudoinflammatory macular dystrophy—rare, initially edema and exudates followed by scarring with pigmentary disturbance and atrophic patches

16. Gaucher disease (glucocerebroside storage disease)—rare, ring-shaped macular lesions, lipid deposits in cornea and conjunctiva

17. Diffuse leukoencephalopathy—rare, white deposits in periphery and macular area

18. Sjögren-Larsson syndrome (oligophrenia-ichthyosis-spastic diplegia syndrome)

19. Angioid streaks (see p. 584)

20. Multiple evanescent white dot syndrome (MEWDS) usually unilateral, predominantly healthy women, vitreitis

21. Acute multifocal placoid pigment epitheliopathy—rare, map-like pigmentary disturbance of posterior pole or more widespread over posterior fundus

Eagle, R.C., et al.: Retinal pigment epithelial abnormalities in fundus flavimaculatus. Ophthalmology, 87:1189, 1980.

Fraunfelder, F.T.: Drug-Induced Ocular Side Effects and Drug Interactions. Philadelphia, Williams & Wilkins, 1996.

Hadden, O.B., and Gass, D.M.: Fundus Flavimaculatus and Stargardt's Disease. Am. J. Ophthalmol., 82:527–539, 1976.

Perkins, E.S., and Dobree, J.H.: The Differential Diagnosis of Fundus Conditions. St. Louis, C.V. Mosby, 1972.

Pigmentary Changes in Macula

1. Hereditary macular degeneration without cerebral or other disease

   A. Best disease (vitelliform macular dystrophy)

   B. Stargardt disease (juvenile flavimaculatus)

   C. Behr syndrome (optic atrophy-ataxia syndrome)

*2. Retinitis pigmentosa

3. Secondary pigmentary retinopathy following trauma or inflammation (see p. 507)

*4. Age-related macular degeneration

* = most important

5. Metabolic disease associated with pigmentary retinopathy
  A. Abetalipoproteinemia (Bassen-Kornzweig syndrome)
  B. Alphalipoprotein deficiency (Tangier syndrome)
  C. Ceroid lipofuscinosis
    (1) Batten-Mayou syndrome
    (2) Dollinger-Bielschowsky syndrome, late infantile (Bielschowsky-Jansky disease)
    (3) Infantile type of neuronal ceroid lipofuscinosis
  D. Hepatic disease
  E. Refsum disease (phytanic acid storage disease)
  F. Tay-Sachs syndrome (gangliosidosis GM_2-type I)
  G. Vitamin A
  H. Mucopolysaccharidosis
    (1) Hunter syndrome (MPS II)
    (2) Hurler syndrome (MPS I-H)
    (3) Sanfilippo-Good syndrome (MPS III)
    (4) Scheie syndrome (MPS I-S)
*6. Drugs, including:

acetophenazine	cisplatin	methdilazine	promethazine
amiodarone(?)	clofazimine	methotrexate	propiomazine
amodiaquine	clonidine(?)	methotrimeprazine	quinacrine(?)
azathioprine	cobalt(?)	minoxidil(?)	quinine
benzatropine(?)	cycrimine(?)	mitotane	sulindac(?)
biperiden(?)	deferoxamine	naproxen	tamoxifen
butaperazine	diethazine	penicillamine	thiethylperazine
carbamazepine	diethylcarbamazine	perazine	thiopropazate
carphenazine	ethambutol(?)	pericyazine	thioproperazine
cephaloridine	ethopropazine	perphenazine	thioridazine
chloramphenicol	fluphenazine	piperacetazine	thiothixene
chloroquine	hydroxychloroquine	prazosin(?)	trifluoperazine
chlorphenoxamine(?)	indomethacin(?)	prochlorperazine	triflupromazine
chlorpromazine	ketoprofen(?)	procyclidine(?)	trihexyphenidyl(?)
chlorprothixene	mesoridazine	promazine	trimeprazine

7. Inflammation
  *A. Toxoplasmosis
   B. Trauma
8. Multifocal necrotizing encephalopathy
9. Dawson disease (subacute sclerosing panencephalitis)
10. Dialinas-Amalric syndrome (deaf mutism—retinal degeneration syndrome)
11. Oculodental syndrome (Peter syndrome)
12. Sorsby syndrome (hereditary macular coloboma syndrome)

Ehrenberg, M., et al.: Pigmentary macular degeneration with multifocal necrotizing encephalopathy. Am. J. Ophthalmol., 92:422–430, 1981.

Fishman, G.A., et al.: X-linked recessive retinitis pigmentosa. Arch. Ophthalmol., 104:1329–1335, 1986.

Fraunfelder, F.T.: Drug-Induced Ocular Side Effects and Drug Interactions. 3rd Ed. Philadelphia, Williams & Wilkins, 1996.

Roy, F.H.: Ocular Syndromes and Systemic Diseases. 2nd Ed. Philadelphia, W.B. Saunders, 1989.

Bull's Eye Macular Lesion—circular area of RPE atrophy surrounding a spared fovea

1. Autosomal dominant benign concentric annular macular dystrophy
2. Ceroid lipofuscinosis
*3. Chloroquine or hydroxychloroquine retinopathy
4. Cone dystrophy
5. Hereditary ataxia
6. Spielmeyer-Vogt syndrome (Batten-Mayou syndrome)
*7. Stargardt disease (or fundus flavimaculatus)
8. Trauma
9. Unknown

Duinkerke-Eerola, et al.: Atrophic maculopathy associated with hereditary ataxia. Am. J. Ophthalmol., 90:846, 1980.

Isenberg, S.J.: The Eye in Infancy. Chicago, Year Book Medical Publishers, 1989.

Weise, E.E., and Yannuzzi, L.A.: Ring maculopathies mimicking chloroquine retinopathy. Am. J. Ophthalmol., 78:204–210, 1974.

Macular Wisps and Foveolar Splinter (Noted in Focal Illumination with Goldmann Contact Lenses, Invisible Ophthalmoscopically)

1. Direct and indirect ocular concussion
2. Following absorption of small prefoveal hemorrhage
3. Foveomacular retinitis
4. Juvenile macular degeneration
5. Old, healed chorioretinitis
6. Retinitis pigmentosa
7. Spontaneous senile posterior vitreous detachment
8. Whiplash injury

Daily, L.: Foveolar splinter and macular wisps. Arch. Ophthalmol., 83:406–411, 1970.

Daily, L.: Further observations on foveolar splinter and macular wisps. Arch. Ophthalmol., 90:102–103, 1973.

Macular Hypoplasia (Incomplete Macular Development Manifested by Decreased Vision)

*1. Albinism
*2. Associated with autosomal dominant aniridia
3. Associated with microcornea and corectopia

* = most important

   4. Associated with myelinated nerve fibers

   5. Forsius-Eriksson syndrome (Aland disease)

   *6. Goldenhar-Gorlin syndrome (oculoauriculovertebral dysplasia)

   7. Krause syndrome (encephalo-ophthalmic dysplasia)

   8. Ring chromosome

   9. Syndrome of foveal hypoplasia and presenile cataract (O'Donnell-Pappas syndrome)—autosomal dominant

   10. Tuomaala-Haapanen syndrome

   11. Waardenburg syndrome (interoculoiridodermatoauditive dysplasia)

Ghose, S., and Mehta, U.: Microcornea with corectopia and macular hypoplasia in a family. Jpn. J. Ophthalmol., 28:126–130, 1984.

Margolis, S., et al.: Retinal and optic nerve findings in Goldenhar-Gorlin syndrome. Ophthalmology, 91:1327–1333, 1984.

Roy, F.H.: Ocular Syndromes and Systemic Diseases. 2nd Ed. Philadelphia, W.B. Saunders, 1989.

Szymanski, K.A., et al.: Genetic studies of ocular albinism in a large Virginia Kindred. Ann. Ophthalmol., 16:183–185, 1984.

Retinal Vascular Tortuosity

   1. Acute malnutrition

   2. Aortic coarctation

   3. Bazzana syndrome (angiospastic ophthalmoauricular syndrome)

   4. Choked disc (see p. 653)

   5. Chronic respiratory insufficiency, such as in cystic fibrosis and familial dysautonomia (Riley-Day syndrome)

   *6. Coats' disease (retinal telangiectasia)

   7. Congenital

   8. Cri du chat syndrome (cat cry syndrome)

   9. Cryoglobulinemia

   10. Down syndrome (trisomy 21)

   11. Eales disease (periphlebitis)

   12. Engelmann syndrome (diaphyseal dysplasia)

   13. Fabry disease (diffuse angiokeratosis)

   *14. Glaucoma, open angle

   15. Granulocytic sarcoma of orbit

   16. Hereditary hemorrhagic telangiectasis (Osler disease)—tortuosity and varicosity

   17. Hypertension

   18. Kenny syndrome (dwarfism, thickened long bone cortex, transient hypocalcemia)

   *19. Leukemia

   20. Lymphogranuloma venereum (Nicolas-Favre disease)

   21. Maroteaux-Lamy syndrome (mucopolysaccharidoses type VI)

   22. Macroglobulinemia

23. Mosse syndrome (polycythemia-hepatic cirrhosis syndrome)

24. Myopia

25. Normal variation with fullness

26. Polycythemia with vessel fullness

27. Retinopathy of prematurity

28. Racemose hemangioma of retina, angiomatosis retinae without obvious tumor formation, or von Hippel-Lindau syndrome (retinocerebral angiomatosis)

29. Reimann syndrome (hyperviscosity syndrome)

*30. Sickle cell disease

31. Visceral larva migrans (nematode ophthalmia syndrome)

Ballantyne, A.J., and Michaelson, I.C.: Textbook of the Fundus of the Eye. 3rd Ed. Baltimore, Williams & Wilkins, 1981.

Davis, J. L., et al.: Granulocytic sarcoma of the orbit. Ophthalmology, 92:1758–1762, 1985.

Roy, F.H.: Ocular Syndromes and Systemic Diseases. 2nd Ed. Philadelphia, W.B. Saunders, 1989.

Wells, C.G., and Kalina, R.E.: Progressive inherited retinal arteriolar tortuosity with spontaneous retinal hemorrhages. Ophthalmology, 92:1015–1024, 1985.

Venous Beading

*1. Diabetes mellitus

2. Loaiasis (Loa loa)

3. Macroglobulinemia (Waldenstrom syndrome)

Schlaegel, T.F.: Essentials of Uveitis. Boston, Little, Brown and Company, 1969.

Ophthalmodynamometry (Blood Pressure of Retinal Artery; Difference between Eyes of about Fifteen Percent of Diastolic Readings is Significant)

1. False-positive or variable readings

    A. Abnormally high or low intraocular pressure or asymmetry between the two eyes

    B. Cardiac abnormalities, such as atrial fibrillation, heart block, or extrasystoles

    C. Marked asymmetry of retinal vessels in the two eyes

    D. Measurements of ophthalmic artery pressure of less than 20g on the instrument

    E. Poor patient cooperation

    F. Variation in systemic blood pressure between readings

2. High ophthalmodynamometry values

    A. Basilar-vertebral occlusion

    B. Bilateral distal internal carotid occlusion—unusual

    C. Progressive intracranial arterial occlusion syndrome

3. Low ophthalmodynamometry values

    A. Both sides reduced with orthostatic hypotension

    *B. Reduced on side of an occluded internal carotid artery

Walsh, F.B., and Hoyt, W.F.: Clinical Neuro-ophthalmology. 4th Ed. Baltimore, Williams & Wilkins, 1985.

* = most important

Pulsation of Retinal Arteriole (High Pulse Pressure)

1. Aortic regurgitation
2. Hyperthyroidism
*3. Intraocular blood pressure higher than diastolic blood pressure but lower than systolic blood pressure

Newell, F.W.: Ophthalmology, Principles and Concepts. 7th Ed. St. Louis, C.V. Mosby, 1992.

Retinal Artery Occlusion (Sudden painless visual loss; on Ophthalmoscopic Examination, a Diffuse Retinal Pallor and a Cherry-Red Spot in Macula Are Noted)

1. Embolism—cardiac or pulmonary sources
    A. Amniotic fluid embolization
    B. Cardiac myxoma
    C. Espildora-Luque syndrome (ophthalmic Sylvian syndrome)
    D. Iatrogenic trauma induced by angiography
    *E. In the elderly—due to atheroma of carotid artery
    F. In young persons—due to postrheumatic vegetations (rheumatic fever), cardiac catheterization, or valvotomy
    G. Moyamoya disease (multiple progressive intracranial arterial occlusion)
    H. Nicolau syndrome (emboli of medication inadvertently introduced into artery)
*2. Atherosclerosis of common carotid artery (ophthalmodynamometry employed for diagnosis)
3. Ischemia
    A. Carotid occlusion or dissection
    B. Essential hypotension
    C. Following orbital floor fractures or repair
    D. Following retinal detachment operation
    E. Generalized shock
    F. Heart failure (rare)
    G. Kahler disease (multiple myeloma)
    H. Knee-chest position
    I. Massive hemorrhage, such as that occurring in hematemesis, gastrointestinal bleeding, or surgical procedures
    J. Migraine
    K. Mosse syndrome (polycythemia-hepatic cirrhosis syndrome)
    L. Orbital hemorrhage following retrobulbar injection
    M. Post scoliosis surgery
    N. Too rapid lowering of blood pressure in hypertensive subjects
4. Inflammation
    A. Abdominal typhus (typhoid fever)
    B. African eye-worm disease (loiasis)

    C. Arteriole vasculitis, such as periarteritis nodosa (Kussmaul disease)

    D. Bacterial endocarditis

    E. Behçet disease (dermatostomato-ophthalmic syndrome)

    F. Diphtheria

    G. Herpes zoster

    H. Metastatic bacterial endophthalmitis

    I. Mucormycosis (phycomycosis)

    J. Pancreatitis

    K. Recurrent toxoplasmic retinochoroiditis

    L. Rocky Mountain spotted fever (spotted fever)

    M. Rubeola (measles)

    N. Subacute bacterial endocarditis

    O. Takayasu disease (pulseless disease)

    *P. Temporal arteritis

    Q. Varicella (chickenpox)

5. Blood disease

    A. After platelet transfusion

    B. Following ocular trauma with secondary glaucoma in youths with sickle-trait hemoglobinopathy

    C. Polycythemia vera (Vaquez-Osler syndrome)

    D. Sickle cell disease

6. Syphilis (acquired lues)

7. Associated factors

    A. Drusen of optic nerve (see p. 621)

    B. Papilledema (see p. 653)

    C. Subdural cerebral hemorrhage

    D. Arteriosclerosis of central retinal artery

    E. Chronic simple glaucoma

8. After dye yellow photocoagulation

9. Complication of retrobulbar block

10. Dego disease (malignant atrophic papulosis)

11. Disseminated lupus erythematosus

12. Fabry-Anderson syndrome (glycosphingolipid lipidosis)

13. Goldenhar-Gorlin syndrome (oculoauriculovertebral dysplasia)

14. Homocystinuria syndrome

15. Hyperhomocystinemia

16. Lyme disease

17. Neoplastic angioendotheliomatosis

18. Polymyalgia rheumatica

19. Protein S deficiency

* = most important

20. Relapsing polychondritis

21. Sneddon disease (livedoreticularis, neurologic abnormalities and labile hypertension)

22. Use of tranexamic acid therapy

Atmaca, L.S., and Ozmert, E.: Optic neuropathy and central retinal artery occlusion in a patient with herpes zoster ophthalmicus. Ann. Ophthal., 24:50–53, 1992.

Butt, Z., et al.: Central retinal artery occlusion in a patient with Marfan's syndrome. Acta. Opthal., 70:281–284, 1992.

Friedberg, M.A., and Micale, A.J.: Monocular Blindness From Central Retinal Artery Occlusion Associated with Chickenpox. Amer. J. Ophthal., 117:117–118, 1994.

Greven, C.M., et al.: Branch retinal artery occlusion after platelet transfusion. Amer. J. Ophthal., 109:105–106,1990.

Grossman, W., and Ward, W.T.: Central retinal artery occlusion after scoliosis surgery with a horseshoe headrest. Spine, 18:1226–1228, 1993.

Johnson, E.V., et al.: Bilateral cavernous sinus thrombosis due to mucormycosis. Arch. Ophthalmol., 106:1089–1092, 1988.

Johnson, M.W., et al.: Idiopathic recurrent branch retinal arterial occlusion. Arch. Ophthalmol., 107:757–758, 1989.

Rao, T.H., et al.: Central retinal artery occlusion from carotid dissection diagnosed by cervical computed tomography. Stroke, 25:1271–1272, 1994.

Roy, F.H.: Ocular Syndromes and Systemic Diseases. 2nd Ed. Philadelphia, W.B. Saunders, 1989.

Russell, S.R., and Folk, J.C.: Branch retinal artery occlusion after dye yellow photocoagulation of an arterial macroaneurysm. Am. J. Ophthalmol., 104:186, 1987.

Stambough, J.L, and Cheeks, M.L.: Central retinal artery occlusion: a complication of the knee-chest position. J. of Spinal Disorders, 5:363–365, 1992.

Wisotsky, B.J., and Engel, H.M.: Transesophageal Echocardiography in the Diagnosis of Branch Retinal Artery Obstruction. Amer. J. Ophthal., 115:653–656, 1993.

Localized Arterial Narrowing

1. Retinal atrophy following:

    A. Degeneration

    B. Inflammation

    C. Trauma

    D. Treatment with diathermy, light or cryopexy

2. Any vascular retinopathy

Nover, A.: The Ocular Fundus: Methods of Examination and Typical Findings. 4th Ed. Philadelphia, Lea & Febiger, 1981.

Perkins, E.S., and Dobree, J.H.: The Differential Diagnosis of Fundus Conditions. St. Louis, C.V. Mosby, 1972.

Retinal Artery Occlusion (Sudden Blindness with Diffuse Retinal Pallor and Cherry-Red Spot in Macula)

	Embolism (Postrheumatic Vegetation)	Common Carotid Artery Atherosclerosis*	Ischemia (Aortic Arch Syndrome)	Inflammation (Temporal Arteritis)*	Sickle Cell Disease*	Lupus Erythematosus
History						
1. Amaurosis fugax	S	U	U			
2. Bilateral			U	S		
3. Common in blacks					U	S
4. Common in females				S		U
5. Common in young adults	U			S		U
6. Diplopia	R			S		
7. Older age			U	U		
8. Orbital and ocular pain		S				
9. Photopsias	S	S	S			
10. Subjective field loss				S		
11. Untreated group A streptococcal pharyngitis	S					
Physical Findings						
1. Acute anterior uveitis	R	R				R
2. Afferent pupillary defect				U		
3. Angioid streaks					S	
4. Arteriosclerotic retinopathy		S				
5. Arteriovenous retinal shunts			U		S	S
6. Bright choroidal plaques		U			S	
7. Cataract		S	S			
8. Conjunctival coma signs					U	
9. Conjunctival hemorrhages—petechial	U					
10. Conjunctival icterus or pallor					S	
11. Conjunctival phlyctenulae						S
12. Corneal ulcer						S
13. Cortical blindness				S		
14. Cotton-wool spots	S	S	S	U	S	S
15. Deep stromal keratitis						S
16. Dilated episcleral vessels		S				
17. Disc neovascularization					R	
18. Episcleritis						S
19. Erythema/scaling of eyelids						U
20. External ophthalmoplegia			S	S		
21. Glaucoma		S	S			
22. Hypertensive retinopathy		S				
23. Hypotony of globe		S		S		
24. Keratoconjunctivitis sicca						S
25. Lid telangiectasis						S
26. Localized yellowish deep choroidal lesions	S					
27. Macular holes					S	

* = most important

Retinal Artery Occlusion (Sudden Blindness with Diffuse Retinal Pallor and Cherry-Red Spot in Macula) *Continued*

	Embolism (Postrheumatic Vegetation)	Common Carotid Artery Atherosclerosis*	Ischemia (Aortic Arch Syndrome)	Inflammation (Temporal Arteritis)*	Sickle Cell Disease*	Lupus Erythematosus
Physical Findings						
28. Occluded arteries		U	S			
29. Optic atrophy		S		S	S	S
30. Optic neuritis						S
31. Papilledema	S			S		S
32. Peripapillary arteriovenous anastomosis			S			
33. Peripheral retinal holes					S	
34. Pseudo Foster-Kennedy syndrome				S		
35. Ptosis				S		R
36. Retinal detachment			S		S	S
37. Retinal hemorrhages		S		U	S	S
38. Retinal microaneurysms		S	S		S	
39. Retinal neovascularization				R	S	
40. Retinal vein occlusion						S
41. Retinal venous dilation		S	S			S
42. Retinitis proliferans				S		
43. Roth spots	U	U				
44. Rubeosis iridis/iris atrophy		S	S		R	
45. Salmon patches in retina					S	
46. Scleritis					S	S
47. Tonic pupil					S	
48. Uveitis						S
49. Vascular tortuosity					S	
50. Vitreous hemorrhage			S		S	
51. White wedge-shaped infarcts in choroid					S	
Laboratory Data						
1. Abnormal ophthalmodynamometry		S	U			
2. Biopsy of temporal artery: fragmentation of the elastic lamina, smooth muscle necrosis, cellular infiltration with lymphocytes, epithelioid cells and giant cells				U		
3. Carotid arteriography		S				
4. Depression of hemoglobin, white blood cells and platelets						U
5. Elevated antistreptolysin titer	S					
6. Elevated C reactive protein	S					
7. Elevated ESR	S			U		
8. Elevated white blood cells	U					
9. False positive STS (serologic test for syphillis)						U
10. Fluorescein angiography abnormal	U	U	U	U	U	S
11. Hemoglobin electrophoresis: presence of HbS					U	
12. L.E. cells positive						U
13. Positive antinulcear antibody trait						U
14. Positive throat culture for group A streptococcus	S					

R = rarely; S = sometimes; and U = usually.

Generalized Arterial Narrowing

1. Local causes

   A. Apparent narrowing

   (1) High hypermetropia—common, small disc, narrow vessels, sometimes pseudopa-pilledema (see p. 653)

   (2) Congenital microphthalmos—rare, hypermetropia, often cataract (see p. 289)

   (3) Aphakia—cataract operation, dislocated lens (see p. 449)

   (4) Hollenhorst syndrome (chorioretinal infarction syndrome)

   (5) Wagner syndrome (hyaloideoretinal degeneration)

   B. Trauma

   (1) Avulsion of optic nerve—rare, secondary optic atrophy

   (2) Fracture involving bony optic canal—rare, secondary optic atrophy

   (3) Following retro-ocular injection—rare secondary optic atrophy

   (4) Orbital hemorrhage following retro-ocular injection or orbital operation—rare, secondary optic atrophy

   (5) Carotid ligation for carotid-cavernous fistula, rare, secondary optic atrophy

   (6) Following angiography—rare, secondary optic atrophy

   (7) Siderosis bulbi—metallic intraocular foreign body

   C. Infection and edema

   (1) Orbital cellulitis—exophthalmos, restricted ocular movements

   (2) Following thyrotropic exophthalmos—ocular muscle paresis, lid retraction

   D. Degenerations, such as progressive cone-rod degeneration

   E. Primary tapetoretinal degenerations, such as retinitis pigmentosa; Hallgren syndrome (retinitis pigmentosa-deafness-ataxia syndrome)

2. Systemic disease

   A. Arteriosclerosis

   (1) In involutionary sclerosis—of population older than years of age, generalized arteriolar narrowing, diminished light reflexes

   (2) In arteriosclerotic disease

   a. Arteriosclerotic central artery occlusion—common arteriovenous crossing signs, focal arteriolar constriction

   *b. Embolus from atheromatous plaque, common, sudden onset, visible white embolus

   B. Hypertensive conditions

   *(1) Essential hypertension—retinal hemorrhages, cotton-wool spots, arteriovenous crossing signs

   *(2) Malignant hypertension—retinal hemorrhages, cotton-wool spots, edema of disc

   (3) Toxemia of pregnancy—rare, sometimes hemorrhages, cotton-wool spots, edema of disc, serous detachment

   (4) Coarctation of aorta—rare, hypertensive changes vary greatly in degree

   (5) Pheochromocytoma—rare, hypertensive changes vary greatly in degree

* = most important

    (6) Adrenal tumor, hyperaldosteronism (adrenal medulla tumor syndrome)—rare, hypertensive changes vary greatly in degree

    (7) Cushing tumor (adrenocortical hyperfunction)—rare, hypertensive changes vary greatly in degree

    (8) Motor neuron disease of cervicothoracic cord hypertension may occur after prolonged artificial pulmonary ventilation

C. Other forms of vascular disease

    (1) Retinal ischemia—hypotension following severe or recurrent bleeding, unilateral blindness in patients

   *(2) Temporal arteritis (cranial arteritis, giant-cell arteritis)—common, years or older; mean age at onset, years; sudden blindness at onset

    (3) Polyarteritis nodosa (Kussmaul disease)—multiple signs involving choroid, retina, cornea, episclera, and ocular muscles

    (4) Proliferative diabetic retinopathy—arterial narrowing occurs in 17% of patients with proliferative diabetic retinopathy, mainly in cicatricial stage

    (5) Cardiac arrest—thread-like arterioles, segmentation of blood column, generalized retinal pallor, pallor of disc, sometimes macular cherry-red spot

    (6) Raynaud disease (idiopathic paroxysmal digital cyanosis)—young adults, more common in women

D. Renal disease

    (1) Acute glomerulonephritis—preceding illnesses, including scarlet fever, streptococcal tonsillitis, otitis media, erysipelas (St. Anthony fire), subacute bacterial endocarditis, polyarteritis nodosa (Kussmaul disease)

    (2) Chronic glomerulonephritis—often asymptomatic and found on routine examination

    (3) Pyelonephritis and pyelitis—commonest causes of renal failure

E. Diseases of the central nervous system

    (1) Migraine

   *(2) Syphilitic neuroretinitis

    (3) Viral neuroretinitis (rare complication)

    (4) Tay-Sachs disease (amaurotic familial idiocy)

    (5) Jansky-Bielschowsky disease (amaurotic familial idiocy, late form)

    (6) Myotonic dystrophy syndrome (Curschmann-Steinert syndrome)

    (7) Retinohypophysary syndrome (Lijo Pavia-Lis syndrome)

    (8) Zellweger syndrome (cerebrohepatorenal syndrome of Zellweger)

F. Toxic causes

    (1) Chloroquine, hydroxychloroquine, quinacrine, amodiaquine

    (2) Lead

    (3) Quinine—rare, may follow large dose (abortifacient) or normal dose in sensitive subjects

G. Other causes

    (1) Caisson syndrome (bends)

    (2) Chédiak-Higashi syndrome (oculocutaneous albinism with recurrent infections; autosomal recessive)

(3) Hunter syndrome (MPS II)

(4) Sanfilippo-Good syndrome (MPS III)

Perkins, E.S., and Dobree, J.H.: The Differential Diagnosis of Fundus Conditions. St. Louis, C.V. Mosby, 1972.

Roy, F.H.: Ocular Syndromes and Systemic Diseases. 2nd Ed. Philadelphia, W.B. Saunders, 1989.

Periarteritis Retinalis Segmentalis (White or Yellow Plaques Arranged in Segments Encircling Arteries like a Cuff, and Localized to One or More Arterial Branches)

*1. Arteriosclerosis secondary to vein obstruction

2. Herpes zoster

3. Hypercholesterolemia

4. Lupus erythematosus (disseminated lupus erythematosus)

5. Metastatic uveitis

6. Periarteritis nodosa (necrotizing angiitis)

*7. Sarcoidosis syndrome

8. Syphilis (acquired lues)

*9. Temporal arteritis (giant-cell arteritis)

*10. Tuberculous retinitis

11. Uveitis, idiopathic

Crouch, E.R., and Goldberg, M.F.: Retinal periarteritis secondary to syphilis. Arch. Ophthalmol., 93:384–387, 1975.

Rask, A.J.: Peri-arteritis retinalis segmentalis. Acta. Ophthalmol., 47:234–237, 1969.

Sheathing of Retinal Veins (White or Gray Envelopes around Veins; Retinal and/or Vitreous Hemorrhage and Exudates May Be Present)

1. Disc only—developmental

2. Disc and retina—papillitis or papilledema

3. Peripheral sheathing

   *A. Acute retinal necrosis

   B. Amebiasis

   C. Behçet disease (dermatostomato-ophthalmic syndrome)

   D. Brucellosis—rare, tortuosity and sheathing of veins, vitreous haze, retinal hemorrhages

   E. Candidiasis

   F. Coccidioidomycosis

   G. Eales disease (periphlebitis)

   H. Diabetes mellitus

   I. Filariasis—hemorrhages and exudates

   J. Hypertension

   K. Infectious mononucleosis—peripheral or central perivascular involvement, venous engorgement and sheathing associated with retinal hemorrhages

   L. Lupus erythematosus

* = most important

M. Non-Hodgkin's lymphoma

N. Onchocerciasis syndrome (river blindness)

O. Rickettsial infections—peripheral or central perivascular involvement, venous engorgement and sheathing associated with retinal hemorrhages

*P. Sarcoidosis

Q. Septicemia and bacteremia—rare, venous engorgement, usually with multiple hemorrhages and focal sheathing

R. Sickle-cell disease

S. Syphilis (secondary) (acquired lues)

T. Tuberculin or Bacille-Calmette-Guérin vaccination—rare, sectorial, or generalized changes

U. Viral infections, including:

   (1) Cytomegalovirus retinitis

   (2) Herpes simplex (likely responsible for acute retinal necrosis)

   (3) Herpes zoster ophthalmicus

   (4) Influenza

   (5) Rift Valley fever

4. Peripheral sheathing without secondary retinopathy—multiple sclerosis

5. Wide and usually dense sheathing of dilated and tortuous veins, suggestive of myelogenous leukemia

Brown, S., et al.: Intraocular lymphoma presenting as retinal vasculitis. Surv. Ophthal., 39:138–140, 1994.

Kohno, T., et al.: Ocular manifestations of adult T-cell leukemia/lymphoma. Ophthalmology, 100:1794–1799, 1993.

Perkins, E.S., and Dobree, J.H.: The Differential Diagnosis of Fundus Conditions. St. Louis, C.V. Mosby, 1972.

Ridley, M.E., et al.: Retinal manifestation of ocular lymphoma. Ophthal., 99:1153–1161, 1992.

Roy, F.H.: Ocular Syndromes and Systemic Diseases. 2nd Ed. Philadelphia, W.B. Saunders, 1989.

Absent Venous Pulsations (Spontaneous Venous Pulsations Absent at Venules on the Disc)

1. Normal individuals

*2. Impending central vein occlusion (see p. 525)

*3. Papilledema (see p. 651)

Ballantyne, A.J., and Michaelson, I.C.: Textbook of the Fundus of the Eye. 3rd Ed. Baltimore, Williams & Wilkins, 1981.

Newell, F.W.: Ophthalmology, Principles and Practice. 7th Ed. St. Louis, C.V. Mosby, 1991.

Central Retinal Vein Occlusion

	External Vein Compression as Central Retinal Artery Atherosclerosis*	Inflammatory Venous Disease as Diabetes Mellitus*	Blood Dyscrasias as Leukemia	Increased Blood Viscosity as Macroglobulinemia	Glaucoma*
History					
1. Amaurosis fugax	U				
2. Common in males				U	
3. Common in persons more than 40 years		U		U	U
4. Common in persons more than 60 years	U				
5. Congenital					S
6. Familial		U	S		S
7. Orbital/ocular pain	S				
8. Photopsias	U				
Physical Findings					
1. Anterior ischemic optic neuropathy	S	S			
2. Arterial occlusions	U				
3. Arteriosclerotic retinopathy	U				
4. Bright plaques	U				
5. Cataract	S	U			S
6. Closed anterior chamber angle					U
7. Conjunctivitis, papillary			U		
8. Corneal edema	S				U
9. Corneal hypesthesia					U
10. Cotton-wool spots		U	U	S	
11. Crystalline deposits in conjunctiva/cornea				U	
12. Dilated episcleral veins	S				
13. Ectropion uvea		S			
14. Elevated intraocular pressure	S		S	U	U
15. Engorgement of conjunctival vessels				U	
16. Extraocular muscle paralysis		S	S		
17. Folds in Descemet membrane					U
18. Glaucomatous cupping					U
19. Hard exudates		U			
20. Hypopyon			S		
21. Iris atrophy	S				U
22. Iris synechiae	S				U
23. Keratoconjunctivitis sicca				U	
24. Macular edema		S	U		
25. Optic atrophy	S	S	S		U
26. Optic neuritis			S		
27. Papilledema		S	S	S	S
28. Retinal detachment			S		
29. Retinal hemorrhages	S	U	U		
30. Retinal microaneurysms	S	U		U	
31. Retinal neovascularization	S	U			
32. Retinal venous dilation	S			U	

* = most important

Central Retinal Vein Occlusion *Continued*

	External Vein Compression as Central Retinal Artery Atherosclerosis*	Inflammatory Venous Disease as Diabetes Mellitus*	Blood Dyscrasias as Leukemia	Increased Blood Viscosity as Macroglobulinemia	Glaucoma*
Physical Findings					
33. Retinal venous thrombosis				U	
34. Rubeosis iridis	S	U			U
35. Visual field defects					U
36. Vitreous hemorrhage	S	S			
37. Vitreous opacities			S		
Laboratory Data					
1. Blood sugar elevated		U			
2. Bone marrow puncture			U	U	
3. Carotid arteriography	S				
4. Fluorescein angiography	U	U	U		
5. Lipid profile	U				
6. Peripheral blood test			U	U	
7. Serum gamma M immunoglobulin elevated				U	
8. Visual field test					U

R = rarely; S = sometimes; and U = usually.

Dilated Retinal Veins (Normally Arteriole-Venule Ratio Is Two to Three; with Increase in this Ratio, the Retinal Veins May Be Dilated)

1. Congenital
    A. Congenital tortuosity of retinal vessels—rare, sometimes associated with coarctation of aorta
    B. Fabry disease (hereditary dystrophic lipidosis)
    C. Hemangioma
    D. Longfellow-Graether syndrome
    E. Ocular fundi in newborns
    F. Racemose (arteriovenous) aneurysm—rare, arteriovenous anastomoses localized to sector of retina
    *G. Retinopathy of prematurity with plus disease
    H. von Hippel-Lindau disease (angiomatosis)—familial in 20% of cases, bilateral in 50%

2. Trauma and inflammation
    A. Anterior uveitis—dilatation of veins, often slight hyperemia of disc
    B. Carotid-cavernous fistula—fracture of base of skull, progressive exophthalmos, bruit
    C. Cavernous sinus thrombosis—rare, proptosis and orbital edema
    *D. Impending obstruction of the central retinal vein
    E. Periphlebitis—sheathing of vessels

3. Cardiovascular disease—dilatation may be present but rarely dominates the fundus picture
    A. Arteriosclerosis
    B. Involutionary sclerosis (later stages)
    C. Secondary to defective arterial flow, such as in:
        (1) Aortic arch syndrome (pulseless disease)
        (2) Cardiac insufficiency
        (3) Congenital heart disease
        (4) Iatrogenic (lowering of blood pressure)
        (5) Severe blood loss
        *(6) Stenosis or occlusion of common carotid
        *(7) Temporal arteritis
        (8) Venous stasis (hypotensive retinopathy of Kearns and Hollenhorst)

4. Respiratory disease—venous dilatation may occur with purplish hue of whole retina; obstruction of venous return from the head, such as in:
    A. Congenital septal defect (Fallot tetralogy)
    B. Emphysema
    C. Hamman-Rich syndrome (diffuse pulmonary fibrosis syndrome)
    D. Heart failure of any type
    E. Kartagener syndrome (sinusitis-bronchiectasis-situs inversus syndrome)
    F. Mechanical compression of chest
    G. Mediastinal tumor obstructing superior vena cava

* = most important

5. Diseases of the central nervous system

   *A. Carotid-cavernous fistula—fractured base of skull; rupture of berry aneurysm, arteriosclerosis

   B. Hemangioma of posterior fossa—rare, papilledema, often grossly dilated veins

   C. Optic nerve lesion—rare, secondary to orbital space-occupying lesion

   *D. Papilledema (see p. 653)

   E. Retrolenticular syndrome (Dejerine-Roussy syndrome)

   *F. Subarachnoid hemorrhage—head injury; subhyaloid hemorrhages near disc, dilated veins, sometimes papilledema

6. Blood diseases

   A. Aplastic anemia—hemorrhages the most striking sign, often spreading around the disc

   B. Cryoglobulinemia—rare, may occur with multiple myeloma, veins dilated, tortuous, and sometimes beaded

   C. Gansslen syndrome (familial hemolytic icterus)

   D. Lymphatic leukemia

   E. Macrocytic anemia of all types—common, retinopathy absent unless hemoglobin below 50%; pale fundus, superficial hemorrhages, cotton-wool spots

      (1) Pernicious anemia

      (2) Steatorrhea

      (3) Celiac disease

      (4) Carcinoma of stomach

   F. Macroglobulinemia—rare; veins dilated tortuous and sometimes beaded, hemorrhages and occasionally microaneurysms

   G. Monocytic leukemia

   H. Myelogenous leukemia

   I. Multiple myeloma (Kahler disease)

   J. Polycythemia rubra vera (primary; Vaquez disease)—common in males; hemorrhages; papilledema may be marked and venous thrombosis may occur

   K. Secondary polycythemia—common; hemorrhages, papilledema and venous thrombosis may occur

   L. Sickle cell disease—dilatation of peripheral veins with retinal, subhyaloid and vitreous hemorrhages

   M. Thrombocytopenic purpura—retinal and subhyaloid hemorrhages near disc, moderate venous dilatation

7. Acute febrile illnesses—rare, occasional dilatation of retinal veins with a few hemorrhages and mild edema of disc

   A. Infectious mononucleosis

   B. Influenza

   C. Rickettsial infections

   D. Septicemia

8. Metabolic diseases

    A. Cystic fibrosis syndrome (fibrocystic disease of pancreas)—venous congestion often swelling of disc

    B. Plasma lecithin

    *C. Diabetic retinopathy—larger veins affected, often beaded

9. Collagen diseases

    A. Polyarteritis nodosa—among other fundus lesions, dilated veins may occur

    B. Sclerosis, progressive systemic (scleroderma)

    C. Systemic lupus erythematosus—cotton-wool spots, occasional hemorrhages, and moderate dilatation of veins

10. Toxic conditions, such as methyl alcohol ingestion

Newell, F.W.: Ophthalmology, Principles and Practice. 7th Ed. St. Louis, C.V. Mosby, 1991.

Perkins, E.S., and Dobree, J.H.: The Differential Diagnosis of Fundus Conditions. St. Louis, C.V. Mosby, 1972.

Roy, F.H.: Ocular Syndromes and Systemic Diseases. 2nd Ed. Philadelphia, W.B. Saunders, 1989.

Central Retinal Vein Occlusion (Characterized by Massive Hemorrhage into Posterior Portion of Eye and Dilated Retinal Veins)

1. External compression of the vein

    A. Atherosclerosis of central retinal artery

    B. Connective tissue strand within the floor of the physiologic excavation

    C. Multiple crossings of the same artery and vein or congenital venous loops or twists in the retinal surface

    D. Pseudotumor cerebri

2. Degenerative or inflammatory venous disease, causing detachment, proliferation, and hydrops

    A. AIDS (HIV retinopathy)

    B. Arterial hypertension

    C. Cardiac decompensation

    *D. Diabetes mellitus (Willis disease)

    E. Ipsilateral internal carotid artery stenosis

    F. Optic disc drusen

    G. Optic nerve inflammation

    H. Systemic granulomatous disease, particularly tuberculosis

3. Thrombosis from venous stagnation

    A. Spasm of corresponding retinal arterioles

    B. Blood dyscrasias

        (1) Emphysema with secondary erythrocytosis

        (2) Homocystinemia

        (3) Increased platelet aggregation

        (4) Leukemias

* = most important

      *(5) Multiple myeloma

      *(6) Polycythemia vera

      (7) Sickle cell disease

  C. Increased viscosity of the blood

      (1) Cystic fibrosis of pancreas

      (2) Following peritoneal dialysis

      (3) Hyperproteinemia

      *(4) Macroglobulinemia

      (5) Use of tranexamic acid

  D. Sudden reduction of systemic blood pressure because of cardiac decompensation, surgical or traumatic shock, or therapy for arterial hypertension

  *E. Glaucoma (pre-existing)

  F. Increase in fibrinolytic inhibitors of blood

  G. Carotid-cavernous sinus fistula

  *H. Syphilis

Allinson, R.W., et al.: Central retinal vein occlusion after heart-lung transplantation. Ann. Ophthal., 25:58–63, 1993.

Archer, D.B., et al.: Classification of branch vein obstruction. Am. Acad. Ophthalmol. Otolaryngol., 78:148–165, 1974.

Ismail, Y., et al.: A rare cause of visual loss in AIDS patients: central retinal vein occlusion. Brit. J. Ophthal., 77:600–601, 1993.

Miller, S.A., and Bresnick, G.H.: Retinal branch vessel occlusion in acute intermittent porphyria. Ann. Ophthalmol., 11:1379, 1979.

Noble, K.G., and Carr, R.E.: Branch vein occlusion. Ophthalmology, 89:86, 1982.

Rath, E.Z., et al.: Risk factors for retinal vein occlusions. A case-control study. Ophthal., 99:509–514, 1992.

Snir, M., et al.: Central venous stasis retinopathy following the use of tranexamic acid. Am. J. Ophthalmol., 111:534–535, 1991.

Wenzler, E.M., et al.: Hyperhomocystinemia in retinal artery and retinal vein occlusion. Amer. J. Ophthal., 115:162–167, 1993.

Dilated Retinal Veins and Retinal Hemorrhages

  1. Carotid-cavernous fistula

  *2. Cavernous sinus fistula syndrome (carotid artery syndrome)

  3. Cavernous sinus thrombosis (hypophyseal-sphenoidal syndrome)

  *4. Central retinal vein occlusion (see p. 525)

  5. Cervical tuberculosis

  6. Choroidal melanoma remote to the neovascularization

  7. Congenital tortuosity and dilation of the retinal vessels

  8. Cryoglobulinemia

  *9. Diabetes mellitus

  10. Intravitreal myiasis

  11. Leukemia

12. Lymphomas

13. Macroglobulinemia (Waldenstrom syndrome)

14. Multiple myeloma (myelomatosis)

15. Ophthalmic vein thrombosis

16. Pappataci fever (phlebotomus fever)

17. Paraproteinemias and dysproteinemias

18. Polycythemia vera

19. Retinal arteritis

*20. Sickle cell disease

*21. Syphilis (acquired lues)

Kalina, R.E., and Kaiser, M.: Familial retinal hemorrhages. Am. J. Ophthalmol., 74:252–255, 1972.

Roy, F.H.: Ocular Syndromes and Systemic Diseases. 2nd Ed. Philadelphia, W.B. Saunders, 1989.

Retinal Hemorrhages (Bleeding that May Be Intraretinal or Preretinal Hemorrhages into the Vitreous, or Subretinal Hemorrhages)

1. Congestion of head and neck, such as in newborns, hanging, or choking

2. Trauma, including electrical injury, hypothermal injury, and child abuse

3. Vascular obstruction, such as cardiorespiratory obesity syndrome, cystic fibrosis syndrome, negative acceleration syndrome, (hydrostatic pressure syndrome), ophthalmoplegic migraine syndrome, papilledema (see p. 653), subarachnoid hemorrhages, superior vena cava syndrome, Symonds syndrome (benign intracranial hypertension), thrombocytopenia, thrombosis and Wernicke syndrome (avitaminosis B_1)

4. Inflammatory conditions, such as Criswick-Schepens syndrome (familial exudative vitreoretinopathy), Loffler syndrome (eosinophilic pneumonitis), perivasculitis, and subacute bacterial endocarditis

*5. Acute febrile and infectious illnesses, including amebiasis ankylostomiasis, aspergillosis, bacterial endocarditis, coccidioidomycosis, cryptococcosis (torulosis), cysticercosis, dengue fever, hydatid cyst (echinococcosis), hydrophobia (rabies), infectious mononucleosis, influenza, Japanese River fever (typhus), lymphogranuloma venereum (Nicolas-Favre disease), metastatic bacterial endophthalmitis, nematode ophthalmia syndrome (toxocariasis), pertussis (whooping cough), Q fever, relapsing fever, trichinellosis, Weil disease (leptospirosis), and yersiniosis

*6. Vascular disease, such as arteriosclerosis, atherosclerosis, arteriovenous fistula, disseminated intravascular coagulation, hypertension, Paget syndrome (hypertensive diencephalic syndrome), progressive systemic sclerosis, pulmonary insufficiency, the retinopathies, particularly diabetic and hypertensive, and when the circulation through the eye is diminished in hypotensive retinopathy, such as in carotid vascular insufficiency syndrome, or pulseless disease (Takayasu syndrome), suprarenal-sympathetic syndrome, temporal arteritis syndrome (cranial arteritis syndrome) and in conditions of extreme cachexia

7. Anemia that may be secondary to drugs, including:

acebutolol	acetaminophen	acetazolamide
acenocoumarin	acetanilid	acetohexamide

* = most important

acetophenazine
actinomycin C
acyclovir
allobarbital
allopurinol
alprazolam
aminopterin
aminosalicylate(?)
aminosalicylic acid(?)
amithiozone
amitriptyline
amobarbital
amodiaquine
amoxicillin
amphotericin B
ampicillin
antazoline
anisindione
antimony lithium thiomalate
antimony potassium tartrate
antimony sodium tartrate
antimony sodium
   thioglycollate
antipyrine
aprobarbital
atenolol
auranofin
aurothioglucose
aurothioglycanide
azatadine
azathioprine
barbital
BCG vaccine
bendroflumethiazide
benzathine penicillin G
benzthiazide
bishydroxycoumarin
bleomycin
brompheniramine
busulfan
butabarbital
butalbital
butallylonal

butaperazine
butethal
cactinomycin
calcitriol
captopril
carbamazepine
carbenicillin
carbimazole
carbinoxamine
carisoprodol
carmustine
carphenazine
cefaclor
cefadroxil
cefamandole
cefazolin
cefonicid
cefoperazone
ceforanide
cefotaxime
cefotetan
cefoxitin
cefsulodin
ceftizoxime
ceftriaxone
cefuroxime
cephalexin
cephaloglycin
cephaloridine
cephalothin
cephapirin
cephradine
chlorambucil
chloramphenicol
chlordiazepoxide
chloroquine
chlorothiazide
chlorpheniramine
chlorpromazine
chlorpropamide
chlorprothixene
chlortetracycline
chlorthalidone

cholecalciferol
cimetidine
cisplatin
clemastine
clindamycin
clofibrate
clonazepam
clorazepate
cloxacillin
colchicine
cyclobarbital
cyclopentobarbital
cyclophosphamide
cycloserine
cyclosporine
cyclothiazide
cyproheptadine
cytarabine
dacarbazine
dactinomycin
dapsone
daunorubicin
deferoxamine
demeclocycline
desipramine
dexbrompheniramine
dexchlorpheniramine
diazepam
diazoxide
dichlorphenamide
dicloxacillin
dicumarol
diethazine
diltiazem
dimercaprol
dimethindene
dimethyl sulfoxide
diphenadione
diphenhydramine
diphenylhydantoin
diphenylpyraline
diphtheria and tetanus toxoids
   and pertussis vaccine
   (adsorbed)

doxorubicin
doxycycline
doxylamine
dromostanolone
droperidol
enalapril
ergocalciferol
erythromycin
ethacrynic acid
ethopropazine
ethosuximide
ethotoin
ethoxzolamide
ethyl biscoumacetate
fenfluramine
fenoprofen
flecainide
floxuridine
fluorouracil
fluoxymesterone
fluphenazine
flurazepam
furosemide
gentamicin
glutethimide
glyburide
gold Au 198
gold sodium thiomalate
gold sodium thiosulfate
griseofulvin
guanethidine
halazepam
haloperidol
heparin
heptabarbital
hetacillin
hexethal
hexobarbital
hydrabamine penicillin V
hydralazine
hydrabamine phenoxymethyl
    penicillin
hydrochlorothiazide

hydroflumethiazide
hydroxychloroquine
hydroxyurea
ibuprofen
imipramine
indapamide
indomethacin
influenza virus vaccine
interferon
isocarboxazid
isoniazid
labetalol
levodopa
lincomycin
lithium carbonate
lomustine
lorazepam
loxapine
maprotiline
measles and rubella virus
    vaccine (live)
measles, mumps and rubella
    virus vaccine (live)
measles virus vaccine (live)
mechlorethamine
mefenamic acid
melphalan
mephenytoin
mephobarbital
meprobamate
mercaptopurine
mesoridazine
methacycline
methaqualone
metharbital
methazolamide
methdilazine
methicillin
methimazole
methitural
methohexital
methotrimeprazine
methotrexate

methsuximide
methyclothiazide
methyldopa
methylene blue
methylphenidate
methylthiouracil
methyprylon
metolazone
metropolol
metrizamide
metronidazole
mexiletine
mianserin
midazolam
minocycline
mitomycin
moxalactam
mumps virus vaccine (live)
nadolol
nafcillin
nalidixic acid
naproxen
nialamide
nifedipine
nitrazepam
nitrofurantoin
nitroglycerin
nortriptyline
oral contraceptives
orphenadrine
oxacillin
oxazepam
oxyphenbutazone
oxytetracycline
paramethadione
penicillamine
pentobarbital
perazine
periciazine
perphenazine
phenacetin
phenelzine
phenformin

phenindione
pheniramine
phenobarbital
phenprocoumon
phensuximide
phenylbutazone
phenytoin
pindolol
piperacetazine
piperazine
pipobroman
poliovirus vaccine
polythiazide
potassium penicillin G
potassium penicillin V
potassium phenethicillin
prazepam
primidone
probarbital
procaine penicillin G
procarbazine
prochlorperazine
promazine
promethazine
propiomazine
propylthiouracil
protriptyline
pyrilamine
pyrimethamine
quinacrine

quinethazone
quinidine
quinine
ranitidine
rifampin
rubella and mumps virus vaccine (live)
rubella virus vaccine (live)
secobarbital
semustine
sodium antimonylgluconate
stibocaptate
stibogluconate
stibophen
streptomycin
sulfonamides
suramin
talbutal
temazepam
testolactone
testosterone
tetracycline
thiabendazole
thiamylal
thiethylperazine
thioguanine
thiopental
thiopropazate
thioproperazine
thioridazine
thiotepa

thiothixene
tocainide
tolazamide
tolazoline
tolbutamide
tranylcypromine
trazodone
triazolam
trichlormethiazide
triethylenemelamine
trifluoperazine
trifluperidol
triflupromazine
trimeprazine
trimethadione
tripelennamine
triprolidine
uracil mustard
urethan
vancomycin
verapamil
vidarabine
vinbarbital
vinblastine
vincristine
vitamin A
vitamin D
vitamin D_2
vitamin D_3
warfarin

8. Vascularized neoplasms, including hereditary hemorrhagic telangiectasia (Rendu-Osler-Weber disease), and periocular and ocular metastatic tumors

9. Drugs, including:

acetylcholine
acid bismuth sodium tartrate
adrenal cortex injection
aldosterone
allopurinol(?)
alseroxylon
aspirin
benoxinate
betamethasone

bismuth carbonate
bismuth oxychloride
bismuth salicylate
bismuth sodium tartrate
bismuth sodium thioglycollate
bismuth sodium triglycollamate
bismuth subcarbonate
bismuth subsalicylate
butacaine

cobalt(?)

cocaine

cortisone

deserpidine

desoxycorticosterone

dexamethasone

dibucaine

dyclonine

epinephrine

ethambutol

fludrocortisone

fluorometholone

fluorouracil

fluprednisolone

glycerin

heparin

hexachlorophene

hydrocortisone

indomethacin

iodide and iodine solution compounds

isosorbide

ketoprofen

lincomycin

mannitol

medrysone

meprednisone

methaqualone

methylphenidate

methylprednisolone

mithramycin

mitotane

oxyphenbutazone

paramethasone

penicillamine

phenacaine

phenylbutazone

piperocaine

plicamycin

pralidoxime

prednisolone

prednisone

proparacaine

radioactive iodides

rauwolfia serpentina

rescinnamine

reserpine

sodium chloride

sodium salicylate

sulfacetamide

sulfachlorpyridazine

sulfacytine

sulfadiazine

sulfadimethoxine

sulfamerazine

sulfameter

sulfamethazine

sulfamethizole

sulfamethoxazole

sulfamethoxypyridazine

sulfanilamide

sulfaphenazole

sulfapyridine

sulfasalazine

sulfathiazole

sulfisoxazole

sulindac

syrosingopine

tamoxifen

tetracaine

triamcinolone

trichloroethylene

urea

urokinase(?)

vitamin A

10. Hematopoietic system such as the anemias, Bing-Neel syndrome (association of macroglobulinemia and central nervous system symptoms), Fanconi syndrome (amino diabetes), Gansslen syndrome (familial hemolytic icterus), Henoch-Schönlein purpura, Herrick syndrome (sickle cell disease), Jacobsen-Brodwell syndrome, leukemias, hemophilia, polycythemia, purpuras, oculo-otoororenoerythropoietic disease, Plummer-Vinson syndrome (sideropenic dysphagia syndrome), Reimann syndrome (hyperviscosity syndrome), Waldenstrom's syndrome (macroglobuline-

mia syndrome), Wiskott-Aldrich syndrome (purpura), also following blood transfusion with incompatibility of blood groups

11. Acosta syndrome (mountain climber syndrome)
12. Amyloidosis
13. Behçet syndrome (dermatostomato-ophthalmic syndrome)
14. Bloch-Sulzberger syndrome (incontinentia pigmenti)
15. Bourneville syndrome (tuberous sclerosis)
16. Following labor induced by oxytocin or dinoprostone in newborns
17. Following use of YAG laser
18. Histiocytosis X (Hand-Schüller-Christian syndrome)
19. HIV-related retinopathy
20. Hodgkin disease
21. Juvenile diabetes—dwarfism-obesity syndrome
22. Macular degeneration, age-related (exudative type)
23. Morning glory syndrome (hereditary central glial anomaly of the optic disc)
24. Mycosis fungoides syndrome (Sezary syndrome)
25. Neuroblastoma
26. Optic nerve drusen (see p. 621)
27. Paget syndrome (osteitis deformans)
28. Plasma lecithin (cholesterol acyltransferase deficiency)
29. Polymyalgia rheumatica
30. Polymyositis dermatomyositis (Wagner-Unverricht syndrome)
31. Porphyria cutanea tarda
32. Purtscher's retinopathy
33. Radiation retinopathy
34. Sarcoidosis syndrome (Schaumman syndrome)
35. Schamberg disease (self-limiting cutaneous vasculitis)
36. Terson syndrome

Fraunfelder, F.T.: Drug-Induced Ocular Side Effects and Drug Interactions. 4th Ed. Philadelphia, William & Wilkins, 1996.

Riffenburgh, R.S., and Sathyavagiswaran, L.: Ocular finding at autopsy of child abuse victims. Ophthalmology, 98:1519–1524, 1991.

Roy, F.H.: Ocular Syndromes and Systemic Diseases. 2nd Ed. Philadelphia, W.B. Saunders, 1989.

Williams, M.C., et al.: Obstetric correlates of neonatal retinal hemorrhage. Obstetrics & Gynecology. 81:688–694, 1993.

Large Hemorrhages in the Fundus of an Infant or Young Child (Suggestive of Increased Intracranial Pressure and Paralysis of Cranial Nerves)

1. Hygroma
*2. Shaken baby syndrome
3. Subarachnoid hemorrhage
4. Subdural hematoma

Lambert, S.R., et al.: Optic nerve sheath and retinal hemorrhages associated with the shaken baby syndrome. Arch. Ophthalmol., 104:1509–1512, 1986.

Nover, A.: The Ocular Fundus: Methods of Examination and Typical Findings. 4th Ed. Philadelphia, Lea & Febiger, 1981.

Retinovitreal Hemorrhage in a Young Adult

    1. Incontinentia pigmenti (Bloch-Sulzberger syndrome)

    2. Congenital x-linked (juvenile) retinoschisis

  *3. Diabetes mellitus

  *4. Sickle cell anemia

    5. Trauma

    6. von-Hippel Lindau syndrome

Duke-Elder, S.: System of Ophthalmology. Vol. X. St. Louis, C.V. Mosby, 1967.

Morse, P.H.: Vitreoretinal Disease—A Manual for Diagnosis and Treatment. 2nd Ed. St. Louis, C.V. Mosby, 1989.

Retinal Hemorrhage with Central White Spot

    1. Collagen disease

    2. Cyanosis retinae—carcinoma of lung

  *3. Diabetes mellitus

    4. Following heart operation

    5. Following uncomplicated pediatric cataract extraction

  *6. Hematopoietic system

      A. Anemias

      B. Leukemia

      C. Multiple myeloma (Kahler disease)

    7. Intracranial hemorrhage (infants)

    8. Septic retinitis

     *A. Candida albicans infection

      B. Kala-azar

      C. Phlebitis

      D. Rheumatic mitral and aortic valvulitis

      E. Rocky mountain spotted fever

     *F. Subacute bacterial endocarditis

      G. Syphilitis aortitis

      H. Viral pneumonia

    9. Vascular disease

* = most important

Retinal Hemorrhage with Central White Spot

	Septic Retinitis—Candida Albicans	Hematopoietic System—Leukemia	Diabetes Mellitus	Vascular Disease—Arteriovenous Fistula	Collagen Disease—Polyarteritis Nodosa	Cyanosis Retinae—Carcinoma of Lung
History						
1. Acute or chronic blood disorder		U				
2. Chronic mucocutaneous candidiasis	S					
3. Congenital				S		
4. Familial			U			
5. In overweight persons			U			
6. Males between ages 20 to 50					U	
7. More in females				S		
8. More in males					U	U
9. Over age 40			U			U
10. Secondary to penetrating or blunt trauma				U		
11. Systemic dissemination in drug addicts, in debilitated patients or immunosuppressed patients	U					
Physical Findings						
1. Asteroid hyalosis				S		
2. Blepharitis	S					
3. Cataract			U	S	S	
4. Cells and flare	U			S	U	
5. Chemosis				S		
6. Conjunctival cicatrization	S					
7. Conjunctival papillary hypertrophy		S				
8. Conjunctival necrosis				S		
9. Conjunctivitis	U				S	
10. Corneal stromal infiltrate	S					
11. Corneal stromal vascularization	S			S		
12. Corneal ulcer					S	
13. Cotton wool spots		U	U		U	
14. Dacryocystitis	S					
15. Darkening of blood column in conjunctival and retinal vessels						U
16. Ectropion uvea			S	U		
17. Eczema of eyelids	S					
18. Edema of eyelids	S			S		
19. Endophthalmitis	U					
20. Engorgement of conjunctival vessels		S				
21. Exophthalmos				S		
22. Exudative detachment of retina	U				U	
23. Glaucoma		S	S	S		
24. Granuloma of eyelids						
25. Hard yellow exudates of retina			U			
26. Hyperemia of eyelids	S					
27. Hyperemia of optic nerve	S					
28. Hypopyon	U	U				
29. Iris atrophy				R		
30. Irregular sheathing of retinal veins			U			
31. Irregularity of arterial caliber						U

Retinal Hemorrhage with Central White Spot *Continued*

	Septic Retinitis—Candida Albicans	Hematopoietic System—Leukemia	Diabetes Mellitus	Vascular Disease—Arteriovenous Fistula	Collagen Disease—Polyarteritis Nodosa	Cyanosis Retinae—Carcinoma of Lung
Physical Findings						
32. Keratitis	S					
33. Lipemia retinalis			S			
34. Macular edema		S	S			S
35. Microaneurysms of retina			U			
36. Optic atrophy		S	S	S	S	
37. Optic neuritis		S	S			
38. Papilledema		S		S		S
39. Papillitis	S					
40 Panophthalmitis	U					
41. Paralysis of extraocular muscles		S	S	S	S	
42. Perivasculitis	S					
43. Phlyctenular keratoconjunctivitis	S					
44. Pseudoretinitis pigmentosa					S	
45. Ptosis				S	S	
46. Retinal atrophy	S					
47. Retinal degeneration					S	
48. Retinal detachment		S	S			
49. Retinal embolism			U			
50. Rubeosis iridis			S			
51. Scleritis					U	
52. Segmental inflammation of retinal arteries					S	
53. Tenonitis					U	
54. Uveitis					U	
55. Vascular engorgement in retina	S	U	U			U
56. Vitreal hemorrhages			U			
57. Vitreous abscess with cellular reaction	S					
58. Vitreous opacities	S	S				
Lab Data						
1. Aqueous and/or vitreous tap for candida isolation	U					
2. Biopsy of temporal artery shows typical arteritic lesion					S	
3. Biopsy of palpable nodules in the neck						S
4. Biopsy of tender muscle positive					S	
5. Blood tests						
—Anemia		U			U	
—Eosinophilia					S	
—E.S.R. elevated					U	
—Hyperglycemia more than 140 mg/L			U			
—Immature abnormal white cells in peripheral blood and bone marrow		U				
—Leukocytosis		U			U	
—Thrombocytopenia					U	
6. Bronchosopy for visualization and biopsy	R					U
7. Carotid arteriography abnormal				U		
8. Cerebral arteriography abnormal				S		
9. Roentgenograms of the skull abnormal				S		

Retinal Hemorrhage with Central White Spot *Continued*

	Septic Retinitis—Candida Albicans	Hemopoietic System—Leukemia	Diabetes Mellitus	Vascular Disease—Arteriovenous Fistula	Collagen Disease—Polyarteritis Nodosa	Cyanosis Retinae—Carcinoma of Lung
Lab Data						
10. Roentgenograms of chest abnormal						S
11. Urinalysis						
—Cylindruria					U	
—Glycosuria			U			
—Hematuria					U	
—Ketonuria			U			
—Proteinuria					U	

R = rarely; S = sometimes; and U = usually.

Mets, M.B., and Del Monte, M.: Hemorrhagic retinopathy following uncomplicated pediatric cataract extraction. Arch. Ophthalmol., 104:975, 1986.

Roy, F.H.: Ocular Syndromes and Systemic Diseases. 2nd Ed. Philadelphia, W.B. Saunders, 1989.

Microaneurysms of Retina (Punctate Red Spots Scattered over Region of Posterior Pole)

1. Aging
2. Aplastic anemia—punctate hemorrhage
3. Associated with cotton-wool spots (see p. 548)
4. Bonnet-Dechaume-Blanc syndrome (cerebroretinal arteriovenous aneurysm syndrome)
5. Choroiditis
6. Chronic uveitis
7. Coats disease (retinal telangiectasia)
*8. Diabetes mellitus
9. Disseminated lupus erythematosus (Kaposi-Libman-Sacks syndrome)
10. Eales disease (periphlebitis)
11. Fabry disease (diffuse angiokeratosis)
*12. Hypertension
13. Hypotensive retinopathy, such as pulseless disease (aortic arch syndrome)
14. Kahler disease (myelomatosis)
15. Leukemias—punctate hemorrhages
16. Loa loa infection
17. Macroglobulinemia (Waldenstrom syndrome)
18. Mauriac syndrome (juvenile diabetes-dwarfism-obesity syndrome)
19. Ocular ischemic syndrome (carotid occlusive disease)
20. Osler hemorrhagic telangiectasia (hereditary hemorrhagic telangiectasis)
21. Pelizaeus-Merzbacher syndrome (aplasia axialis extracorticalis congenita)
22. Reimann syndrome (hyperviscosity syndrome)
*23. Retinoblastoma
24. Sickle cell hemoglobin C disease
25. Skin divers
26. Subacute bacterial endocarditis
27. Venous occlusion—occlusion of central retinal vein or one of its branches (see p. 525)

Polkinghorne, P.J., et al.: Ocular fundus lesions in divers. Lancet. Dec., 1381–1383, 1988.

Roy, F.H.: Ocular Syndromes and Systemic Diseases. 2nd Ed. Philadelphia, W.B. Saunders, 1989.

Sanders, R.J., et al.: Foveal avascular zone diameter and sickle cell disease. Arch. Ophthalmol., 109:812–816, 1991.

* = most important

Microaneurysms of Retina

	Diabetes Mellitus*	Hypertensive Retinopathy*	Central Retinal Vein Occlusion	Blood Disorder as Leukemia	Hypotensive Retinopathy as Pulseless Disease	Retinoblastoma*	Leber Miliary Aneurysm	Subacute Bacterial Endocarditis	Eales Disease	Fabry Disease	Osler Hemorrhagic Teleangiectasia
History											
1. Acute or chronic blood disorder				U							
2. Elevated blood pressure		U									
3. Familial	U			S		S					
4. Hereditary				S		S	U			U	U
5. Japanese extraction					U						
6. Lipoid storage disorders										U	
7. More in females					U						
8. More in males									U		
9. More than 40 years	U										
10. Occurs in children/youth					U	U	S		U		
11. Occurs in middle to older age			U		S			U			
Physical Findings											
1. Asteroid hyalosis	S										
2. Cataract	U				U					U	
3. Central retinal artery occlusion										U	
4. Choroiditis								S			
5. Corneal opacity										U	
6. Cotton-wool spots	U	U	U	U	U						
7. Endophthalmitis						U					
8. Ectropion uvea	U										
9. Exophthalmos						S					
10. Extraocular muscle paralysis	S	S	S			U				U	
11. Filamentary keratitis											U
12. Glaucoma	S		U	S		U					
13. Hard yellow exudates	U										
14. Heterochromia iridis						U					
15. Hyphema						U					
16. Hypopyon				S		U					
17. Hypotony	S										
18. Iris atrophy					S						
19. Keratoconus							S				
20. Leukokoria						U					
21. Lid edema						U			U		
22. Lipemia retinalis	U										
23. Macular edema	S			S							
24. Mydriasis						U					
25. Nystagmus							S				
26. Optic nerve atrophy	S			S	S						
27. Optic neuritis				S				S			
28. Papilledema		U	S		S			U		U	
29. Papillary hypertrophy of conjunctiva				U							

Microaneurysms of Retina *Continued*

	Diabetes Mellitus*	Hypertensive Retinopathy*	Central Retinal Vein Occlusion	Blood Disorder as Leukemia	Hypotensive Retinopathy as Pulseless Disease	Retinoblastoma*	Leber Miliary Aneurysm	Subacute Bacterial Endocarditis	Eales Disease	Fabry Disease	Osler Hemorrhagic Teleangiectasia
Physical Findings											
30. Retinal detachment		S		S						U	
31. Retinal hemorrhages	U	U	U	U							R
32. Retinal neovascularization	U		U						U		
33. Roth spots				U				U			
34. Retinal pigmentation (bone corpuscle or salt and pepper-like)							U				
35. Rubeosis iridis	U		U			U					
36. Small retinal angiomas											U
37. Star-shaped angiomas of the palpebral conjunctiva											U
38. Varicosities of palpebral and bulbar conjunctiva										U	
39. Vitreal hemorrhages	S	U					U		U		
40. Vitreous opacities				U				U			
Laboratory Data											
1. Angiographic brain studies					U						
2. Biopsy of tumor						S					
3. Blood culture								U			
4. Computed tomographic scan						U					
5. Chest roentgenogram									U		
6. ELISA for tuberculosis									U		
7. Fluorescein angiography	S	U	U	S	U				U		S
8. Glucose tolerance test or random blood sugar	U										
9. Lipid profile										U	
10. Ocular ultrasonography							U				
11. Ophthalmodynamometry					U						
12. Purified protein derivative									U		
13. Ultrasound of carotids					U						
14. Venereal disease reaction level					U						
15. Visual fields			U								
16. White blood cell count, hemoglobin, hematocrit				U							

R = rarely; S = sometimes; and U = usually.

* = most important

Macroaneurysms of Retinal Arteries (Found within First Three Orders of Bifurcation of Arterioles; Frequently Associated with Localized Hemorrhage and Exudation)

1. Congenital
*2. Generalized arteriosclerosis
*3. Hypertension
4. Idiopathic
5. Following open heart surgery

Kuhn, F.: Retinal emboli after open heart surgery. Arch. Ophthalmol., 107:317, 1989.

Robertson, D.M.: Macroaneurysm of the retinal arteries. Trans. Am. Acad. Ophthalmol. Otolaryngol., 77:55–67, 1973.

Schatz, H.: Essential Fluorescein Angiography: A Compendium of Classical Cases. San Anselmo, Calif., Pacific Press, 1982.

Retinal Neovascularization (Growth of abnormal new blood vessels into the vitreous)

1. Anemia
2. Behçet syndrome (dermatostomato-ophthalmic syndrome)
*3. Central retinal vein occlusion (see p. 525)
*4. Diabetes mellitus
5. Eales disease (periphlebitis)
6. Ehlers-Danlos syndrome (fibrodysplasia elastica generalisata)
7. Hypertension (malignant and essential)
8. Leukemia
9. Lupus erythematosus
10. Macroglobulinemia (Waldenstrom syndrome)
11. Retinal detachment with hemorrhage
*12. Sickle cell disease
13. Syphilis (acquired lues)
14. Trauma
15. von Hippel-Lindau syndrome (retinocerebral angiomatosis)
16. Werlhof disease (hemophilia and thrombocytopenic purpura)

L'Esperance, F.A., and James, W.A.: Diabetic Retinopathy; Clinical Evaluation and Management. 2nd Ed. St. Louis, C.V. Mosby, 1982.

Roy, F.H.: Ocular Syndromes and Systemic Diseases. 2nd Ed. Philadelphia, W.B. Saunders, 1989.

Predisposition to Rhegmatogenous Retinal Detachment

1. Aphakia (see p. 453)
2. High myopia
3. Chorioretinitis
4. Peripheral retinal degeneration
    A. Vitreous base excavation

      *B. Retinal hole

      C. Retinoschisis

      D. Cystic retinal tuft

      E. Zonular traction tuft

      F. Meridional folds

      G. Partial-thickness retinal tear

     *H. Full-thickness retinal tear

      *I. Lattice degeneration

5. Trauma—blunt and perforating, including operation for strabismus

6. Angiomatosis retinae

Feman, S.S., et al.: Rhegmatogenous retinal detachment due to macular hole. Arch. Ophthalmol., 91:371–372, 1974.

Nicholson, D.H., et al.: Rhegmatogenous retinal detachment in angiomatosis retinae. Am. J. Ophthalmol., 101:187–189, 1986.

Tasman, W., and Shields, J.A.: Disorders of the Peripheral Fundus. New York, Harper and Row, 1980.

Retinal Detachment (Location and Morphologic Classification)

1. Equator

      A. Myopic type—equatorial horseshoe tear

      B. Equatorial type associated with lattice degeneration

2. Ora serrata

      A. Aphakic, with multiple small breaks often in nasal periphery

      B. Dialysis in young, lower temporal quadrant, often bilateral

      C. Giant dialysis, often bilateral

3. Posterior pole

      A. Macular breaks, rare

      B. Other breaks at posterior pole, from cellular proliferation in inner retinal surface

Benson, W.E.: Retinal Detachment, Diagnosis and Management. 2nd Ed. New York, J.B. Lippincott, 1988.

Bonnett, M.: Microsurgery of Retinal Detachment. New York, Masson, 1980.

Folk, J.C., and Burton, T.C.: Bilateral phakic retinal detachment. Ophthalmology, 89:815, 1982.

Syndromes and Diseases Associated with Retinal Detachment

1. Exudative

      A. Systemic disease

         (1) Abdominal typhus

         (2) Aspergillosis

         (3) Atopic dermatitis

         (4) Blood diseases

            a. Dysproteinemias

* = most important

       b. Leukemia

       c. Sickle cell disease

  (5) Boutonneuse fever (rickettsia)

  (6) Candidiasis

  (7) Coenurosis

  (8) Cryoglobulinemia

  (9) Cryptococcosis

(10) Cysticercosis

(11) Disseminated intravascular coagulation

(12) Extreme venous congestion, such as occurs during choking

(13) Goldsheider syndrome (epidermolysis bullosa)

(14) Goodpasture syndrome (chronic relapsing pulmonary hemosiderosis)

(15) Gronblad-Strandberg syndrome (systemic elastodystrophy)

(16) Histiocytosis X (Hand-Schüller-Christian syndrome)

(17) Homocystinuria syndrome

(18) Hurler syndrome (MPS I-H)

(19) Hydatid cyst

(20) Hypertension—grade IV

(21) Krause syndrome (congenital encephalo-ophthalmic dysplasia)

*(22) Lupus erythematosus

(23) Polyarteritis nodosa (Kussmaul disease)

(24) Reese syndrome (D trisomy)

(25) Regional enteritis

(26) Relapsing polychondritis

(27) Renal disease, including chronic glomerulonephritis or uremia

(28) Rheumatic fever

(29) Rift Valley fever

(30) Sturge-Weber syndrome (meningocutaneous syndrome)

(31) Temporal arteritis syndrome (cranial arteritis syndrome)

(32) Toxemia of pregnancy

B. Ocular disease

  (1) Acute retinal necrosis

  (2) Choroidal or retinal tumor

       a. Hemangioma

       b. Melanoma

       c. Metastasis—including that from breast, lung, and stomach

       d. Retinoblastoma

  (3) Dominant myopia and retinal detachment

  (4) Familial exudative vitreoretinopathy

(5) Harada disease and Vogt-Koyanagi syndrome

(6) Lymphoid hyperplasia of the uveal tract

(7) Morning glory syndrome (hereditary central glial anomaly of the optic disk)

(8) Norrie disease (atrophia oculi congenita)—x-linked

(9) Optic nerve pit

(10) Postinflammation of the orbit or sinuses, or cyclitis

(11) Retina, congenital nonattachment and falciform folds—autosomal recessive

(12) Schwartz syndrome (glaucoma associated with retinal detachment)

(13) Scleritis (especially posterior scleritis)

(14) Sympathetic ophthalmia

(15) Toxocara infection

(16) Uveal effusion syndrome

C. Associated with retinal or choroidal vascular disease

(1) Coats disease (retinal telangiectasia)

   a. In juvenile

   b. In adult

(3) Central serous choroidopathy

(4) Detached pigment epithelium

(5) Eales disease (periphlebitis)

(6) Hollenhorst syndrome (chorioretinal infarction syndrome)

(7) Incontinentia pigmenti

(8) Osteoporosis-pseudoglioma syndrome

(9) Post irradiation

(10) Subpigment epithelium hemorrhage

(11) von Hippel Lindau disease (retinocerebral angiomatosis)

D. Drugs, including:

chymotrypsin(?)	hydrocortisone	oxygen	pilocarpine
cortisone	isoflurophate(?)	oxyphenbutazone	prednisolone
demecarium(?)	methylphenidate	penicillamine	
dexamethasone	methyl prednisolone	phenylbutazone	
echothiophate	neostigmine(?)	physostigmine(?)	

2. Traction

  *A. Pull of adherent and degenerated vitreous

  B. Organized vitreous band

(1) After vitreous hemorrhage

   a. Spontaneous

   b. Traumatic

(2) Hypertensive retinopathy

(3) Posthemorrhagic proliferative retinopathy

(4) Sickle cell retinopathy

* = most important

    C. Postneovascularization of vitreous

      *(1) Diabetic retinopathy, proliferative

      (2) Eales disease (periphlebitis)

      (3) Ehler Danlos syndrome (fibrodysplasia elastica-generalisata)

      (4) Fibrinoid syndrome

      *(5) Retinopathy of prematurity

      (6) Severe uveitis

    D. Congenital deformities, such as retinal dysplasia, coloboma, persistence of fetal vascular system, and pit of optic nerve

    E. Penetrating injury

   *F. Proliferative vitreoretinopathy

    G. Puckering syndrome

    H. Retinal disinsertion syndrome

    I. Retinopathy of prematurity

    J. Warburg syndrome

3. Rhegmatogenous

    A. Accommodation spasm, including strong miotics

    B. Alport syndrome (neuropathy and deafness)

    C. Apert syndrome (acrocephalosyndactylism syndrome)

    D. Equatorial or anterior choroiditis

    E. FOAR syndrome

    F. Following YAG laser capsulotomy

    G. Hereditary ocular vitreoretinal degeneration and skeletal abnormality (cleft palate)

    H. Juxtapapillary microholes

    I. Knobloch syndrome (retinal detachment and occipital encephalocele)—autosomal recessive

    J. Marchesani syndrome

    K. Marfan syndrome (arachnodactyly dystrophia mesodermalis congenita)

    L. Marshall (D) syndrome

    M. Meckel syndrome

    N. Myopia, including staphyloma—autosomal dominant or recessive

    O. Retinal degeneration at periphery

      (1) Presenile or myopic type

      (2) Lattice and paving-stone types—autosomal dominant

    P. Retinal detachment—autosomal dominant or x-linked

    Q. Retinoschisis—adult or juvenile

    R. Spondyloepiphyseal dysplasia, congenital

    S. Stickler syndrome (hereditary progressive arthro-ophthalmopathy)

    T. Trauma

      (1) Direct injury—perforating wound and foreign body

      (2) Indirect injury

      (3) Post cataract operation

          a. Sunset syndrome

          b. Vitreous tug syndrome

      (4) Battered baby syndrome (Silverman syndrome)

    *U. Viral retinitis

      (1) Acute retinal necrosis

      (2) Cytomegalovirus retinitis

    V. Vitreous degeneration

    W. Wagner syndrome (hyaloideoretinal degeneration)

Alio, J.L., et al.: Retinal Detachment as a Potential Hazard in Surgical Correction of Severe Myopia with Phakic Anterior Chamber Lenses. Amer. J. Ophthal., 115:145–148, 1993.

Benson, W.E.: Retinal Detachment, Diagnosis and Management. 2nd Ed. New York, J.B. Lippincott, 1988.

Fraunfelder, F.T.: Drug-Induced Ocular Side Effects and Drug Interactions. 4th Ed. Philadelphia, Williams & Wilkins, 1996.

Isenberg, S.J.: The Eye in Infancy. Chicago, Year Book Medical Publishers, 1989.

Jabs, D.A , et al.: Retinal detachments in patients with cytomegalovirus retinitis. Arch. Ophthalmol., 109:794–800, 1991.

McKusick, V.A.: Mendelian Inheritance in Man. 9th Ed. Baltimore, Johns Hopkins University Press, 1994.

Ober, R.R., et al.: Rhegmatogenous retinal detachment after neodymium-YAG laser capsulotomy in phakic and pseudophakic eyes. Am. J. Ophthalmol., 101:81–89, 1986.

Pau, H.: Differential Diagnosis of Eye Diseases. 2nd Ed. New York, Thieme Med. Pub., 1988.

Roy, F.H.: Ocular Syndromes and Systemic Diseases. 2nd Ed. Philadelphia, W.B. Saunders, 1989.

Retinal Folds

    1. Proliferative retinal folds—inner layer outstrips outer layer

    2. Traction folds

        A. Associated with remnants of hyaloid artery

        B. Secondary to vitreous traction

      *C. Retinopathy of prematurity (cicatricial form)

    3. Falciform retinal fold (congenital retinal septum)

        A. Familial exudative vitreoretinopathy

        B. Isolated

        C. Trisomy syndrome

        D. Warburg syndrome

    4. Chronic uveitis

    5. Parasite

    6. Occult intraocular foreign body

  *7. Shaken baby syndrome

    8. Terson syndrome

Isenberg, S.J.: The Eye in Infancy. Chicago, Year Book Medical Publishers, 1989.

Keithahn, M.A., et al.: Retinal folds in Terson syndrome. Ophthal., 100:1187–1190, 1993.

Larrison, W.I., et al.: Posterior retinal folds following vitreoretinal surgery. Arch. Ophthal., 111: 621–625, 1993.

* = most important

Cotton-wool Spots

	Malignant Hypertension	Toxemia of Pregnancy	Collagen Disease (Lupus Erythematosus)	Diabetes Mellitus	Anemic Conditions (Hypotensive Retinopathy)	Infective Conditions (Subacute Bacterial Endocarditis)	Traumatic Conditions (Purtscher Retinopathy)	Renal Disease (Renal Failure)	Blood Disease (Severe Anemia)
History									
1. Absence of renal function								U	
2. Accidents associated with sudden rise in blood pressure and congestion of head and chest							U		
3. Acute massive blood loss					U				
4. After thirty-second week of pregnancy		U							
5. Decreased blood pressure					U				S
6. Elevated blood pressure	U	U				U		U	
7. Familial	U			U					S
8. Pericarditis caused by staphylococcus epidermidis						U			
9. More in females		U	U						
10. After age 40				U					
11. Young persons	U	U	U						
Physical Findings									
1. Altered visual acuity		U		S	U				
2. Arteriosclerosis	U			S					
3. Asteroid hyalosis				S					
4. Band keratopathy								S	
5. Cataract				U					
6. Choroiditis						S			
7. Conjunctival calcium deposits								S	
8. Conjunctival petechiae						S			
9. Conjunctival phlyctenulae			S						
10. Corneal ulcer			S						
11. Cortical blindness								S	
12. Deep stromal keratitis			S						
13. Episcleritis			S						
14. Erythema or scaling of lids			S						
15. Floaters in aqueous and vitreous						S			
16. Hard yellow exudates	S			U					
17. Ischemic optic neuropathy			S	S					U
18. Keratoconjunctivitis sicca			S						
19. Lipemia retinalis				U					
20. Macular edema				S					
21. Macular star	S								
22. Microaneurysms of retina				U					
23. Optic atrophy			S	S					
24. Optic disc edema	S	S		S					
25. Optic neuritis			S			S			
26. Palpebral conjunctival pallor									U
27. Papillitis						S			
28. Posterior and macular serous detachment							U		

Cotton-wool Spots *Continued*

	Malignant Hypertension	Toxemia of Pregnancy	Collagen Disease (Lupus Erythematosus)	Diabetes Mellitus	Anemic Conditions (Hypotensive Retinopathy)	Infective Conditions (Subacute Bacterial Endocarditis)	Traumatic Conditions (Purtscher Retinopathy)	Renal Disease (Renal Failure)	Blood Disease (Severe Anemia)
Physical Findings									
29. Preretinal hemorrhage						S			
30. Retinal artery occlusion			S			R			
31. Retinal arteriolar narrowing	U	U							
32. Retinal detachment		S	S						
33. Retinal edema	U						U	U	
34. Retinal hemorrhages	U	U	S		U	S	U		U
35. Retinal neovascularization				S					
36. Retinal venous dilation	S		S	U	S		U		
37. Roth spot					U	S			
38. Rubeosis iridis				U					
39. Scleritis			S						
40. Telangiectasis of lids			S						
41. Third nerve paresis				S					
42. Uveitis			S						
43. Vascular sheathing				S					U
Laboratory Data									
1. Blood culture positive for staphylococcus epidermidis						U			
2. BUN elevated								U	
3. Depression of hemoglobin, white cells and platelets			U		U				U
4. Fluorescein angiography									
Dilated capillaries at margin of lesion with aneurysm dilations	U								
Varicose looping and corkscrew coiling	U								
5. Glycosuria				U					
6. Hypercalcemia								U	
7. Hyperglycemia				U					
8. Hyponatremia								U	
9. Lupus erythematosus cell positive			U						
10. Positive immunofluorescence test (for antinuclear antibodies)			U						
11. Proteinuria		U						U	
12. Roentgenogram multiple bone fractures							U		

R = rarely; S = sometimes; and U = usually.

Cotton-Wool Spots (Soft Exudates) (fluffy, white, focal infarcts in the nerve fiber layer)

1. Acute pancreatitis
2. Anemic conditions
   A. Cirrhosis of the liver
   B. Following cardiac surgery
   C. Gastric ulcer syndrome
   D. Hypotensive retinopathy
   E. Ligation of the carotid artery
   F. Severe primary and secondary anemias
   G. Severe systemic blood loss
3. Blood disease
   A. Aplastic anemia
   B. Dysproteinemia
   C. Leukemia
   D. Multiple myeloma (myelomatosis)
   E. Pernicious anemia (vitamin B_{12} deficiency)
   F. Waldenstrom syndrome (macroglobulinemia syndrome)
4. Carbon monoxide poisoning
5. Carcinomatous cachexia
6. Collagen diseases
   A. Dermatomyositis (polymyositis dermatomyositis)
   B. Diffuse scleroderma
   C. Disseminated lupus erythematosus (systemic lupus erythematosus)
   D. Polyarteritis nodosa (necrotizing angiitis)
   E. Rheumatoid arthritis with scleromalacia perforans or polymyalgia rheumatica
*7. Diabetic retinopathy
8. Hodgkin disease
9. Infective conditions
   *A. Human immunodeficiency virus infection (HIV)
   B. Pneumonia
   C. Rheumatic fever
   D. Rift Valley fever
   E. Rocky mountain spotted fever (spotted fever)
   F. Roth septic retinitis
   G. Subacute bacterial endocarditis
10. Microemboli following cardiac operation
11. Primary amyloidosis (idiopathic amyloidosis)
12. Primary open-angle glaucoma
13. Purtscher retinopathy (fat embolism syndrome)
14. Renal disease

15. Serum disease

16. Suprarenal-sympathetic syndrome (pheochromocytoma syndrome)

17. Takayasu syndrome (aortic arch syndrome)

18. Toxemic retinopathy of pregnancy

*19. Untreated malignant hypertension

Brezin A., et al.: Cotton-wool spots and AIDS related complex. International Ophthal., 14:37–41, 1990.

Jabs, D.A., et al.: Severe retinal vaso-occlusive disease in systemic lupus erythematosus. Arch. Ophthalmol., 104:558–563, 1986.

Mausour, A.M., et al.: Cotton-wool spots in acquired immunodeficiency syndrome compared with diabetes mellitus, systemic hypertension, and central retinal vein occlusion. Arch. Ophthalmol., 106:1074–1077, 1988.

Roy, F.H.: Ocular Syndromes and Systemic Diseases. 2nd Ed. Philadelphia, W.B. Saunders, 1989.

* = most important

Hard Exudates (Yellowish-White Discrete Masses Deep in Retina)

	Diabetes Mellitus*	Hypertensive Disease*	Coats' Disease	Essential Hypercholesterolemic Xanthomatosis
History				
1. Bilateral	U	S		U
2. Congenital			U	
3. Elevated blood pressure		U		
4. Familial	U			U
5. More in males			S	
6. Occurs in persons up to 10 years old			U	
7. Occurs in persons 11 to 40 years old	S		R	R
8. Occurs in persons more than 40 years old		U		S
Physical Findings				
1. Anterior uveitis			U	
2. Cataract—coronary				U
3. Cataract—vesicular and posterior subcapsular cataract	U			
4. Conjunctivitis				U
5. Corneal arcus	S			U
6. Cotton-wool spots	U	U		
7. Glaucoma	S		S	
8. Lipid rings around microaneurysms				U
9. Macular edema	S	U	U	
10. Optic disc edema		S		
11. Optic nerve atrophy	S		U	
12. Retinal detachment	S	S	U	
13. Retinal hemorrhages		U	S	
14. Retinal microaneurysms	U	U	U	
15. Retinal telangiectatic vessels			S	
16. Retinal vein occlusion	S	S	U	U
17. Retinal vein sheathing	U	U		
18. Rubeosis iridis	S		U	
19. Vitreous hemorrhage	S	U	U	
Laboratory Data				
1. Elevated blood sugar	U			
2. Elevated lipid profile, including cholesterol and triglyceride	S	S		U
3. Phosphorus 32 uptake elevation			U	
4. Retinal angiography	S	U	U	U
5. Ultrasound, ocular	R		U	

R = rarely; S = sometimes; and U = usually.

Hard Exudates (Yellowish-White Discrete Masses Deep in Retina)

1. Circinate retinopathy
2. Coats disease (retinal telangiectasia)
*3. Diabetes mellitus
*4. Exudative age related macular degeneration
*5. Hypertensive disease
6. Radiation induced
7. Retinal arterial macroaneurysm

Berman, D.H., and Friedman, E.A.: Partial absorption of hard exudates in patients with diabetic end-stage renal disease and severe anemia after treatment with erythropoietin. Retina, 14:1–5, 1994.

Haik, B.G., et al.: Radiation and chemotherapy of parameningeal rhabdomyosarcoma involving the orbit. Ophthalmology, 93:1001–1009, 1986.

Roy, F.H.: Ocular Syndromes and Systemic Diseases. 2nd Ed. Philadelphia, W.B. Saunders, 1989.

Retinal Exudate and Hemorrhage

1. Capillary telangiectasis of retina (Reese)
2. Coats disease (retinal telangiectasia)
*3. Diabetes mellitus
4. Eales disease (periphlebitis)
5. Multiple retinal aneurysms (Leber syndrome)
6. Racemose hemangioma of the retina
7. von Hippel-Lindau, with absence of visible angioma (retinocerebral angiomatosis)

Ballantyne, A.J., and Michaelson, I.C.: Textbook of the Fundus of the Eye. 3rd Ed. Baltimore, Williams & Wilkins, 1981.

Michelson, J.B., et al.: Ocular reticulum cell sarcoma. Arch. Ophthalmol., 99:1409, 1981.

Retinitis or Pseudoretinitis Pigmentosa (Pigment May Be Bone Corpuscular Dots or Heaped-up Masses; Salt and Pepper Fundus)

1. Retinitis pigmentosa
    A. Abetalipoproteinemia(Bassen-Kornzweig syndrome)
    B. Alstrom disease (cataract and retinitis pigmentosa)
    C. Cockayne syndrome (dwarfism with retinal atrophy and deafness)
    D. Diallinas-Amalric syndrome (deaf-mutism-retinal degeneration syndrome)
    E. Hallgren syndrome (retinitis pigmentosa-deafness-ataxia syndrome)
    F. Hypotrichosis, syndactyly and retinitis pigmentosa—autosomal recessive
    G. Hunter syndrome (MPS II)
    H. Hurler syndrome (MPS I)
    I. Infantile phytanic acid storage disease
    J. Jeune syndrome
    *K. Kearns-Sayre syndrome (ophthalmoplegic retinal degeneration syndrome)
    L. Laurence-Moon-Bardet-Biedl syndrome (retinitis pigmentosa-polydactyly-adiposogenital syndrome)

* = most important

   M. Metaphyseal chondrodysplasia with retinitis pigmentosa—autosomal recessive

   N. Microcephaly with chorioretinopathy

   O. Multiple sulfatase deficiency

   P. Muscular atrophy, ataxia, retinitis pigmentosa, diabetes mellitus—autosomal dominant

   Q. Olivopontocerebellar atrophy, type III

   R. Pallidal degeneration, progressive with retinitis pigmentosa—autosomal recessive

 *S. Refsum syndrome (phytanic acid storage disease)

   T. Retinitis pigmentosa alone (usually autosomal recessive but may be autosomal dominant or sex linked)

   U. Retinitis pigmentosa associated with myopia, keratoconus, and/or glaucoma

   V. Retinitis pigmentosa, congenital deafness—sex linked

  W. Retinitis pigmentosa inversa (predominant—pigmentation around the disc and macula) and deafness—autosomal recessive

   X. Retinitis pigmentosa, nerve deafness, mental retardation, and hypogonadism—autosomal recessive

   Y. Retinitis pigmentosa, PPRPE type (with preserved para-arteriole retinal pigment epithelium)—autosomal recessive

   Z. Retinitis pigmentosa, spastic quadriplegia, and mental retardation—autosomal recessive

 AA. Rud syndrome

 BB. Sanfilippo disease (MPS III)

 CC. Scheie disease (MPS IS)

 DD. Spielmeyer-Vogt syndrome (cerebroretinal degeneration)

 EE. Usher syndrome (hereditary retinitis pigmentosa-deafness syndrome)

2. Senile changes—degenerative pigmentation
3. Vascular lesion, such as occlusion of arteriole
4. Inflammatory

   A. Behçet disease (oculobuccogenital syndrome)

   B. Chickenpox virus

   C. Cytomegalic inclusion disease

   D. Dawson disease (inclusion-body encephalitis)

   E. Fetal varicella effects

   F. Focal dermal hypoplasia (Goltz syndrome)

   G. Harada disease (Vogt-Koyanagi-Harada syndrome)

   H. Hypomelanosis of Ito

   I. Influenza virus

   J. Nematode endophthalmitis (visceral larva migrans syndrome)

   K. Onchocerciasis (river blindness)

   L. Polyarteritis nodosa (Kussmaul disease)

   M. Rubella (German measles)

N. Rubeola (measles)

*O. Syphilis

*P. Toxoplasmosis

Q. Typhoid fever (enteric fever)

R. Vaccinia

5. Toxic

A. Accidental intraocular injection of depot corticosteroids

B. Chloroquine and Atabrine

C. Diaminodiphenoxyalkanes—possible drug for treatment of schistosomiasis

D. Indomethacin

E. Phenothiazines

(1) Chlorpromazine

(2) Thioridazine (Mellaril)

F. Pregl solution (Septojod-formerly used for treatment of puerperal sepsis)

G. Quinine

H. Sparsomycin

6. Acute lymphocytic leukemia

7. Cryogenic "pigmentary fall-out"—following use of cryosurgery for retinal detachment

8. Cystinosis syndrome (Lignac-Fanconi syndrome)

9. External ophthalmoplegias

*10. Gardner Syndrome (congenital hypertrophy of the retinal pigment epithelium and familial intestinal polyposis)

11. Hagberg-Santavuori syndrome (neuronal ceroid lipofuscinosis)

12. Hallervorden-Spatz syndrome (pigmentary degeneration of globus pallidus)

13. Hereditary ataxias (Friedrich and Marie)

14. Leber congenital amaurosis

15. Lens dislocated into vitreous

16. Mucolipidoses IV (ML IV)

17. Myotonic dystrophy syndrome (Curschmann-Steinert syndrome)

18. Pelizaeus-Merzbacher syndrome (aplasia axialis extracorticalis congenita)

19. Pellagra (ariboflavinosis)

20. Progressive cone-rod degeneration

21. Renal disorders, including familial juvenile nephronophthisis (medullary cystic disease)

22. Rud syndrome (hypophyseal deficiency)

23. Sjögren-Larsson syndrome (oligophrenia-ichthyosis-spastic diplegia syndrome)

24. Tapetal-like reflex syndrome

25. Trauma, including blunt, penetrating, obstetrical, and radiotherapy, Frenkel syndrome (ocular contusion syndrome)

26. Waardenburg syndrome (interoculoiridodermatoauditive dysplasia)

* = most important

Retinal Bone Corpuscular Dots

	Retinitis Pigmentosa	Senile Degeneration	Vascular (Arterial Occlusion)	Inflammatory (Rubella)	Toxic (Chloroquine)	Cystinosis	Trauma (Blunt)	Progressive Cone-rod Degeneration	Myotonic Dystrophy
History									
1. Amaurosis fugax			S						
2. Children						U			
3. Common in males	U								
4. Glare					U				
5. Hereditary	U					U		U	U
6. Older age group		U							
7. Lacrimation						S			
8. Night blindness	U								
9. Onset, about 20 years									U
10. Photophobia						U			
11. Rubela infection, first trimester				U					
12. Trauma							U		
Physical Findings									
1. Angle recession							S		
2. Bull's eye or doughnut retinal lesion					U			U	
3. Buphthalmos				S					
4. Cataracts	S					U	S		U
5. Conjunctival hemorrhage							S		
6. Conjunctivitis				S					
7. Corneal haziness				S		U			
8. Crystals located in conjunctiva, cornea						U			
9. Cystoid macular edema	R								
10. Disc drusen	S								
11. Disc hamartoma	S								
12. Epithelial corneal edema							S		R
13. Glaucoma	S			S					
14. Hyphema							S		
15. Hypotony							S		
16. Iris atrophy				S					
17. Keratopathy				S	U				R
18. Keratoconus	R								
19. Loss of corneal sensitivity									U
20. Macular degeneration	R	U						U	U
21. Macular red spot									U
22. May progress to blindness	U				S				
23. Megalocornea				S					
24. Microcornea				S					
25. Microphthalmos	R			S					
26. Minute whitish corneal dots in whorl pattern					U				
27. Myopia	U								
28. Neovascular retinal proliferation			S						
29. Nystagmus	R		U					S	
30. Optic disc atrophy/pallor	U			S				U	R
31. Peripheral retinal drusen		U							

Retinal Bone Corpuscular Dots *Continued*

Physical Findings

	Retinitis Pigmentosa	Senile Degeneration	Vascular (Arterial Occlusion)	Inflammatory (Rubella)	Toxic (Chloroquine)	Cystinosis	Trauma (Blunt)	Progressive Cone-rod Degeneration	Myotonic Dystrophy
32. Progressive external ophthalmoplegia	R								S
33. Ptosis	R								U
34. Pupil dilated and fixed							S		
35. Retinal arteriosclerosis		U							
36. Retinal hemorrhage							S		
37. Retinal vessel attenuation	U	U	S		S			S	
38. Retrobulbar hemorrhage							S		U
39. Sheathing of retinal vessels	R			R	S				
40. Silver wire or chalky-white arterioles				U	S				
41. Spherophakia				R					
42. Strabismus	R			S					
43. Uveitis				S					
44. Vitreous opacities	U								

Laboratory Data

	Retinitis Pigmentosa	Senile Degeneration	Vascular (Arterial Occlusion)	Inflammatory (Rubella)	Toxic (Chloroquine)	Cystinosis	Trauma (Blunt)	Progressive Cone-rod Degeneration	Myotonic Dystrophy
1. Color vision abnormalities	U				S			U	
2. Cystine in conjunctival biopsy, cultured skin fibroblasts or polymorphonuclear leukocytes						U			
3. Dark adaptation abnormal	U								
4. Electro-oculogram	U				U			S	
5. Electroretinogram	U				U			U	
6. Fluorescein angiography							R		
Bull's eye lesion					U			U	
Diffuse hyperfluorescence scattered spicules of pigment, dye leakage from cystoid macular edema may be present	U	S		S			S		
Peripheral arteriolar occlusion			U						
7. Fluorescent rubella antibody test				U					
8. Hemoglobin electrophoresis			U						
9. Leukopenia				U				U	
10. Red blood cell count elevated			U						
11. Rubella virus hemagglutination inhibition				U					
12. Serum immunoglobulin G concentration reduced									U
13. Visual field abnormal	U	R	S		S			U	

R = rarely; S = sometimes; and U = usually.

Bateman, J.B., and Philippart, M.: Ocular features of the Hagberg-Santavuori syndrome. Am. J. Oph-
    thalmol., 102:262–271, 1986.

Bloome, M.A., and Garcia, C.A.: A Manual of Retinal and Choroidal Dystrophies. East Norwalk,
    Conn., Appleton-Century-Crofts, 1982.

Carr, R.E., and Noble, K.G.: Retinitis pigmentosa. Ophthalmology, 88:199, 1981.

Isenberg, S.J.: The Eye in Infancy. Chicago, Year Book Medical Publishers, 1989.

McKusick, V.A.: Mendelian Inheritance in Man. 9th Ed. Baltimore, Johns Hopkins University Press,
    1994.

Roy, F.H.: Ocular Syndromes and Systemic Diseases. 2nd Ed. Philadelphia, W.B. Saunders, 1989.

Lesions Confused with Retinoblastoma

1. Anomalous optic disc
2. Anteriorly dislocated lens with secondary glaucoma
*3. Coats disease (retinal telangiectasia)
4. Coloboma of choroid and optic disc (see p. 615)
5. Congenital corneal opacity
6. Congenital rubella syndrome (Gregg syndrome)
7. Cysts in a remnant of the hyaloid artery
8. Developmental retinal cyst
9. Glioma of the retina
10. Hematoma under retinal pigment epithelium
11. High myopia with advanced chorioretinal degeneration
12. Juvenile (x-linked) retinoschisis
13. Juvenile xanthogranuloma (nevoxanthoendothelioma)
*14. Larval granulomatosis (Toxocara canis)
15. Medullation of nerve fiber layer
16. Metastatic endophthalmitis
17. Norrie disease (atrophia oculi congenita)
18. Oligodendroglioma of the retina
19. Organization of intraocular hemorrhage
*20. Persistent hyperplastic primary vitreous
21. Retinal detachment due to choroidal or vitreous hemorrhage
22. Retinal dysplasia (massive retinal fibrosis)
*23. Retinopathy of prematurity
24. Retrolental membrane associated with Bloch-Sulzberger syndrome (incontinentia pigmenti)
25. Rhegmatogenous and falciform retinal detachment
26. Secondary glaucoma
27. Sex-linked microphthalmia
28. Tapetoretinal degeneration
29. Trisomy 13 (Patau syndrome)
*30. Toxoplasmosis (ocular toxoplasmosis)

31. Traumatic chorioretinitis
*32. Tumors other than retinoblastoma
33. Uveitis in secondary retinal detachment
34. "White-with-pressure" sign

* = most important

Single Dark Fundus Lesion

	Retinal Detachment	Retinoschisis (Senile)	Macular Degeneration (Exudative)	Chorioretinitis ie Ocular Histoplasmosis	Intraocular Foreign Body	Coats' Disease	Ocular Metastatic Tumors	Choroidal Detachment	Melanocytoma of Optic Nerve	Malignant Melanoma
History										
1. Affects both sexes equally		U		U						
2. Aphakic, myopic and traumatized eyes	U									
3. Bilateral		U					S			
4. Diagnosed between two to ten years of age						U				
5. Discovery may be at birth						U				
6. Discovered in middle age									U	
7. During or immediately following an operation								U		
8. Familial blindness	S									
9. Hereditary	S		S							
10. History of ocular trauma					U			U		
11. History of scleritis or episcleritis								U		
12. More in blacks and other dark complexioned people									U	
13. Most are young adults				U	U					
14. Most common in females									U	
15. Most common in males					U	U				
16. Ocular pain							U			S
17. Onset in advanced age			U			S				
18. Onset in juvenile period			S							
19. Over 50 years of age			S							
20. Unilateral in 90%						U			U	
21. Wide age range	U			U						
Physical Findings										
1. Abnormal afferent pupillary reaction	S	S			U			S	U	
2. Anterior chamber flat					S			U		
3. Atrophic macular degeneration								U		
4. Atrophic scar around nerve head			U	U						
5. Blood vessels narrowed and yellow					U		R			U
6. Cataract	S				S	U				
7. Cholesterol crystals of retina								U		
8. Choroidal elevations of periphery										
9. Choroiditis				U						
10. Conjunctival and episcleral injection								U		
11. Corneal striae and aqueous flare								U		
12. Dark smooth multilobulated elevations								U		
13. Elevation of the retina	U	U							U	
14. Enlargement of blind spot									S	
15. Extraocular muscle paralysis							S			
16. Exudative and atrophic retinal reaction			U							
17. Glaucoma						U	S			
18. Hazy vitreous					S			U		
19. Impairment of central vision			U		S					
20. Iris discolored (green in copper, yellow in iron)					U					
21. Iritis	S									
22. Loss of vision	S		U		U			S	U	U
23. Low intraocular pressure	U							U		

Single Dark Fundus Lesion *Continued*

	Retinal Detachment	Retinoschisis (Senile)	Macular Degeneration (Exudative)	Chorioretinitis ie Ocular Histoplasmosis	Intraocular Foreign Body	Coats' Disease	Ocular Metastatic Tumors	Choroidal Detachment	Melanocytoma of Optic Nerve	Malignant Melanoma
Physical Findings										
24. Macular edema				U						
25. Macular hemorrhages			S	S						
26. Microaneurysms in retina						U				
27. Neovascular glaucoma						S				
28. Optic nerve swelling							S			S
29. Retinal detachment	U	S				S	R	R		U
30. Retinal exudates						U				
31. Retinal folds or striae	S						U			
32. Retinal hemorrhages			U							
33. Retina is wrinkled and gray	U									
34. Retinal ischemia						U				
35. Retinal neovascularization				U						
36. Retinal tears or holes	U	S								
37. Retinal telangiectasia						U				
38. Rubeosis iridis							S			
39. Sensory retinal detachment						S				
40. Serous elevation overlying mass in retina							U			
41. Shifting subretinal fluid							U	S		
42. Splitting of the neurosensory retina		U								
43. Subretinal hemorrhages							S			
44. Tortuosity of retinal vessels	U									
45. Uveitis							U			
46. Vitreal hemorrhage						S	S			S
47. Vitreous cells	S									
48. Vitreous green or yellow and liquid					U					
49. Yellow macular deposits					U					
Laboratory Data										
1. A scan										U
2. B scan	U				U		U			U
3. 32 P test							U			U
4. Fluorescein angiography										U

R = rarely; S = sometimes; and U = usually.

Howard, G.M.: Erroneous clinical diagnoses of retinoblastoma and uveal melanoma. Trans. Am. Acad. Ophthalmol. Otolaryngol., 73:199–203, 1969.

Nicholson, D.H., and Green, W.R. (eds.): Pediatric Ocular Tumors. New York, Masson, 1981.

Single White Lesion of Retina

*1. Amelanotic melanoma

2. Astrocytoma of tuberous sclerosis

3. Degeneration of retinal pigment epithelium

4. Diktyoma

5. Glioma of optic nerve

6. Hamartomas of the optic disc of retinitis pigmentosa

7. Metastatic or direct extension of a tumor

8. Neurofibroma of von Recklinghausen syndrome

*9. Retinoblastoma

*10. Toxocara canis

Nicholson, D.H., and Green, W.R. (eds.): Pediatric ocular Tumors, New York, Masson, 1981.

Robertson, D.M.: Hamartomas of the optic disc with retinitis pigmentosa. Am. J. Ophthalmol., 74:526–531, 1972.

Pale Fundus Lesions

1. Generalized pallor

   A. Albinism—photophobia; defective vision; absence of pigment in iris, retina, and choroid

   B. Chediak-Higashi syndrome (oculocutaneous albinism with recurrent infections)

   C. Waardenburg syndrome (embryonic fixation syndrome)

   D. Choroideremia—rare; night blindness; contraction of visual fields; degeneration of pigment epithelium in periphery with exposure of choroidal vessels

   E. Myopia—thinning of retina and choroidal crescent at disc

   F. Retinal ischemia

      (1) Occlusion of retinal arteries (see p. 512)

      (2) Spasm of retinal arteries—angiospasm: quinine, lead poisoning, migraine, or Raynaud disease

      (3) Anemia

   *G. Vascular retinopathies—hypertension, edema, hemorrhages, swelling of disc

   H. Leukemia

   I. The lipidoses

      (1) Congenital, rare

      (2) Infantile (Tay-Sachs disease)

      (3) Late infantile—(Jansky-Bielschowsky syndrome)—2 to 4 years of age

      (4) Juvenile—(Spielmeyer-Vogt syndrome)—5 to 8 years of age; optic atrophy

      (5) Adult—(Kuf disease)—15 to 25 years of age; eyes may be normal or show some pigmented macular changes

    J. Gaucher disease (glucocerebroside storage disease)

    K. Hereditary dystrophic lipidosis (Fabry disease)

    L. Hyperlipemia

        (1) Diabetes—rare, yellowish retinal and choroidal vessels

        (2) Essential hyperlipemic xanthomatosis—rare, yellowish retinal and choroidal vessels

    M. Oguchi disease

2. Localized pale areas

    A. Medullated nerve fibers (see p. 562)

    *B. Retinopathy of prematurity

    C. Localized retinal edema

        (1) Inflammation

        (2) Trauma

        (3) Vascular lesions

    D. Retinal detachment and schisis (see p. 541)

    *E. Retinoblastoma

    F. Coats disease (retinal telangiectasia)

    G. Coloboma (see p. 505)

    H. Normal fundus features—pale streaks mark site of ciliary nerves

    I. Atrophic areas—diathermy, light coagulation, or cryosurgery

    J. Scattered retinal exudates

        (1) Preretinal—severe posterior uveitis; discrete white spots, often most marked along vessels adjacent to a patch of choroiditis

        (2) Retinal

            a. Purtscher compression syndrome—cotton-wool spots

            b. Fat emboli

            c. Hemangiomatosis—yellow exudates

          *d. Hypertensive retinopathy—cotton-wool and hard exudates

            e. Toxemia of pregnancy

            f. Hypotensive retinopathy

            g. Pulseless disease (Takayasu syndrome)

            h. Arterial occlusion

            i. Blood loss—cotton-wool spots

            j. Anemia (all types)

            k. Leukemia

            l. Purpura

           m. Macroglobulinemia (Waldenstrom syndrome)

            n. Hodgkin disease—soft exudates

          *o. Diabetes—cotton-wool and hard exudates

            p. Hypercholesterolemia—lipid deposits

            q. Systemic lupus erythematosus (disseminated lupus erythematosus)

* = most important

r. Dermatomyositis—cotton-wool spots

s. Polyarteritis nodosa (Kussmaul disease)

t. Scleroderma (progressive systemic sclerosis)

u. Vitamin A deficiency—small white spots along course of retinal vessels

v. Retinal capillariosis—yellowish-white spots in substance of retina

w. Leber congenital retinal aplasia—bilateral blindness, multiple white specks

x. Female carrier of retinitis pigmentosa—brilliant silvery reflex with shining yellow spots deep to retinal vessels

3. Dystrophic conditions

A. Gyrate atrophy—rare, irregular atrophic areas with visual defects and night blindness

B. Choroidal sclerosis—rare, diffuse peripapillary or central choroidal atrophy with larger choroidal vessels prominent

C. Infarction or occlusion of ciliary arteries—rare, embolism (air, fat), injury, atrophic area with prominent choroidal vessels

D. Pseudoinflammatory macular dystrophy—rare, fourth to sixth decades, central edema, hemorrhage and exudate, bilateral and symmetrical

E. Helicoid peripapillary chorioretinal atrophy—rare, congenital and adult forms, star-shaped atrophic areas radiating from disc

F. Retinitis punctata albescens—rare, onset in second and third decades, multiple discrete whitish dots which may appear crystalline, night blindness and field defects in progressive type

G. Fundus flavimaculatus—rare, onset in second and third decades, yellow flecks deep in the retina

H. Geographic choroiditis—rare, map-like pigmentary disturbance at posterior pole or more widespread over posterior fundus

I. Doyne honeycomb dystrophy—rare; middle age and older; drusen at posterior pole, with pigmentary or cystoid macular changes

J. Progressive bifocal chorioretinal atrophy—atrophy temporal to disc, extending later; night blindness in late stage

Ballantyne, A.J., and Michaelson, I.C.: Textbook of the Fundus of the Eye. 3rd Ed. Baltimore, Williams & Wilkins, 1981.

Bloome, M.A., and Garcia, C.A.: Manual of Retinal and Choroidal Dystrophies. East Norwalk, CT, Appleton-Century-Crofts, 1981.

Perkins, E.S., and Dobree, J.H.: The Differential Diagnosis of Fundus Conditions. St. Louis, C.V. Mosby, 1972.

Medullated Nerve Fibers (Opaque White Patch Usually Adjacent to and May Cover Disc; Localized to One Sector of Disc; Peripapillary or Arcuate with a Peripheral, Feathered Edge)

*1. Isolated finding

2. Autosomal recessive or dominant inheritance

3. Associated with:

A. Aplasia of macula

    B. Coloboma of optic nerve or choroid (see p. 613)

    C. Conus of disc

    D. Cranial dysostosis (oxycephaly, dolichocephaly, brachycephaly, and craniofacial dysostosis)

    E. Hyaloid remnants

    F. Macular colobomas (see p. 505)

    G. Myopia

    *H. Neurofibromatosis

Ballantyne, A.J., and Michaelson, I.C.: Textbook of the Fundus of the Eye. 3rd Ed. Baltimore, Williams & Wilkins, 1981.

Pigmented Fundus Lesions

1. Diffuse pigmentation

    A. Negroid fundus—accentuation of fundus pigmentation

    B. Melanosis bulbi—rare, pigmentation of external eye and fundus

    C. Nevus of Ota

    D. Waardenburg syndrome (embryonic fixation)

2. Single pigmented lesions

    A. Flat lesions

        (1) Benign melanoma—bluish, gray, or black lesion

        (2) Pigmented scar—patch of dense pigment, usually atrophic area in center

        (3) Fuchs dark spot—dark spot in macular region

      *(4) Macular degeneration (exudate, age-related)

    B. Raised lesions

        (1) Simple detachment (see p. 541)

          a. Macular, such as in central serous retinopathy

          b. Associated with uveitis, such as that associated with Vogt-Koyanagi-Harada syndrome

          c. Hemorrhagic macrocyst

      *(2) Malignant melanoma—raised pigmented lesion with secondary detachment, abnormal vessels

        (3) Choroidal hemorrhage—trauma, spontaneous in patients with vascular disease, high myopia

      *(4) Exudative macular lesion—common, old age, subretinal exudate

        (5) Hemangioma of choroid—rare, raised grayish tumor near disc, secondary detachment later

      *(6) Metastatic tumor—flattish tumor with little pigment, primary in breast, or lung

        (7) Chorioretinitis

        (8) Foreign body

        (9) Coats disease (retinal telangiectasia)

3. Multiple pigmented lesions

* = most important

A. Scattered focal lesions

*(1) Congenital melanosis—cat's paw patches of pigment in one sector of fundus (may be part of Gardner's syndrome)

(2) Postinflammatory—flat pigment with areas of atrophy

(3) Hypertensive retinopathy—hypertensive vascular changes with scattered pigmentation

(4) Siegrist streaks—rare, chain of pigment spots along sclerosed choroidal vessel

(5) Paravenous retinochoroidal atrophy—paravenous pigmentation with chorioretinal atrophy

(6) Incontinentia pigmenti (Bloch-Sulzberger syndrome)

(7) Chorioretinal scars from cryosurgery

B. Widely disseminated pigmentary changes

(1) Genetic conditions

a. Typical retinitis pigmentosa—attenuation of retinal vessels, optic atrophy (myopia, posterior polar cataract, keratoconus)

b. Atypical retinitis pigmentosa—rare, little or no pigment, pigment in clumps

c. Retinitis pigmentosa syndromes

1. Cockayne syndrome (dwarfism with retinal atrophy and deafness)

2. Hallgren syndrome (retinitis pigmentosa-deafness-ataxia syndrome)

3. Kearn syndrome (ophthalmoplegic retinal degeneration syndrome)

4. Laurence-Moon-Biedl syndrome (retinitis pigmentosa polydactyly-adiposo-genital syndrome)

5. Leber congenital retinal aplasia syndrome

6. Lignac-Fanconi syndrome (cystinosis syndrome)

7. Myotonic dystrophy syndrome (dystrophia myotonica syndrome)

8. Pelizaeus-Merzbacher syndrome (aplasia axialis extracorticalis congenital)

(2) Infectious conditions—secondary retinitis pigmentosa

*a. Syphilis (congenital)—pepper-and-salt pigmentation, interstitial keratitis

b. Syphilitic neuroretinitis—rare, retinitis pigmentosa

c. Rubella—cataract, secondary retinitis pigmentosa (nonprogressive)

d. Vaccinia—rare, retinitis pigmentosa, history of vaccination

(3) Metabolic disturbances

a. Refsum syndrome (phytanic acid storage disease)

b. Bassen-Kornzweig syndrome (familial hypolipoproteinemia)

(4) Toxic conditions, such as chloroquine, phenothiazine derivatives; usually central pigmentation; cornea and lens change

4. Ciliary body and choroid

A. Tumors

(1) Hemangioma

(2) Malignant melanoma

*(3) Metastatic carcinoma, such as that from the lungs, breast, testis, kidney, prostate gland, bladder

(4) Nevus

(5) Neurilemmoma

(6) Neurofibroma

B. Detachment—serous or hemorrhagic

*C. Lymphoma and leukemias

D. Peripheral giant cysts

5. Vitreous body

A. Hemorrhage

B. Abscess

6. Staphyloma of sclera

Perkins, E.S., and Dobree, J.H.: The Differential Diagnosis of Fundus Conditions. St. Louis, C.V. Mosby, 1972.

Zinn, K., and Marmor, M. (eds.): The Retinal Pigment Epithelium. Harvard University Press, 1979.

Cholesterol Emboli of Retina (Hollenhorst Plaques) (Bright-yellow Plaques Often Observed at Bifurcation of Arterioles, Indicative of Generalized Atherosclerosis and Should Signal Ophthalmologist to Measure Retinal Artery Pressures and Refer Patient for General Medical Evaluation)

1. Abdominal aortic aneurysms

*2. Aortic stenosis

3. Arteriography showing occlusions in one or more cervical arteries

4. Atrial fibrillation

5. Bleeding duodenal or gastric ulcer

*6. Bruits in one or both carotid arteries

*7. Calcification of internal carotids (Doppler ultrasonography)

8. Congestive heart failure

9. Coronary heart disease with myocardial infarct or angina

*10. Diabetes mellitus

11. New or old strokes or transient attacks of cerebral ischemia

12. Peripheral atherosclerosis obliterans, popliteal or femoral aneurysms

13. Renal artery occlusions

*14. Retinal arterial occlusions

15. Torsion and calcification of aorta (roentgenogram)

16. Vocal cord paralysis (aortic arch aneurysm)

Pfaffenbach, D.D., and Hollenhorst, R.W.: Morbidity and survivorship of patients with embolic cholesterol crystals in the ocular fundus. Am. J. Ophthalmol., 75:66–72, 1973.

Wylie, E.J., and Ehrenfeld, W.K.: Extracranial Occlusive Cerebrovascular Disease: Diagnosis and Management. Philadelphia, W.B. Saunders, 1970.

Retinal Microemboli

1. Platelet-fibrin—mural or "tail" thrombus in carotid occlusion

*2. Cholesterol-lipid croding atheroma in carotid bifurcation

* = most important

3. Calcific or fibrinoid

   A. Calcific valvular disease dislodged spontaneously following cardiac catheterization, or angiography, or prolapse of mitral valve

   B. Rheumatic heart disease

   C. Myocardial disease

   D. Septic emboli

4. Foreign bodies

   A. Silicone or cloth particles covered cardiac valves

   B. Talc or cornstarch emboli from drug addicts

   C. Mercury

   D. Secondary to retrobulbar or intranasal methyl prednisolone acetate

5. Tumors

   A. Cardiac myxomas

   B. Metastic tumors including malignant melanomas and breast carcinomas

6. Fat emboli from fracture of the long bones

7. Air emboli from crushing injuries of the chest

Fraunfelder, F.T., and Roy, F.H.: Current Ocular Therapy. 4th Ed. Philadelphia, W.B. Saunders, 1995.

Williams, I.M., et al.: Brain and retinal microemboli during cardiac surgery. Ann. of Neurology, 30:736–737, 1991.

Lipemia Retinalis (Arterioles and Venules are Similar in Color and Appear Orange-Yellow to White)

1. Primary hyperlipoproteinemia

   A. Type I—familial fat-induced hyperlipoproteinemia (hyperchylomicronemia)

   B. Type III—familial hyper-beta- and hyper-pre-beta-lipoproteinemia (carbohydrate-induced hyperlipemia)

   C. Type IV—familial hyper-pre-beta-lipoproteinemia (carbohydrate-induced hyperlipemia)

   D. Type V—familial hyperchylomicronemia with hyper-pre-beta-lipoproteinemia (mixed hyperlipemia)

*2. Diabetes mellitus with hyperlipemia

3. Secondary hyperlipoproteinemia

   A. Biliary obstruction

   B. Chronic pancreatitis

   C. Chronic renal failure

   D. Coats disease in adults (retinal telangiectasia)

   E. Glycogen storage disease

   F. Hypergammaglobulinemia

   G. Hypothyroidism (cretinism)

   H. Idiopathic hypercalcemia

   I. Insulin-deficient diabetes mellitus (Willis disease)

*J. Malignant neoplasms

K. Nephrotic syndrome (lipoid nephrosis)

L. Progressive lipodystrophy

Martinez, K.R., et al.: Lipemia retinalis. Arch. Ophthal., 110:1171, 1992.

Spaeth, G.L.: Ocular manifestations of the lipidoses. In Tasman, W. (ed.): Retinal Diseases in Children. New York, Harper & Row, 1971.

Hemorrhagic or Serous Exudates Beneath Pigment Epithelium

1. Angioid streaks (see p. 584)

2. Best macular degeneration (vitelliruptive macular dystrophy)

3. Coats disease (retinal telangiectasia)

4. Doyne honeycomb macular degeneration

*5. Histoplasmosis (histoplasmosis choroiditis)

*6. Macular drusen in age-related macular degeneration

7. Myopia

8. Solid neoplasms

9. Trauma

Gitter, K.A., et al.: Traumatic hemorrhagic detachment of retinal pigment epithelium. Arch. Ophthalmol., 79:729–732, 1968.

Retinal Vascular Tumors and Angiomatosis Retinae Syndromes

1. Associated with pheochromocytoma

2. Blue rubber bleb nevus syndrome (Bean syndrome)

3. Bonnet-Dechaune-Blanc syndrome (neuroretinal angiomatosis syndrome)

4. Cavernous retinal hemangioma-intraretinal angiomas

*5. Coats disease (retinal telangiectasia)

6. Racemose angioma—with arteriovenous anomalies of central nervous system (Wyburn-Mason syndrome)

7. Retinal telangiectasis (Leber military aneurysms)—telangiectasia retinae of Reese

8. Sturge-Weber syndrome (meningocutaneous syndrome)

*9. von Hippel-Lindau syndrome (retinocerebral angiomatosis retinae)

Crompton, J.L., and Taylor, D.: Ocular lesion in the blue rubber nevus syndrome. Ophthalmology, 65:133–137, 1981.

Geeraets, W.J.: Ocular Syndromes. 3rd Ed. Philadelphia, Lea & Febiger, 1976.

* = most important

Retinal Vascular Tumors

	Retinal Telangiectasia	Cavernous Retinal Hemangioma	Wynburn Mason Syndrome	Coats' Disease	Von Hippel-Lindau Syndrome	Sturge-Weber Syndrome	Pheochromocytoma
History							
1. Bilateral	S		S	S	S		
2. Congenital	U	U	R	U	R	U	
3. Greater in males	S	S			S		
4. Occurs during second to third decades					U		
5. Occurs before fourth decade			U				
6. Occurs during fourth to sixth decades							U
7. Onset during first decade of life	U	U		U			
Physical Findings							
1. Third, fourth, and sixth nerve palsies			S				
2. Angiomatosis of iris					S		
3. Choroidal hemangioma						U	
4. Conjunctival telangiectasia						S	
5. Glaucoma	R			S	S	S	
6. Optic atrophy							
7. Papilledema			S				U
8. Port-wine lid stain						S	
9. Ptosis			R				
10. Pulsatile exophthalmos			S				
11. Retinal hemorrhage	U		S	U	S		S
12. Soft exudates of retina	S		S	S	S		S
13. Telangiectatic retinal vessels	U	U		U	S	U	S
14. Total retinal detachment	R			U	S	S	
15. Uveitis	R			S			
Laboratory Data							
1. Computed tomographic scan of head			U				
2. Cerebral angiography			U			S	R
3. Fluorescein angiography	S	S	U	S	U	S	S
4. Ocular ultrasound	R	S	R	U	U	U	U
5. Urinary catecholamine and vanillylmandelic acid							U
6. Visual field test	S	S	U	S	U	S	S

R = rarely; S = sometimes; and U = usually.

Traumatic Retinopathies

	Purtscher Retinopathy	Commotio Retinae	Traumatic Asphyxia	Fat Emoblism
Type of trauma	Chest compression	Local	Chest	Fractures
Accompanying signs	None	None	Cyanosis	Chest, cerebral, and cutaneous signs
Onset of systemic picture	None	None	Immediate	Symptom-free, 48-hour interval
Initial vision	Variable	20/200	Variable	Occasionally reduced
Duration of loss of vision	Several weeks	Days	Several weeks	Several weeks
Ultimate vision	Normal	Normal	Variable	Normal
External eye	Normal	Contused	Hemorrhage	Normal or petechiae
Fundus picture	Exudates and hemorrhage	Retinal edema	Normal or hemorrhage	Exudate, edema, and hemorrhages
Onset of fundus abnormalities	Within 1 to 2 days	A few hours	Immediate or a few hours	After 1 to 2 days

Retinal "Sea-Fans" (Vasoproliferative Lesions with a Characteristic Fan-Shaped Appearance; "Parachute" Lesion)

1. Aortic arch syndrome (pulseless disease)
2. Carotid-cavernous fistula (carotid artery syndrome)
*3. Central and branch retinal vein occlusion (see p. 525)
4. Chronic myelocytic leukemia
*5. Diabetes mellitus
6. Eales disease (periphlebitis)
7. Facioscapulohumeral muscular dystrophy (FSH syndrome)
8. Incontinentia pigmenti I (Block-Sulzberger syndrome)
9. Familial exudative vitreoretinopathy (Criswick-Schepens syndrome)
10. Hemoglobin C trait
11. Leukemia
12. Longstanding retinal detachment
13. Lupus erythematosus
14. Macroglobulinemia
15. Multiple sclerosis
16. Polycythemia vera (erythremia)
*17. Retinopathy of prematurity
18. Sarcoidosis syndrome
*19. Sickle cell disease
20. Talc and cornstarch emboli
21. Uveitis, including pars planitis

Garoon, I., et al.: Vascular tufts in retrolental fibroplasia. Ophthalmology, 87:1129, 1980.

Gurwin, E.B., et al.: Retinal telangiectasis in facioscapulohumeral muscular dystrophy with deafness. Arch. Ophthalmol., 103:1695–1707, 1985.

Jampol, L.M., and Goldberg, M.H.: Peripheral proliferative retinopathies. Surv. Ophthalmol., 25:1–14, 1980.

Rodgers, R., et al.: Ocular involvement in congenital leukemia. Am. J. Ophthalmol., 101:730–732, 1986.

Roy, F.H.: Ocular Syndromes and Systemic Diseases. 2nd Ed. Philadelphia, W.B. Saunders, 1989.

Tasman, W., and Shields, J.A.: Disorders of the Peripheral Fundus. New York, Harper and Row, 1980.

Retinal Vessels Displaced Temporally

1. Familial vitreoretinopathy
2. Hamartomas
3. Inflammation
4. Myopia with lattice-like retinal degeneration
*5. Retinopathy of prematurity
*6. Sickle cell disease (drepanocytic anemia)
7. Trauma

Ballantyne, A.J., and Michaelson, I.C.: Textbook of the Fundus of the Eye. 3rd Ed. Baltimore, Williams & Wilkins, 1991.

Nover, A.: The Ocular Fundus: Methods of Examination and Typical Findings. 4th Ed. Philadelphia, Lea & Febiger, 1981.

Retinal Vessels Displaced Nasally

1. Axial myopia

*2. Glaucoma

3. Inflammation

4. Trauma

Ballantyne, A.J., and Michelson, I.C.: Textbook of the Fundus of the Eye. 3rd Ed. Baltimore, Williams & Wilkins, 1981.

Nover, A.: The Ocular Fundus: Methods of Examination and Typical Findings. 4th Ed. Philadelphia, Lea & Febiger, 1981.

Peripheral Fundus Lesions

1. Pale raised lesions

    A. Vitreous opacities—white fluffy or discrete opacities, associated with pars planitis or sarcoid uveitis

    B. Retinopathy of prematurity—retinal edema and dense white lesions with neovascularization

    C. Toxocariasis (nematode ophthalmia syndrome)—vitreous opacities with peripheral granuloma

    D. Leprosy (Hansen disease)—peripheral exudates with anterior uveal involvement

    E. Vitreoretinal dystrophies—bands in vitreous with retinoschisis or retinal detachment

    F. Angiomatosis—retinal tumor with enlarged, feeding vessels

    *G. Retinoblastoma—raised creamy-white fluffy lesion without inflammatory signs

2. Flat lesions

    A. Coloboma—pale area with pigmented edge in region of fetal cleft

    B. Chorioretinitis

        (1) Disseminated, congenital syphilis—pepper-and-salt or larger confluent lesions

        (2) Toxoplasmosis—pigmented scars of old lesions

        (3) Cytomegalic inclusion disease—localized chorioretinitis or general peripheral infiltration

        *(4) Histoplasmosis—peripheral punched-out lesions with or without pigmentation

    C. Peripheral degenerations

        (1) Senile changes—of eyes older than years of age, depigmented areas with pigmented margins (cobblestone degeneration)

        (2) Secondary pigmentary degeneration—peripheral pigmentary changes similar to senile type or to retinitis pigmentosa

* = most important

(3) Cystoid degeneration—multiple cystic spaces and thin areas in peripheral retina

*(4) Lattice degeneration—lacework of white lines with depigmented and pigmented patches

(5) Cystinosis (cystine storage aminoaciduria dwarfism syndrome)—granular rings of pigment in periphery of fundus, similar to cobblestone degeneration

D. Equatorial linear pigment disturbance

(1) Ophthalmomyiasis internal

(2) Histoplasmosis syndrome

E. Retinitis

*(1) Acute retinal necrosis

*(2) Cytomegalovirus retinitis

3. Dark raised lesions

A. Choroidal detachment (see p. 591)

(1) Spontaneous—slowly progressive detachment, no inflammatory signs

*(2) Postoperative—intraocular operation; particularly for cataract and glaucoma; shallow anterior chamber; leaking wound

(3) Exudative

a. Inflammatory—shallow anterior chamber, myopia, and peripheral detachment

b. Vascular—nephritis, hypertension, toxemia of pregnancy, polyarteritis nodosa, leukemia

*c. Tumors—intraocular tumors; tumors of orbit and lacrimal gland

d. Traumatic—contusion injuries, perforating wounds, hypotony, anterior chamber may be shallow or deep if perforation occurs posteriorly

B. Exudative retinal detachment (see p. 541)

*(1) Secondary to general disease with retinopathy—hypertension, toxemia of pregnancy, leukemia, dysproteinemia, polyarteritis nodosa, rickettsial arteritis, venous congestion, talc and cornstarch emboli

(2) Secondary to local disease of the eye—inflammatory signs with exudative detachment, Harada disease, sympathetic ophthalmitis, scleritis, tenonitis, choroidal tumor, and ophthalmomyiasis

C. Simple detachment—myopia in two thirds of patients, trauma, may follow cataract extraction or discission for congenital cataract

D. Cysts

(1) Ciliary body—larger cysts usually push iris forward; rarely, cyst extends backward to be seen ophthalmoscopically

(2) Pars plana—may enlarge and appear as a multilocular reddish-brown cyst

E. Scleral indentation—retinal detachment operation

F. Neoplasms of ciliary body

(1) Benign epithelioma—brown spot to mm in diameter on surface of ciliary body

*(2) Other tumors—diktyoma, leiomyoma, reticuloses, neurofibroma, malignant melanoma, rare, usually present as a mass protruding through root of iris, may cause glaucoma, dark bulge seen ophthalmoscopically, lens changes adjacent to tumor

G. Neoplasms of choroid

(1) Congenital melanosis—cat's paw patches of pigment in one sector of fundus

(2) Choroidal nevus—flat bluish-gray or black lesion

*(3) Malignant melanoma—raised, pigmented lesion with secondary detachment

(4) Secondary metastatic—rare, primary lesion in breast, lung, etc.

4. Vascular lesions

A. Periphlebitis (Eales disease) common; young adults; sheathing of peripheral veins; hemorrhages in new vessels and later retinal detachment (see p. 541)

*B. Perivasculitis secondary to uveitis—perivascular infiltration, particularly in pars planitis, sarcoidosis, Behçet disease, and toxoplasmosis

C. Systemic diseases

(1) Rickettsia—engorgement of veins, retinal edema, hemorrhages, and exudates

(2) Multiple sclerosis (disseminated sclerosis)—sheathing of veins (see p. 519)

(3) Polyarteritis nodosa (necrotizing angiitis)—hemorrhages, exudates, and serous detachment of retina (see p. 541)

(4) Tuberculin or Bacille-Calmette-Guérin inoculation—rare, sheathing of peripheral veins with hemorrhages

*(5) Sickle cell retinopathy (Herrick syndrome)—dilatation of peripheral veins, hemorrhages, and connective tissue sheets in periphery, new vessel formation

Mason, G.I.: Bilateral ophthalmomyiasis interna. Am. J. Ophthalmol., 91:65–70, 1981.

Perkins, E.S., and Dobree, J.H.: The Differential Diagnosis of Fundus Conditions. St. Louis, C.V. Mosby, 1972.

Tasman, W., and Shields, J.A.: Disorders of the Peripheral Fundus. New York, Harper and Row, 1980.

Retinal Disease Associated with Corneal Problems

1. Abdominal typhus (enteric fever)—corneal ulcer, retinal detachment, central retinal artery emboli

2. Acanthamoeba—keratitis, pannus, corneal ring abscess, retinal perivasculitis

3. African eyeworm disease—keratitis, central retinal artery occlusion, macular hemorrhages

4. Amyloidosis—amyloid corneal deposits, corneal dystrophy, retinal hemorrhages

5. Anderson-Warburg syndrome (oligophrenia-microphthalmos syndrome)—corneal opacification, malformed retina with retina pseudotumors

6. Angioedema (hives)—central serous retinopathy, corneal edema

*7. Anterior segment ischemia syndrome—corneal edema midperiphery retinal hemorrhages

8. Apert syndrome (acrodysplasia)—exposure keratitis, retinal detachment

9. Arteriovenous fistula—bullous keratopathy, retinal hemorrhages

10. Aspergillosis—corneal ulcer, keratitis, retinal hemorrhages, retinal detachment

11. Atopic dermatitis—keratoconus and retinal detachment

12. Avitaminosis C—retinal hemorrhages, keratitis, corneal ulcer

13. Bacillus cereus—ring abscess of cornea, necrosis of retina

14. Bang disease (brucellosis)—keratitis, chorioretinitis, macular edema

* = most important

15. Behçet syndrome (dermatostomata-ophthalmic syndrome)—keratitis, posterior corneal abscess, retinal vascular changes

16. Bietti disease (Bietti marginal crystalline dystrophy)—marginal corneal dystrophy, retinitis punctate albescens

17. Candidiasis—keratitis, corneal ulcer, retinal atrophy, retinal detachment

*18. Carotid artery syndrome—corneal ulcer, loss of corneal sensation, retinal edema, engorgement of retinal veins

19. Chickenpox (varicella)—corneal ulcer, corneal opacity, retinitis, hemorrhagic retinopathy

20. Chloroquine—corneal epithelial pigmentation, macular lesions

21. Chronic granulomatous disease of childhood—keratitis, destructive chorioretinal lesions

22. Cockayne syndrome (dwarfism with retinal atrophy and deafness)—pigmentary degeneration, band keratopathy, corneal dystrophy

23. Crohn disease (granulomatous ileocolitis)—marginal corneal ulcers, keratitis, macular edema, macular hemorrhages

24. Cryoglobulinemia—deep corneal opacities, venous stasis

25. Cystinosis (aminoaciduria)—crystals in cornea and pigment in retina

26. Dengue fever—keratitis, corneal ulcer, retinal hemorrhages

27. Diffuse keratoses syndrome—corneal nodular thickening in the stroma worse in fall, retinal phlebitis

28. Diphtheria—keratitis, corneal ulcer, central artery occlusion

29. Disseminated lupus erythematosus (Kaposi-Libman-Sacks syndrome)—keratitis, keratoconjunctivitis sicca, corneal ulcer, central retinal vein occlusion, retinal detachment

30. Ehlers-Danlos syndrome (cutis hyperelastica)—keratoconus, and retinitis pigmentosa

31. Electrical injury—corneal perforation, retinal edema, retinal hemorrhages, pigmentary degeneration, retinal holes, dilatation of retinal veins

32. Fabry disease (diffuse angiokeratosis)—whorl-like changes in cornea, central retinal artery occlusion, tortuosity of retinal vessels

33. Goldscheider syndrome (epidermolysis bullosa)—bullous keratitis with opacities, retinal detachment

34. Gronblad-Strandberg syndrome (systemic elastodystrophy)—angioid streaks of the retina, macular hemorrhages, retinal detachment, keratoconus

35. Hamman-Rich syndrome (alveolar capillary block syndrome)—keratomalacia ischemic retinopathy, cystic macular changes

36. Heerfordt syndrome (uveoparotid fever)—band keratopathy, retinal vasculitis

37. Hennebert syndrome (luetic otitic nystagmus syndrome)—interstitial keratitis, disseminated syphilitic chorioretinitis

38. Histiocytosis X (Hand-Schüller-Christian syndrome)—retinal hemorrhage, retinal detachment, bullous keratopathy, corneal ulcer, pannus

39. Hodgkin disease—keratitis, retinal hemorrhages

40. Hollenhorst syndrome (chorioretinal infarction syndrome)—hazy cornea, serous retinal detachment, pigmentary retinopathy

41. Hunter syndrome (mucopolysaccharidoses [MPS] II)—splitting or absence of peripheral Bowman membrane, stromal haze, pigmentary retinal degeneration, narrowed retinal vessels

42. Hurler-Scheie syndrome (MPS IH-S)—corneal clouding, pigmentary retinopathy

43. Hurler syndrome (gargoylism)—diffuse corneal haziness, retinal pigmentary changes, megalocornea, retinal detachment

44. Hydatid cyst (echinococcosis)—keratitis, abscess of cornea, retinal detachment, retinal hemorrhages

45. Hyperlipoproteinemia—arcus juvenilis, lipemia retinalis, xanthomata of retina

46. Hyperparathyroidism—band keratopathy, vascular engorgement of retina

47. Hypovitaminosis A—keratomalacia with perforation, corneal opacity, retinal degeneration

48. Idiopathic hypercalcemia (blue diaper syndrome)—band keratopathy, optic atrophy, papilledema

49. Indomethacin—corneal deposits, reduced retinal sensitivity

50. Influenza—keratitis, retinal hemorrhage

51. Japanese River fever (typhus)—keratitis, retinal hemorrhages

52. Juvenile rheumatoid arthritis (Still disease)—band keratopathy, macular edema

53. Kahler disease (multiple myeloma)—crystalline deposits of cornea, central retinal artery occlusion, retinal microaneurysms

54. Kussmaul disease (periarteritis nodosa)—retinal detachment, pseudoretinitis pigmentosa, corneal ulcer

55. Leber tapetoretinal dystrophy syndrome (retinal aplasia)—keratoconus, salt-and-pepper or "bone corpuscle" pigmentation, yellowish-brown or gray macular lesions

56. Lubarsch-Pick syndrome (primary amyloidosis)—amyloid corneal deposits, retinal hemorrhages

*57. Lymphogranuloma venereum disease (Nicolas-Favre disease)—keratitis, pannus, corneal ulcer, keratoconus, tortuosity of retinal vessels, retinal hemorrhages

58. Marfan syndrome (arachnodactyly dystrophia mesodermalis congenita)—keratoconus, retinitis pigmentosa

59. Meckel syndrome (dysencephalia splanchnocystic syndrome)—sclerocornea, microcornea, retinal dysplasia

60. Meningococcemia—keratitis, retinal endophlebitis

61. Mikulicz-Radeski syndrome (dacryosialoadenopathy)—keratoconjunctivitis, retinal candlewax spots

62. ML IV (mucolipidosis IV)—corneal clouding, corneal opacities, retinal atrophy

63. Morbilli (measles-rubeola)—keratitis, corneal ulcer, pigmentary retinopathy, central retinal artery occlusion

64. Mucormycosis (phycomycosis)—corneal ulcer, striate keratopathy, retinitis, central retinal artery thrombosis

65. Mycosis fungoides syndrome (malignant cutaneous reticulosis syndrome)—keratoconjunctivitis, retinal edema, retinal hemorrhage

* = most important

66. Myotonic dystrophy syndrome—corneal epithelial dystrophy, loss of corneal sensitivity, tapetoretinal degeneration, macular red spot, macular degeneration, chorioretinitis

*67. Neurofibromatosis (von Recklinghausen syndrome)—nodular swelling nerves, hamartoma of retina

68. Norrie disease (atrophia oculi congenita)—malformation of sensory cells of retina, corneal nebulae

69. Oculodental syndrome (Peter's syndrome)—corneoscleral staphyloma, megalocornea, corneal marginal opacities, macular pigmentation

70. Onchocerciasis syndrome—punctate keratitis, sclerosing keratitis, chorioretinitis, retinal degeneration

71. Paget syndrome (osteitis deformans)—corneal ring opacities, retinal hemorrhages, pigmentary retinopathy, macular changes resembling Kuhnt-Junius degeneration

72. Phenothiazine—epithelial and endothelial pigment, retinal pigmentation

73. Pierre-Robin syndrome (micrognathia-glossoptosis)—retinal disinsertion, megalocornea

74. Plasma lecithin (cholesterol acyltransferase deficiency)—corneal stromal opacities, retinal hemorrhages

75. Porphyria cutanea tarda—keratitis, retinal hemorrhages, cotton-wool spots, macular edema

76. Postvaccinial ocular syndrome—corneal vesicles, and marginal ulcers, chorioretinitis, central serous retinopathy, central retinal vein thrombosis

77. Progressive systemic sclerosis—marginal corneal ulcers with cicatrization, cotton-wool spots, retinal hemorrhages

78. Radiation—corneal ulcer, punctate keratitis, keratoconjuctivitis sicca, retinal hemorrhage, macular degeneration, macular holes with vascularization

*79. Refsum syndrome (phytanic acid oxidase deficiency)—band keratopathy, retinitis pigmentosa

80. Relapsing fever—interstitial keratitis, retinal hemorrhage

81. Relapsing polychondritis—corneal ulcer, retinal detachment, retinal artery thrombosis, keratoconjunctivitis sicca

82. Renal failure—cotton-wool spots, band keratopathy

83. Rendu-Osler syndrome (hereditary hemorrhagic telangiectasis)—intermittent filamentary keratitis, small retinal angiomas, retinal hemorrhages

84. Retinal disinsertion syndrome—bilateral keratoconus, retinal detachment

*85. Retinoblastoma—corneal neovascularization, retinal tumor

86. Rothmund syndrome (telangiectasia-pigmentation cataract syndrome)—corneal lesions, retinal hyperpigmentation

87. Rubella syndrome (Gregg syndrome)—microcornea, pigmentary retinal changes

88. Sabin-Feldman syndrome—microcornea, chorioretinitis or atrophic degenerative chorioretinal changes

89. Sanfillipo-Good syndrome (mucopolysaccharidosis III)—slight narrowing of retinal vessels, acid mucopolysaccharide deposits in cornea.

*90. Schaumann syndrome (sarcoidosis syndrome)—mutton fat keratitic precipitates, keratitis sicca, band-shaped keratitis, inflammatory retinal exudates

91. Scheie syndrome (mucopolysaccharidoses I-S)—diffuse to marked corneal clouding, tapetoretinal degeneration

92. Schwartz syndrome (glaucoma associated with retinal detachment)—retinal detachment, microcornea

93. Shy-Gonatas syndrome (orthostatic hypotension syndrome)—keratopathy, corneal ulcer, lattice-like white opacities in the area of Bowman membrane, retinal pigmentary degeneration

94. Smallpox—keratitis, congenital corneal clouding, chorioretinitis

95. Stannus cerebellar syndrome (riboflavin deficiency)—corneal vascularization, superficial diffuse keratitis, corneal opacities, brownish retinal patches

96. Stickler syndrome (hereditary progressive arthroophthalmopathy)—keratopathy, chorioretinal degeneration, total retinal detachment

97. Sturge-Weber syndrome (neuro-oculocutaneous angiomatosis)—retinal detachment, increased corneal diameter with cloudiness

*98. Syphilis (acquired lues)—keratitis, retinal hemorrhages, retinal proliferation

*99. Temporal arteritis syndrome (Hutchinson-Horton-Magath-Brown syndrome)—retinal detachments, narrowing of retinal vessels, central retinal artery occlusion, corneal hypesthesia

100. Trisomy 13 (Patau syndrome)—malformed cornea, retinal dysplasia

*101. Tuberculosis—keratitis, pannus, corneal ulcer, retinitis

102. Ullrich syndrome (dyscraniopygophalangy)—cloudy cornea, corneal ulcers, chorioretinal coloboma

103. Ultraviolet radiation—photokeratitis, band keratopathy, herpes simplex keratitis, recurrent corneal erosions, retinal degeneration

104. Vaccinia—keratitis, pannus, corneal perforation, central serous retinopathy, pseudoretinitis pigmentosa

105. van Bogaert-Scherer-Epstein (primary hyperlipidemia)—arcus juvenilis of the cornea, lipid keratopathy, retinopathy with yellowish deposits

106. Vitreous tug syndrome—vitreous strands attached to corneal wound or scar, circumscribed retinal edema, posterior retinal detachment

107. von Gierke disease (glycogen storage disease type I)—corneal clouding, discrete nonelevated, yellow flecks in macula

108. Waardenburg syndrome (embryonic fixation syndrome)—microcornea, cornea plana, hypopigmentation and hypoplasia of retina

109. Wagner syndrome (hyaloideoretinal degeneration)—corneal degeneration, band-shaped keratopathy, hyaloideoretinal degeneration, narrowing of retinal vessels, retinal detachment, avascular preretinal membranes

110. Waldenstrom syndrome (macroglobulinemia syndrome)—crystalline corneal deposits, keratoconjunctivitis sicca, retinal venous thrombosis, retinal microaneurysms, cotton-wool spots

111. Weil disease (leptospirosis)—keratitis, retinitis

112. Werner syndrome (progeria of adults)—bullous keratitis, paramacular retinal degeneration

113. Wiskott-Aldrich syndrome (sex-linked draining ears, eczematoid dermatitis, bloody diarrhea)—corneal ulcers, retinal hemorrhages

* = most important

114. Yersinosis—corneal ulcer, retinal hemorrhages

115. Zellweger syndrome (cerebrohepatorenal syndrome)—corneal opacities, narrowing of retinal vessels, retinal holes without detachment, tapetoretinal degeneration

116. Zieve syndrome (hyperlipemia hemolytic anemia-icterus syndrome)—cloudy cornea, corneal ulcers, retinal lipemia

Arffa, R.C.: Grayson's Disease of the Cornea. 3rd Ed. St. Louis, Mosby–Yearbook, 1991.

Roy, F.H.: Ocular Syndromes and Systemic Diseases. 2nd Ed. Philadelphia, W.B. Saunders, 1989.

Retinal Lesions Associated with Deafness

1. Alport syndrome (hereditary familial congenital hemorrhagic nephritis)

2. Alstrom disease—retinitis pigmentosa (see p. 551)

3. Choroideremia, obesity, and congenital deafness

4. Cockayne syndrome (dwarfism with retinal atrophy and deafness)

5. Dialinas-Amalric syndrome (deaf-mutism-retinal degeneration syndrome)

*6. Harada syndrome (Vogt-Koyanagi-Harada syndrome)

7. Hallgren syndrome (retinitis pigmentosa-deafness-ataxia syndrome)

8. Hunter syndrome (mucopolysaccharidoses [MPS] II)

9. Laurence-Moon-Bardet-Biedl syndrome (retinitis pigmentosa-polydactyly adiposogenital syndrome)

10. Norrie disease—mental retardation, X-linked retinal malformation, and hearing loss

*11. Refsum syndrome (phytanic acid storage disease)

12. Retinal vessel changes, muscular dystrophy, mental retardation, and hearing loss

13. Rubella (German measles)—cardiac disorders, cataract, salt-and-pepper pigmentation

14. Sanfilippo syndrome (MPS III, autosomal recessive)

*15. Syphilis—acquired or congenital

16. Usher syndrome (hereditary retinitis pigmentosa—deafness syndrome)

17. Waardenburg syndrome (embryonic fixation syndrome)

Ayazi, S.: Choroideremia obesity, and congenital deafness. Am. J. Ophthalmol., 92:63–69, 1981.

Millay, R.H., et al.: Ophthalmologic and systemic manifestations of Alstrom's disease. Am. J. Ophthalmol., 102:482–490, 1986.

Roy, F.H., et al.: Ocular manifestations of congenital rubella syndrome. Arch. Ophthalmol., 75:601, 1966.

Epiretinal Membranes—Membranes that Grow on Inner Surface of Retina

*1. After retinal photocoagulation, cryotherapy, or reattachment of retina

2. Following blunt or penetrating injuries

*3. Idiopathic

4. Nonproliferative retinal vascular disorders

*5. Proliferative retinopathies (see p. 540)

6. Rhegmatogenous retinal detachment (see p. 541)

7. Sickle cell disease, including sickle cell C, sickle cell S, and sickle cell B with thalassemia

8. Vitreous hemorrhage (see p. 474)

Carney, M.D., and Jampol, L.M.: Epiretinal membranes in sickle cell retinopathy. Arch. Ophthalmol., 105:214–217, 1987.

Cherfan, G.M., et al.: Nuclear sclerotic cataract after vitrectomy for idiopathic epiretinal membranes causing macular pucker. Amer. J. Ophthal., 111:434–438,1991.

Kao, S.F., et al.: Subretinal fibrosis following cyclocryotherapy. Arch. Ophthalmol., 105:214–217, 1987.

Lansing, M.B., et al.: The effect of pars plana vitrectomy and transforming growth factor-beta without epiretinal membrane peeling on full-thickness macular holes. Ophthal., 100:871–872, 1993.

Linear Streaks Pattern in Fundus

*1. Angioid streaks (see p. 586)

2. Bird-shot retinochoroidopathy

3. Choroidal rupture

4. Demarcation lines

*5. Presumed ocular histoplasmosis syndrome—peripheral, parallel to equator

6. Migrating parasites

    A. Botfly larvae

    B. Trematodes

*7. Retinal and choroidal detachment

*8. Snail-track configuration of lattice degeneration

Fountain, J.A., and Schloegel, T.F.: Linear streaks of the equator in the presumed ocular histoplasmosis syndrome. Arch. Ophthalmol., 99:246, 1981.

Yellow-Orange Lesions of Subretinal Fundus

*1. Acute inflammatory lesions of pigment epithelium, choriocapillaris, and choroid

*2. Detachment of retinal pigment epithelium

3. Isolated pocket of subretinal fluid

4. Subretinal fluid following scleral buckling procedure

Avirs, L.R., and Hilton, G.F.: Lesions simulating serous detachments of the pigment epithelium. Arch. Ophthalmol., 98:1427–1429, 1980.

Lobes, L.R., and Grand, M.G.: Subretinal lesions following scleral buckling procedure. Arch. Ophthalmol., 98:680–683, 1980.

Talc Retinopathy—Drug Addicts Who Inject Drugs Intravenously

1. Optic disc neovascularization (see p. 624)

2. Peripheral retinal neovascularization (see p. 540)

3. Vitreous hemorrhage (see p. 474)

O'Brien, R.J., and Schroedl, B.L.: Talc retinopathy. Optometry & Vision Science, 68:54–57, 1991.

Tse, D.T., and Ober, R.R.: Talc retinopathy. Am. J. Ophthalmol., 90:624–640, 1980.

* = most important

Crystalline Retinopathy

1. Bietti crystalline dystrophy (Bietti disease)
2. Cystinosis (cystine storage-aminoaciduria-dwarfism syndrome)
3. Gyrate atrophy with hyperornithemia (ornithine ketoacid aminotransferase deficiency)
4. Hyperoxaluria (oxalosis)
5. Nitrofurantoin therapy
6. Sjögren-Larson syndrome (oligophrenia-ichthyosis-spastic diplegia syndrome)
*7. Talc emboli
*8. Tamoxifen retinopathy

Ibanez, H.E., et al.: Crystalline retinopathy associated with long-term nitrofurantoin therapy. Arch. Ophthal., 112:304–305, 1994.

Meredith, T.A., et al.: Ocular involvement in primary hyperoxaluria. Arch. Ophthalmol., 102: 584–587, 1984.

Zak, T.A., and Buncic, R.: Primary hereditary oxalosis retinopathy. Arch. Ophthalmol., 101:78–80, 1983.

Pulfrich Stereo-Illusion Phenomenon (Central Serous Elevation of the Macula with Abnormal Latency of the Visual-Evoked Potential)

*1. Optic nerve disease—demyelinating optic neuropathy
2. Media opacity
3. Anisocoria
4. Macular disease

Greenberg, H.S.: Visual-evoked responses. J. Clin. Neuro. Ophthalmol., 1:273, 1981.

Hofeldt, A.J., et al.: Pulfrich stereo-illusion phenomenon in serous sensory retinal detachment of the macula. Am. J. Ophthalmol., 100:576–580, 1985.

Parafoveal Telangiectasia (Retinal Microvascular Anomaly Involving the Parafoveal Capillary Network as well as Immediately Adjacent Vascular Bed, Best Demonstrated by Fluorescein Angiography)

*1. Carotid artery obstruction
*2. Diabetes mellitus usually bilateral
*3. Idiopathic
4. Localized form of Coats disease, usually unilateral
5. Small branch venular occlusion
6. Small retinal capillary hemangioma, usually unilateral
7. Roentgenogram, irradiation

Gass, J.D., and Oyakawa, T.: Idiopathic Juxtafoveal Telangiectasia. Arch. Ophthalmol., 100:769, 1982.

Millay, R.H., et al.: Abnormal glucose metabolism and parafoveal telangiectasia. Am. J. Ophthalmol., 102:363–370, 1986.

Hereditary Pediatric Retinal Degenerations

1. Acquired

    A. Juvenile retinitis pigmentosa

    B. Early onset retinitis pigmentosa

        (1) Autosomal dominant

        (2) Autosomal recessive

        (3) X-linked recessive

2. Congenital

    A. Complicated Leber congenital amaurosis

        (1) Multiple neurologic abnormalities

        (2) Others

        (3) Saldino-Mainzer syndrome

        (4) Senior-Loken syndrome (tubulointerstitial nephropathy syndrome)

        (5) Zellweger syndrome (cerebrohepatorenal syndrome of Zellweger)

    B. Uncomplicated Leber congenital amaurosis

Foxman, S.G., et al.: Classification of congenital and early onset retinitis pigmentosa. Arch. Ophthalmol., 103:1502–1506, 1985.

Nickel, B., and Hoyt, C.S.: Leber's congenital amaurosis. Arch. Ophthalmol., 100:1089–1092, 1982.

Reticular Pattern of Dark Lines in Fundus

1. Granular pigmentary pattern of the peripheral fundus
2. Multiple drusen of peripheral fundus
3. Reticular degeneration of the pigment epithelium (peripheral)
4. Reticular pattern dystrophy of posterior fundus (Sjögren reticular dystrophy, Mesker macroreticular dystrophy, pattern dystrophy of the retinal pigment epithelium, Doyne honeycomb reticular degeneration)
5. Tapetochoroidal hypopigmentation

Gass, J.D.M., et al.: Drusen and disciform macular detachment and degeneration. Arch. Ophthalmol., 90:206–217, 1973.

Lewis, H., et al.: Reticular degeneration of the pigment epithelium. Ophthalmology, 92:1485–1495, 1985.

Retinal Pigment Epithelial Tears (Flat, Uniform, Crescent-shaped Area of Exposed Choroid of Pigment Epithelial Elevation)

1. Acute retinal necrosis
*2. After laser photocoagulation
3. Along margin of retinal detachment
*4. Associated with pigment epithelial detachments
5. Spontaneous
6. Trauma

Fox, G.M., and Blumenkranz, M.: Giant retinal pigment epithelial tears in acute retinal necrosis. Amer. J. Ophthal., 116:302–306, 1993.

* = most important

Krishan, N.R., et al.: Diagnosis and pathogenesis of retinal pigment epithelial tears. Am. J. Ophthalmol., 100:698–707, 1985.

Levin, L.A., et al.: Retinal pigment epithelial tears associated with trauma. Amer. J. Ophthal., 112: 396–400, 1991.

Schoeppner, G., et al.: The risk of fellow eye visual loss with unilateral retinal pigment epithelial tears. Am. J. Ophthalmol., 108:683–685, 1989.

Retinal Pigment Epithelial Folds

1. Choroidal folds (see p. 584)
2. Pigment epithelial detachment
3. Retinal pigment epithelial tears (rips)
4. Retinal striae
*5. Subretinal neovascularization

Schatz, H., et al.: Retinal pigment epithelial folds associated with retinal pigment epithelial detachment in macular degeneration. Ophthal., 97:658–665, 1990.

Schoeppner, G., et al.: The risk of fellow eye visual loss with unilateral retinal pigment epithelial tears. Am. J. Ophthalmol., 108:683–685, 1989.

Mizuo Phenomenon (Change of Color of the Fundus from Red in the Dark-Adapted State to Golden Immediately or Shortly After the Onset of Light)

1. Oguchi disease
2. X-liked juvenile retinoschisis
3. X-linked recessive cone dystrophy

de Jong, P.T.V., et al.: Mizuo phenomenon in X-linked retinoschisis. Arch. Ophthalmol., 109:1104–1108, 1991.

Mizuo, G.A.: A new discovery in dark adaptation in Oguchi's disease. Acta. Soc. Ophthalmol. Jpn., 17:1148–1150, 1913.

Choroid

VINAY N. DESAI, M.D.

Contents

Angioid Streaks (Rupture of Bruch Membrane with Brownish Lines around Disc and Radiating toward Periphery)

	Senile (Actinic) Elastosis	Pseudoxanthoma Elasticum (Gronblad-Strandberg Syndrome)	Fibrodysplasia Hyperplastica (Ehlers-Danlos Syndrome)	Osteitis Deformans (Paget Disease)	Cardiovascular Disease with Hypertension	Sickle Cell Disease	Dwarfism	Acromegaly	Pituitary Tumor	Epilepsy	Lead Poisoning	Thrombocytopenic Purpura	Facial Angiomatosis	Previous Choroidal Detachment	Francois Dycephalic Syndrome	Ocular Melanocytosis
History																
1. Autosomal dominant			U	U												
2. Autosomal recessive		U					U									
3. Congenital																U
4. Develop with age/exposure to sun	U															
5. Elevated blood pressure					U											
6. Familial	U														U	
7. Hereditary		U	U	U		U							U			
8. Metamorphopsia									U							
9. Micropsia									U							
10. More in blacks						U										
11. More in children												S				
12. More in males				U												
13. More in whites																U
14. Ocular/periocular trauma														U		
15. Onset after 40 years				U				U								
16. "Pica" in children											U					
17. Severer in females				U												
18. Unilateral														U		U
Physical Findings																
1. Anterior synechiae														U		
2. Bilateral microphthalmos															U	
3. Black sunbursts, retina						U										
4. Blue sclera		U													S	
5. Buphthalmos													U			
6. Cataract		S					U								U	
7. Chalk-white vessels of retina						U										
8. Chorioretinal hyperpigmentation								S							U	
9. Choroidal coloboma														S		
10. Choroidal detachment		U												U		
11. Choroidal hemangioma													U			
12. Cotton-wool spots					U											
13. Decreased intraocular pressure									S					U		
14. Descemet wrinkles		S	S													
15. Exophthalmos		S							S						S	
16. Extraocular muscle paralysis			U								U					
17. Gaze paresis										U						
18. Hemianopia									U						U	
19. High myopia			S						S							
20. Holes in periphery/macula						U	U									
21. Hyaloid/vitreous anterior displacement														U		
22. Increased intraocular pressure					U									U	S	
23. Increased pigment episclera/sclera/uvea																U
24. Keratoconus		U	S													

Angioid Streaks (Rupture of Bruch Membrane with Brownish Lines around Disc and Radiating toward Periphery) *Continued*

	Senile (Actinic) Elastosis	Pseudoxanthoma Elasticum (Gronblad-Strandberg Syndrome)	Fibrodysplasia Hyperplastica (Ehlers-Danlos Syndrome)	Osteitis Deformans (Paget Disease)	Cardiovascular Disease with Hypertension	Sickle Cell Disease	Dwarfism	Acromegaly	Pituitary Tumor	Epilepsy	Lead Poisoning	Thrombocytopenic Purpura	Facial Angiomatosis	Previous Choroidal Detachment	François Dycephalic Syndrome	Ocular Melanocytosis
Physical Findings																
25. Macular hemorrhages		U			S								U			
26. Malignant melanoma																S
27. Microcornea			U												U	
28. Nevus of ota																U
29. Nystagmus									U						U	
30. Optic atrophy		S		S			U		U				S		S	
31. Optic neuritis										U	U					
32. Optic nerve cupping					S								S			
33. Papilledema					U				U		U	U				
34. Peripheral artery occlusion						U										
35. Port-wine stain of face													U			
36. Ptosis									U	S						
37. Retinal atrophy					U											
38. Retinal degeneration										S						
39. Retinal detachment		U	U													
40. Retinal edema					U											
41. Retinal hemorrhage					U	U					U	U				
42. Shiny dots in macula											U					
43. Skin papules	U	S	S													
44. Strabismus		U							U						S	
45. Vascular sheathing											U					
46. Visual field defects		U		U					U							
47. Vitreous hemorrhage		U			S	U										
Laboratory Data																
1. Bones, roentgenogram			S	U			U	U								
2. Computed tomographic scan							U	S	U	S			U		S	
3. Cerebral angiography									S				U			
4. Electroencephalogram										U						
5. Fluorescein angiography		S	S										U	U		U
6. Hemoglobin electrophoresis						U										
7. Lipid profile tests					U											
8. Peripheral blood test (hemoglobin, hematocrit, red blood cell, and platelet counts)					U							U				
9. Pituitary panel, including prolactin, growth hormone, adrenocorticotropic hormone, follicle-stimulating hormone, luteinizing hormone, thyroid-stimulating hormone									U							
10. Pneumoencephalogram									S							
11. Serum alkaline phosphatase				U												
12. Skin biopsy	U	U	U													
13. Skull roentgenogram							S	U	U	U						
14. Ultrasonography, ocular														U	S	R
15. Urinary calcium levels			S	U												

R = rarely; S = sometimes; and U = usually.

Angioid Streaks (Ruptures of Bruch Membrane Characterized Ophthalmoscopically by Brownish Lines Surrounding the Disc and Radiating toward the Periphery)

1. AC hemoglobinopathy
2. Acanthocytosis (abetalipoproteinemia, Bussen-Kornzwerg syndrome)
3. Acromegaly
4. Beta thalassemia minor
5. Calcinosis
6. Chronic congenital idiopathic hyperphosphatasemia
7. Cardiovascular disease with hypertension
8. Cooley anemia
9. Diffuse lipomatosis
10. Dwarfism
11. Epilepsy
12. Facial angiomatosis
13. Fibrodysplasia hyperelastica (Ehlers-Danlos syndrome)
14. François dyscephalic syndrome (Hallermann-Streiff syndrome)
15. Hereditary spherocytosis
16. Lead poisoning
17. Ocular melanocytosis
18. Optic disc drusen
19. Osteitis deformans (Paget disease)
20. Pituitary tumor
21. Previous choroidal detachment
*22. Pseudoxanthoma elasticum (Grönblad-Strandberg syndrome)
23. Senile (actinic) elastosis of the skin
24. Sickle cell disease (Herrick syndrome)
25. Thrombocytopenic purpura

Aessopos, A, et al.: Angioid streaks in sickle-thalassemia. Amer. J. Ophthal., 117:589–592, 1994.

Mansour, A.M.: Is there an association between optic disc drusen and angioid streaks? Graefes Archives for Clinical and Experimental Ophthal., 230:595–596, 1992.

Mansour, A.M.: Systemic Associations of Angioid Streaks. International Ophthalmology Clinics, 31: 61–68, 1991.

McBrayer, G.M., et al.: Angioid streaks and AC hemoglobinopathy—a newly discovered association. J. Amer. Optometric Assoc., 64: 250–253, 1993.

Roy, F.H.: Ocular Syndromes and Systemic Diseases. 2nd Ed. Philadelphia, W.B. Saunders, 1989.

Choroidal Folds (Folds of Posterior Pole, at Level of Choroid, with Hruby Lens and Pattern of Alternating Light Lines on Fluorescein Angiography)

1. Choroidal tumor, such as a melanoma
2. Disciform degeneration
3. Exophthalmos

4. Graves disease (Basedow syndrome)

5. High hyperopia

6. Idiopathic—no underlying pathologic state

7. Infection of paranasal sinuses

8. Longstanding orbital inflammation

9. Massive cranioorbital hemangiopericytoma

*10. Ocular hypotony (see p. 367)

11. Orbital mass

12. Papilledema (see p. 653)

13. Posteriorly located choroidal detachment

14. Postoperative condition, such as scleral buckle

15. Primary retinal detachment

16. Subretinal neovascularization

17. Uveitis

Friberg, T.R., and Grove, A.S.: Choroidal folds and refractive errors associated with orbital tumors. Arch. Ophthalmol., 101:598–603, 1983.

Shields, J.A., et al.: Clinicopathologic correlation of choroidal folds: secondary to massive cranioorbital hemangiopericytoma. Ophthal Plastic & Reconstructive Surgery, 8:62–68, 1992.

* = most important

Choroidal Detachment (Solid Appearance, Smooth Surface and Normal Retinal Vessels with Unchanged Color)

	Inflammatory Disease as Harada Disease	Vascular Disease as Diabetes Mellitus	Neoplastic Disorder as Malignant Melanoma	Ocular Trauma as Blunt Trauma	Acute Ocular Hypotony	Spontaneous Detachment with Uveal Effusion as Nonrhegmatogenous Retinal Detachment
History						
1. Bilateral	U	U				
2. Common in males				U		U
3. Familial		U				
4. Japanese/Italian extraction	U					
5. Occurs in persons 11 to 40 years		S				
6. Occurs in young adults	U	U				
7. Ocular pain					S	
8. Surgery					U	
9. Virus infection	U					
10. Visual distortion			S			S
Physical Findings						
1. Acute diffuse exudative choroiditis	U					U
2. Cataracts	S		U		S	
3. Cyclodialysis cleft					S	
4. Corneal abrasions				S		
5. Corneal arcus		S				
6. Cotton-wool spots		U				
7. Choroidal folds					S	
8. Choroidal nevus			S			
9. Choroidal rupture				U	S	S
10. Decreased intraocular pressure				S	U	U
11. Endothelial corneal damage				S		
12. Extraocular muscle paralysis			S			
13. Exudative iridocyclitis	U					S
14. Glaucoma	U	S	S	S		
15. Hyphema				S		
16. Hypermetropia			U			
17. Increased lid pigmentation			S			
18. Iridodialysis				S		
19. Macular edema					S	
20. Macular hemorrhage	S					
21. Optic nerve atrophy		S	S	S		
22. Oribital mass			S			
23. Papilledema	U		S			
24. Phthisis bulbi	S					
25. Pigmentary retinopathy	U		S			
26. Pigmentary iris degeneration					S	
27. Pigmented/amelanotic choroidal mass			U			
28. Poliosis	U					
29. Recessed chamber angle				S		
30. Retinal detachment	U	S	U	S		U
31. Retinal edema	U					S
32. Retinal folds					U	

Choroidal Detachment (Solid Appearance, Smooth Surface and Normal Retinal Vessels with Unchanged Color) *Continued*

	Inflammatory Disease as Harada Disease	Vascular Disease as Diabetes Mellitus	Neoplastic Disorder as Malignant Melanoma	Ocular Trauma as Blunt Trauma	Acute Ocular Hypotony	Spontaneous Detachment with Uveal Effusion as Nonrhegmatogenous Retinal Detachment
Physical Findings						
33. Retinal hemorrhage			S	S′		
34. Retinal microaneurysms		U				
35. Retinal vein occlusion		S				
36. Scleral rupture				S	S	
37. Shallow anterior chamber					S	
38. Subluxed lens				S		
39. Sympathetic ophthalmitis	U					
40. Uveitis	U					
41. Vitreous detachment				S		S
42. Vitreous hemorrhage			S	S		
43. Vitreous opacities	U					
44. White lashes	U					
Laboratory Data						
1. Abnormal blood sugar		U				
2. Computed tomographic scan of globe			S	S		
3. Fluorescein angiography	U	U	U	U		S
4. Phosphorus 32 uptake elevated			U			
5. Ultrasonography, globe	S		S	U	U	U

R = rarely; S = sometimes; and U = usually.

Lesions Confused with Malignant Melanoma

1. Ciliary body and choroid
   - A. Angioid streaks (see p. 586)
   - B. Choroiditis
   - C. Coats disease
   - D. Detachment
   - E. Leukemia and lymphoma
   - F. Limited choroidal hemorrhage
   - G. Lymphoid hyperplasia
   - H. Nodular hyperplasia
   - I. Sclerouveitis
   - J. Tumors
     - (1) Hemangioma
     - (2) Melanocytoma
     - (3) Meningioma
     - (4) Metastic carcinoma
     - (5) Neurilemmoma
     - (6) Neurofibroma
     - (7) Nevus
   - K. Uveal effusion
2. Optic nerve head
   - A. Congenital crater
   - B. Melanocytoma
3. Retina
   - A. Chorioretinitis
   - B. Ciliary body and choroid
   - C. Disciform macular degeneration
   - D. Foreign body
   - E. Hemorrhagic macrocyst of retina
   - F. Lesions of pigment epithelium
   - G. Retinal detachment
     - (1) Macular
     - (2) More extensive
   - H. Retinoschisis
4. Vitreous body
   - A. Abscess
   - B. Hemorrhages

Morgan, C.M., and Gragoudas, E.S.: Limited choroidal hemorrhage mistaken for a choroidal melanoma. Ophthalmology, 94:41–46, 1987.

Saraux, H.: Strabismus and Tumors of the Uvea. Basel, Switzerland, Karger, 1981.

Shields, J.A., and Shields, C.L.: Intraocular Tumors: A Text and Atlas. W.B. Saunders Co., Philadelphia, 1992.

Strempel, I.: Rare choroidal tumors simulating a malignant melanoma. Ophthalmologica, 202: 110–114, 1991.

Choroidal Hemorrhage

1. Acute choroiditis
*2. After glaucoma filtering procedure (especially with Sturge-Weber syndrome)
3. Choroidal vascular aneurysm
4. Choroidal vascular sclerosis, such as senile macular degeneration with hemorrhage (disciform degeneration of the macula)
5. General diseases
    A. Arteriosclerosis
    B. Blood dyscrasias
        (1) Leukemia
        (2) Pernicious anemia
        (3) Purpura
        (4) Thrombocytopenia
    C. Diabetes mellitus (Willis disease)
    D. Ehlers-Danlos syndrome (fibrodysplasia elastica generalisata)
    E. Paget disease (osteitis deformans)
    F. Valsalva maneuver
6. Myopia—accompanied by choroidal atrophy
7. Papilledema—rare

Boker, T., and Steinmetz, R.: Hyperopia and Choroidal Neovascularization. Ophthal.,: 101:972, 1994.

Dhir, S.P., et al.: Choroidal vascular aneurysm with massive choroidal hemorrhage. Ann. Ophthal. 24:182–184, 1992.

Piper, J.G., et al.: Perioperative choroidal hemorrhage at pars plana vitrectomy. A case-control study. Ophthal., 100:699–704, 1993.

Roy, F.H.: Ocular Syndromes and Systemic Diseases. 2nd Ed. Philadelphia, W.B. Saunders, 1989.

VanMeurs, J.C., and van der Bosch, W.A.: Suprachoroidal hemorrhage following a Valsalva maneuver. Arch. Ophthal., 111:1025–1026, 1993.

Choroidal Detachment (May Be Differentiated from Retinal Detachment and Tumor by Solid Appearance, Smooth Surface, and Appearance of Normal Retinal Vessels with Color Unchanged and Good Transillumination)

*1. Acute ocular hypotony (see p. 367)
    A. Myopia
    B. Operative or perforating wounds, including those required for surgical treatment of cataract, glaucoma, grafting of cornea, and retinal detachment
    C. Severe uveitis with severe visual loss, intense ocular pain, unusually low tension, and extremely deep anterior chamber in women
    D. YAG laser cyclophotocoagulation

* = most important

2. Inflammatory disease

   A. Acute sinusitis

   B. Chronic cyclitis

   C. Harada disease (Vogt-Koyanagi-Harada syndrome)

   D. Orbital abscess

   E. Orbital pseudotumor

   F. Scleritis and tenonitis

   G. Sympathetic ophthalmia

3. Neoplastic disease

   A. Intraocular tumor, such as metastatic or malignant melanoma

   B. Leukemia

   C. Orbital tumor

4. Spontaneous detachment associated with uveal effusion, such as nonrhegmatogenous retinal detachment, shifting subretinal fluid, and peripheral annular choroidal detachment affecting males almost exclusively

5. Trauma

   A. Complication of scleral buckling retinal detachment surgery

   B. Contusion of globe without perforation

   C. Following perforation injury, including that because of perforating corneal ulcer

   D. Phthisical eye with traction of organized inflammatory tissue

6. Vascular disease

   A. Diabetes mellitus (Willis disease)

   B. Disseminated intravascular coagulation

   C. Hypertension

   D. Leukemia

   E. Multiple myeloma (Kahler disease)

   F. Nephritis

   G. Oral acetazolamide

   H. Periarteritis nodosa (Kussmaul disease)

   I. Syphilitic vascular disease

   J. Toxemia of pregnancy

Allinson, R.W., et al.: Recurrent hemorrhagic choroidal detachment associated with disseminated intravascular coagulation. Annal. Ophthal., 24:72–74, 1992.

Fan, J.T., et al.: Transient myopia, angle-closure glaucoma, and choroidal detachment after oral acetazolamide. Amer. J. Ophthal., 115:813–814, 1993.

Kurtz, S., et al.: Orbital pseudotumor presenting as acute glaucoma with choroidal and retinal detachment. German J. Ophthal., 2:61–62, 1993.

Lakhanpal, V.: Experimental and clinical observations on massive suprachoroidal hemorrhage. Transactions of the Amer. Ophthal. Society, 91:545–652, 1993.

Magruder, G.B., and Harbin, T.S.: Ciliochoroidal detachment associated with stretched ciliary processes. Am. J. Ophthalmol., 106:357–359, 1988.

Roy, F.H.: Ocular Syndromes and Systemic Diseases. 2nd Ed. Philadelphia, W.B. Saunders, 1989.

Wang, M.L., et al.: Total choroidal detachment complicating dural arteriovenous sinus fistula. Ophthalmic Surgery, 24:856–857, 1993.

Conditions Simulating Posterior Uveitis or Choroiditis

1. Angioid streaks (see p. 586)
2. Central serous retinopathy
   A. Central serous retinopathy and exudative chorioretinopathy associated with systemic vasculitis
   B. Central serous retinopathy associated with crater-like holes in the optic disc
   C. Choroidal
   D. Chorioretinal
   E. Retinal
3. Chorioretinopathy with hereditary microcephaly
4. Circinate retinopathy
5. Congenital macular dysplasia
6. Doyne homogeneous retinal degeneration
7. Drug-induced macular disease
   A. Chloroquine (Aralen)
   B. Indomethacin (Indocin)
   C. Thioridazine (Mellaril)
8. Drusen because of
   A. Disease (vascular, inflammatory, or neoplastic)
   B. Heredity (primary degeneration)
   C. Senility
9. Fundus flavimaculatus
10. Helicoid peripapillary chorioretinal degeneration
11. Hemangioma of the choroid
12. Idiopathic hyperlipemia
13. Ischemic ocular inflammation
14. Ischemic optic neuropathy (vascular pseudopapillitis)
15. Jensen disease (juxtapapillary retinopathy)
16. Macular degeneration
17. Malignant melanoma
18. Metastatic carcinoma
19. Night-blinding retinochoroidopathies
    A. Predominantly choroidal heredodegenerations
       (1) Choroidal sclerosis
       (2) Choroideremia
       (3) Fuchs spot
       (4) Gyrate atrophy of choroid
       (5) Myopic retinopathy and choroidopathy

    B. Predominantly taperetinal heredodegenerations

      (1) Retinitis pigmentosa group

      (2) Retinitis punctata albescens

20. Opacities of the macular retina

    A. Cotton-wool patches (see p. 548)

    B. Glial scars

    C. Hemorrhage

    D. Hemosiderin

    E. Inspissated exudates

    F. Lipoid deposits

    G. Pigment epithelium

      (1) Pigment epithelium migration

      (2) Pigment epithelium secretion

      (3) Pigment epithelium seeds

      (4) Proliferation in response to demand for phagocytes

      (5) Proliferation with formation of cuticular masses

      (6) Proliferation with metaplasia

      (7) Simple proliferation

21. Peripheral chorioretinal atrophy

22. Pigmentary perivenous—chorioretinal degeneration

23. Primary familial amyloidosis

24. Relapsing polychondritis

25. Retinal perforation during surgical treatment for strabismus

26. Retinal vasculitis

    A. Involvement of central retinal vein (papillophlebitis)

    B. Retinal periarteritis

    C. Retinal periphlebitis

27. Retinoblastoma

28. Sickle cell retinopathy

29. Solar burns

30. Sorsby pseudoinflammatory (hemorrhagic) macular degeneration

31. Vitreous hemorrhage (see p. 474)

Schlaegel, T.F.: Essentials of Uveitis. Boston, Little, Brown and Co., 1969.

Suran, A., et al.: Immunology of the Eye, Workshop III. Immunologic Aspects of Ocular Disease: Infection, Inflammation and Allergy. Oxford, England, IRL Press, 1981.

Choroiditis (Posterior Uveitis)

1. Anterior and posterior uveitis

    A. Herpes viruses

    B. Peripheral uveitis (cyclitis)

      C. Sarcoidosis syndrome (Schaumann syndrome)

      D. Syphilis (acquired lues)

      E. Toxoplasmosis

      F. Tuberculosis

      G. Unknown

      H. Vogt-Koyanagi-Harada syndrome (uveitis-vitiligo-alopecia-poliosis syndrome)

2. Acquired immune deficiency syndrome

3. Acute posterior multifocal placoid pigment epitheliopathy

4. Behcet's disease

5. Birdshot choroidopathy

6. Candidiasis

7. Cryptococcosis

8. Cytomegalovirus inclusion disease

9. Coccidioidomycosis

10. Epstein-Barr virus

11. Lyme disease

12. Histoplasmosis

13. Multiple evanescent white dot syndrome

14. Multiple sclerosis

15. Pneumocystis carinii

16. Punctate inner choroidopathy

17. Sarcoidosis syndrome (Schaumann syndrome)

18. Serpiginous choroidopathy

19. Syphilis (acquired lues)

20. Systemic lupus erythematosus

21. Toxocariasis

*22. Toxoplasmosis

23. Unknown

24. Varicella zoster

Kerrison, J.R., et al.: Retinal pathologic changes in multiple sclerosis. Retina, 14:445–451, 1994.

Kraus, M., et al.: Uveitis-Pathophysiology and Therapy. 2nd Ed. New York, Thieme, 1986.

Schubert, H.D., et al.: Cytologically proven seronegative Lyme choroiditis and vitreitis. Retina 14:39–41, 1994.

Seregard, S.: Retinochoroiditis in the acquired immune deficiency syndrome. Findings in consecutive post-morten examinations. Acta. Ophthal., 72:223–228, 1994.

Conditions Simulating Posterior Uveitis in Children

1. Coats syndrome (retinal telangiectasia)

2. Cockayne disease (dwarfism with retinal atrophy and deafness)

3. Cystinosis syndrome (Lignac-Fanconi syndrome)

4. Hypogammaglobulinemia

* = most important

5. Idiopathic hyperlipemia

6. Leukemia

7. Massive retinal fibrosis

*8. Retinoblastoma

Freidman, A.H., et al.: An Atlas of Uveitis, Diagnosis and Management. Baltimore, Williams & Wilkins, 1982.

Kraus, M., et al.: Uveitis—Pathophysiology and Therapy. 2nd Ed. New York, Thieme, 1986.

Schlaegel, T.F.: Essentials of Uveitis. Boston, Little, Brown and Company, 1969, pp. 71–75.

Choroiditis (Posterior Uveitis) in Children

1. Ankylosing spondylitis

2. Anterior and posterior uveitis

    A. Sarcoidosis syndrome (Schaumann syndrome)

    B. Sympathetic ophthalmia

    C. Vogt-Koyanagi-Harada syndrome

3. Arteritis

4. Behçet disease (dermatostomato-ophthalmic syndrome)

5. Chorioretinitis of unknown cause

    A. Disseminated chorioretinitis

    B. Juxtapapillary chorioretinitis

6. Cytomegalovirus inclusion disease (cytomegalovirus)

7. Diffuse unilateral subacute neuroretinitis

8. Herpes simplex chorioretinitis

9. Human immunodeficiency virus retinopathy

10. Inability of leukocytes to kill micro-organisms

11. Intermediate uveitis

12. Juvenile psoriatic arthritis

13. Juvenile rheumatoid arthritis

14. Nematode (Toxocara) retinochoroiditis

15. Reiter disease (idiopathic blennorrheal arthritis syndrome)

16. Reticulum cell sarcoma of brain

17. Rubella

18. Subacute sclerosing panencephalitis

19. Syphilitic retinochoroiditis

*20. Toxoplasmic retinochoroiditis

21. Tuberculosis

Kanski, J.J., and Shun-Shin, A.: Systemic uveitis syndrome in childhood: An analysis of cases. Ophthalmology, 91:1247–1251, 1984.

Kraus, M., et al.: Uveitis-Pathophysiology and Therapy. New York. 2nd Ed. Thieme, 1986.

Okada, A.A., and Foster, C.S.: Posterior Uveitis in the Pediatric Population. International Ophthalmology Clinics, 32:121–152, 1992.

Syndromes and Diseases Associated with Uveitis

1. Arthralgia
    A. Hilding syndrome (destructive iridocyclitis and multiple joint dislocations)
    B. Histoplasmosis
    C. Whipple disease (intestinal lipodystrophy)
2. Arthritis
    A. Ankylosing spondylitis
    B. Behçet syndrome (dermatostomato-ophthalmic syndrome)
    C. Bleu's syndrome
    D. Familial histiocytic dermatoarthritis syndrome
    E. Felty syndrome (rheumatoid arthritis with hypersplenism)
    F. Gonorrhea
    G. Juvenile rheumatoid arthritis (Still disease)
    H. Leprosy (Hansen disease)
    I. Mucocutaneous lymph node syndrome
    J. Progressive systemic sclerosis
    K. Psoriatic arthritis
    L. Reiter syndrome (polyarthritis enterica)
    M. Rheumatoid arthritis (adult)
    N. Sarcoidosis syndrome (Schaumann syndrome)
    O. Sporotrichosis
    P. Ulcerative colitis
    Q. Van Metre peripheral polyarthritis or monoarthritis
    R. Whipple disease (intestinal lipodystrophy)
    S. Yersiniosis
3. Cataract
    A. Acrodermatitis chronica atrophicans
    B. Andogsky syndrome (dermatogenous cataract)
    C. Anterior segment ischemia syndrome
    D. Arteriovenous fistula
    E. Atopic dermatitis
    F. Carotid artery syndrome (carotid vascular insufficiency syndrome)
    G. Cerebral palsy
    H. Chickenpox
    I. Cockayne syndrome (dwarfism with retinal atrophy and deafness)
    J. Cytomegalic inclusion disease
    K. Electrical injury
    L. Familial histiocytic dermatoarthritis syndrome
    M. Hallermann-Streiff-François syndrome (dyscephalic mandibulo-oculo facial syndrome)

* = most important

   N. Herpes simplex

   O. Herpes zoster

   P. Hilding syndrome (destructive iridocyclitis and multiple joint dislocations)

   Q. Histiocytosis X (Hand-Schüller-Christian syndrome)

   R. Hodgkin disease (lymph node disease)

   S. Homocystinuria syndrome

   T. Hypervitaminosis D

   U. Influenza

   V. Juvenile rheumatoid arthritis (Still disease)

   W. Kussmaul disease (periarteritis nodosa)

   X. Leptospirosis (Weil disease)

   Y. Listerellosis

   Z. Malaria

  AA. Measles (rubeola)

  BB. Moniliasis (idiopathic hypoparathyroidism)

  CC. Myotonic dystrophy syndrome

  DD. Oculo-oto-ororenoerythropoietic disease

  EE. Passow syndrome (syringomyelia)

  FF. Radiation

  GG. Relapsing polychondritis

  HH. Rubella syndrome

   II. Sarcoidosis syndrome (Schaumann syndrome)

   JJ. Stevens-Johnson syndrome (erythema multiforme exudativum)

  KK. Stickler syndrome (hereditary progressive arthro-ophthal-myopathy)

  LL. Toxocariasis (visceral larva migrans syndrome)

  MM. Toxoplasmosis

  NN. Werner syndrome (progeria of adults)

  OO. Yersiniosis

4. Conjunctivitis

   A. Acanthamoeba

   B. Actinomycosis

   C. African eyeworm disease

   D. Amebiasis

   E. Andogsky syndrome (dermatogenous cataract)

   F. Angular conjunctivitis

   G. Ascariasis

   H. Atopic dermatitis

   I. Bacillary dysentery (shigellosis)

   J. Bacterial endocarditis

   K. Behçet syndrome (dermatostomato-ophthalmic syndrome)

    L. Boutonneuse fever (Rickettsia, Marseilles fever)

    M. Brucellosis

    N. Candidiasis

    O. Charlin syndrome (nasal nerve syndrome)

    P. Chlamydia

    Q. Coccidioidomycosis

    R. Coenurosis

    S. Cogan syndrome (nonsyphilitic interstitial keratitis)

    T. Crohn disease (granulomatous ileocolitis)

    U. Cytomegalic inclusion disease

    V. Disseminated lupus erythematosus (Kaposi-Libman-Sacks syndrome)

    W. Epidermic keratoconjunctivitis

    X. Escherichia coli

    Y. Felty syndrome (rheumatoid arthritis with hypersplenism)

    Z. Hemophilus aegyptius

  AA. Herpes simplex

  BB. Herpes zoster

  CC. Hodgkin disease

  DD. Infectious mononucleosis

  EE. Influenza

  FF. Kussmaul disease (periarteritis nodosa)

  GG. Leptospirosis (Weil disease)

  HH. Listerellosis

   II. Lymphogranuloma venereum

   JJ. Measles (rubeola)

  KK. Meningococcemia

  LL. Metastatic bacterial endophthalmitis

 MM. Mikulicz-Radecki syndrome (dacryosialoadenopathy)

  NN. Moniliasis (idiopathic hypoparathyroidism)

  OO. Moraxella lacunata

  PP. Mucocutaneous lymph node syndrome

  QQ. Mumps

  RR. Mycosis fungoides syndrome (Sezary syndrome)

  SS. Nocardiosis

  TT. Ocular vaccinia

  UU. Pneumococcus

  VV. Polymyositis dermatomyositis

 WW. Progressive systemic sclerosis (scleroderma)

  XX. Psoriatic arthritis

  YY. Q fever

    ZZ. Radiation

  AAA. Reiter syndrome (polyarthritis enterica)

  BBB. Relapsing fever

  CCC. Rocky Mountain spotted fever

  DDD. Rubella syndrome

   EEE. St. Anthony fire (erysipelas)

   FFF. Seborrheic dermatitis

  GGG. Sporotrichosis

  HHH. Staphylococcus

    III. Stevens-Johnson syndrome (erythema multiforme exudativum)

   JJJ. Streptococcus

  KKK. Syphilis (acquired lues)

   LLL. Trichinellosis

 MMM. Tuberculosis

  NNN. Vaccinia

  OOO. Xeroderma pigmentosum

   PPP. Yersiniosis

5. Cornea

   A. Acanthamoeba

   B. Acrodermatitis chronic atrophicans

   C. Actinomycosis

   D. African eyeworm disease

   E. Andogsky syndrome (dermatogenous cataract)

   F. Angioedema (Quincke disease)

   G. Angular conjunctivitis (Morax-Axenfeld bacillus)

   H. Ankylosing spondylitis

   I. Anterior segment ischemia syndrome

   J. Arteriovenous fistula

   K. Atopic dermatitis

   L. Bee sting of the cornea

   M. Behçet syndrome (dermatostomato-ophthalmic syndrome)

   N. Brucellosis (Bang disease)

   O. Candidiasis

   P. Charlin syndrome (nasal nerve syndrome)

   Q. Chickenpox

   R. Chlamydia

   S. Cockayne syndrome (dwarfism with retinal atrophy and deafness)

   T. Cogan syndrome (I) (nonsyphilitic interstitial keratitis)

   U. Crohn disease (granulomatous ileocolitis)

   V. Cystinosis syndrome

   W. Cytomegalic inclusion disease

   X. Disseminated lupus erythematous (Kaposi-Libman-Sacks syndrome)

   Y. Electrical injury

   Z. Epidemic keratoconjunctivitis

  AA. Escherichia coli

  BB. Felty syndrome (rheumatoid arthritis with hypersplenism)

  CC. Gonorrhea

  DD. Hemophilus aegyptius

  EE. Herpes simplex

  FF. Herpes zoster

  GG. Hilding syndrome (destructive iridocyclitis and multiple joint dislocations)

  HH. Histiocytosis X (Hand-Schüller-Christian syndrome)

  II. Hodgkin disease (lymph node disease)

  JJ. Homocystinuria syndrome

  KK. Hypervitaminosis D

  LL. Hypothermal injury

 MM. Influenza

  NN. Japanese River fever (mite borne typhus)

  OO. Juvenile rheumatoid arthritis (Still disease)

  PP. Juvenile xanthogranuloma (nevoxanthoendothelioma)

  QQ. Kussmaul disease (periarteritis nodosa)

  RR. Leprosy (Hansen disease)

  SS. Leptospirosis (Weil disease)

  TT. Lewis syndrome (tuberoserpiginous syphilid of Lewis)

  UU. Listerellosis

  VV. Lockjaw

 WW. Lymphogranuloma venereum

  XX. Malaria

  YY. Measles (rubeola)

  ZZ. Meningococcemia

 AAA. Mikulicz-Radecki syndrome (dacryosialoadenopathy)

 BBB. Moniliasis-idiopathic hypoparathyroidism (Addison syndrome)

 CCC. Moraxella lacunata

DDD. Mumps

 EEE. Mycosis fungoides syndrome (Sezary syndrome)

 FFF. Myotonic dystrophy syndrome

GGG. Nocardiosis

HHH. Ocular vaccinia

  III. Onchocerciasis syndrome

  JJJ. Passow syndrome (status dysraphicus)

KKK. Plague

LLL. Pneumococcus

MMM. Postvaccinial ocular syndrome

NNN. Progressive systemic sclerosis (scleroderma)

OOO. Psoriasis

PPP. Psoriatic arthritis

QQQ. Radiation

RRR. Reiter syndrome (polyarthritis enterica)

SSS. Relapsing fever

TTT. Relapsing polychondritis

UUU. Rheumatoid arthritis (adult)

VVV. Rubella syndrome

WWW. St. Anthony fire (erysipelas)

XXX. Sarcoidosis syndrome (Schaumann syndrome)

YYY. Seborrheic dermatitis

ZZZ. Sporotrichosis

AAAA. Staphylococcus

BBBB. Stevens-Johnson syndrome (erythema multiforme exudativum)

CCCC. Stickler syndrome (hereditary progressive arthro-ophthal-mopathy)

DDDD. Streptococcus

EEEE. Syphilis

FFFF. Thelaziasis

GGGG. Toxoplasmosis

HHHH. Tuberculosis

IIII. Vaccinia

JJJJ. Werner syndrome (progeria of adults)

KKKK. Xeroderma pigmentosum

LLLL. Yersiniosis

6. Diarrhea

   A. Amebiasis

   B. Bacillary dysentery

   C. Chlamydia

   D. Crohn disease (granulomatous ileocolitis)

   E. Escherichia coli

   F. Listerellosis

   G. Psoriatic arthritis

   H. Regional enteritis (ulcerative colitus)

   I. Rubella syndrome

   J. Staphylococcus

   K. Ulcerative colitis (regional enteritis)

L. Whipple disease (intestinal lipodystrophy)

M. Yersiniosis

7. Disc neovascularization

    A. Ischemic uveitis of Knox

    B. Papillophlebitis

8. Exophthalmus (proptosis)

    A. Actinomycosis

    B. Angioedema

    C. Arteriovenous fistula

    D. Coenurosis

    E. Cryptococcosis

    F. Disseminated lupus erythematosus (Kaposi-Libman-Sacks syndrome)

    G. Hallermann-Streiff-François syndrome (dyscephalic mandibulo-oculo facial syndrome)

    H. Herpes zoster

    I. Histiocytosis X (Hand-Schüller-Christian syndrome)

    J. Juvenile xanthogranuloma (nevoxanthoendothelioma)

    K. Kussmaul disease (periarteritis nodosa)

    L. Mumps

    M. Polymyositis dermatomyositis

    N. Relapsing polychondritis

    O. Streptococcus

    P. Trichinellosis

    Q. Werner syndrome (progeria of adults)

9. Exudative detachment

    A. Acute retinal necrosis syndrome

    B. Bacterial endocarditis

    C. Boutonneuse fever (Rickettsia, Marseilles fever)

    D. Cryptococcosis

    E. Histiocytosis X (Hand-Schüller-Christian syndrome)

    F. Japanese River fever (typhus)

    G. Kussmaul disease (periarteritis nodosa)

    H. Mycosis fungoides syndrome

    I. Oculo-oto-ororenoerythopoietic disease

    J. Pappataci fever (sandfly fever)

    K. Periocular and ocular metastatic tumors

    L. Progressive systemic sclerosis (scleroderma)

    M. Rheumatic fever

    N. Rocky Mountain spotted fever

    O. Sarcoidosis syndrome (Schaumann syndrome)

    P. Schwartz syndrome (glaucoma associated with retinal detachment)

    Q. Stickler syndrome (hereditary progressive arthro-ophthal-mopathy)

    R. Toxocariasis (visceral larva migrans syndrome)

    S. Toxoplasmosis

    T. Weber-Christian syndrome (subcutaneous inflammatory lesions)

10. Glaucoma

    A. Acanthamoeba

    B. Angioedema

    C. Arteriovenous fistula

    D. Acariasis

    E. Atopic dermatitis

    F. Behçet syndrome (dermatostomato-ophthalmic syndrome)

    G. Brucellosis (late manifestation) (Bang disease)

    H. Carotid artery syndrome

    I. Coats disease (retinal telangiectasia)

    J. Coccidioidomycosis

    K. Coenurosis

    L. Electrical injury

    M. Escherichia coli

    N. Familial histiocytic dermatoarthritis syndrome

    O. Hallermann-Streiff-François syndrome (dyscephalic mandibulo-oculo facial syndrome)

    P. Homocystinuria syndrome

    Q. Juvenile rheumatoid arthritis (Still disease)

    R. Juvenile xanthogranuloma (nevoxanthoendothelioma)

    S. Leprosy (Hansen disease)

    T. Listerellosis

    U. Measles (rubeola)

    V. Oculo-oto-ororenoerythropoietic disease

    W. Onchocerciasis syndrome

    X. Periocular and ocular metastatic tumors

    Y. Pneumococcus

    Z. Posner-Schlossman syndrome (glaucomatocyclitic crisis)

    AA. Pseudouveitis, glaucoma, hyphema syndrome (PUGH syndrome)

    BB. Radiation

    CC. Relapsing polychondritis

    DD. Rubella syndrome

    EE. Sarcoidosis syndrome (Schaumann syndrome)

    FF. Schwartz syndrome (glaucoma associated with retinal detachment)

    GG. Staphylococcus

    HH. Stickler syndrome (hereditary progressive arthro-ophthalmopathy)

    II. Streptococcus

    JJ. Trichinellosis

    KK. Uveitis, glaucoma, hyphema syndrome (UGH syndrome)

    LL. Weber-Christian syndrome (subcutaneous inflammatory lesions)

11. Hepatomegaly

    A. Cytomegalic inclusions disease

    B. Toxocariasis (visceral larva migrans syndrome)

    C. Toxoplasmosis

12. Influenza-like disease

    A. Acanthamoeba

    B. Amebiasis

    C. Bacillary dysentery

    D. Boutonneuse fever (rickettsia, Marseilles fever)

    E. Brucellosis (Bang disease)

    F. Chickenpox

    G. Chlamydia

    H. Escherichia coli

    I. Gonorrhea

    J. Hemophilus aegyptius

    K. Histoplasmosis

    L. Influenza

    M. Japanese River fever (mite-borne typhus)

    N. Leptospirosis (Weil disease)

    O. Malaria

    P. Measles (rubeola)

    Q. Meningococcemia

    R. Mumps

    S. Pappataci fever (sandfly fever)

    T. Plague (bubonic plague)

    U. Pneumococcus

    V. Q fever

    W. Relapsing fever

    X. Rocky Mountain spotted fever

    Y. Staphylococcus

    Z. Streptococcus

    AA. Toxoplasmosis

    BB. Tuberculosis

13. Iris neovascularization, such as Knox ischemic ocular inflammation (rubeosis iridis)

14. Jaundice

    A. Leptospirosis

15. Meningism (meningitis)
    A. Acanthamoeba
    B. Behçet syndrome (dermatostomato-ophthalmic syndrome)
    C. Cryptococcosis
    D. Gonorrhea
    E. Herpes simplex
    F. Histoplasmosis
    G. Leptospirosis (Weil disease)
    H. Listerellosis
    I. Meningococcemia
    J. Sympathetic ophthalmia
    K. Toxoplasmosis
    L. Tuberculosis
16. Microphthalmia
    A. Cytomegalic inclusion disease
    B. Hallermann-Streiff-François syndrome (dyscephalic mandibulo-oculo facial syndrome)
    C. Mumps
    D. Rubella syndrome
    E. Toxoplasmosis
17. Nodules in the leg
    A. Histoplasmosis
    B. Sarcoidosis syndrome (Schaumann syndrome)
    C. Ulcerative colitis
18. Optic neuritis (papillitis)
    A. Angioedema
    B. Behçet syndrome (dermatostomato-ophthalmic syndrome)
    C. Boutonneuse fever (rickettsia, Marseilles fever)
    D. Brucellosis (Bang disease)
    E. Candidiasis
    F. Chickenpox
    G. Cytomegalic inclusion disease
    H. Disseminated lupus erythematosus (Kaposi-Libman-Sacks syndrome)
    I. Electrical injury
    J. Felty syndrome (rheumatoid arthritis with hypersplenism)
    K. Herpes zoster
    L. Hodgkin disease (lymph node disease)
    M. Infectious mononucleosis
    N. Influenza
    O. Juvenile rheumatoid arthritis (Still disease)

    P. Leptospirosis

    Q. Malaria

    R. Measles

    S. Meningococcemia

    T. Mikulicz-Radecki syndrome (dacryosialoadenopathy)

    U. Mumps

    V. Ocular vaccinia

    W. Onchocerciasis syndrome

    X. Pappataci fever (sandfly fever)

    Y. Postvaccinial ocular syndrome

    Z. Q fever

  AA. Reiter syndrome (polyarthritis enterica)

  BB. Regional enteritis (ulcerative colitis)

  CC. Rocky Mountain spotted fever

  DD. Sarcoidosis syndrome (Schaumann syndrome)

  EE. Stevens-Johnson syndrome (erythema multiforme exudativum)

  FF. Streptococcus

  GG. Sympathetic ophthalmia

  HH. Syphilis (acquired lues)

   II. Toxocariasis (visceral larva migrans syndrome)

   JJ. Toxoplasmosis

  KK. Trichinellosis

  LL. Tuberculosis

 MM. Vaccinia

19. Papilledema

    A. Angioedema

    B. Arteriovenous fistula

    C. Acariasis

    D. Bacterial endocarditis

    E. Behçet syndrome (dermatostomato-ophthalmic syndrome)

    F. Brucellosis (Bang disease)

    G. Chickenpox

    H. Coccidioidomycosis

    I. Cryptococcosis

    J. Cysticercosis

    K. Disseminated lupus erythematosus (Kaposi-Libman-Sacks syndrome)

    L. Histiocytosis X (Hand-Schüller-Christian syndrome)

    M. Hodgkin disease (lymph node disease)

    N. Hypervitaminosis D

    O. Malaria

P. Moniliasis—idiopathic hypoparathyroidism (Addison disease)

Q. Mycosis fungoides syndrome (Sezary syndrome)

R. Papillophlebitis

S. Pappataci fever (sandfly fever)

T. Passow syndrome (status dysraphicus)

U. Periocular and ocular metastatic tumors

V. Progressive systemic sclerosis

W. Sarcoidosis syndrome (Schaumann syndrome)

X. Syphilis

Y. Trichinellosis

Z. Whipple disease (intestinal lipodystrophy)

20. Paralysis of extraocular muscle

A. African eyeworm disease

B. Arteriovenous fistula

C. Bacterial endocarditis

D. Brucellosis

E. Cerebral palsy

F. Chickenpox

G. Coccidioidomycosis

H. Cysticercosis

I. Disseminated lupus erythematosus

J. Electrical injury

K. Herpes simplex

L. Herpes zoster

M. Hodgkin disease (lymph node disease)

N. Hypothermal injury

O. Infectious mononucleosis

P. Influenza

Q. Kussmaul disease (periarteritis nodosa)

R. Lockjaw (tetanus)

S. Malaria

T. Measles (rubeola)

U. Meningococcemia

V. Multiple sclerosis

W. Mumps

X. Ocular vaccinia

Y. Passow syndrome (status dysraphicus)

Z. Periocular and ocular metastatic tumors

AA. Reiter syndrome (polyarthritis enterica)

BB. Relapsing fever

CC. Relapsing polychondritis

DD. Rocky Mountain spotted fever

EE. Streptococcus

FF. Syphilis (acquired lues)

GG. Trichinellosis

21. Perivenous sheathing

A. Acanthamoeba

B. Amebiasis

C. Boutonneuse fever (rickettsia, Marseilles fever)

D. Brucellosis (Bang disease)

E. Candidiasis

F. Coccidioidomycosis

G. Metastatic bacterial endophthalmitis

H. Metastatic fungal endophthalmitis

I. Multiple sclerosis

J. Myotonic dystrophy syndrome

K. Ocular vaccinia

L. Onchocerciasis syndrome

M. Plague

N. Postvaccinial ocular syndrome

O. Q fever

P. Sarcoidosis syndrome (Schaumann syndrome)

Q. Syphilis (acquired lues)

R. Toxocariasis (visceral larva migrans syndrome)

S. Toxoplasmosis

T. Tuberculosis

U. Vaccinia

V. Weber-Christian syndrome (subcutaneous inflammatory lesions)

22. Pneumonitis

A. Chlamydia

B. Cytomegalic inclusion disease

C. Plague (Bubonic plague)

D. Pneumococcus

E. Rubella syndrome

F. Toxocariasis

G. Whipple disease (intestinal lipodystrophy)

23. Prostatitis

A. Gonococcosis

B. Whipple disease (intestinal lipodystrophy)

24. Salt-and-pepper fundus

A. Choroideremia in males

    B. Cockayne disease (dwarfism with retinal atrophy and deafness)

    C. Cystinosis

    D. Prenatal influenza

    E. Prenatal syphilis

25. Skin lesions

    A. Acrodermatitis chronica atrophicans

    B. African eyeworm disease

    C. Andogsky syndrome (dermatogenous cataract)

    D. Angioedema

    E. Atopic dermatitis

    F. Behçet syndrome (dermatostomato-ophthalmic syndrome)

    G. Chickenpox

    H. Disseminated lupus erythematosus (Kaposi-Libman Sacks syndrome)

    I. Familial histiocytic dermatoarthritis syndrome

    J. Herpes simplex

    K. Herpes zoster

    L. Histiocytosis X (Hand-Schüller-Christian syndrome)

    M. Juvenile xanthogranuloma (nevoxanthoendothelioma)

    N. Leprosy (Hansen disease)

    O. Lewis syndrome (tuberoserphiginous syphilid of Lewis)

    P. Listerellosis

    Q. Measles (rubeola)

    R. Moraxella lacunata

    S. Mucocutaneous lymph node syndrome

    T. Mycosis fungoides syndrome (Sezary syndrome)

    U. Polymyositis dermatomyositis

    V. Postvaccinial ocular syndrome

    W. Psoriasis

    X. Psoriatic arthritis

    Y. St. Anthony fire (erysipelas)

    Z. Schistosomiasis (bilharziasis)

    AA. Seborrheic dermatitis

    BB. Sporotrichosis

    CC. Staphylococcus

26. Stomatitis

    A. Behçet syndrome (dermatostomato-ophthalmic syndrome)

    B. Disseminated systemic histoplasmosis—not the ocular form

    C. Herpes simplex

    D. Lewis syndrome (tuberoserphiginous syphilid of Lewis)

    E. Reiter syndrome (polyarthritis enterica)

F. Regional enteritis

G. Ulcerative colitis

27. Tonsillitis

A. Whipple disease (intestinal lipodystrophy)

28. Trauma (nonpenetrating)

Bunchman, T.E., and Bloom, J.N.: A syndrome of acute interstitial nephritis and anterior uveitis. Pediatric Nephrology, 7: 520–522, 1993.

Friedman, A.H., et al.: An Atlas of Uveitis, Diagnosis and Management. Baltimore, Williams & Wilkins, 1982.

Harvey, A.S., et al.: Chronic encephalitis (Rasmorsen's syndrome) and ipsilateral uveitis. Annals of Neurology, 32:826–829, 1992.

James, D.G.: A comparison of Blau's syndrome and sarcoidosis. Sarcoidosis, 11:100–101, 1994.

Kraus, M., et al.: Uveitis-Pathophysiology and Therapy. 2nd Ed. New York, Thieme, 1986.

Peyman, G.A., et al.: Principles and Practice of Ophthalmology. Philadelphia, W. B. Saunders, 1980.

Rosenbaum, J.T., et al.: Uveitis precipitated by nonpenetrating ocular trauma. Am. J. Ophthalmol., 112:392–395, 1991.

Roy, F.H.: Ocular Syndromes and Systemic Diseases. 2nd Ed. Philadelphia, W. B. Saunders, 1989.

Schlaegel, T.F.: Essentials of Uveitis. Boston, Little, Brown & Company, New York, 1983.

Chorioretinitis Juxtapapillaris (Large, Irregular Opaque Mass that Protrudes Three to Four Diopters and Obscures the Retinal Vessels Is Seen Near the Disc; May Be Confused with Acute Optic Neuritis or a Tumor)

1. Acanthamoeba keratitis of fellow eye

2. Bird-shot retinochoroidopathy

3. Coccidioides immitis

4. Histoplasmosis

5. Sarcoidosis syndrome (Schaumann syndrome)

6. Syphilis (acquired lues)

7. Toxoplasmosis

8. Tuberculosis

Eide, N., and Skjeldal, O.: Juxtapapillary chorioretinitis in neurosyphilis. Acta. Ophthalmol. (Copenh.), 62:351–358, 1984.

Haessler, F.H.: Eye Signs in General Disease. Springfield, Ill., Charles C Thomas, 1960, p. 98.

John, K.J., et al.: Chorioretinitis in the contralateral eye of a patient with acanthamoeba keratitis. Ophthalmology, 95:635–639, 1988.

Soubrane, G., et al.: Birdshot retinochoroidopathy and subretinal new vessels. Br. J. Ophthalmol., 67:461–470, 1983.

Woods, A.C.: Endogenous Inflammations of the Uveal Tract. Baltimore, Williams & Wilkins, 1961.

Characteristics of Granulomatous and Nongranulomatous Inflammation in Posterior Uvea

Symptomatology	Granulomatous Uveitis	Nongranulomatous Uveitis	
		Acute, Self-limited Insult	Chronic or Often Repeated Insult
Anterior ocular changes	Sometimes epithelioid or "mutton-fat" keratotic deposits; often Koeppe nodules	Usually none	None in early irreversible in stage; terminal stages
Vitreous changes	Usually heavy vitreous blurring; heavy veil-like opacities	Slight to intense general blurring; fine muscae or string-like fibrinous opacities	Slowly increasing blue with heavy opacities in terminal stages
Retinal and subretinal edema	Usually slight or moderate and localized around exudates; intense only when there is a secondary allergic reaction	Marked and generalized, with blurring of neuro-retinal vascular bed	Low grade at onset; may become intense in later stages
Choroidal exudates	Heavy massive exudates— edges may be blurred by surrounding retinal and subretinal edema	No heavy massive exudates; occasionally localized areas of deeper infiltration	Great tendency to localized deep ill-defined infiltrates (lymphocyte, etc.)
Secondary retinal involvement	Almost invariable with retinal destruction	None or limited to pigment and neuroepithelium	None in early stage; irreversible in later stages with involvement of neuro-epithelium
Residual organic damage in retina and choroid	Heavy glial scars with massive pigment heaping which often surrounds the lesion	No fine granular changes in pigment epithelium but damage to neuroepithelium and occasionally superficial gliosis	Fine granular change in early stages; superficial gliosis in terminal stages

Choroidal Neovascularization (New Vessel Formation from Choriocapillaris through Defect in Bruch Membrane; Suggested by Fluorescein Angiography)

1. Choroidal neovascular ingrowth at the margin of the optic nerve head

    A. Angioid streaks (see p. 586)

    B. Hyaline bodies of optic nerve head

    C. Idiopathic choroidal neovascularization

    D. Macular drusen

    E. Multiple evanescent white dot and acute idiopathic blind spot enlargement syndrome

    F. Optic nerve coloboma

    G. Peripapillary choroiditis

    H. Presumed ocular histoplasmosis syndrome

    I. Pseudotumor cerebri (Symond syndrome)

    J. Serpiginous choroiditis

2. Choroidal neovascular in-growth through breaks in Bruch membrane in the macular area

3. Acute posterior multifocal placoid pigment epitheliopathy

    A. Angioid streaks (see p. 586)

    B. Behçet syndrome (dermatostomato-ophthalmic syndrome) Best disease

    C. Bird-shot retinochoroidopathy

    D. Choroidal rupture

    E. Choroidal tumors

    F. Chronic uveitis

    G. Foveomacular dystrophy

    H. Fundus flavimaculatus

    I. Idiopathic choroidal neovascularization

    *J. Macular drusen

    K. Morning glory syndrome

    L. Myopic degeneration

    M. Parafoveal telangiectasis

    N. Photocoagulation of macular lesions with argon laser

    O. Presumed ocular histoplasmosis syndrome

    P. Osteogenesis imperfecta (van der Hoeve syndrome)

    Q. Retinitis pigmentosa

    R. Rubella syndrome (Gregg syndrome)

    S. Sarcoidosis syndrome (Schaumann syndrome)

    T. Scars from previous deep macular hemorrhage

    U. Senile disciform macular degeneration (Kuhnt-Junius disease)

    V. Serpiginous choroiditis

* = most important

W. Sorsby's fundus dystrophy

X. Tilted disc syndrome

Y. Toxocariasis

Z. Toxoplasma retinochoroiditis

AA. Trauma

BB. Vein occlusion

CC. Vogt-Koyanagi-Harada syndrome (uveitis-vitiligo-alopecia-poliosis syndrome)

Brodsky, M.C., et al.: Subretinal neovascular membrane in an infant with a retinochoroidal oloboma. Arch. Ophthal., 109:1650–1651, 1991.

Callanan, D., and Gass, J.D.: Multifocal choroiditis and choroidal neovascularization associated with the multiple evanescent white dot and acute idiopathic blind spot enlargement syndrome. Ophthal., 99:1678–1685, 1992.

Dailey, J.R., et al.: Peripapillary choroidal neovascular membrane associated with an optic nerve coloboma. Arch. Ophthal., 111:441–442, 1993.

Feist, R.M, et al.: Choroidal neovascularization in a patient with adult foveomacular dystrophy and a mutation in the retinal degeneration slow gene. Amer. J. Ophthal., 118:259–260, 1994.

Giuffre, G.: Chorioretinal degenerative changes in the tilted disc syndrome. Int. Ophthalmol., 15: 1–7, 1991.

Holz, F.G., et al.: Recurrent choroidal neovascularization after laser photocoagulation in Sorsby's fundus dystrophy. Retina, 14:329–334, 1994.

Roy, F.H.: Ocular Syndromes and Systemic Diseases. 2nd Ed. Philadelphia, W. B. Saunders, 1989.

Ruby, A.J, et al.: Choroidal neovascularization associated with choroidal hemangiomas. Arch. Ophthal., 110:658–661, 1992.

Ischemic Infarcts of Choroid (Elschnig Spots) (When Healed, May Show Small, Disseminated Yellowish Scars with Central Pigment Deposits and May Be Associated with Retinal Separation when Acute)

1. Chronic glomerulonephritis

2. Collagen disease, such as scleroderma

*3. Malignant hypertension

4. Toxemia of pregnancy

Klein, B.A.: Ischemic infarcts of choroid (Elschnig spots). Am. J. Ophthalmol., 66:1069–1074, 1968.

Venecia, G., et al.: The eye in accelerated hypertension—Elschnig's spots in nonhuman primates. Arch. Ophthalmol., 98:913, 1980.

Chorioretinal and Choriovitreal Neovascularization—New Vessel Formation from Choroid into Retina and/or Vitreous Usually Occurring after Photocoagulation or Following:

1. Atrophic scars in the presumed ocular histoplasmosis syndrome

2. Central serous chorioretinopathy

*3. Diabetes mellitus (Willis disease)

4. Diseases of the retinal pigment epithelium

5. Eales' disease (periphlebitis)

6. Leber's syndrome (optic atrophy—amaurosis pituitary syndrome)

7. Sarcoidosis syndrome (Schaumann syndrome)

8. Sickle cell disease (Herrick syndrome)

Chandra, S.R., et al.: Choroidovitreal neovascular ingrowth after photocoagulation for proliferative diabetic retinopathy. Arch. Ophthalmol., 98:1593, 1980.

Dizon-Moore, R.V., et al.: Chorioretinal and choriovitreal neovascularization. Arch. Ophthalmol., 99:842, 1981.

Uveal Effusion—Leaking of Fluid from Choriocapillaris into Choroid and/or Subretinal Space

1. Hydrostatic

   A. Dural arteriovenous fistula

   *B. Hypotony, wound leak

   C. Nanophthalmos

2. Idiopathic

3. Inflammatory

   A. After panretinal photocoagulation

   B. HIV

   C. Scleritis, infected scleral buckle

   D. Trauma, intraocular surgery

   E. Uveitis, sympathetic ophthalmia, Harada disease

Morita, H., et al.: Recurrence of nanophthalmic uveal effusion. Ophthalmologica, 207:30–36, 1993.

Nash, R.W., and Lindquist, T.D.: Bilateral angle-closure glaucoma associated with uveal effusion: presenting sign of HIV. Surv. Ophthal., 36:255–258, 1992.

Choroid Coloboma

1. Aicardi syndrome

2. Basal cell nevus syndrome (Gorlin syndrome)

3. Cat-eye syndrome (partial G-trisomy)

4. CHARGE association among coloboma, heart anomaly, choanal atresia, retardation, genital and ear anomalies

5. Doubtful association

   A. Crouzon syndrome (dysostosis craniofacialis)

   B. Ellis-Van Crevald syndrome (chondroectodermal dysplasia)

   C. Hallerman Steiff syndrome (dyscephalic mandibulo-oculo facial)

   D. Incontinentia pigmenti I (Block-Sulzberger syndrome)

   E. Kartagener syndrome (bronchiectasis-dextrocardia-sinusitis)

   F. Laurence-Moon-Bardet-Biedl syndrome (retinitis pigmentosa-polydactyl-adiposogenital syndrome)

   G. Pierre-Robin syndrome (micrognathia-glossoptosis syndrome)

   H. Stickler syndrome (hereditary progressive arthro-ophthalmopathy)

   I. Tuberous sclerosis (Bourneville syndrome)

6. Goldenhar syndrome (oculoauriculovertebral dysplasia)

* = most important

7. Goltz syndrome (focal dermal hypoplasia syndrome)

8. Isolated, sporadic

9. Joubert syndrome with bilateral chorioretinal coloboma (coloboma, chorioretinal with cerebellar vermis aplasia)

10. Klinefelter syndrome (gynecomastia-aspermatogenesis syndrome)

11. Lenz microphthalmia syndrome

12. Linear sebaceous nevus syndrome

13. Median facial cleft syndrome

14. Meckel syndrome (dysencephalia splanchnocystic syndrome)

15. Retinal astrocytoma

16. Retinal dysplasia

17. Retinoblastoma

18. Rubinstein-Taybi syndrome (broad thumbs syndrome)

19. Triploidy

*20. Trisomy (Edward syndrome)

21. Trisomy (Patau syndrome)

22. Turner syndrome

23. Warburg syndrome

24. 13q syndrome

Epstein, R.J., et al.: Uveal colobomas and Klinefelter syndrome. Am. J. Ophthalmol., 98:241–243, 1984.

Isenberg, S.J.: The Eye in Infancy. Chicago, Year Book Medical Publishers, 1989.

Ward, J.R., et al.: Upperlimb defect associated with developmental delay, unilateral poorly developed antihelix, hearing deficit, and bilateral choroid coloboma: a new syndrome. J. Medical Genetics, 29:589–591, 1992.

Choroidal Ischemia (Decreased Choroidal Perfusion Demonstrated by Fluorescein Angiography)

1. Arteritic anterior ischemic optic neuropathy

2. Disseminated intravascular coagulation

*3. Hypertension, severe

4. Renal failure

5. Systemic lupus erythematosus

6. Toxemia of pregnancy

7. Thrombotic thrombocytopenic purpura

Kinyoun, J.L., and Kalina, R.E.: Visual loss from choroidal ischemia. Am. J. Ophthalmol., 101:650–656, 1986.

Kishi, S., et al.: Fundus lesions in malignant hypertension. Arch. Ophthalmol., 103:1189, 1985.

Slavin, M.L., and Barondes, M.J.: Visual loss caused by choroidal ischemia preceding anterior ischemic optic neuropathy in giant cell arteritis. Amer. J. Ophthal., 117:81–86, 1994.

Pars Planitis (Peripheral Uveitis) (Inferior Exudates in Peripheral Retina, Ora, Pars Plana, and Peripheral Vitreous, Vitreous Ray and Cells, Posterior Cortical Cataract, Perivasculitis, Partial Thrombosis of Central Retinal Vein, Glaucoma, Peripheral Retinal Hemorrhages, and Retinal Detachment May Be Present)

1. Dental infection
2. Hereditary
*3. Idiopathic
4. Multiple sclerosis (disseminated sclerosis)
5. Nematodiases
6. Rheumatic disease
7. Sarcoidosis syndrome (Schaumann syndrome)
8. Sinus infection
9. Streptococcal hypersensitivity
10. Syphilis (acquired lues)
11. Toxoplasmosis
12. Ulcerative colitis (inflammatory bowel disease)

Duinkerke-Eerola, K.U., et al.: Pars planitis in father and son. Ophthal. Pediatrics & Genetics, 11:305–308, 1990.

Josephberg, R.G., et al.: A fluorescein angiographic study of patients with pars planitis and peripheral exudation (snowbanking) before and after cryopexy. Ophthal., 101:262–1266, 1994.

Phillips, W.B., et al.: Pars planitis presenting with vitreous hemorrhage. Ophthal. Surg., 24:630–631, 1993.

Zierhut, M., and Foster, C.S.: Multiple sclerosis, sarcoidosis and other diseases in patients with pars planitis. Developments in Ophthalmology, 23:41–47, 1992.

Differential Diagnosis of Pars Planitis

	Chronicity	Vitreous Opacities	Retinal Edema	Fluorescein Leakage	Organized Vitreous	Distinguishing Features
Acute nongranulomatous iritis	−	±	±	±	−	Acute red eye
Acute recurrent cyclitis	+	+	+	+	+	Localized area of inflammation in ciliary body
Nematode	+	+	+	+(?)	+	Nodular focus and dragged retina, one eye
Irvine-Gass syndrome	+	+	+	+	±	Usually postoperative
Behçet syndrome	+	+	+	+(?)	+	Retinal vasculitis
Peripheral toxoplasmosis	±	+	±	±	±	Localized area of inflammation
Sarcoidosis	+	+	+	+	+	Other ocular signs of sarcoidosis

* = most important

Optic Nerve

FERENC KUHN, M.D., AND TAMAS HALDA, Ph.D.

Contents

Blurred Optic Nerve Heads

	Vision	Visual Fields	Retinal Veins	Color of Nerve Head	Retinal Hemorrhages	Peripapillary Retinal Edema	Vitreous Cells	Symmetry of Nerve Heads	Comments
1. Early papilledema	Normal	Normal (except blind spot enlargement)	Slightly distended; early loss of spontaneous pulsations	Pink	±	±	−	Often asymmetric	Headaches
2. Advanced papilledema	Normal or, at times, somewhat reduced	Normal (except blind spot enlargement)	Distended without spontaneous pulsations	Very pink to pale	+	+	−	Often symmetric	Sixth nerve palsies are additional clue to increased pressure
3. Hyperopia and physiologic variants	Normal	Normal	Normal	Normal	−	−	−	Often symmetric	Fundus seen with + lens; central disc cupping usually present
4. Optic neuritis	Impaired	Central scotoma ± peripheral loss	Distended ± spontaneous pulsations	Pink	±	±	±	Usually unilateral	Precipitous onset; may have pain with ocular motility
5. Optic nerve tumor	Normal or markedly reduced	Normal or markedly reduced	Normal or distended	May be pigmented if disc tumor contains melanin; very pink to pale	±	±	−	Usually unilateral	May involve only the orbital or intracranial optic nerve, and not the intraocular portion; primary nerve tumors are rarely observed on the disc
6. Optic nerve avulsion	Blind eye	−	Sludged	Pale	±	−	±	Contralateral eye normal	Contre-coup or direct trauma

Blurred Optic Nerve Heads Continued

	Vision	Visual Fields	Retinal Veins	Color of Nerve Head	Retinal Hemorrhages	Peripapillary Retinal Edema	Vitreous Cells	Symmetry of Nerve Heads	Comments
7. Hyaline bodies of nerve head parents	Normal	Normal or a variety of field cuts	Normal	Normal	– (Very rarely +)	–	–	Often symmetric hyaline bodies sometimes seen at disc margins in one eye only	Often familial (examine and siblings)
8. Hypotony of eye (after trauma)	Slightly impaired	Usually normal	Distended	Pink ±	±	Peripheral edema	–	Unilateral	Soft eye; commotio retinae

Paton, D., and Goldberg, M.F.: Injuries of the Eye, the Lids, and the Orbit. Philadelphia, W.B. Saunders, 1968.

Cilio-optic Vein—Vein Appears at Disc Edge and Dips into Optic Nerve to Anastomose with Branches of Central Retinal Vein

1. Congenital
2. Neurofibromatosis (von Recklinghausen syndrome)
3. Sturge-Weber syndrome (meningocutaneous syndrome)

Zaret, C.R., et al.: Cilio-optic vein associated with phakomatosis. Ophthalmology, 87:330–334, 1980.

Drusen of Optic Nerve (White or Yellow Conglomerate Translucent Bodies in Optic Nerve; May Cause Field Defects)

1. Alport syndrome (hereditary nephritis)
2. Angioid streaks (pseudoxanthoma elasticum; Gronblad-Strandberg syndrome)
3. Associated with corneal dystrophy
4. Diabetes mellitus (Willis disease)
5. Friedreich ataxia
6. Glaucoma
7. Hereditary—autosomal dominant
8. High myopia
9. Idiopathic
10. Meningioma (unusual)
11. Pituitary tumor (unusual)
12. Retinal vein occlusion
13. Retinitis pigmentosa
14. Systemic lupus erythematosus (SLE)
15. Status dysraphicus syndrome (Passow syndrome)
16. Syphilis (acquired lues)
17. Tuberous sclerosis (Bourneville syndrome)
18. Wilson's disease (hepatolenticular degeneration)

Chern, S., et al.: Central retinal vein occlusion associated with drusen of the optic disc. Annal Ophthal., 23:66–69, 1991.

Newell, F.W.: Ophthalmology, Principles and Concepts. 7th Ed. St. Louis, C.V. Mosby, 1991.

Roy, F.H.: Ocular Syndromes and Systemic Diseases. 2nd Ed. Philadelphia, W.B. Saunders, 1989.

Walsh, F.B., and Hoyt, W.F.: Clinical Neuro-ophthalmology. 4th Ed. Baltimore, Williams & Wilkins, 1985.

Fluid Enlargement of Retrobulbar Optic Nerve and/or Sheath (Demonstrated by Computed Tomographic Scanning and Echography)

1. Arachnoiditis
2. Basilar artery aneurysm
3. Bilateral temporal lobe cysts
4. Central retinal vein occlusion (see p. 525)
5. Facial trauma
6. Iliojejunal bypass
7. Occipital intradural arteriovenous malformation

8. Optic nerve meningioma

9. Optic nerve sheath cyst

10. Pseudotumor cerebri

11. Subdural hematoma

12. Trauma (intrasheath hemorrhage of optic nerve)

13. Uveal meningeal syndrome

Hupp, S.L. and Glaser, J.S.: Optic nerve sheath decompression. Arch. Ophthalmol., 105::386–389, 1987.

Hyperemia of Disc

1. Central retinal vein thrombosis (see p. 525)

2. Hemangioma

3. Hypermetropia

4. Hypertensive retinopathy

5. Ischemic optic neuropathy

6. Neovascularization

7. Optic neuritis (see p. 641)

8. Papilledema (see p. 651)

9. Polycythemia vera (Vaquez disease)

10. von Hippel-Lindau disease (retinocerebral angiomatosis)

Duke-Elder, S., and Scott, G.I.: System of Ophthalmology. Vol. 12. St. Louis, C.V. Mosby, 1971.

Ischemic Optic Neuropathy (Anterior Form is Occlusive Disease of Optic Nerve Head and Retrolaminar Region of the Optic Nerve; Posterior Form is Occlusion of One or More Nutrient Arteries to Rest of Optic Nerve; Onset Usually Sudden, Painless Unilateral Visual Loss and Visual Field Defect)

1. Compression

   A. Orbital hemorrhage (trauma)

   B. Thyroid disease (Graves' disease)

2. Drugs

   A. Sumatriptan

   B. Vigabatrin

3. Systemic diseases (often in combination)

   A. Arteriosclerosis

   B. Atherosclerosis

   C. Cerebrovascular disease

   D. Diabetes mellitus

   E. Gastrointestinal ulcer

   F. Hyperparathyroidism

   G. Hypertension, nocturnal hypotension

   H. Ischemic heart disease

   I. Sickle cell disease

4. Vasculitis

   A. Churg-Strauss syndrome (allergic granulomatosis and angiitis)

B. Collagen diseases

C. Giant cell (temporal) arteritis

5. Miscellaneous

A. Acute anemia

B. Anemia combined with hypotension

C. Carotid artery disease

D. Fabry's disease (angiokeratoma corporis diffusum)

E. Migraine

F. Radiation

G. Retinal artery occlusion

H. Tobacco

I. Various vascular disorders (e.g., cavernous sinus thrombosis)

Chung, S.M., et al.: Nonarteritic ischemic optic neuropathy. the impact of tobacco use. Ophthal., 101:779–782, 1994.

Coppeto, J.R., and Greco, T.P.: Autoimmune ischemic optic neuropathy associated with positive rheumatoid factor and transient nephrosis. Ann. Ophthal., 24:434–438, 1992.

Gadkari, S.S., et al.: Traumatic ischemic optic neuropathy. Ann. Ophthal., 24:434–438, 1991.

Hayreh, S.S.: Systemic diseases associated with nonarteritic anterior ischemic optic neuropathy. Amer. J. Ophthal., 112:925–931, 1994.

Katz, D.M., et al.: Ischemic optic neuropathy after lumbar spine surgery. Arch. Ophthal., 112:925–931, 1994

Maskin, S.L., et al.: Bipolaris Hawaiiensis-caused phaeohyphomycotic orbitopathy. Ophthalmology, 96:175–179, 1989.

Perlman, J.I., et al.: Retrobulbar ischemic optic neuropathy associated with sickle cell disease. J. Neuro-Ophthal., 14:45–48, 1994.

Sharma, R., and Desai, S.: Postpartum hemorrhage producing acute ischemic optic neuropathy. Asia-Oceania J. Obs. & Gynaecol., 19:249–251, 1993.

Slavin, M.L., and Barondes, M.J.: Ischemic optic neuropathy in sickle cell disease. Am. J. Ophthalmol., 105:212–214, 1988.

Linear Hemorrhage on Optic Disc

1. Diabetes mellitus

2. Drusen of optic nerve

3. Glaucoma

4. Ischemic optic neuropathy

A. Altitudinal field loss

B. Dense arcuate field loss

C. Sector-shaped field loss

5. Isolated finding

6. Leukemia

7. Systemic hypertension

Drance, S.M., et al.: Studies of factors involved in the production of low tension glaucoma. Arch. Ophthalmol., 90:457, 1973.

Jonas, J.B., and Xu, L.: Optic Disk Hemorrhages in Glaucoma. Amer. J. Ophthal., 118:1–8, 1994.

Shihab, Z.M., et al.: The significance of disc hemorrhage in open-angle glaucoma. Ophthalmology, 89:211, 1982.

Neovascularization of Optic Disc (Growth of Blood Vessels onto Optic Disc)

1. Anemia
2. ARMD (age-related macular degeneration)
3. Arterial insufficiency
4. Behçet disease (oculobuccogenital syndrome)
5. Buerger diseases (thromboangiitis obliterans)
6. Coats disease (retinal telangiectasia)
7. Choroidal rupture
8. Diabetes mellitus
9. Drusen of optic nerve head
10. Eales disease (periphlebitis)
11. Geographic helicoid peripapillary choroidopathy
12. Glaucoma, chronic uncontrolled
13. Hereditary drusen of Bruch membrane
14. von Hippel-Lindau's disease (retinocerebral angiomatosis)
15. Hypertensive retinopathy, advanced
16. Incontinentia pigmenti achromians (hypomelanosis of Ito syndrome)
17. Infection
    A. Endophthalmitis
    B. Congenital rubella syndrome (Gregg's syndrome)
    C. Histoplasmosis
    D. Toxoplasmosis
18. Intraocular inflammation
    A. Rheumatoid arthritis
    B. Sarcoidosis syndrome (Schaumann syndrome)
    C. Uveitis (unspecified)
19. Myopia, severe
20. Norrie disease (fetal iritis syndrome)
21. Pseudotumor cerebri (Symond syndrome)
22. Retinal vein occlusion (see p. 525)
23. Retinitis pigmentosa
24. Retinopathy of prematurity (ROP)
25. Sickle cell disease (Herrick syndrome)
26. Takayasu disease (Aortic arch syndrome)
27. Trauma
28. Tumors
    A. Benign
        (1) von Hippel-Lindau's disease
        (2) Juxtapapillary capillary hemangioma
        (3) Nevus
    B. Malignant
        (1) Choroidal melanoma

    (2) Leukemia

    (3) Lymphoma

    (4) Metastatic tumors

29. Vogt-Koyangi-Harada syndrome (uveitis-vitiligo-alopecia-poliosis)

Bovino, J.A., et al.: Optic disk neovascularization and rubeosis iridis after surgical resection of the optic nerve. Am. J. Ophthalmol., 106:231–232, 1988.

Roy, F.H.: Ocular Syndromes and Systemic Diseases. 2nd Ed. Philadelphia, W.B. Saunders, 1989.

To, K.W., et al.: Bilateral optic disc neovascularization in association with retinitis pigmentosa. Cand. J. Ophthal., 26:152–155, 1991.

Neuroretinitis (Inflammation of optic nerve and adjacent retina)

1. Cat scratch disease

2. Herpes simplex

3. Idiopathic

4. Mumps (epidemic parotitis)

5. Nematode

6. Salmonella

7. Syphilis

8. Toxocara canis

9. Toxoplasmosis

Fish, R.H., et al.: Toxoplasmosis Neuroretinitis. Ophthal., 100:1177–1182, 1993.

King, M.H., et al.: Leber's Idiopathic Stellate Neuroretinitis. Ann. Ophthal., 23:58–60, 1991.

Optic Nerve Atrophy

1. Chromosome disorders

    A. Angelman's syndrome (happy puppet syndrome; microdeletion of chromosome 15q 11–13)

    B. Chromosome deletion (long arm) syndrome (de Grouchy's syndrome)

    C. Crying cat syndrome (cri du chat syndrome; deletion of short arm of chromosome 5)

    D. Patau's syndrome (trisomy syndrome)

    E. Subacute sclerosing panencephalitis (Dawson's disease)

2. Demyelinating and degenerative diseases

    A. Arylsulfatase A deficiency syndrome (ADL, metachromatic leukodystrophy)

    B. Devic's syndrome (optical myelitis)

    C. Hereditary motor sensory neuropathy (HMSN I; Charcot-Marie-Tooth syndrome)

    D. Hereditary optic atrophy (Behr's syndrome)

    E. Multiple sclerosis

3. Dermatological disorders

    A. Keratodermia palmaris et plantaris

    B. McCune-Albright syndrome (fibrosus dysplasia)

    C. Naegeli's syndrome (reticular pigmented dermatosis)

D. Porphyria cutanea tarda

E. Pseudoxanthoma elasticum (Gronblad-Strandberg syndrome)

F. Wrinkly skin syndrome

4. Drugs, poisons and vaccines

acetophenazine

acetylsalicylic acid

allobarbital

amobarbital

antimony lithium thiomalate

antimony potassium tartrate

antimony sodium tartrate

antimony sodium thioglycollate

aprobarbital

aspirin

auranofin(?)

aurothioglucose(?)

aurothioglycanide(?)

barbital

benzathine penicillin G

bromide(?)

bupivacaine(?)

butabarbital

butalbital

butallylonal

butaperazine

butethal

calcitriol

carbamazepine

carbon dioxide

carphenazine

cephaloridine(?)

chloramphenicol(?)

chloroprocaine(?)

chlorpromazine

cholecalciferol

cisplatin

colchicine

cortisone

cyclobarbital

cyclopentobarbital

diethazine

ethambutol

ethopropazine

etidocaine(?)

fluorometholone

fluphenazine

glutethimide

gold Au 198

gold sodium thiomalate(?)

gold sodium thiosulfate(?)

heptabarbital

hexethal

hexobarbital

hydrabamine phenoxymethyl penicillin

ibuprofen

interferon

isocarboxazid(?)

isoniazid

lidocaine(?)

mephobarbital

mepivacaine(?)

mesoridazine

methaqualone(?)

metharbital

methdilazine

methitural

methohexital

methotrimeprazine

methyl alcohol

methylene blue

methyprylon

mitotane

nalidixic acid

nadolol(?)

naproxen(?)

penicillamine

pentobarbital

perazine

pericyazine

perphenazine

phenelzine(?)

phenobarbital

phenoxymethyl penicillin

piperacetazine

potassium penicillin G

potassium penicillin V

potassium phenethicillin

prilocaine(?)

primidone

probarbital

procaine(?)

procaine penicillin G

procarbazine

prochlorperazine

promazine

promethazine

propiomazine

propoxycaine(?)

quinine

secobarbital

sodium antimonylgluconate

sodium salicylate

stibocaptate

stibogluconate

stibophen

sulfacetamide

sulfachlorpyridazine

sulfacytine

sulfadimethoxine

sulfamerazine

sulfameter

sulfamethazine

sulfamethizole

sulfamethoxazole

sulfamethoxypyridazine

sulfanilamide

sulfaphenazole

sulfapyridine

sulfasalazine

sulfathiazole

sulfisoxazole

sulthiame

talbutal

tamoxifen

thiamylal

thiethylperazine

thiopental

thiopropazate

thioproperazine

thioridazine

tranylcypromine(?)

trifluoperazine

triflupromazine

trimeprazine

vaccines—influenza

vinbarbital

vitamin D,(retinol)

vitamin D_2(ergocalciferol)

vitamin D_3(cholecalciferol)

5. Endocrine

   A. Cretinism (hypothyroidism)

   B. Cushing's syndrome (adrenocortical syndrome)

   C. Diabetes mellitus

   D. DIDMOAD (diabetes mellitus and insipidus with optic atrophy and deafness) syndrome; Wolfram's syndrome, Marquardt-Loriaux syndrome)

   E. Frohlich's syndrome (dystrophia adiposogenitalis)

   F. Hyperparathyroidism

   G. Hypophosphatasia (phosphoethanolaminuria)

   H. Juvenile diabetes mellitus (Mauriac's syndrome)

   I. Pituitary gigantism syndrome (Launois' syndrome)

    J. Simmonds' syndrome (hypopituitarism syndrome)

    K. Retinohypophysary syndrome (Lijo Pavia-Lis syndrome)

    L. Zollinger-Ellison syndrome (polyglandular adenomatosis syndrome)

6. Granulomatoses

    A. Sarcoidosis

    B. Tuberculosis

    C. Wegener's syndrome (Wegener's granulomatosis)

7. Infectious

    A. African eye worm disease (loiasis)

    B. Anthrax

    C. Congenital cytomegalic inclusion disease

    D. Congenital rubella syndrome (Gregg's syndrome)

    E. Cysticercosis

    F. Deerfly fever (tularemia)

    G. Encephalitis

    H. Encephalomeningitis

    I. Echinococcosis (hydatid cyst)

    J. Lyme disease (borreliosis, relapsing fever)

    K. Malaria

    L. Meningitis

    M. Measles (morbilli)

    N. von Mikulicz-Radecki's syndrome (dacryosialoadenopathy)

    O. Mumps (epidemic parotitis)

    P. Mycoplasma pneumoniae

    Q. Onchocerciasis syndrome (river blindness)

    R. Rocky Mountain spotted fever

    S. Syphilis (congenital or acquired)

    T. Toxoplasmosis

    U. Yellow fever

8. Inherited

    A. Congenital optic atrophy (autosomal dominant or recessive)

    B. Jensen's syndrome (opticoacustic nerve atrophy with dementia; X-linked)

    C. Juvenile optic atrophy (autosomal dominant)

    D. Metaphyseal dysplasia, anetoderma and optic atrophy (autosomal recessive)

    E. Optic atrophy, cataract and neurologic disorder (dominant)

    F. Optic atrophy, non-Leber type, early onset (x-linked)

    G. Optic atrophy, polyneuropathy, and deafness (x-linked)

    H. Optic atrophy, spastic paraplegia syndrome (x-linked)

    I. Optic atrophy, spasticparaplegia, dementia (autosomal dominant)

    J. Optic atrophy, nerve deafness, and distal neurogenic amyotrophy (recessive)

K. Optic atrophy with demyelinating of central nervous system (autosomal dominant)

L. Optic atrophy hypoplasia, familial, bilateral (autosomal dominant)

9. Inherited metabolic disorders

A. Leukodystrophies

(1) Adrenoleukodystrophy (ALD)

(2) Canavan's disease (spongy degeneration of the nervous system)

(3) Cockayne's syndrome

(4) Homocystinuria syndrome

(5) Krabbe's disease

(6) Maple syrup urine disease

(7) Menkes' disease (kinky-hair syndrome)

B. Peroxisome abnormalities

(1) Defective biogenesis:

a. infantile Refsum's syndrome (heredopathia atactica polyneuritiformis)

b. neonatal adrenoleukodystrophy (ALD) (adrenal cortical atrophy, patchy brain demyelination)

c. Zellweger's syndrome (cerebro-hepato-renal syndrome)

(2) Refsun's syndrome (heredopathia atactica polyneuritiformis

(3) Rhizomeric chondrodysplasia punctata

(4) Single enzyme deficiency

a. primary hyperoxaluria type I

b. x-linked adrenoleukodystrophy (ALD)

C. Storage disorders

(1) Lipoidoses

a. Generalized gangliosidosis

1. Gangliosidosis Gm2, type

2. Generalized gangliosidosis Gm type

3. Juvenile gangliosidosis Gm type

b. sphingolipidoses (arylsulfatase A deficiency syndrome

1. Arylsulfatase A deficiency syndrome (metachromatic leukodystrophy)

(a) Late infant form: Greenfield's disease

(b) Adult form: Bogaert-Nijssen-Peiffer syndrome

(c) Austin's disease (multiple sulfatase deficiency

(d) Fabry's disease (angiokeratoma corporis diffusum)

(e) Krabbe's disease (globoid cell leukodystrophy)

(f) Niemann-Pick syndrome (essential lipoid histiocytosis)

(g) Tay-Sachs syndrome (hexosaminidase deficiency)

(2) Glucose-phosphate dehydrogenase deficiency (von Gierke's disease)

(3) Mucolipidoses IV (ML IV)

    (4) Mucopolysaccharidoses or lysosomal storage diseases

      a. Mucopolysaccharidosis I-H (Hurler's syndrome; chondroosteodystrophy or lipochondrodystrophy)

      b. Mucopolysaccharidosis I-S (Scheie's syndrome)

      c. Mucopolysaccharidosis II (Hunter's syndrome)

      d. Mucopolysaccharidosis III (Sanfilippo's syndrome)

      e. Mucopolysaccharidosis IV (Morquio's syndrome)

      f. Mucopolysaccharidosis VI (Maroteaux-Lamy syndrome)

    (5) Neural ceroid lipofuscinosis

      a. Infantile type: Haltia-Santavuori disease

      b. Late infantile type: Jansky-Bielschowsky disease (internuclear ophthalmoplegia)

      c. Juvenile type: Batten's disease (Spielmeyer-Vogt-Sjögren syndrome; cerebro retinal degeneration)

    (6) Other disorders involving lipids

      a. Bassen-Kornzweig syndrome(familial hypolipoproteinemia)

      b. Refsum's syndrome (heredopathia atactica polyneuritiformis)

10. Local

    A. Aphakic cystoid macula edema (ACME; Irvine-Gass syndrome)

    B. Birdshot chorioretinopathy

    C. Coats' disease

    D. Drusen of optic nerve

    E. Glaucoma

    F. Vascular occlusion

11. Mental and psychomotor deficiency, retardation

    A. Drummond's syndrome (idiopathic hypercalcemia)

    B. Familial dysautonomia (Riley-Day syndrome)

    C. Hallervorden-Spatz syndrome

    D. Hallgren's syndrome (retinitis-pigmentosa-deafness-ataxia syndrome)

    E. Kloepfer's disease

    F. Rubinstein-Taybi syndrome

12. Miscellaneous

    A. Albinism

    B. Anemia

    C. Arachnoidal adhesion, e.g. caused by tabes

    D. Bloch-Sulzberger disease (incontinentia pigmenti)

    E. Bobble-head doll syndrome (massive dilatation of third ventricle)

    F. Bonnet-Dechaume-Blanc syndrome (neuroretinoangiomatosis)

    G. Brown-Sequard syndrome

    H. Cerebellar ataxia (Louis-Bar syndrome)

    I. Cerebral palsy

    J. Cystic fibrosis syndrome

    K. Foster-Kennedy syndrome (basal-frontal syndrome)

    L. Histiocytosis X eosinophil granuloma (Hand-Schuller-Christian syndrome)

    M. Incipient prechiasmal optic nerve compression syndrome

    N. Laurence-Moon-Bardet-Biedl syndrome (retinitis pigmentosa-polydactyly-adiposogenital syndrome.

    O. Leber's syndrome

    P. Oculodental syndrome (Peter's syndrome)

    Q. Opticcochleodental degeneration syndrome

    R. Peliazeus-Merzbacher disease (aplasia axialis extracorticalis congenita)

    S. Posthypoxic syndrome

    T. Pseudotumor cerebri

    U. Rieger's syndrome

    V. Russell's syndrome

    W. Status dysraphicus syndrome (Passow's syndrome)

    X. Sphenomaxillary fossa syndrome (pterygopalatine fossa syndrome)

    Y. Wagner's disease (hereditary vitreoretinal degeneration)

13. Nutritional deficiency

    A. Avitaminosis B (Wernicke's syndrome, beriberi)

    B. Avitaminosis B (pellagra)

    C. Garland's syndrome (central nervous system deficiency)

    D. (?) Infantile neuroaxonal dystrophy (possible vitamin E deficiency, Seitelberger's disease II)

    E. Kwashiorkor syndrome (hypoproteinemia syndrome)

    F. (?) Oculo-oro-genital syndrome (avitaminosis B with possible avitaminosis A)

14. Orbital

    A. Hutchinson-Pepper syndrome (metastatic infraorbital neuroblastoma)

    B. Rollet's syndrome (orbital apex syndrome)

    C. Superior orbital fissure syndrome (Rochon-Duvigneaud syndrome)

15. Rheumatoid

    A. von Bechterew-Stumpelld syndrome (ankylosing spondylitis)

    B. Behcet's disease (oculobuccogenital syndrome)

    C. Polymyalgia rheumatica

    D. Systemic lupus erythematosus (SLE)

16. Skeletal disorders

    A. Achondroplasia

    B. Albers-Schonberg syndrome (osteopetrosis)

    C. Anencephaly

    D. Apert's syndrome (acrocephalosyndactylism syndrome)

    E. Brachmann-de Lange syndrome

F. Camurati-Engelmann syndrome (progressive diaphyseal dysplasia)

G. Chondrodystrophia calcificans congenita (Conradi's syndrome)

H. Cloverleaf skull syndrome (Kleeblattschädel deformity)

I. Craniometaphyseal dysplasia (Pyle's syndrome)

J. Craniostenosis

  (1) Oxycephaly

  (2) Plagiocephaly

  (3) Scaphalocephaly

  (4) Trigonocephaly

K. Crouzon's syndrome (dysotosis craniofacialis)

L. Enchondromatosis syndrome (Ollier's syndrome)

M. Generalized gangliosidosis Gm type

N. Greig's syndrome (hypertelorism ocularis)

O. Hallermann-Steiff-Francois syndrome (oculomandibulofacial dyscephaly)

P. Hutchinson-Gilford progeria syndrome (progeria)

Q. Marchesani's syndrome

R. McCune-Albright syndrome (fibrosus dysplasia)

S. Metaphyseal dysplasia, anetoderma, and optic atrophy

T. Microcephaly

U. Osteogenesis imperfecta (van der Hoeve's syndrome)

V. Paget's syndrome (osteitis deformans)

W. Primary hyperoxaluria type (osteodystrophy hydrocephalus)

X. Zellweger's syndrome (cerebrohepatorenal syndrome)

17. Trauma

A. Direct and indirect optic nerve trauma

B. Electrical injury

C. Mechanical injury/surgical trauma (orbital floor fracture, malar fractures, Krönlein lateral orbitotomy)

D. Ocular contusion

E. Optic nerve evulsion

F. Radiation

18. Tumors

A. Craniopharyngiomas

B. Ectopic pinealomas

C. Gliomas

D. Hemangiomas

E. Meningiomas

F. Nasopharyngeal carcinomas

G. Neuroblastomas

H. Pituitary adenomas

      I. von Recklinghausen's syndrome (neurofibromatosis)

      J. Tumors extending into fourth ventricle and cerebellum causing papilledema

19. Vascular

     A. Aneurysm of internal carotid artery (foramen lacerum syndrome)

     B. Arteriosclerosis

     C. Cavernosus sinus thrombosis (Foix's syndrome)

     D. Giant cell (temporal arteritis)

     E. Hollenhorst's syndrome (chorioretinal infarction syndrome)

     F. Kussmaul's disease (necrotizing angiitis)

     G. Occlusion of the carotid artery

     H. Sickle cell disease (Herrick's syndrome)

     I. Takayasu's syndrome (aortic arch syndrome)

Boniuk, M., et al.: Hemangiopericytoma of the meninges of the optic nerve. Ophthalmology, 92:1780–1787, 1985.

Fraunfelder, F.T.: Drug-Induced Ocular Side Effects and Drug Interactions. 4th Ed. Philadelphia, Williams & Wilkins, 1996.

Kline, L.B., et al.: Radiation optic neuropathy. Ophthalmology, 92:1118–1126, 1985.

McKusick, V.A.: Mendelian Inheritance in Man. 9th Ed. Baltimore, Johns Hopkins University Press, 1994.

Newman, N.W., et al.: Bilateral optic neuropathy and osteolytic sinusitis: Complications of cocaine abuse. J.A.M.A., 259:72–74, 1988.

Rizzo, J.F., et al.: Optic atrophy in familial dysautonomia. Am. J. Ophthalmol., 102:463–467, 1986.

Roy, F.H.: Ocular Syndromes and Systemic Diseases. 2nd Ed. Philadelphia, W.B. Saunders, 1989.

Sorcinelli, I., et al.: Cherry-red spot, optic atrophy and corneal cloudings in a patient suffering from GM gangliosidosis type I. Metabolic, Pediatric and Systemic Ophthalmol., 10:62, 1987.

Optic Nerve Atrophy and Deafness

1. Adult form of arylsulfatase A deficiency (Bogaert-Nijssen-Peiffer syndrome; optic-ocochleodentale degeneration)

2. Camuati-Engelmann syndrome (progressive diaphyseal dysplasia)

3. Hereditary motor sensory neuropathy (HMSN I; Charcot-Marie-Tooth syndrome)

4. Congenital rubella syndrome (German measles, Gregg's syndrome)

5. Cockayne syndrome (dwarfism with retinal atrophy and deafness)

6. Craniometaphyseal dysplasia (Pyle's syndrome)

7. DIDMOAD syndrome (optic atrophy, sensorineural deafness, diabetes mellitus and diabetes insipidus)

8. Dominant inheritance—congenital deafness and progressive optic nerve atrophy

9. Friederich's ataxia (optic atrophy, ataxia and progressive hearing loss)

10. Generalized gangliosidosis Gm type

11. Hallgren syndrome (retinitis pigmentosa-deafness-ataxia syndrome)

12. Juvenile diabetes mellitus

13. Krabbe syndrome (infantile globoid [II] cell leukodystrophy)

14. Mucolipidosis IV

15. Mucopolysaccharidosis I-H (Hurler's syndrome)

16. Mucopolysaccharidosis II (Hunter's syndrome)

17. Mucopolysaccharidosis IV (Morquio's syndrome)

18. (?) Mucopolysaccharidosis (Maroteaux-Lamy syndrome)

19. (?) Niemann-Pick syndrome (essential lipoid histiocytosis)

20. Osteogenesis imperfecta

21. Recessive: nerve deafness, optic atrophy, and distal neurogenic amyotrophy

22. Refsum syndrome (phytanic acid oxidase deficiency)

23. Rosenberg-Chutorian syndrome

24. Sylvester disease

25. Treft's syndrome

Emery, J.M., et al.: Krabbe's disease. Am. J. Ophthalmol., 74:400–406, 1972.

Konigsmark, B.W., et al.: Dominant congenital deafness and progressive optic nerve atrophy. Arch. Ophthalmol., 91:99–103, 1974.

Pilley, S.F., and Thompson, H.S.: Familial syndrome of diabetes insipidus, diabetes mellitus, optic atrophy and deafness (DIDMOOD syndrome) in childhood. Br. J. Ophthalmol., 60:294–298, 1976.

Roy, F.H.: Ocular Syndromes and Systemic Diseases. 2nd Ed. Philadelphia, W.B. Saunders, 1989.

Shields, J.A., et al: Pigmented Adenoma of the Optic Nerve Head Simulating a Melanocytoma. Ophthalmology, 99:1705–1709, 1992.

Syndromes and diseases associated with optic atrophy

1. Achondroplasia

2. Acquired lues (syphilis)

3. African eye worm disease (loiasis)

4. Albers-Schonberg syndrome (osteopetrosis)

5. Albinism

6. Albright syndrome (fibrous dysplasia)

7. Anemia

8. Anencephaly

9. Aneurysm of internal carotid artery syndrome (foramen lacerum syndrome)

10. Anthrax

11. Apert syndrome (acrocephalosyndactylism syndrome)

12. Arachnoidal adhesion, including tabes

13. Arteriosclerosis

14. Arylsulfatase A deficiency syndrome (metachromatic leukodystrophy)

15. Avitaminosis B_2 (pellagra)

16. Bassen-Kornzweig syndrome (familial hypolipoproteinemia)

17. Batten-Mayou syndrome (cerebroretinal degeneration)

18. Behçet syndrome (oculobuccogenital syndrome)

19. Behr syndrome (optic atrophy-ataxia)

20. Bielschowsky-Jansky disease (internuclear ophthalmoplegia)

21. Bloch-Sulzberger disease (incontinentia pigmenti)

22. Bobble-Head Doll syndrome

23. Bonnet-Dechaume-Blanc syndrome (neuroretinoangiomatosis)

24. Brown-Marie syndrome (hereditary ataxia syndrome)

25. Brown-Sequard syndrome (lesion of spinal cord)

26. Carbon monoxide

27. Central nervous system deficiency—bitemporal pallor because of deficient diet (Garland syndrome)

28. Cerebral palsy

29. Cerebellar ataxia

30. Charcot-Marie-Tooth syndrome (progressive neuritic muscular syndrome)

31. Chondrodystrophia calcificans congenita (Conradi syndrome)

32. Chromosome deletion (long-arm) syndrome (de Grouchy syndrome)

33. Coats disease (retinal telangiectasia)

34. Cockayne syndrome (dwarfism with retinal atrophy and deafness)

35. Congenital cytomegalic inclusion disease

36. Congenital optic atrophy—autosomal dominant or recessive

37. Congenital syphilis

38. Craniometaphyseal dysplasia (Pyle syndrome)

39. Craniostenosis (including oxycephaly, Scaphalocephaly, trigonocephaly and plagiocephaly)

40. Cretinism (hypothyroidism)

41. Cri du chat syndrome (crying cat syndrome)

42. Crouzon syndrome (dysostosis craniofacialis)

43. Cushing syndrome (adrenocortical syndrome)

44. Cystic fibrosis syndrome (fibrocystic disease of pancreas)

45. Cysticercosis

46. Dawson disease (subacute sclerosing panencephalitis)

47. Deerfly fever (tularemia)

48. de Lange syndrome (congenital muscular hypertrophy-cerebral syndrome)

49. Devic syndrome (optical myelitis)

50. Diabetes mellitus

51. Didmoad-Wolfram syndrome (diabetes mellitus and insipidus with optic atrophy and deafness)—autosomal recessive

52. Diencephalic syndrome (Penfield syndrome)

53. Disseminated lupus erythematosus (Kaposi-Libman-Sacks syndrome)

54. Dollinger-Bielschowsky syndrome (lipidosis)

55. Drugs, including:

acetophenazine	aminosalicylate(?)
allobarbital	aminosalicylic acid(?)
alseroxylon(?)	amobarbital

amodiaquine
antimony lithium thiomalate
antimony potassium tartrate
antimony sodium tartrate
antimony sodium thioglycollate
antipyrine
aprobarbital
aspirin
barbital
betamethasone
bromide(?)
bromisovalum
broxyquinoline
bupivacaine(?)
butabarbital
butalbital
butallylonal
butaperazine
butethal
calcitriol
carbromal
carphenazine
chloramphenicol
chloroprocaine(?)
chloroquine
chlorpromazine
cholecalciferol
clindamycin
cobalt(?)
cocaine
cortisone
cyclobarbital
cyclopentobarbital
cycloserine(?)
dapsone
deferoxamine
deserpidine(?)
dexamethasone
dextrothyroxine(?)
diethazine
digitalis(?)
diiodohydroxyquin
ergocalciferol

ergonovine(?)
ergot(?)
ergotamine(?)
ethambutol
ethopropazine
etidocaine(?)
ferrocholinate(?)
ferrous fumarate(?)
ferrous gluconate(?)
ferrous succinate(?)
ferrous sulfate(?)
fluorometholone
fluphenazine
gentamicin
heptabarbital
hexachlorophene
hexamethonium
hexethal
hexobarbital
hydrocortisone
hydroxychloroquine
iodide and iodine solutions and compounds
iodoquinol
iodochlorhydroxyquin
iron dextran(?)
iron sorbitex
isoniazid
levothyroxine(?)
lidocaine(?)
liothyronine
liotrix(?)
medrysone
mephobarbital
mepivacaine(?)
mesoridazine
metharbital
methdilazine
methitural
methohexital
methotrexate(?)
methotrimeprazine
methyl alcohol
methylene blue

methylergonovine(?)

methysergide(?)

methylprednisolone

nitroglycerin(?)

oral contraceptives

oxyphenbutazone

pentobarbital

perazine

pericyazine

perphenazine

phenobarbital

phenylbutazone

piperacetazine

polysaccharide iron complex(?)

prednisolone

prilocaine(?)

primidone

probarbital

procaine(?)

prochlorperazine

promazine

promethazine

propiomazine

propoxycaine(?)

propoxyphene

quinine

radioactive iodides

rauwolfia serpentina(?)

rescinnamine(?)

reserpine(?)

secobarbital

sodium antimonylgluconate

sodium salicylate

stibocaptate

stibogluconate

stibophen

streptomycin

sulfacetamide(?)

sulfachlorpyridazine(?)

sulfacytine(?)

sulfadiazine(?)

sulfadimethoxine(?)

sulfamerazine(?)

sulfameter(?)

sulfamethazine

sulfamethizole(?)

sulfamethoxazole(?)

sulfamethoxypyridazine

sulfanilamide(?)

sulfaphenazole

sulfapyridine(?)

sulfasalazine(?)

sulfathiazole(?)

sulfisoxazole(?)

suramin

syrosingopine(?)

talbutal

thiamylal

thiethylperazine

thiopental

thiopropazate

thioproperazine

thioridazine

thyroglobulin(?)

thyroid(?)

tobramycin

trichloroethylene

trifluoperazine

triflupromazine

trimeprazine

tryparsamide

vinbarbital

vinblastine

vincristine

vitamin A

vitamin D

vitamin D_2

vitamin D_3

56. Drummond syndrome (idiopathic hypercalcemia)
57. Drusen of optic nerve
58. Dyschondroplasia syndrome (Ollier syndrome)
59. Electrical injury

60. Encephalitis, acute
61. Engelmann syndrome (diaphyseal dysplasia)
62. Exfoliation syndrome
63. Foix syndrome (cavernous sinus thrombosis)
64. Foster-Kennedy syndrome (basal-frontal syndrome)
65. Friedreich ataxia (optic atrophy and sensorineural deafness)—recessive
66. Frohlich syndrome (dystrophia adiposogenitalis)
67. Galactosyl ceramide lipidosis (globoid cell leukodystrophy)
68. Gangliosidosis GM 1, type
69. Generalized gangliosidosis (infantile)
70. Greig syndrome (hypertelorism ocularis)
71. Glaucoma
72. Glucose-phosphate dehydrogenase deficiency (von Gierke disease)
73. Gronblad-Strandberg syndrome (systemic elastodystrophy)
74. Hallermann-Streiff-François syndrome (oculomandibulofacial dyscephaly)
75. Hallervorden-Spatz syndrome (pigmentary degeneration of globus pallidus)
76. Hallgren syndrome (retinitis-pigmentosa deafness-ataxia syndrome)
77. Happy puppet syndrome (puppet children)
78. Herrick syndrome (sickle-cell disease)
79. Histiocytosis X (Hand-Schüller-Christian syndrome)
80. Hollenhorst syndrome (chorioretinal infarction syndrome)
81. Homocystinuria syndrome
82. Hutchinson syndrome (progeria)
83. Hydatid cyst
84. Hydrocephalus chondrodystrophicus congenita (Kleeblattschädel syndrome)
85. Hyperparathyroidism
86. Hypophosphatasia (phosphoethanolaminuria)
87. Incipient prechiasmal optic nerve compression syndrome
88. Infantile neuroaxonal dystrophy (Seitelberger disease II)
89. Infantile type of neuronal ceroid lipofuscinosis
90. Infections such as basal meningitis, infectious encephalomeningitis (especially measles epidemic parotitis), congenital neurosyphilis (rare before 2 years of age), and toxoplasmosis
91. Irvine syndrome (spontaneous rupture of vitreous face with vitreous adhesions to the wound followed by macular edema)
92. Jensen syndrome (opticoacoustic nerve atrophy with dementia)—x-linked
93. Juvenile diabetes—rare
94. Juvenile optic atrophy—autosomal dominant
95. Keratodermia palmaris et plantaris
96. Kloepfer disease

97. Krabbe disease (meningocutaneous syndrome)

98. Kussmaul disease (necrotizing angiitis)

99. Kwashiorkor (hypoproteinemia syndrome)

100. Laurence-Moon-Bardet-Biedl syndrome (retinitis pigmentosa-polydactyly-adiposo-genital syndrome)

101. Leber syndrome (optic atrophy-amaurosis-pituitary syndrome)

102. Leigh disease (subacute necrotizing encephalomyelopathy)

103. Leukemia

104. Malaria

105. Maple syrup urine disease (branched chain ketoaciduria)

106. Marchesani syndrome (brachymorphy with spherophakia)

107. Maroteoux-Lamy disease (mucopolysaccharidoses [MPS] VI)

108. Marquardt-Loriaux syndrome

109. Measles (Morbilli)

110. Menkes disease (kinky hair disease)

111. Metachromatic leukodystrophy (Greenfield disease)

112. Metaphyseal dysplasia, anetoderma and optic atrophy—autosomal recessive

113. Microcephaly

114. Mikulicz-Radecki syndrome (dacryosiaioadenopathy)

115. Mucolipidosis IV (ML IV)

116. Mucopolysaccharidosis IH (Hurler syndrome)

117. Mucopolysaccharidosis IS (Scheie syndrome)

118. Mucopolysaccharidosis II (Hunter syndrome)

119. Mucopolysaccharidosis IV (Morquio syndrome)

120. Multiple sclerosis (disseminated sclerosis)

121. Mumps

122. Naegeli syndrome (reticular pigmented dermatosis)

123. Neimann-Pick syndrome (essential lipoid histiocytosis)

124. Occlusion of carotid artery

125. Oculodental syndrome (Peter syndrome)

126. Oculo-oro-genital syndrome (riboflavin deficiency syndrome)

127. Onchocerciasis syndrome (river blindness)

128. Optic atrophy, cataract and neurologic disorder—dominant

129. Optic atrophy, nerve deafness, and distal neurogenic amyotrophy—recessive

130. Optic atrophy, non-Leber type, with early onset—x-linked

131. Optic atrophy, polyneuropathy and deafness—x-linked

132. Optic atrophy, spastic paraplegia syndrome—x-linked

133. Optic atrophy with demyelinating of central nervous system—autosomal dominant

134. Optic nerve hypoplasia, familial, bilateral—autosomal dominant

135. Opticocochleodental degeneration syndrome

136. Orbital operation, such as following orbital floor fracture, reduction of malar fractures and Krönlein lateral orbitotomy
137. Osteogenesis imperfecta (van der Hoeve syndrome)
138. Paget syndrome (osteitis deformans)
139. Passow syndrome (syringomyelia)
140. Peliazeus-Merzbacher disease (aplasia axialis extracorticalis congenita)
141. Pituitary gigantism syndrome (Launois syndrome)
142. Polymyalgia rheumatica
143. Porphyria cutanea tarda
144. Posthypoxic encephalopathy syndrome
145. Radiation
146. Refsum syndrome (phytanic acid oxidase deficiency)
147. Relapsing fever
148. Retinohypophysary syndrome (Lijo Pavia-Lis syndrome)
149. Rieger syndrome (hypodontia and iris dysgenesis)
150. Riley-Day syndrome (congenital familial dysautonomia)
151. Rochon-Duvigneaud syndrome (superior orbital fissure syndrome)
152. Rocky Mountain spotted fever
153. Rollet syndrome (orbital apex-sphenoidal syndrome)
154. Rosenberg-Chutorian syndrome
155. Rubella syndrome (German measles)
156. Rubinstein-Taybi syndrome (broad thumb syndrome)
157. Russell syndrome
158. Sabin-Feldman syndrome
159. Sanfilippo disease (MPS III)
160. Scaphocephaly syndrome
161. Schaumann syndrome (sarcoidosis syndrome)
162. Schilder syndrome (encephalitis periaxialis diffusa)
163. Simmonds syndrome (hypopituitarism syndrome)
164. Spastic paraplegia, optic atrophy, dementia—autosomal dominant
165. Sphenomaxillary fossa syndrome (pterygopalatine fossa syndrome)
166. Spielmeyer-Vogt syndrome (cerebroretinal degeneration)
167. Spongy degeneration of the white matter
168. Suprarenal—sympathetic syndrome (adrenal medulla tumor syndrome)
169. Sylvester disease
170. Symond syndrome (benign intracranial hypertension)
171. Takayasu syndrome (aortic arch syndrome)
172. Tay-Sachs syndrome (hexosaminidase deficiency)
173. Temporal arteritis syndrome (Hutchinson-Horton-Magath-Brown syndrome)
174. Toxins, including: lead, chronic cyanide intoxication such as from eating cassava, thallium (used for treatment of scalp fungi)

175. Trauma, evulsion of optic nerve, and ocular contusion

176. Treft syndrome

177. Trisomy D syndrome (Patau syndrome)

178. Tuberculosis

179. Tumors including: craniopharyngiomas, ectopic pinealomas, gliomas, hemangiomas, meningiomas, nasopharyngeal carcinomas, neuroblastomas, pituitary adenomas, and tumors extending into fourth ventricle and cerebellum causing papilledema

180. Tunbridge-Paley disease

181. Vaccinia

182. Vascular accident

183. von Bechterev-Stumpell syndrome (ankylosing spondylitis)

184. von Recklinghausen syndrome (neurofibromatosis)

185. Wagner syndrome (hyaloideoretinal degeneration)

186. Wegener syndrome (Wegener granulomatosis)

187. Wernicke syndrome (thiamine deficiency)

188. Wrinkly skin syndrome

189. Yellow fever

190. Zellweger syndrome (cerebrohepatorenal syndrome)

191. Zollinger-Ellison syndrome (polyglandular adenomatosis syndrome)

Boniuk, M., et al.: Hemangiopericytoma of the meninges of the optic nerve. Ophthalmology, 92:1780–1787, 1985.

Fraunfelder, F.T.: Drug-Induced Ocular Side Effects and Drug Interactions. 4th Ed. Philadelphia, Williams & Wilkins, 1996.

Kline, L.B., et al.: Radiation optic neuropathy. Ophthalmology, 92:1118–1126, 1985.

McKusick, V.A.: Mendelian Inheritance in Man. 9th Ed. Baltimore, Johns Hopkins University Press, 1994.

Newman, N.W., et al.: Bilateral optic neuropathy and osteolytic sinusitis: Complications of cocaine abuse. J.A.M.A., 259:72–74, 1988.

Rizzo, J.F., et al.: Optic atrophy in familial dysautonomia. Am. J. Ophthalmol., 102:463–467, 1986.

Roy, F.H.: Ocular Syndromes and Systemic Diseases. 2nd Ed. Philadelphia, W.B. Saunders, 1989.

Sorcinelli, I., et al.: Cherry-red spot, optic atrophy and corneal cloudings in a patient suffering from GMgangliosidosis type I. Metabolic, Pediatric and Systemic Ophthalmol., 10:62, 1987.

Optic Nerve Hypoplasia

1. Chromosome disorders

    A. Down's syndrome (trisomy 21)

    B. Deletion of long chromosome (13)

    C. Edward's syndrome (trisomy 18)

    D. Patau's syndrome (trisomy 13)

    E. Ring chromosome mosaicism

2. Idiopathic

3. Neurological conditions

    A. Anencephaly

    B. Basal encephalocele

    C. Behavioral problems

    D. Cerebellar atrophy

    E. Cerebral atrophy

    F. Cerebral infarcts

    G. Cerebral palsy

    H. Colpocephaly

    I. Congenital suprasellar tumors

    J. Congenital third, fourth and sixth nerve palsies and up-gaze palsies

    K. Encephaloceles

    L. Hydranencephaly

    M. Hydrocephaly

    N. Mental retardation

    O. Perinatal encephalopathy

    P. Porencephaly

4. Ocular conditions

    A. Albinism

    B. Aniridia

    C. Astigmatism

    D. Blepharophimosis

    E. Colobomas (optic disc and chorioretinal)

    F. High myopia

    G. Microphthalmos

    H. Retinal vascular tortuosity

5. Systemic conditions

    A. Aicardi syndrome

    B. Albinism

    C. Chondrodysplasia punctata

    D. Cleft lip and palate

    E. Diabetes mellitus (maternal)—segmental optic nerve hypoplasia in infant

    F. Duane retraction syndrome

    G. Fetal alcohol syndrome

    H. Goldenhar-Gorlin syndrome

    I. Hemifacial atrophy

    J. Hypertelorism

    K. Intrauterine infections—including cytomegalovirus and hepatitis

        (1) Cytomegalovirus

        (2) Hepatitis

    L. Inherited (autosomal dominant or recessive)

    M. Klippel-Trenaunay-Weber syndrome

    N. Meckel syndrome

    O. Median cleft face syndrome

    P. de Morsier syndrome (septo-optic dysplasia)

    Q. Osteogenesis imperfecta

    R. Potter syndrome

    S. Syndrome of nevus sebaceus of Jadassohn

6. Toxins (maternal use of)

    A. Alcohol

    B. Lysergic acid diethylamide (LSD)

    C. Phencyclidine (PCP)

    D. Phenytoin

    E. Quinine

    F. Tobacco

Brodsky, M.C., et al.: Congenital optic disc anomalies (Review) Surv. Ophthal., 32:89–112, 1994.

Lambert, S.R., et al.: Optic nerve hypoplasia (Review). Surv. of Ophthalmol., 32:1–9, 1987.

Chismire, K.J., and Witkop, G.S.: Angle dysgenesis in a patient with blepharophimosis syndrome. Amer. J. Ophthal., 117:676–677, 1994.

Isenberg, S.J.: The Eye in Infancy. Chicago, Year Book Medical Publishers, Inc., 1989.

Zeki, S.M., and Dutton, G.N.: in children. Br. J. Ophthalmol., 74:300–304, 1990.

Zeki, S.M.: and astigmatism: a new association. Brit. J. Ophthal., 74:297–299, 1990.

Optic Neuritis (Papillitis and Retrobulbar Neuritis) Characterized by: Progressive loss of vision and possibly complete amaurosis; pain in or behind eye, especially on lateral movement; Marcus Gunn pupillary phenomenon; and centralor paracentral scotoma.

1. Demyelinating and degenerative diseases

    A. Adrenoleukodystrophy

    B. Hereditary ataxia (Brown-Marie syndrome)

    C. Multiple sclerosis

    D. Opticomyelitis (Devic's disease)

2. Drugs, poisons, vaccines

    A. Drugs, including:

acetohexamide	aprobarbital
acetyldigitoxin	barbital
alcohol	bromisovalum
allobarbital	broxyquinoline
aminosalicylate	bupivacaine(?)
aminosalicylic acid(?)	butabarbital
amiodarone(?)	butalbital
amitriptyline	butallylonal
amobarbital	butethal

calcitriol(?)

caramiphen

carbromal

carmustine

chloral hydrate(?)

chloramphenicol

chloroprocaine(?)

chlorpropamide(?)

cholecalciferol

cisplatin

clindamycin

clophene(?)

cyclobarbital

cyclopentobarbital

cycloserine(?)

deferoxamine

desipramine

deslanoside

dextrothyroxine(?)

diethylpropion(?)

digitalis

digitoxin

digoxin

diiodohydroxyquin

diphtheria and tetanus toxoids (adsorbed)

diphtheria and tetanus toxoids and pertussis vaccine (adsorbed)

diphtheria toxoid (adsorbed)

disulfiram

ergocalciferol(?)

ergonovine

ergotamine

ethambutol

ethchlorvynol

ethionamide

etidocaine(?)

etretinate

fenoprofen

ferrocholinate(?)

ferrous fumarate(?)

ferrous gluconate(?)

ferrous succinate

ferrous sulfate(?)

fluorouracil(?)

gitalin

glyburide

heptabarbital

hexethal

hexobarbital

ibuprofen

imipramine

indomethacin(?)

influenza virus vaccine

iodide and iodine solutions and compounds

iodochlorhydroxyquin

iodoquinol

iron dextran(?)

iron sorbitex(?)

isocarboxazid(?)

isoniazid

isotretinoin

kanamycin(?)

lanatoside C

levothyroxine(?)

lidocaine

liothyronine(?)

liotrix(?)

lidocaine

measles and rubella virus vaccine (live)

measles, mumps and rubella virus vaccine (live)

mephobarbital

mepivacaine(?)

metharbital

methitural

methohexital

methyl alcohol

methylergonovine

methysergide

metronidazole(?)

minoxidil(?)

mumps virus vaccine (live)

naproxen

nialamide(?)

nitrofurantoin(?)

nortriptyline

nystatin

oral contraceptives

ouabain

oxyphenbutazone

penicillamine

pentobarbital

phenobarbital

phenylbutazone

piroxicam(?)

poliovirus vaccine(?)

polysaccharide-iron complex(?)

prilocaine(?)

primidone

probarbital

procaine(?)

procarbazine

propoxycaine(?)

protriptyline

quinacrine

quinidine

rabies immune globulin

rabies vaccine

radioactive iodides

rifampin(?)

rubella and mumps virus vaccine (live)

rubella virus vaccine (live)

secobarbital

smallpox vaccine

streptomycin

sulfacetamide

sulfachlorpyridazine

sulfacytine

sulfadiazine

sulfadimethoxine

sulfamerazine

sulfameter

sulfamethizole

sulfamethoxazole

sulfamethoxypyridazine

sulfanilamide

sulfaphenazole

sulfapyridine

sulfasalazine

sulfathiazole

sulfisoxazole

sulindac(?)

talbutal

tamoxifen(?)

tetanus immune globulin(?)

tetanus toxoid(?)

thiamylal

thiopental

thyroglobulin(?)

thyroid(?)

tolazamide

tolbutamide

trichloroethylene

tryparsamide

vinbarbital

vinblastine

vincristine

vitamin D

vitamin D_2(?)

vitamin D_3(?)

B. Poisons (inhalation, skin absorption or ingestion): alcohol, arsenicals (inorganic, gaseous, or organic), carbon disulfide, carbon tetrachloride, chlorodinitrobenzene and dinitrobenzene, copper, dinitrotoluene, Lysol solution, mercury, methyl bromide, methyl alcohol, siderosis (exogen: IOFB or endogen: iron metabolism disorders), tobacco, toluene (methyl benzene), trichlorethylene, tricresil phosphate, venoms (e.g., bee sting), vinyl benzene (styrene)

C. Vaccines and toxoids: Bacille Calmette-Guerin (BCG) vaccination, diphtheria toxoid (absorbed), diphtheria and tetanus toxoids (absorbed), influenza virus vaccine, measles and/or mumps and /or rubella live vaccine, poliovirus vaccine, rabies immune globulin, rabies vaccine, smallpox vaccine, tetanus immune globulin (?), tetanus toxoid (?)

3. Infection and inflammation
   A. Bacterial
      (1) Anthrax
      (2) Botulism (toxin from clostridium botulinum)
      (3) Brucellosis (undulant fever)
      (4) Diphtheria
      (5) Endocarditis
      (6) Leptospirosis (Weil syndrome)
      (7) Lyme disease (borreliosis, relapsing fever)
      (8) Mycoplasma pneumoniae
      (9) Pertussis (whooping cough)
     (10) Streptococcus (scarlet fever)
     (11) Syphilis (acquired lues)
     (12) Tuberculosis
     (13) Typhoid fever (abdominal typhus)
   B. Fungal
      (1) Candidiasis
      (2) Coccidioidomycosis
      (3) Mucormycosis
      (4) Torulosis (cryptococcus)
   C. Viral
      (1) AIDS (acquired immune deficiency syndrome)
      (2) Bornholm disease (epidemic pleurodynia)
      (3) Chickenpox (varicella)
      (4) Epidemic keratoconjunctivitis
      (5) Equine encephalitis
      (6) Hepatitis A,B,C
      (7) Infectious mononucleosis
      (8) Influenza
      (9) Measles (rubeola)
     (10) Mumps
     (11) Pappataci fever (sandfly fever)
     (12) Poliomyelitis
     (13) Smallpox
     (14) Yellow fever
   D. Protozoan
      (1) Malaria
      (2) Toxoplasmosis
      (3) Trypanosomiasis
   E. Rickettsial

      (1) Boutonneuse fever rickettsia (Marseilles fever)

      (2) Japanese river fever (typhus)

      (3) Q fever

      (4) Rocky Mountain spotted fever

   F. Orbit

      (1) Herpes zoster

      (2) Infections of the gasserian ganglion

      (3) von Mikulicz-Radecki's syndrome (dacryosialoadenopathy)

      (4) Rollet's syndrome (orbital apex syndrome)

      (5) Tolosa-Hunt syndrome (painful ophthalmoplegia)

   G. Helminth infestations

      (1) Acanthamoeba

      (2) Echinococcosis (hydatid cyst)

      (3) Onchocerciasis (river blindness)

      (4) Toxocariasis (nematode ophthalmia syndrome)

      (5) Trichinellosis

   H. Spread from sphenoid and posterior ethmoidal sinuses

    I. Postinfectious

      (1) Guillain-Barre syndrome (acute infectious neuritis)

      (2) Reye's syndrome (acute encephalopathy syndrome)

      (3) Subacute sclerosing panencephalitis (Dawson's disease)

      (4) Vogt-Koyanagi-Harada syndrome (uveitis-vitiligo-alopecia-poliosis syndrome)

4. Non-infectious arteritis, hypersensitivity vasculitis

   A. Involving small vessels

      (1) Drugs

      (2) Henoch-Schonlein

   B. Involving small and medium sized vessels

      (1) Polyarteritis nodosa (Kussmaul's disease)

      (2) Necrotizing granulomatous arthritis

         a. Sarcoidosis

         b. Wegener's granulomatosis (Wegener's syndrome)

      (3) Buerger's disease (thromboangiitis obliterans)

      (4) Localized arteritis

         a. Idiopathic

         b. Polyarteritis nodosa

   C. Involving large, medium and small vessels

      (1) Arteritis in collagen vascular disease

         a. Behcet's disease (oculobuccogenital syndrome)

         b. Progressive systemic sclerosis (PSS; scleroderma)

         c. Rheumatoid arthritis

         d. Systemic lupus erythematosus (SLE)

      (2) Giant cell (temporal) arteritis

      (3) Takayasu's syndrome (aortic arch syndrome)

  D. Idiopathic paroxysmal digital cyanosis (Raynaud's disease)

  E. Multiple myeloma (Kahler's disease)

5. Others

  A. Chorioretinitis

  B. Cystic fibrosis syndrome

  C. Hutchinson-Gilfor (progeria) syndrome

  D. Hysteria

  E. McCune-Albright syndrome (fibrous dysplasia)

  F. Naegeli's syndrome (melanophoric nevus)

  G. Paget's disease (osteitis deformans)

  H. Parkinson's syndrome (paralysis agitans)

  I. Relapsing polychondritis

  J. Stevens-Johnson syndrome (erythema multiforme exudativum)

  K. Uveitis including sympathetic ophthalmia

6. Systemic diseases

  A. Endocrine

      (1) Diabetes mellitus

      (2) Hypoparathyroidism

      (3) Hyperthyroidism (Basedow's syndrome)

      (4) Hyperthyroidism

      (5) Juvenile diabetes-dwarfism-obesity syndrome (Mauriac's syndrome)

      (6) Lactation

      (7) Pregnancy

      (8) Puberty

      (9) Retinohypophysary syndrome (Lijo Pavia-Lis syndrome)

  B. Nutritional diseases

      (1) Beriberi (vitamin B deficiency)

      (2) Carcinomatosis

      (3) Hyperemesis gravidarum

      (4) Pellagra (vitamin B deficiency)

  C. Rheumatic disease, arthritis

      (1) Felty's syndrome

      (2) Juvenile rheumatoid arthritis (Still's disease)

      (3) Polymyalgia rheumatica

      (4) Reiter's syndrome (polyarthritis enterica)

      (5) Rheumatoid arthritis

  D. Miscellaneous

      (1) Amyloidosis (Lubarsch-Pick syndrome)

(2) Chronic glomerulonephritis with secondary renal hypertension or pyelonephritis

(3) Emphysema

(4) Hepatic failure

(5) Hypertension

(6) Porphyria

7. Trauma

    A. Mechanical

    B. Radiation

        (1) Electromagnetic

            a. High voltage/lighting

            b. Microwave

            c. Laser burn

            d. X-ray

        (2) Radioactive source

            a. α-Ruthenium

            b. β-betatron

            c. γ-cobalt

            d. pisotope

8. Tumors

    A. Craniopharyngioma

    B. Hemangiopericytoma of optic nerve

    C. Myeloproliferative diseases

        (1) Hodgkin's disease

        (2) Leukemia

        (3) Lymphoma

    D. Neuroblastoma

Beck, R.W., et al.: Fellow Eye Abnormalities in Acute Unilateral Optic Neuritis. Ophthalmology, 100:691–698, 1993.

Cappaert, W.E., and Kiprov, R.V.: Craniopharyngioma presenting as unilateral central visual loss. Ann. Ophthalmol., 13:703, 1981.

Fraunfelder, F.T.: Drug-Induced Ocular Side Effects and Drug Interactions. 4th Ed. Philadelphia, Williams & Wilkins, 1996.

Glaser, J.S.: Neuro-Ophthalmology. 2nd Ed. Philadelphia, J.B. Lippincott Co., 1989.

Kerty, E., et al.: Chiasmal optic neuritis. Acta. Ophthalmologica, 69:135–139, 1991.

Song, H.S., and Wray, S.H.: Bee sting optic neuritis. A case report with visual evoked potentials. J. Clinical Neuro-Ophthal., 11:45–59, 1991.

Straussberg, R., et al.: Epstein-Barr virus infection associated with encephalitis and optic neuritis J. Pediatric Ophthal. & Strabismus, 30:262–263, 1993.

Yen, M.Y., and Liu, J.H.: Bilateral optic neuritis following bacille Calmette-Guerin (BCG) vaccination. J. Clin. Neuro-Ophthal., 11:246–249, 1991.

(Neuritis) Papillitis and Retrobulbar Neuritis

	Multiple Sclerosis	Temporal Arteritis	Sinusitis	Diabetes Mellitus	Hyperthyroidism	Chronic Glomerulonephritis	Paget's Disease	Fibrocystic Disease of Pancreas	Oral Contraceptives
History									
1. Familial				U					
2. Greater in children						S			
3. Greater in elderly									
4. Greater in females					S				
5. Greater in men							U		
6. Greater in young individuals	U		U						
7. Greater over age 40				U					
8. Headache, tender temporal arteries and jaw claudication		U							
9. Hereditary						S	U	U	
10. Oral contraceptive history									U
11. Orbital ache (deep)									
12. Possible early viral infection	S								
Physical Findings									
1. Angioid streaks							S		
2. Anisocoria	U			S					
3. Asteroid hyalosis				S					
4. Blue sclera				S			S		
5. Cataract							S		
6. Central retinal artery occlusion		U							
7. Convergent weakness	S			S					
8. Corneal ring opacities							U		
9. Cotton wool spots		U		U		U			
10. Decreased or absent pupillary reaction to light	U	S							
11. Dilation of retinal veins				U		U		U	
12. Diplopia	S								S
13. Discoloration of upper eyelids					S				
14. Extropion uvea				R					
15. Exophthalmos					U		S		
16. Gaze palsy	S								
17. Glaucoma					R	R			
18. Hard yellow exudates				U					
19. Hypotony of the globe			S	R					
20. Hippus of pupil	U								
21. Impaired fixation on extreme lateral gaze	R				S				
22. Iritis		S							
23. Irregular sheathing of retinal veins				S					
24. Ischemic optic neuropathy		U		S				U	
25. Ischemic retinopathy	R			U					
26. Keratitis					S				
27. Keratoconjunctivitis sicca									S
28. Lid lag					U				
29. Lid trembling on gentle closure					U				
30. Lipemia retinalis				U					
31. Macular degeneration							S	S	

(Neuritis) Papillitis and Retrobulbar Neuritis *Continued*

Physical Findings

	Multiple Sclerosis	Temporal Arteritis	Sinusitis	Diabetes Mellitus	Hyperthyroidism	Chronic Glomerulonephritis	Paget's Disease	Fibrocystic Disease of Pancreas	Oral Contraceptives
32. Macular edema				U					
33. Marcus Gunn pupil sign	U	U							
34. Microaneurysms of retina				U					
35. Myopia									S
36. Myokymia	S								
37. Neuroretinal edema				S	U	S			
38. Nystagmus	U								
39. Ophthalmoplegia		S							
40. Optic atrophy	S			S			S	S	
41. Pain and tenderness of the brows			U						
42. Paralysis of 3rd or 6th nerve	S			S			S		
43. Photophobia					S				
44. Prolapse of lacrimal gland					U				
45. Pseudo-Foster Kennedy syndrome	R	U							
46. Ptosis	S	S							
47. Reduced blinking					S				
48. Retinal hemorrhages		S		U		U	S	S	
49. Retinal periphlebitis	R								
50. Retinal neovascularization				S					
51. Retraction of upper lid					U				
52. Rubeosis iridis				S					
53. Scleritis		S							
54. Shallow orbits					S				
55. Swelling of eyelids					U				
56. Tearing, excessive					S				
57. Tonic pupil		U							
58. Uveitis	S								
59. Vitreal hemorrhages					S				R
60. Xerosis of conjunctiva								S	

Lab Data

	Multiple Sclerosis	Temporal Arteritis	Sinusitis	Diabetes Mellitus	Hyperthyroidism	Chronic Glomerulonephritis	Paget's Disease	Fibrocystic Disease of Pancreas	Oral Contraceptives
1. CT scan of optic foramina and parasellar areas abnormal									
2. Dense, expanded bones on X ray							U		
3. E.S.R. elevated		U							
4. Fluorescein angiography abnormal	R	U		U					
5. Glycosuria				U					
6. Hematuria						U			
7. Hyperglycemia				U					
8. Ketonuria				U					
9. Proteinuria				R		U			
10. T4, radio T3 resin uptake and radioiodine uptake elevated					U				
11. Temporal artery biopsy with cellular infiltration and giant cells		U							
12. Urinary hydroxyproline elevated							U		

R = rarely; S = sometimes; U = usually.

Pseudo-optic Neuritis (Lesions that Mimic Optic Neuritis)

1. Congenital retinoschisis
2. Hematoma
3. Ischemic optic neuropathy
4. Papilledema (see p. 653)
5. Retinal lesions that also exhibit metamorphopsia, e.g. serous or angiospastic retinopathy
6. Tumors

     A. Disc

        (1) Gliomas

        (2) Meningiomas

        (3) Metastatic carcinoma

        (4) Neurofibromas

     B. Expanding lesions of anterior and middle cranial fossa producing central scotoma

        (1) Craniopharyngiomas

        (2) Ectopic pinealomas

        (3) Meningiomas

        (4) Metastatic carcinomas

        (5) Myeloproliferative diseases

          a. Hodgkin disease

          b. Lymphomas

          c. Plasmocytoma

        (6) Nasopharyngeal carcinomas

        (7) Pituitary adenomas

Huber, A.: Eye Symptoms in Brain Tumors. 2nd Ed. St. Louis, C.V. Mosby, 1971.

Roy, F.H.: Ocular Syndromes and Systemic Diseases. 2nd Ed. Philadelphia, W.B. Saunders, 1989.

Opticociliary Shunts—Tortous, Ectatic Channels from Optic Nerve to Choroid

1. Arachnoid cyst of the optic nerve
2. Central retinal vein occlusion (see p. 525)
3. Chronic atrophic papilledema
4. Drusen of the optic nerve
5. Optic nerve glioma
6. Primary nerve sheath meningioma
7. Sickle cell trait
8. Spheno-orbital meningioma

Dowhan T.P., et al.: Optociliary shunts and sickle retinopathy in a woman with sickle cell trait. Annal. Ophthal., 22:66–69, 1990.

Zaret, C. R., et al.: Cilio-Optic vein associated with phakomatosis. Ophthalmology, 87:330–336, 1980.

Papilledema (Swelling of Optic Disc)

1. Drugs, poisons and vaccines

    A. Drugs (capitalized indicate drugs also causing pseudotumor cerebri):

acetophenazine

ADRENAL CORTEX INJECTION

ALDOSTERONE

allobarbital

AMPHOTERICIN B

AMIODARONE

amobarbital

antimony lithium thiomalate

antimony potassium tartrate

antimony sodium tartrate

antimony sodium thioglycollate

aprobarbital

aspirin

auranofin(?)

aurothioglucose(?)

aurothioglycanide(?)

AZATHIOPRINE

barbital

benzathine penicillin G

bromide(?)

bupivacaine(?)

butabarbital

butalbital

butallylonal

butaperazine

butethal

calcitriol

carbamazepine

carbon dioxide

carphenazine

cephaloridine(?)

CHLORAMBUCIL

chloramphenicol(?)

chloroprocaine(?)

chlorpromazine

CHLORTETRACYCLIN

cholecalciferol

cisplatin

colchicine

CORTISONE

cyclobarbital

cyclopentobarbital

DANAZOL

DEMECLOCYCLINE

DESOXYCORTICOSTERONE

DEXAMETHASONE

DEXTROTHYROXINE

diethazine

DOXYCYCLINE

ELTROXIN

ethambutol

ethopropazine

etidocaine(?)

FLUDROCORTISONE

fluorometholone

fluphenazine

FLUPREDNISOLONE

GENTAMYCIN

glutethimide

gold Au 198

gold sodium thiomalate(?)

gold sodium thiosulfate(?)

heptabarbital

HEXCHLOROPHENE

hexethal

hexobarbital

hydrabamine phenoxymethyl penicillin

HYDROCORTISONE

IBUPROFEN

INDOMETHACIN

INSULIN-LIKE GROWTH FACTOR I

interferon

isocarboxazid(?)

isoniazid

ISOTRETINOIN

KETOPROFEN

LEVODOPA

LEVOTHYROXINE

lidocaine
LIOTHYRONINE
LITHIUM CARBONATE
LITHIUM CITRATE
MANGANESE
mephobarbital
mepivacaine(?)
MEPREDNISONE
mesoridazine
METHACYCLINE
methaqualone(?)
metharbital
methdilazine
methitural
methohexital
methotrimeprazine
methyl alcohol
methylene blue
METHYLPREDNISOLONE
methyprylon
mitotane
NALIDIXIC ACID
nadolol(?)
naproxen(?)
NORPLANT
NITROFURANTOIN
NITROGLYCERIN
ofloxacin
ORAL CONTRACEPTIVES
OXYTETRACYCLINE
PARAMETHASONE
penicillamine
pentobarbital
perazine
PERHEXILINE
pericyazine
perphenazine
phenelzine(?)
phenobarbital
phenoxymethyl penicillin
PHENYLPROPANOLAMINE
PHENYTOIN
piperacetazine

POTASSIUM PENICILLIN G
POTASSIUM PENICILLIN V
POTASSIUM PHENETHICILLIN
PREDNISOLONE
PREDNISONE
prilocaine(?)
primidone
probarbital
procaine(?)
PROCAINE PENICILLIN G
procarbazine
prochlorperazine
promazine
promethazine
propiomazine
propoxycaine(?)
PYRIDOXINE
quinine
RETINOIDS
secobarbital
sodium antimonylgluconate
sodium salicylate
stibocaptate
stibogluconate
stibophen
sulfacetamide
sulfachlorpyridazine
sulfacytine
sulfadimethoxine
sulfamerazine
sulfameter
sulfamethazine
sulfamethizole
sulfamethoxazole
sulfamethoxypyridazine
sulfanilamide
sulfaphenazole
sulfapyridine
sulfasalazine
sulfathiazole
sulfisoxazole
sulthiame
talbutal

tamoxifen
TETRACYCLINE
thiamylal
thiethylperazine
thiopental
thiopropazate
thioproperazine
thioridazine
THYROGLOBULIN
THYROID

tranylcypromine(?)
trifluoperazine
triflupromazine
trimeprazine
vinbarbital
VITAMIN A (RETINOL)
vitamin D (calcitriol)
vitamin D_2 (ergocalciferol)
vitamin D_3 (cholecalciferol)

B. Poisons (inhalation, skin absorption or ingestion)

   (1) carbon dioxide

   (2) lead

   (3) methyl alcohol

C. Vaccines

   (1) diphtheria-tetanus toxoids-pertussis vaccine (absorbed)

   (2) influenza virus vaccine

   (3) measles and/or mumps and / or rubella live vaccine

2. Intracranial causes—usually bilateral

A. Tumors

  *(1) Frontal lobe lesion—mental changes (apathy, euphoria, and social behavioral changes); normal visual field if confined to frontal lobe; most likely tumors are medulloblastoma, meningioma, astrocytoma, glioblastoma, or metastasis from lung or breast

  *(2) Temporal lobe lesions—formed hallucinations, superior homonymous quadrantanopia, or homonymous hemianopia, ipsilateral mydriatic fixed pupil and oculomotor paresis, and contralateral facial palsy; most likely tumors are medulloblastoma, meningioma, astrocytoma, glioblastoma, or metastasis from lung or breast

  *(3) Parietal lobe lesions—visual agnosia such as alexia or dyslexia, complete homonymous hemianopia, or inferior homonymous quadrantanopia, disturbances of trigeminal nerve, including decreased corneal sensation, and positive (asymmetric response) optokinetic nystagmus; most likely caused by

     a. Astrocytoma

     b. Glioblastoma

     c. Medulloblastoma

     d. Meningioma

     e. Metastasis from lung or breast

   (4) Occipital lobe lesions—unformed visual hallucinations and homonymous congruous visual field defect; most likely caused by

     a. Astrocytoma

     b. Glioblastoma

     c. Hemangioma

* = most important

    d. Meningioma

    e. Metastasis from lung or breast

(5) Third ventricle and sellar lesions—visual field of bitemporal hemianopia or unilateral blindness and contralateral temporal hemianopia; most likely tumors are craniopharyngioma

(6) Fourth ventricle and cerebellum lesions—ataxia, asynergy, dysmetria, hypotonia, and acquired jerk nystagmus, usually horizontal and more pronounced in lateral gaze; most likely caused by

    a. Astrocytoma

    b. Hemangioblastoma

    c. Medulloblastoma

    d. Metastasis from lung or breast

(7) Cerebellar-pontine angle tumor such as Cushing syndrome II (acoustic neuroma syndrome)

(8) Base skull tumor such as Garcin syndrome (half-base syndrome)

(9) Chiasmal tumor such as Frohlich syndrome (dystrophia adiposogenitalis)

(10) Neuroblastoma

(11) Russell's syndrome (diencephalic syndrome)

(12) Zollinger-Ellison syndrome (polyglandular adenomatosis syndrome)

B. Decreased intracranial capacity, such as in acrocephalosyndactyly (Apert disease), Arnold-Chiari syndrome (cerebellomedullary malformation syndrome), craniofacial dysostosis (Crouzon disease), craniostenosis, hypertelorism, and tower skull (oxycephaly)

C. Pseudotumor cerebri (Symonds syndrome)—bilateral papilledema and increased intracranial pressure but negative neurologic and general physical findings

(1) Addison disease (adrenal cortical insufficiency)

(2) Autosomal dominant endosteal hyperostosis

(3) Drugs including:

adrenal cortex injection	doxycycline
aldosterone	etretinate
amiodarone	fludrocortisone
benzathine penicillin G	fluprednisolone
betamethasone	gentamicin
chlorambucil	griseofulvin
chlortetracycline	hexachlorophene
cortisone	hydrabamine penicillin V
danazol	hydrocortisone
demeclocycline	ibuprofen(?)
desoxycorticosterone	indomethacin
dexamethasone	isotretinoin
diphtheria and tetanus toxoids and pertussis vaccine (adsorbed)	ketoprofen
	levodopa(?)

levothyroxine

lithium carbonate

meprednisone

manganese

methacycline

methylprednisolone

minocycline

nalidixic acid

nitrofurantoin

nitroglycerin

oral contraceptives

oxytetracycline

paramethasone

PERHEXILINE

phenylpropanolamine

phenytoin

potassium penicillin G

potassium penicillin V

potassium phenethicillin

prednisolone

prednisone

procaine penicillin G

tetracycline

triamcinolone

vitamin A

    (4) Frankl-Hochwart syndrome (pineal-neurologic-ophthalmic syndrome)

    (5) Glomus jugulare tumor

    (6) Iron deficiency anemia

    (7) Menarche

    (8) Pregnancy

    (9) Thrombosis of the sagittal or lateral sinus, such as that following otitis media in children

    (10) Yersinia pseudotuberculosis

3. Neurologic disorders

  A. Cerebral palsy

  B. Foster-Kennedy syndrome

    (1) Aneurysm of internal carotid, anterior cerebral, or anterior communicating artery

    (2) Arteriosclerotic plaques of internal carotid or anterior cerebral arteries

    (3) Chiasmal arachnoiditis secondary to trauma, spinal anesthesia, or syphilis

    (4) Craniopharyngioma with forward extension

    (5) Frontal lobe tumors or abscess

    (6) Glioma of the intracranial portion of optic nerve

    (7) Internal hydrocephalus because of tumor of posterior fossa

    (8) Old unilateral optic nerve atrophy (e.g., consecutive ischemic optic neuropathies)

    (9) Olfactory groove, sphenoid ridge and suprasellar meningioma

  C. High cerebrospinal fluid protein content and defective absorption (e.g., Guillain-Barre syndrome (acute infectious neuritis))

  D. Muscular dystrophy

  E. Parkinson syndrome (shaking palsy)

  F. Status dysraphicus syndrome (Passow's syndrome, syringomyelia)

  G. Subdural or subarachnoid hemorrhage

4. Miscellaneous

  A. Abscess

    B. Angioedema

    C. Brown-Sequard syndrome

    D. Camurati-Engelmann syndrome (progressive diaphyseal dysplasia)

    E. Chediak-Higashi syndrome (anomalous leukocytic inclusions with constitutional stigma)

    F. Churg-Strauss syndrome (allergic granulomatosis and angiitis)

    G. Citrullinemia (late onset)

    H. Degos' syndrome (malignant atrophic papulosis)

    I. Fabry's disease (angiokeratoma corporis diffusum)

    J. Hydrocephalus

    K. Kenny's syndrome

    L. McCune-Albright syndrome (fibrosus dysplasia)

    M. Nocturnal hypoventilation

    N. Pelizaeus-Merzbacher syndrome (aplasia axialis extracorticalis congenita)

    O. Polymyalgia rheumatica

    P. Primary hyperoxaluria type

    Q. Renal insufficiency

5. Ocular cause—usually unilateral

    A. Acute glaucoma

    B. Aphakic cystoid macula edema (ACME; Irvine-Gass syndrome)

    C. Central retinal vein or artery occlusion

    D. Hypotony, including that following intraocular surgery

    E. Inflammatory

      (1) Birdshot retinochoroideopathy

      (2) Gumma of nerve head

      (3) Juxtapapillary choroiditis

      (4) Neuroretinitis (see p. 551)

      (5) Retinal vasculitis

      (6) Rocky Mountain spotted fever

      (7) Sarcoidosis

      (8) Tuberculoma of nerve head

      (9) Uveitis

    (10) Vasculitis

    F. Trauma

    G. Tumors

      (1) Glioma

      (2) Hemangioma

      (3) Melanocytoma

      (4) Melanotic sarcoma

      (5) Neurofibromatosis (von Recklinghausen disease)

      (6) Periocular and ocular metastatic tumors

    (7) Secondary carcinoma

    (8) Tuberous sclerosis

6. Orbital cause—usually unilateral, may have exophthalmos

    A. Aneurysm of the ophthalmic artery

    B. Orbital abscess

    C. Rollet's syndrome (orbital apex syndrome)

    D. Scaphocephaly syndrome (craniofacial dysostosis)

    E. Sinusitis

    F. Superior orbital fissure syndrome (Rochon-Duvigneaud syndrome)

    G. Trauma

    H. Tumors

      (1) Benign

        a. Cystic adenoma

        b. Dermoid cyst

        c. Osteopetrosis (Albers-Schonberg disease)

        d. Paget's disease

      (2) Malignant

        a. Fibrosarcoma

        b. Glioma

        c. Hutchinson-Pepper syndrome

        d. Lacrimal gland

        e. Lymphosarcoma

        f. Myosarcoma

        g. Osteosarcoma

        h. Secondary metastasis and extension from nasopharynx or sinuses

      (3) Orbital invasion by intracranial tumor, e.g., chordoma

7. Systemic diseases—usually bilateral

    A. Blood dyscrasias

      (1) Iron-deficiency anemias

      (2) Pernicious anemia

      (3) Thrombocytopenic purpura

    B. Carbohydrate metabolisms disorders

      (1) Diabetes mellitus

      (2) Mucolipidoses III

      (3) Mucopolysaccharidoses II (Hunter's syndrome)

      (4) Mucopolysaccharidoses VI (Maroteaux-Lamy syndrome)

    C. Cardiopulmonary insufficiency

      (1) Chronic bronchitis

      (2) Congenital heart disease

      (3) Cystic fibrosis of lungs

      (4) Pickwickian syndrome

      (5) Pulmonary emphysema

D. Collagen diseases
  (1) Polyarteritis nodosa
  (2) Progressive systemic sclerosis (PSS; scleroderma)
  (3) Relapsing polychondritis
  (4) Systemic lupus erythematosus (SLE)

E. Endocrine
  (1) Addison disease (adrenal cortical insufficiency)
  (2) Diabetes mellitus (Willis disease)
  (3) Hyperparathyroidism
  (4) Hyperthyroidism (Basedow syndrome)
  (5) Hypothyroidismus
  (6) Hypocalcemia
  (7) Hypoparathyroidism
  (8) Hypophosphatasia
  (9) Idiopathic hypercalcemia (Drummond syndrome)
  (10) Menses
  (11) Pituitary deficiency
  (12) Pregnancy
  (13) Pseudohypoparathyroidism syndrome
  (14) Suppression of adrenal function from prolonged use of steroids
  (15) Suprarenal—sympathetic syndrome

F. Giant cell (temporal arteritis)

G. Hypertension/arteriosclerosis

H. Infectious (rare usually optic neuritis)
  (1) AIDS (acquired immunodeficiency syndrome)
  (2) Anterior poliomyelitis
  (3) Bang disease (brucellosis)
  (4) Chickenpox
  (5) Coccidioidomycosis
  (6) Echinococcosis (hydatid cyst)
  (7) Encephalitis
  (8) Infectious mononucleosis
  (9) Lyme disease (borreliosis, relapsing fever)
  (10) Malaria
  (11) Meningitis
  (12) Mycoplasma pneumoniae
  (13) Parasitic infections, e.g., cysticercosis and cryptococcus
  (14) Parinaud syndrome (divergence paralysis)
  (15) Pertussis (whooping cough)
  (16) Presumed ocular histoplasmosis

(17) Psittacosis

(18) Sandfly fever (Pappataci fever)

(19) Trichinellosis

(20) Whipple's disease (intestinal lipodystrophy)

I. Postinfectious

(1) Guillain-Barre syndrome (acute infectious neuritis)

(2) Reye's syndrome (acute encephalopathy syndrome)

(3) Subacute sclerosing panencephalitis (Dawson's disease)

(4) Vogt-Koyanagi-Harada syndrome (uveitis-vitiligo-alopecia-poliosis)

J. Myeloproliferative diseases

(1) Histiocytosis X (lipoid granuloma)

(2) Hodgkin's disease

(3) Leukemia

(4) Multiple myeloma

(5) Mycosis fungoides (Sezary's syndrome)

(6) Polycythemia vera

K. Paraproteinemias

(1) Cryoglobulinemia

(2) Macroglobulinemia

(3) Mediterranean fever

(4) POEMS syndrome (polyneuropathy, organomegaly, endocrinopathy, M protein, and skin changes)

L. Nutritional diseases

(1) Beriberi (thiamine deficiency)

(2) Pellagra (niacin deficiency)

(3) Plummer-Vinson syndrome (deficiency of vitamin B complex and iron)

(4) Vitamin B_{12} deficiency

M. Sarcoidosis (Heerford's syndrome, Schaumann's syndrome)

8. Trauma

A. Battered/shaken baby syndrome

B. Cerebral hemorrhage

C. Purtscher's syndrome

9. Vascular malformations

A. Arteriovenous fistula

B. Aneurysms

(1) Bonnet-Dechaume-Blanc syndrome (neuroretinoangiomatosis)

(2) Foramen lacerum syndrome (aneurysm of internal carotid artery syndrome)

(3) Superior vena cava syndrome

C. Cavernous sinus thrombosis (Foix's syndrome)

Beck, R.W., et al.: Optic disc edema in the presumed ocular histoplasmosis. Ophthal., 91:183, 1984.

Cohen, S.M., and Keltner, J.L.: Thrombosis of the lateral transverse sinus with papilledema. Arch. Ophthal., 11:274–275, 1993.

Collins, M.L.Z., et al.: Optic nerve head swelling and optic atrophy in the systemic mucopolysaccharidoses. Ophthalmology, 97:1445–1449, 1991.

Fraunfelder, F.T.: Drug-Induced Ocular Side Effects and Drug Interactions. 4th Ed. Philadelphia, Williams & Wilkins, 1996.

Garrity, J.A., et al.: Optic nerve sheath decompression for visual loss in patients with acquired immunodeficiency syndrome and cryptococcal meningitis with papilledema. Amer. J. Ophthal., 116:472–478, 1993.

Glaser, J.S.: Neuro-Ophthalmology. 2nd Ed. Philadelphia, J.B. Lippincott Co., 1989.

Hardten, D.R., et al.: Papilledema and intraspinal lumbar paraganglioma. J. Clinical Neuro-Ophthal., 12:158–162, 1992.

Roy, F.H.: Ocular Syndromes and Systemic Diseases. 2nd Ed. Philadelphia, W.B. Saunders, 1989.

Unilateral Papilledema (Swelling of Optic Disc)

	Hypotony	Acute Glaucoma*	Ocular Inflammation as Sarcoid	Retinoblastoma	Central Retinal Vein Occlusion*	Central Retinal Artery Occlusion*	Ocular Trauma	Orbital Benign Tumor as Paget Disease	Orbital Malignant Tumor as Lacrimal Gland	Orbital Infection as Abscess
History										
1. Common in blacks		U	U				S			
2. Common in females			U	S		R				
3. Common in males		S					U		U	S
4. Common over fourth decade		U			S	U		U		
5. Familial		S		S						
6. Hereditary				S				U		
7. Lacrimation							S	S	S	
8. Ocular pain	U						S		S	U
9. Painless				U						
10. Trauma/surgery	U						U			S
Physical Findings										
1. Anterior/posterior synechiae	S	U	S				S			
2. Associated with neurofibromatosis				R						
3. Blue sclera							R	S		
4. Cataract	S	U	S				U	S		
5. Chemosis of conjunctiva		U							S	U
6. Cherry-red spot of macula						U				
7. Choroidal detachment	U									
8. Choroidal folds	U		S	S					S	S
9. Choroidal rupture							S			
10. Closed anterior chamber angle		U								
11. Cotton-wool spots					S					
12. Cyclodialysis cleft	S									
13. Dacryoadenitis			S							
14. Dacryocystitis			S							
15. Decreased intraocular pressure	U				S		S			
16. Disc pallor				S						
17. Endothelial corneal damage							S			
18. Epithelial corneal edema		U					S			
19. Exophthalmos			S	S			S	S	S	
20. Extraocular muscle paralysis			S	S				S	S	U
21. Folds in Bowman Descemet membrane	U	U								
22. Globe displacement								R	S	
23. Hard exudates					S					
24. Hypermetropia				S						
25. Hyphema							S			
26. Hypopyon			R							
27. Increased intraocular pressure		U	S	S	S	S	R	S		S
28. Involvement of trigeminal nerve									S	S
29. Iridodialysis							S			
30. Keratopathy	U	S								S
31. Macular edema	S				S	S	R			S
32. Macular hemorrhage			R		S		S			
33. Marcus-Gunn pupil				S			S			

Unilateral Papilledema (Swelling of Optic Disc) *Continued*

	Hypotony	Acute Glaucoma*	Ocular Inflammation as Sarcoid	Retinoblastoma	Central Retinal Vein Occlusion*	Central Retinal Artery Occlusion*	Ocular Trauma	Orbital Benign Tumor as Paget Disease	Orbital Malignant Tumor as Lacrimal Gland	Orbital Infection as Abscess
Physical Findings										
34. Milky appearance of retina						U	S			
35. Nystagmus				S						
36. Optic neuritis			S							S
37. Orbital mass				U					U	
38. Orbital myositis								R	S	
39. Panophthalmitis									R	
40. Pigmentary iris degeneration	S	U								
41. Pigmentary retinopathy							S	S		
42. Pseudoretinitis pigmentosa							S			
43. Pupil dilated and fixed		U	S			S	S			
44. Recessed chamber angle							S			
45. Retinal detachment			S				S			
46. Retinal folds	U									
47. Retinal hemorrhages			S		U	R	U	S		
48. Retinal microaneurysms					S					
49. Retinal neovascularization					S					
50. Retinal tractional tear							S			
51. Rubeosis iridis					S	R				
52. Scleral rupture							S			
53. Shallow anterior chamber	U	U								
54. Shallow orbits								S		
55. Strabismus				S						
56. Subluxed lens	S						S			
57. Uveitis	S		S	R						S
58. Visual field defects		U		S	U	U	S			
59. Vitreous hemorrhage			S				S			
Laboratory Data										
1. Abnormal glucose tolerance test					S					
2. Biopsy of inferior forniceal follicles			U							
3. Computed tomography of orbit				U			U	S	U	
4. Cerebrospinal fluid protein level elevated			U							S
5. Chest roentgenogram			U						S	S
6. Fluorescein angiography	S				U	U	U	S	R	S
7. Lipid profile elevated					S					
8. Orbit roentgenogram			S	U				S	R	S
9. Visual field test		U		S			S			
10. Ultrasonography	S		S	U			U	S	S	S

R = rarely; S = sometimes; and U = usually.

Bilateral Papilledema (Swelling of Optic Disc)

	Frontal Lobe Tumor as Meningioma	Temporal Lobe Tumor as Medulloblastoma	Parietal Lobe Tumor as Astrocytoma	Occipital Lobe Tumor as Glioblastoma	Third Ventricle and Sellar Tumor as Craniopharyngioma	Fourth Ventricle and Cerebellum Tumor as Hemangioblastoma	Infection as Meningitis	Pseudotumor Cerebri	Blood Dyscrasias	Hypertension	Cystic Fibrosis	Hyperthyroidism	Diabetes Mellitus	Collagen Disorders as Polyarteritis Nodosa
History														
1. Common in children		U	U		R	U	S		S		U			
2. Common in females	U							U				U		
3. Common in males			U		R	R		S						U
4. Congenital				U							U			
5. Familial										R	S	U	U	
6. Hereditary						R					U			
7. Occurs in blacks								U						
8. Occurs in whites								U			U			
9. Visual hallucinations		S		U										
10. Visual object agnosia				S										
Physical Findings														
1. Associated with neurofibromatosis	S													
2. Cataract													U	S
3. Cotton-wool spots									S	S			S	S
4. Edema of lids/conjunctiva	S											S		S
5. Exophthalmos	S	S	S			S								S
6. Extraocular muscle paralysis	U	S			S	S	S	S	S			S		S
7. Glaucoma						S				S			S	
8. Hypermetropia	S													
9. Infrequent blinking												U		
10. Intraorbital bleeding										U				
11. Keratitis	S					S	S					U		S
12. Lid lag												U		
13. Macular edema									S	S		U		
14. Marcus-Gunn pupil	S					S								
15. Nystagmus	S	S	U			S								S
16. Optic neuritis		S		S	S		U			S	S	R		
17. Opticocilary venous shunts	S													
18. Orbital mass	U					S				U				
19. Orbital myositis				S										
20. Peripheral retinal neovascularization										S			S	
21. Ptosis						S				R				S
22. Retinal angioma						U								
23. Retinal detachment						S				S	S		S	R
24. Retinal hemorrhages										S	S	S	U	
25. Retinal microaneurysms										S	S		U	
26. Venous sheathing										S	R		S	R
27. Retinal vein occlusion											S		S	S
28. Retraction of upper lid												U		
29. Rubeosis iridis													S	
30. Scleritis														S

Bilateral Papilledema (Swelling of Optic Disc) *Continued*

	Frontal Lobe Tumor as Meningioma	Temporal Lobe Tumor as Medulloblastoma	Parietal Lobe Tumor as Astrocytoma	Occipital Lobe Tumor as Glioblastoma	Third Ventricle and Sellar Tumor as Craniopharyngioma	Fourth Ventricle and Cerebellum Tumor as Hemangioblastoma	Infection as Meningitis	Pseudotumor Cerebri	Blood Dyscrasias	Hypertension	Cystic Fibrosis	Hyperthyroidism	Diabetes Mellitus	Collagen Disorders as Polyarteritis Nodosa
Physical Findings														
31. Superficial strawberry hemangioma						S								
32. Strabismus						S								
33. Tremor of closed eyelids												U		
34. Uveitis							R		R					S
35. Visual field defects	S	S	U	U	U			U						S
36. Vitreous hemorrhage									S	S			S	
Laboratory Data														
1. Angiography, cerebral	R	R	R	R	R	R		R						
2. Biopsy, muscle														U
3. Blood cell count							U		U					U
4. Blood sugar elevated													U	
5. Bone marrow puncture									U					
6. Computed tomography	U	U	U	U	U	U						U		
7. Cerebral spinal fluid							U	U	U					
8. Chest roentgenogram											U			
9. Fluorescein angiography						S				U			U	
10. Lipid profile										U			S	
11. Sed rate							U							S
12. Ultrasonography, orbit	S					S						U		
13. MRI	U	U	U	U	U	U	S	U	R					

R = rarely; S = sometimes; and U = usually.

Pseudopapilledema (May Be Mistaken for Swelling of Optic Nerve)

1. Arteriovenous aneurysms (racemose aneurysms) of the retina (Wyburn-Mason syndrome)
2. Bergmeister papilla
3. Cervico-oculo-acousticus syndrome
4. Down's syndrome
5. Drusens of optic nerve (see p. 601)
6. Epipapillary membrane and Bergmeister papilla
7. Fuchs's coloboma (partial)
8. Hematoma
9. High hyperopia or astigmatism
10. Juvenile diabetes mellitus (Mauriac's syndrome)
11. Medullated nerve fibers (opaque nerve fibers)
12. Normal variant
13. Opacities or haziness of the media, especially nuclear sclerosis of the lens
14. Optic neuritis or papillitis (see p. 643)
15. Peripapillary retinal hemangioma
16. Sarcoidosis (Schaumann's syndrome)
17. Tilted disc (partial)
18. Tortuosity and anomalous early branching of the retinal vessels
19. Tumors of disc
    A. Gliomas
    B. Meningiomas
    C. Metastatic
    D. Neurinoma
    E. Neurofibroma

Catalano, R.A., and Simon, J.W.: Optic disk elevation in Down's syndrome. Am. J. Ophthalmol., 110:28–32, 1990.

Duke-Elder, S., and Scott, G.I.: System of Ophthalmology. Vol. 12. St. Louis, C.V. Mosby, 1971, pp. 76–78.

Perkins, E.S., and Dobree, J.H.: The Differential Diagnosis of Fundus Conditions. St. Louis, C.V. Mosby, 1972.

Peripapillary Subretinal Neovascularization

1. Excessive laser treatment
2. Optic disc drusens
3. Optic nerve coloboma
4. Presumed histoplasmosis syndrome
5. Presumed sarcoidosis
6. Serpiginous peripapillary choroiditis

Gragoudas, E.S., and Regan, C.D.J.: Peripapillary subretinal neovascularization in presumed sarcoidosis. Arch. Ophthalmol., 99:1194, 1981.

Jampol, L.M., and Goldbaum, M.H.: Peripheral proliferative retinopathies. Surv. Ophthalmol., 25:1, 1980.

Yedavally, S., and Frank, R.N.: Peripapillary subretinal neovascularization associated with coloboma of the optic nerve. Arch. Ophthal., 111:552–553, 1993.

Pigmented Tumors of Optic Disc

1. Drusen
2. Bourneville's syndrome (tuberous sclerosis)
3. Hemangioma of the disc with hemorrhages and secondary pigmentation
4. Malignant melanoma
5. Melanocytomas
6. Metastases

Apple, D.J., et al.: Congenital anomalies of the optic disc. Surv. Ophthalmol., 27:3, 1982.

Pseudoglaucomatus Atrophy of Optic Disc (Cupping of Nerve Head with Optic Atrophy and Field Defects Simulating True Glaucoma but without Ocular Hypertension)

1. Arteriosclerosis
2. Congenital anomalies of the optic disc
    A. Branching of vessels behind the lamina, so that the individual branches appear at the disc margins
    B. Coloboma within the nerve sheath
    C. Congenital coloboma of the optic disc
    D. Morning glory anomaly
    E. Oblique insertion of the optic nerve
    F. Traction of the disc with bowing of the scleral crescent
3. Giant cell (temporal) arteritis
4. Optic pit
5. Patients using digitalis
6. Reduced blood supply to optic nerve, e.g., acute hypotension, blood loss (severe) carotid insufficiency, gastrointestinal bleeding, ischemic optic neuropathy, myocardial infarction, pernicious anemia
7. Schnobel's cavernous atrophy
8. Syphilitic optic nerve atrophy
9. Tumors arising near the chiasm

Abedin, S., et al.: Progressive low-tension glaucoma. Ophthalmology, 89:1, 1982.

Jonas, J.B., et al.: Pseudoglaucomatous physiologic large cups. Am. J. Ophthalmol., 107:137–144, 1989.

Kolker, A.E., and Hetherington, J.: Becker-Schaffer's Diagnosis and Therapy of the Glaucomas. 6th Ed. St. Louis, C.V. Mosby, 1989.

Maisel, J.M., et al.: Large optic disks in the Marshallese population. Am. J. Ophthalmol., 107:145–150, 1989.

Sebag, J., et al.: Optic disc cupping in arteritic anterior ischemic optic neuropathy resembles glaucomatous cupping. Ophthalmology, 93:357–361, 1986.

Vaughan, D., et al.: General Ophthalmology. 12th Ed. Norwalk, Conn., Appleton & Lange, 1989.

Temporally Displaced Disc (Dragged Disc)

1. Abnormal tortuous retinal vessels temporally
2. Ectopic macula
3. Retinopathy of prematurity (ROP)
4. Temporally displaced vessels (see p. 568)

Gow, J., and Oliver, G.L.: Familial exudative vitreoretinopathy. Arch. Ophthalmol., 86:150–155, 1971.

Visual Field Defects

EDWARD G. BUCKLEY, M.D.

Contents

Pseudo visual field defect

1. Facial contour

    A. Prominent nose

    B. Bushy projecting eyebrows

    C. High cheekbones

    D. Ptosis or blepharochalasis

    E. Sunken globes

    F. Fracture of orbit

2. Corneal opacities

3. Lenticular opacities, especially if miotics are used, will depress fields and exaggerate existing scotomas

4. Aphakia without lens or with convex lens; little distortion with contact lens or intraocular lens

5. Dull patient, patient may be mentally defective, have toxemia, arteriosclerosis, cerebral tumor, brain abscess, or increased intracranial pressure

6. Pupillary size

    A. Decrease in miotic field, especially with opacities of ocular media

7. Uncorrected refractive errors—correct for distance testing

8. Head tilting when the head is tilted toward the left shoulder, the right blind spot is elevated; when the head is tilted toward the right shoulder, the right blind spot is lowered

9. Environmental artifacts

    A. Reduction in illumination of screen and test objects magnifies field defect

    B. Variation in size of test object changes field defect

    C. Standard distance of patient from screen

    D. Attention of patient

    E. Technique of examiner

10. Psychologic artifacts

    A. Patient's misunderstanding of test

    B. Tiring of patient by prolonged testing

    C. Malingering—isopters at different distances are inconsistent

    D. Hysteria—spiral field defects may be found

11. Frames of glasses and segments of multifocal lenses

12. Colored contact lenses

Insler, M.S., et al.: Visual field constriction caused by colored contact lenses. Arch. Ophthalmol., 106:1680–1682, 1988.

Meyer, D.R., et al.: Evaluating the Visual Field Effects of Blepharoptosis Using Automated Static Perimetry. Ophthalmology, 100:651–659, 1993.

Differential Diagnosis of Eye Diseases. 2nd ed. New York, Thieme Med. Pub., 1988.

Bilateral Central Scotomas (Bilateral Macular Defects with Decreased Visual Acuity; Scotomas May Be Central or Centrocecal)

1. Bilateral macular lesions such as cysts or those due to hemorrhage, edema, degeneration, detachment, hole, or infection (see p. 501 or 541)

2. Bilateral optic nerve lesions

    A. Papilledema with macular edema (see p. 493)

    B. Papillitis (see p. 643)

    C. Retrobulbar neuritis (see p. 643)

3. Diabetes mellitus

4. Familial optic atrophies (see p. 625)

5. Hyperbaric oxygen

6. Migraine—forerunner of visual aurae

*7. Nutritional deficiency, such as thiamine or Vitamin B_{12} deficiency

8. Pernicious anemia

9. Occipital cortex lesions

* = most important

10. Toxic agents

    A. Aromatic amino- and nitro-compounds—aniline, nitrobenzene, trinitro-toluene

    B. Carbon disulfide

    C. Drugs, including:

acetophenazine

acetyldigitoxin

adrenal cortex injection

alcohol

aldosterone

allobarbital

aluminum nicotinate(?)

aminosalicylic acid(?)

amobarbital

amodiaquine

aprobarbital

aspirin

barbital

betamethasone

bromide

bromisovalum

butabarbital

butalbital

butallylonal

butaperazine

butethal

caramiphen(?)

carbromal

carphenazine

chloramphenicol

chloroquine

chlorpromazine

chlorpropamide(?)

clomiphene

cobalt(?)

cortisone

cyclobarbital

deslanoside

desoxycorticosterone

dexamethasone

diethazine

digitalis

digitoxin

digoxin

disulfiram

emetine

epinephrine

ergot

ethambutol

ethchlorvynol

ethopropazine

fludrocortisone

fluorometholone

fluphenazine

fluprednisolone

gitalin

heptabarbital

hexethal

hexobarbital

hydrocortisone

hydroxychloroquine

ibuprofen

indomethacin(?)

iodide and iodine solutions and compounds

isoniazid

lanatoside C

lithium carbonate

medrysone

mephobarbital

mesoridazine

metharbital

methdilazine

methitural

methohexital

methotrimeprazine

methylprednisolone

methysergide

morphine(?)

niacinamide(?)

nicotinic acid(?)

nicotinyl alcohol(?)

opium

oral contraceptives

ouabain
oxygen
paramethadione
paramethasone
pentobarbital
perazine
pericyazine
perphenazine
phenobarbital
piperacetazine
prednisolone
prednisone
primidone
probarbital
prochlorperazine
promazine
promethazine
propiomazine
quinacrine
quinidine
quinine
radioactive iodides
secobarbital
sodium salicylate
streptomycin
sulfacetamid

sulfachlorpyridazine
sulfadiazine
sulfadimethoxine
sulfamerazine
sulfameter
sulfamethizole
sulfamethoxazole
sulfamethoxypyridazine
sulfanilamide
sulfaphenazole
sulfisoxazole
talbutal
thiamylal
thiethylperazine
thiopental
thiopropazate
thioproperazine
thioridazine
thyroid(?)
triamcinolone
trichloroethylene
trifluoperazine
triflupromazine
trimeprazine
trimethadione
vinbarbital

   D. Ethyl alcohol

   E. Halogenated hydrocarbons—methyl chloride, methyl bromide, iodoform, trichloroethylene

   F. Metals—lead, thallium (inorganic), arsenic

   G. Methyl alcohol

   H. Tobacco

Fraunfelder, F.T.: Drug-Induced Ocular Side Effects and Drug Interactions. Philadelphia, Williams & Wilkins, 1996.

Harrington, D.O., and Drake, M.V.: The Visual Fields: Text and Atlas of Clinical Perimetry. 6th ed. St. Louis, C.V. Mosby, 1990.

Enlargement of Blind Spot

   1. Blind spot syndrome (multiple evernescent white dot syndrome [MEWS])

   2. Coloboma of the optic nerve

   3. Drugs, including:

adrenal cortex injection
aldosterone
betamethasone

carbon dioxide
chlortetracycline
cortisone

demeclocycline
desoxycorticosterone
dexamethasone

doxycycline	medrysone	prednisone
ergot	methacycline	quinacrine
fludrocortisone	methylprednisolone	tetracycline
fluorometholone	minocycline	triamcinolone
fluprednisolone	oxytetracycline	trichloroethylene
hydrocortisone	paramethasone	vitamin A
indomethacin(?)	prednisolone	

3. Drusen of the optic nerve (see p. 619)

4. Glaucoma

5. Inferior conus

6. Inverted disc or nasally directed scleral canal

7. Juxtapapillary choroiditis

8. Medullated nerve fibers

9. Multifocal choroiditis

10. Multifocal evanescent white-dot syndrome

*11. Papilledema (pseudotumor cerebri) (see p. 653)

12. Papillitis (see p. 643)

13. Progressive myopia with a temporal crescent

14. Senility—senile halo

Fraunfelder, F.T.: Drug-Induced Ocular Side Effects and Drug Interactions. Philadelphia, Williams & Wilkins, 1996.

Kahn, H.A., and Milton, R.C.: Alternative definitions of open angle glaucoma. Arch. Ophthalmol., 98:2172, 1980.

Khorram, K.D., et al.: Blind spot enlargement as a manifestation of multifocal choroiditis. Arch. Ophthalmol., 109:1403–1416, 1991.

Singh, K., et al.: Acute idiopathic blind spot enlargement. Ophthalmology, 98:497–502, 1991.

Arcuate (Cuneate) Scotoma (Scotoma Follows the Lines of the Nerve Fibers in the Retina with the Narrow End at the Blind Spot and Broad End at Horizontal Raphe)

1. Acute bleeding episode

2. Branch artery occlusion

3. Branch vein occlusion

4. Chorioretinitis juxtapapillaris

5. Coloboma of the disc

6. Drusen of optic nerve

*7. Glaucoma

8. High myopia

9. Inferior conus

10 Ischemic optic neuropathy

11. Myelinated nerve fibers

Greve, E.L., and Verriest, G.: Fourth International Visual Field Symposium. The Hague, Netherlands, Dr. Junk, 1981.

Harrington, D.O., and Drake, M.V.: The Visual Fields: Text and Atlas of Clinical Perimetry. 6th ed. St. Louis, C.V. Mosby, 1990.

Unilateral Sector-shaped Defects (Narrow End of Scotoma Characteristically Touches the Physiologic Blind Spot)

1. Optic disc involvement

   A. Glaucoma (early stages primarily on nasal side)

   B. Papillitis

   C. Secondary optic atrophy after choked disc (more on nasal side)

2. Retina

   A. Branch artery occlusion (see p. 512)

   B. Juxtapapillary chorioretinitis

3. Optic nerve—between disc and chiasm

   A. Aneurysm

   B. Drusen

   C. Tumor

Hart, W.M., and Becker, B.: The onset and evolution of glaucomatous visual field defects. Ophthalmology, 89:268, 1982.

Spekreijse, H., and Apkarian, P.A.: Visual Pathways. The Hague, Netherlands, Dr. Junk, 1981.

Peripheral Field Contraction (Central Vision Present; Patient May Complain of Poor Night Vision)

1. Choroiditis—periphery of fundus

*2. Chronic atrophic papilledema (pseudotumor cerebri)

3. Bilateral homonymous hemianopia (if the macular sparing in one homonymous hemianopia is larger than that in the other homonymous hemianopia, the spared central portion of the field has small vertical steps, above and below fixation, where the two areas of macular sparing do not quite coincide)

   A. Cortical blindness with damage to occipital lobe and macular recovery

      (1) Anoxia

      (2) Carbon monoxide poisoning

      (3) Cardiac arrest

      (4) Cerebral angiography

      (5) Exsanguination

      (6) Trauma

   B. Stroke of infarction of occipital lobe

4. Drugs, including:

acetophenazine	amodiaquine
acridine	aprobarbital
alcohol	arsenic
allobarbital	aspirin
amobarbital	barbital

* = most important

bromisovalum
butalbital
butallylonal
butaperazine
butethal
carbon dioxide
carbon monoxide
carbromal
carisoprodol
carphenazine
chloramphenicol
chloroquine
chlorpromazine
chlorpropamide(?)
clomiphene
cobalt
cortisone
cyclobarbital
deslanoside
desoxycorticosterone
dexamethasone
diethazine
digitalis
digoxin
disulfiram
emetine
epinephrine
ergot
ethambutol
ethchlorvynol
ethopropazine
ethylhydrocupreine
filax mas
fludrocortisone
fluorometholone

fluphenazine
fluprednisolone
gitalin
heptabarbital
hexamethonium
hexethal
hexobarbital
hydrocortisone
hydroxychloroquine
ibuprofen
indomethacin
iodide and iodine solutions and compounds
isoniazid
lanatoside C
lithium carbonate
medrysone
mephobarbital
mesoridazine
metharbital
methdilazine
methitural
methohexital
methotrimeprazine
methylprednisolone
methysergide
morphine(?)
niacinamide(?)
nicotinic acid(?)
nicotinyl alcohol(?)
opium
oral contraceptives
ouabain
oxygen
paramethadione
omas

5. Drusen of optic disc

6. Frontal lobe tumors

7. General apathy in a lackadaisical subject

*8. Glaucoma

9. Hysteria and malingering

10. Many conditions in which night blindness occurs (see p. 729)

11. Optic atrophy (see p. 625)

12. Papillitis (see p. 643)

13. Retinitis—periphery of fundus

14. Retinitis pigmentosa

15. Unilateral concentric constriction, excluding diseased retina or glaucoma suggests lesion of optic nerve and chiasm

    A. Meningioma of tuberculum sellae, sphenoid ridge, or the olfactory groove

    B. Tumor of optic nerve

Fraunfelder, F.T.: Drug-Induced Ocular Side Effects and Drug Interactions. Philadelphia, Williams & Wilkins, 1996.

Harrington, D.O., and Drake, M.V.: The Visual Fields: Text and Atlas of Clinical Perimetry. 6th ed. St. Louis, C.V. Mosby, 1990.

Pau, H.: Differential Diagnosis of Eye Diseases. 2nd ed. New York, Thieme Med. Pub., 1988.

Altitudinal Hemianopia (Defective Vision or Blindness in the Upper or Lower Horizontal Half of the Visual Field; May be Unilateral or Bilateral; Unilateral Field Defect Is Prechiasmal)

1. Anemia—produces bilateral inferior altitudinal hemianopia

*2. Anterior ischemic optic neuropathy

3. Bilateral branch retinal artery occlusion

4. Fusiform aneurysms (arteriosclerotic or congenital)—may produce inferior altitudinal hemianopia by pressure against the lateral halves of the optic chiasm or nerve

5. Herpes zoster

6. Lesion that presses the chiasm upward against the superior margin of the optic foramen

7. Occipital lobe lesions

    A. Hypoxia

    B. Stroke

8. Olfactory groove meningioma extending postero-inferior to compress the intracranial portion of the optic nerve

9. Optic nerve lesion

    A. Anterior ischemia optic neuropathy

    B. Coloboma

    C. Glaucoma

    D. Optic neuritis

    E. Papilledema

    *F. Trauma

    G. Tumor

10. Sclerotic plaques of internal carotid artery or anterior cerebral arteries—pressure of plaques on optic nerve results in inferior altitudinal hemianopia

Anderson, D.R.: Perimetry with and without Automation. 2nd ed. St. Louis, C.V. Mosby, 1986.

Harrington, D.O., and Drake, M.V.: The Visual Fields: A Text and Atlas of Clinical Perimetry. 6th ed. St. Louis, C.V. Mosby, 1990.

Miyashita, K., et al.: Superior altitudinal hemianopia and herpes zoster. Annals of Ophthalmology, 25:20–23, 1993.

Binasal Hemianopia (Defects in Nasal Half of Visual Fields; Usually Incomplete; Due to Lateral Involvement of Chiasm; Presupposes Bilateral Lesions)

1. Bilateral occipital lesion (thrombosis)
2. Chiasmic arachnoiditis, postneuritic optic atrophy, and bilateral retrobulbar neuritis of multiple sclerosis
3. Damage to chiasm
4. Drusen of optic nerve (see p. 621)
5. Fusiform aneurysms—arteriosclerotic or congenital—of internal carotid artery
6. Glaucoma
7. Meningiomas, especially from the lesser wing of the sphenoid bone
8. Nasal quadrant peripheral depression of glaucoma—bilateral and reasonably symmetrical
9. Pituitary tumor with third ventricle dilatation pushing laterally
10. Retinal damage
11. Severe exsanguination
12. Sclerotic plaques of internal carotid artery or anterior cerebral arteries
13. Symmetric lesions in the temporal halves of both retinas, such as severe retinal edema associated with diabetic retinopathy
14. Trauma

Cox, T.A., et al.: Unilateral nasal hemianopia as a sign of intracranial optic nerve compression. Am. J. Ophthalmol., 92:230–232, 1981.

Harrington, D.O., and Drake, M.V.: The Visual Fields: Text and Atlas of Clinical Perimetry. 6th ed. St. Louis, C.V. Mosby, 1990.

Pau, H.: Differential Diagnosis of Eye Diseases. 2nd ed. New York, Thieme Med. Pub., 1988.

Bitemporal Hemianopia (Defects in Temporal Half of Visual Field; Usually Incomplete; Due to Pressure on the Optic Chiasm)

1. Chiasmal lesions
   A. Congenital defect as de Morsier syndrome (septo-optic dysplasia)
   B. Inflammatory lesions
      *(1) Basal meningitis, including: chronic chiasmal syphilitic, tuberculous, actinomycotic, and cysticercal arachnoiditis
      (2) Chiasmal neuritis
   C. Tumors of the chiasm
      *(1) Primary tumors, including: gliomas in childhood
      *(2) Secondary tumors (rare), including: meningiomas, retinoblastoma, pinealoma, and ependymoma
   D. Vascular lesions
      (1) Arterial compression
      (2) Arteriosclerosis
      (3) Ectasia of the intracranial carotid arteries
      *(4) Intracranial aneurysms, such as congenital, endocardial emboli, traumatic, atheromatic, or syphilitic, especially intrasellar aneurysms
      (5) Thrombosis of the carotid artery

2. Perisellar lesions

   A. Parasellar tumors

      (1) Injuries to the chiasmal pathway, such as from trauma

     *(2) Meningioma of the sphenoid ridge

      (3) Migraine

      (4) Sudden onset without apparent cause

         a. Arteriosclerotic or giant-cell arteritic occlusion of nutrient vessels of the chiasm in elderly patients

         b. Disseminated sclerosis

      (5) Tumors of the basal meninges

      (6) Tumors of the sphenoid bone including osteochondroma, sarcoma, anaplastic carcinoma

   B. Presellar tumors

     *(1) Meningioma of the olfactory groove

      (2) Neuroblastoma of the olfactory groove

   C. Suprasellar tumors

      (1) Chordoma

     *(2) Craniopharyngioma—manifestations may include diabetes insipidus, infantilism, and calcification of hypophyseal-pituitary region

      (3) Epidermoids

      (4) Lymphoblastoma

      (5) Pinealoma

     *(6) Suprasellar meningioma

      (7) Teratoma

      (8) Tumors of the frontal lobe, including: porencephaly (cystic cavity in brain substance) and glioma

      (9) Tumors of the third ventricle and internal hydrocephalus, such as glioma and epidymoma

3. Pituitary lesions

   A. Pituitary hyperplasia

   B. Pituitary tumors

      (1) Adenoma

         a. Acidophilic adenoma—varies from gigantism to acromegaly

         b. Basophilic adenoma—hyperadrenalism (Cushing disease), Nelson syndrome

         c. Chromophobe adenoma—varies from no endocrine symptoms to panhypopituitarism; most common type of pituitary tumor, Frohlich syndrome

      (2) Adenocarcinoma (rare)

      (3) Metastatic tumors as from breast (rare)

Lao, et al.: Vascular architecture of the human optic chiasma and bitemporal hemianopia. Chinese Medical Sciences Journal, 9:38–44, 1994.

Roy, F.H.: Ocular Syndromes and Systemic Diseases. 2nd ed. Philadelphia, W.B. Saunders, 1989.

* = most important

Slavin, M.L.: Bitemporal hemianopia associated with dolichoectasia of the intracranial carotid arteries. J. Clinical Neuro-Ophthalmology, 10:80–81, 1990.

Homonymous Quadrantanopia (One Quadrant Involved in Upper or Lower and Right or Left Visual Fields; Etiology May Include Tumor, Vascular Lesion or Infection)

1. Superior homonymous quadrantanopia

    A. Inferior lip of the calcarine fissure—congruous

    B. Temporal lobe—incongruous

2. Inferior homonymous quadrantanopia

    A. Anton syndrome (denial—visual hallucination)

    B. Superior radiation in parietal lobe—incongruous

    C. Upper lip of the calcarine fissure in the occipital lobe—congruous

Bosley, T.M., et al.: Neuro-imaging and positron emission tomography of congenital homonymous hemianopsia. Am. J. Ophthalmol., 111:413–418, 1991.

Ellenberger, C.: Perimetry: Principles, Technique and Interpretation. New York, Raven Press, 1980.

Harrington, D.O., and Drake, M.V.: The Visual Fields: Textbook and Atlas of Clinical Perimetry. 6th ed. St. Louis, C.V. Mosby, 1990.

Crossed Quadrantanopia (Upper Quadrant of One Visual Field is Along with the Lower Quadrant of Opposite Visual Field)

*1. Asymmetrical homonymous hemianopia, such as vascular lesion of the upper lip of the calcarine area on one side and the lower lip of the opposite calcarine cortex

2. Chiasm compression from lesion below compressing it against contiguous arterial structure

3. Glaucoma

4. Inflammatory lesion, such as choroiditis juxtapapillaris

Harrington, D.O., and Drake, M.V.: The Visual Fields: Text and Atlas of Clinical Perimetry. 6th ed. St. Louis, C.V. Mosby, 1990.

Homonymous Hemianopia (Hemianopia Affecting Right or Left Halves of Visual Fields; Lesion is Posterior to Optic Chiasm)

1. Optic tract lesions—visual conduction system posterior to optic chiasm and anterior to lateral geniculate body; lesion demonstrates incongruous field defect on side opposite to defect, often with decreased vision, optic atrophy and afferent pupil.

    A. Demyelinative disease—retrobulbar, multiple sclerosis, and Schilder disease

    B. Migraine

    C. Pituitary adenomas and craniopharyngiomas (most common); nasopharyngeal carcinomas, chordomas, infundibulomas, and gliomas (less common)

    D. Saccular aneurysms of internal carotid or posterior communicating artery

    E. Trauma

2. Temporoparietal lesions—temporal lobe lesions are manifest initially in the upper visual fields, whereas lesions of the parietal lobe are first manifest in the lower visual fields

A. Diffuse demyelinative diseases
  (1) Krabbe type (Sturge-Weber-Krabbe syndrome)
  (2) Metachromatic leukoencephalopathy
  (3) Pelizaeus-Merzbacher type (aplasia axialis extracorticalis congenita)
  (4) Progressive multifocal leukoencephalopathy
  (5) Schilder type (encephalitis periaxialis diffusa)
  (6) Spongy degeneration of the brain (Canavan disease)

B. Migraine

C. Tumor—gradual onset of symptoms—lesions include intrinsic astrocytoma and glioblastoma, extrinsic meningioma, and lung metastasis

D. Vascular lesions—sudden onset
  (1) Embolism—may be associated with rheumatic or arteriosclerotic heart disease, bacterial endocarditis, myocardial infarction, or septic focus in lungs
  (2) Occlusion—middle cerebral occlusion affects primarily the arm and face; anterior cerebral occlusion affects primarily the leg
  (3) Subdural hematoma—spontaneous or following trauma
  (4) Thrombosis—premonitory symptoms include unilateral blackouts in one eye

E. Trauma (surgical)

3. Occipital lesions—congruous field defect and macular sparing most likely

A. Demyelinative disease
  (1) Creutzfeldt-Jakob disease
  (2) Krabbe type (Sturge-Weber-Krabbe syndrome)
  (3) Metachromatic leukoencephalopathy
  (4) Pelizaeus-Merzbacher type (aplasia axialis extracorticalis congenita)
  (5) Progressive multifocal leukoencephalopathy
  (6) Schilder type (encephalitis periaxialis diffusa)
  (7) Spongy degeneration of the brain (Canavan disease)

B. Migraine

C. Poisons, such as carbon monoxide, digitalis, mescal, opium, lysergic acid diethylamide

D. Trauma
  (1) Direct—penetrating missiles and depressed bone fragments
  (2) Indirect—general concussion syndrome
  (3) Temporal lobectomy

E. Tumors—gradual onset of symptoms—lesions, include: intrinsic astrocytoma and glioblastoma, extrinsic meningioma, and lung metastasis

F. Vascular lesion—sudden onset
  (1) Arteriovenous anomalies
  (2) Aneurysms (rare)
  (3) Occlusion of posterior cerebral artery—thrombotic or embolic
  (4) Subclavian steal syndrome, with reversal of blood flow through the vertebral artery

* = most important

Anderson, D.R., et al.: Optic tract injury after anterior temporal lobectomy. Ophthalmology, 96:1065–1070, 1989.

Harrington, D.O., and Drake, M.V.: The Visual Fields: Text and Atlas of Clinical Perimetry. 6th ed. St. Louis, C.V. Mosby, 1990.

Lewis, R.A., et al.: Visual loss in migraine. Ophthalmology, 96:321–326, 1989.

Roy, F.H.: Ocular Syndromes and Systemic Diseases. 2nd Ed. Philadelphia, W.B. Saunders, 1989.

Tychsen, L., and Hoyt, W.F.: Relative afferent pupillary defect in congenital occipital hemianopia. Am. J. Ophthalmol., 100:345–346, 1985.

Vargas, M.E., et al.: Homonymous field defect as the first manifestation of Creutzfeldt-Jakob disease. Amer. J. Ophthal., 119:497–504, 1995.

Spiral Field Defects

*1. Hysteria

2. Radiation therapy in or about the retina, optic nerve, and anterior visual pathways

Fitzgerald, C.R., et al.: Radiation therapy in and about the retina, optic nerve, and anterior visual pathway. Arch. Ophthalmol., 99:611–623, 1981.

Double Homonymous Hemianopsia (Peripheral Constriction with Small Vertical Steps Above and Below Fixation due to Lesions of Occipital Area and Probable Involvement of Striate Cortex of Both Occipital Lobes)

1. Bilateral central retinal artery occlusion

2. Bilateral central retinal vein occlusion

3. Bilateral vascular lesions involving a calcarine fissure

4. Increased intracranial pressure with shift of uncal portion of temporal lobe down over edge of tentorium with compression of posterior cerebral arteries and infarction in calcarine cortex.

5. Partial recovery from cortical blindness (see p. 704) from trauma, anoxia, carbon monoxide poisoning, cerebral angiography, cardiac arrest, exsanguination and other similar conditions.

6. Severe end stage glaucoma

7. Severe trauma with massive brain damage as in depressed fracture of occiput.

Harrington, D.O., and Drake, M.V.: The Visual Fields: Text and Atlas of Clinical Perimetry. 6th ed. St. Louis, C.V. Mosby, 1990.

General Signs and Symptoms

Visual Disturbance

G.A. CIOFFI, M.D.

Contents

*Acquired Myopia (Error of Refraction, in which Parallel Rays of Light Focus in Front of Retina Usually Producing Blurred Distant Vision and Clear Near Vision)

*1. Conditions such as diabetes mellitus or nuclear sclerotic cataract in which there is increased index of refraction of lens

*2. Refractive myopia—increased curvature of the refracting surfaces because of:

    A. Ciliary muscle spasm

        (1) Functional—adolescence, hysteria

        (2) Miotics such as carbachol, demecarium, echothiophate, isoflurophate, neostigmine, and physostigmine

        (3) Trauma—ocular contusion or anterior dislocation of the lens

        (4) Mushroom (Amanita muscaria) poisoning

    B. Lens hydration changes—diabetes mellitus, dysentery, or toxemia of pregnancy

    C. Drug reaction—probably because of ciliary body edema including:

acetazolamide	doxycycline	methylprednisolone
acetophenazine	droperidol(?)	metolazone
adrenal cortex injection	echothiophate	minocycline
alcohol	ethopropazine	morphine
aldosterone	ethosuximide	neostigmine
aspirin	ethoxzolamide	opium
bendroflumethiazide	fludrocortisone	oral contraceptives
benzthiazide	fluphenazine	oxygen
betamethasone	fluprednisolone	oxytetracycline
betaxolol	haloperidol(?)	paramethasone
butaperazine	hyaluronidase	penicillamine
carbachol	hydrochlorothiazide	perazine
carphenazine	hydrocortisone	pericyazine
chlorothiazide	hydroflumethiazide	perphenazine
chlorpromazine	ibuprofen	phenformin
chlortetracycline	indapamide	phensuximide
chlorthalidone	isoflurophate	physostigmine
cimetidine(?)	isosorbide dinitrate	pilocarpine
clofibrate	isotretinoin	piperacetazine
codeine	levobunolol	polythiazide
cortisone	meprednisone	prednisolone
cyclothiazide	mesoridazine	prednisone
demecarium	methacholine	prochlorperazine
demeclocycline	methacycline	promazine
desoxycorticosterone	methazolamide	promethazine
dexamethasone	methdilazine	propiomazine
dichlorphenamide	methotrimeprazine	quinethazone
diethazine	methsuximide	sodium salicylate
digitalis(?)	methyclothiazide	spironolactone

sulfacetamide	sulfamethoxypyridazine	thioproperazine
sulfachlorpyridazine	sulfanilamide	thioridazine
sulfacytine	sulfaphenazole	timolol
sulfadiazine	sulfapyridine	triamcinolone
sulfadimethoxine	sulfasalazine	trichlormethiazide
sulfamerazine	sulfathiazole	trifluoperazine
sulfameter	sulfisoxazole	trifluperidol(?)
sulfamethazine	tetracycline	triflupromazine
sulfamethizole	thiethylperazine	trimeprazine
sulfamethoxazole	thiopropazate	

    D. Elongated globe

    E. Paralysis of accommodation for distance (sympathetic paralysis)—young patient with unilateral Homer syndrome or migraine

    F. Retinopathy of prematurity (retrolental fibroplasia)

    G. Congenital glaucoma

    H. Albinism

    I. Gyrate atrophy (ornithine ketoacid aminotransferase deficiency)

    J. Hypoparathyroidism

    K. Malaria

    L. Inherited

        (1) Cochlear deafness with myopia and intellectual impairment—autosomal recessive

        (2) Epiphyseal dysplasia of femoral heads, myopia, deafness—autosomal recessive

        (3) Epiphyseal dysplasia, multiple, with myopia and conductive deafness—autosomal dominant

        (4) Microcornea and cataract—autosomal dominant

        (5) Microphthalmos with myopia and corectopia—autosomal dominant

        (6) Myopia—autosomal recessive or dominant or less often X-linked

        (7) Night blindness, congenital stationary with myopia (nyctalopia-myopia)—X-linked

        (8) Night blindness with high-grade myopia—autosomal recessive

        (9) Pingelopese blindness (total color blindness with myopia, achromatopsia with myopia)—autosomal recessive

    M. With scleral buckling surgery

3. Syndromes associated with myopia

    A. Aberfeld syndrome (congenital blepharophimosis)

    B. Achard syndrome (Marfan syndrome with dysostosis mandibulofacialis)

    C. Alport syndrome (hereditary familial congenital hemorrhagic nephritis)

    D. Bloch-Sulzberger syndrome

    E. Chromosome partial deletion (long-arm) syndrome

    F. Cohen syndrome

    G. Cri-du-chat syndrome

* = most important

H. de Lange syndrome (congenital muscular hypertrophy cerebral syndrome)

I. Down syndrome (trisomy syndrome)

J. Ehlers-Danlos syndrome (fibrodysplasia elastica generalisata)

K. Fetal alcohol syndrome

L. Forsius-Eriksson syndrome (Aland disease)

M. Gansslen syndrome (familial hemolytic icterus)

N. Haney-Falls syndrome (congenital keratoconus posticus circumscriptus)

O. Homocystinuria

P. Hypomelanosis of Ito syndrome

Q. Kartagener syndrome (sinusitis, bronchiectasis, situs inversus syndrome)

R. Kneist syndrome

S. Laurence-Moon-Bardet-Biedl syndrome (retinitis pigmentosa-polydactyly-adiposogenital syndrome)

T. Marchesani syndrome (brachymorphy with spherophakia)

U. Marfan syndrome (arachnodactyly dystrophia mesodermalis congenita)

V. Marshall syndrome (atypical ectodermal dysplasia)

W. Matsoukas syndrome (oculo-cerebro-articulo-skeletal syndrome)

X. Myasthenia gravis (Erb-Goldflam syndrome)

Y. Noonan syndrome (male Turner syndrome)

Z. Obesity-cerebral-ocular-skeletal anomalies syndrome

AA. Oculodental syndrome (Peter syndrome)

BB. Pierre-Robin syndrome (micrognathia-glossoptosis syndrome)

CC. Pigmentary ocular dispersion syndrome

DD. Rubinstein-Taybi syndrome (broad thumbs syndrome)

EE. SED congenita (spondyloepiphyseal dysplasia, congenital type)—autosomal dominant

FF. Scheie syndrome

GG. Schwartz syndrome (glaucoma associated with retinal detachment)

HH. Siemens syndrome (hereditary ectodermal dysplasia syndrome)—autosomal recessive

II. Stickler syndrome (hereditary progressive arthro-ophthalmopathy)—autosomal dominant

JJ. Trisomy 20p syndrome

KK. Trisomy syndrome

LL. Toumaala-Haapanen syndrome (unknown etiology similar to pseudohypoparathyroidism)

MM. Van Bogaert-Hozoy syndrome (similar to Rubinstein-Taybi syndrome)

NN. Wagner syndrome (hyaloideoretinal degeneration)

OO. Weil-Marchesani syndrome (brachymorphy with spherophakia)

PP. Wrinkly skin syndrome

QQ. XXXXY syndrome (hypogenitalism, limited elbow pronation, low dermal finger tip ridge count)

4. Transient myopia

    A. Chemical agents and disease

  *B. Diabetes

  *C. After surgery

    D. Trauma

Crysberg, J.R.M., et al.: Features of a syndrome with congenital cataract and hypertrophic cardiomyopathy. Am. J. Ophthalmol., 102:740–749, 1986.

Fraunfelder, F.T.: Drug-Induced Ocular Side Effects and Drug Interactions. 4th ed. Philadelphia, Williams & Wilkins, 1996.

Gordon, R.A., et al.: Myopia associated with retinopathy of prematurity. Ophthalmology, 93:1593–1598, 1986.

Isenberg, S.J.: The Eye in Infancy. Chicago, Year Book Medical Publishers, 1989.

Lerner, B.C., et al.: Transient myopia and accommodative paresis following retinal cryotherapy and panretinal photocoagulation. Am. J. Ophthalmol., 97:704–708, 1984.

McKusick, V.A.: Mendelian Inheritance in Man. 9th Ed. Baltimore, Johns Hopkins University Press, 1994.

Roy, F.H.: Ocular Syndromes and Systemic Diseases. 2nd Ed. Philadelphia, W.B. Saunders, 1989.

Walsh, F.B., and Hoyt, W.F.: Clinical Neuro-ophthalmology. Vol. I. 4th Ed. Baltimore, Williams & Wilkins, 1985.

Acquired Hyperopia (Farsightedness, Error of Refraction, in which Parallel Rays of Light Focus behind Retina, Usually Producing Clear Distant Vision and Blurred Near Vision)

  1. Aarskog syndrome (facial-digital-genital syndrome)

  2. Adie syndrome (tonic pupil)

 *3. Aphakia

  4. Best syndrome (vitelliform dystrophy)

 *5. Diabetes mellitus (poorly controlled to controlled)

  6. Down syndrome (mongolism)

  7. Drugs including:

antihistamines	sulfachlorpyridazine(?)	sulfanilamide(?)
cannabis	sulfadiazine(?)	sulfaphenazole(?)
chloroquine	sulfadimethoxine(?)	sulfapyridine(?)
ergot	sulfamerazine	sulfasalazine(?)
imipramine	sulfameter(?)	sulfathiazole(?)
meprobamate	sulfamethazine	sulfisoxazole(?)
phenothiazines	sulfamethizole	tolbutamide(?)
parasympatholytic drugs	sulfamethoxazole	
penicillamine	sulfamethoxypyridazine(?)	

  8. Flat cornea

  9. Gorlin-Chaudhry-Moss syndrome (multiple basal cell nevi syndrome)

*10. Hyperopia—refractive or axial

 11. Hypoglycemia

 12. Kenny syndrome (nanophthalmos with hyperopia)

* = most important

13. Leber congenital amaurosis

14. Lesions causing internal ophthalmoplegia with paralysis of accommodation

15. Macular edema

16. Orbital tumor with extraocular globe pressure and retinal striae

17. Post surgical correction of myopia (RK, ALK, PRK)

*18. Presbyopia

19. Rubinstein-Taybi syndrome

20. Sorby syndrome (hereditary macular coloboma syndrome)

20. Toxin of Clostridium botulinum

21. Trauma to the eye with posterior dislocation of the lens, macular edema, or ciliary body contusion

Fraunfelder, F.T.: Drug-Induced Ocular Side Effects and Drug Interactions. 4th Ed. Philadelphia, Williams & Wilkins, 1996.

John, M.E.: High Hyperopia after Radial Keratotomy. J. Cataract Refract. Surg., 19:446–448, 1993.

Isenberg, S.J.: The Eye in Infancy. Chicago, Year Book Medical Publishers, 1989.

Larsen, J.L., et al.: Unusual cause of short stature. Am. J. Med., 78:1025–1032, 1985.

Newell, F.W.: Ophthalmology, Principles and Concepts. 8th Ed. St. Louis, C.V. Mosby, 1992.

Pau, H.: Differential Diagnosis of Eye Diseases. 2nd Ed. New York, Thieme Med. Pub., 1988.

Roy, F.H.: Ocular Syndromes and Systemic Diseases. 2nd Ed. Philadelphia, W.B. Saunders, 1989.

Dysmegalopsia—Optical Illusions of Size

1. Macropsia (objects appear larger)

    *A. Miotics

    *B. Spasm of accommodation (see p. 466)

    C. Use of excessive plus lenses

2. Metamorphopsia (objects appear distorted)

    A. Cerebral

        (1) Drug intoxications

        (2) Epilepsy

        (3) Focal lesions such as thrombosis of right middle cerebral artery

        *(4) Migraine

        (5) Parietal lobe lesion, including tumor and vascular lesion

        (6) Schizophrenia

    B. Hysteria

    C. Ocular

        (1) Astigmatism

        *(2) Macular lesions, including: orbital tumor with macular striae and macular edema, inflammation or heterotopia

        (3) Posterior vitreous separation and residual vitreoretinal macular traction

        (4) Retinal detachment

    D. Paget disease (osteitis deformans)

3. Micropsia (objects appear smaller)

    A. Accommodative paralysis and subnormal accommodation (see p. 467)

    B. Atropinization

    C. Botulism

    D. Diphtheria

   *E. Presbyopia

    F. Use of excessive minus lenses

    G. Use of scopolamine

4. Teleopsia (objects appear farther away than they actually are)

    A. Bilateral parietal lesion

    B. Parietal lesion in nondominant hemisphere

Pau, H.: Differential Diagnosis of Eye Diseases. 2nd Ed. New York, Thieme Med. Pub., 1988.

Walsh, F.B., and Hoyt, W.F.: Clinical Neuro-ophthalmology. Vol.1. 4th Ed. Baltimore, Williams & Wilkins, 1985.

Bilateral Transient Loss of Vision (Transient Darkening of Vision)

 *1. Circulatory disturbances when bending over or straining (postural hypotension)

  2. Essential hypotension

    A. Arteriosclerosis

    B. Chronic hypotension

   *C. Fatigue

    D. Hormonal disorders

    E. Hunger

    F. Vitamin deficiency

  3. Fainting with vasomotor collapse

  4. Heart failure

  5. Transurethral resection of the prostate

Creel, D.J., et al.: Transient blindness associated with transurethral resection of the prostate. Arch. Ophthalmol., 105:1537–1539, 1987.

Pau, H.: Differential Diagnosis of Eye Diseases. 2nd Ed. New York, Thieme Med. Pub., 1988.

Amaurosis Fugax (Transient Monocular Blackout of Vision)

  1. Amaurosis fugax syndrome

  2. Arteriosclerosis, hypertension, and hypertensive crisis

  3. Canalis opticus syndrome: functional—hysteria, neurasthenia

 *4. Cerebrovascular insufficiency

    A. Arterial aneurysms

    B. Congenital or acquired arteriovenous malformations

    C. Fibromuscular hyperplasia

    D. Post-traumatic acute and chronic arterial occlusion

* = most important

E. Takayasu syndrome (pulseless disease)

*F. Unilateral occlusive carotid disease

5. Functional—hysteria, neurasthenia

6. Hematologic causes

    A. Emboli

        (1) Infective, such as subacute bacterial endocarditis

        (2) Gas in dysbarism

    B. Idiopathic thrombocytosis

    C. Multiple myeloma (Kahler disease)

    D. Polycythemia (Vaquez disease)

    E. Severe anemia

    F. Sickle cell disease (Herrick syndrome)

7. Hypotension of fundus

    A. Cardiac arrhythmia

    B. Impending vascular occlusion, retinal vasospasm associated with systemic vasospastic disease (migraine)

    C. Increased intracranial pressure, such as from intracranial tumors that interfere with vascular supply to the optic nerve

    D. Increased venous pressure

        (1) Impending central retinal vein occlusion (see p. 653)

        (2) Intermittent elevation of intraocular pressure (glaucoma)

    E. Negative G-force in pilots—circular maneuver with head toward the center of the circle

    F. Orbital vascular insufficiency with giant-cell arteritis

    G. Papilledema—lasts for to seconds (see p. 653)

    H. Positive G-force in pilots—circular maneuver with feet toward center of circle

8. Large vitreous floater

9. Ornithine transcarbamoylase deficiency

10. Pituitary tumor

11. Polymyalgia rheumatica

12. Quinine poisoning

13. Raynaud disease (paroxysmal digital cyanosis)

14. Retrobulbar anesthesia

15. Spontaneous bleeding from a normal-appearing iris

16. Taveras syndrome (progressive intracranial arterial occlusion syndrome)

17. Uhthoff symptom—vision decreased with exercise or ocular hyperthermia can occur with:

    A. Friedreich ataxia

    B. Insufficiency of posterior cerebral arteries

    C. Intrasellar and parasellar tumor

    D. Multiple sclerosis (disseminated sclerosis)

18. Uremic amaurosis—with eclampsia

19. Wasp sting

Bishara, S.A., et al.: Immediate contralateral amaurosis after retrobulbar anesthesia. Annals of Ophthal., 22:63–65, 1990.

Cohen, G.R., et al.: Clinical significance of transient visual phenomena in the elderly. Ophthalmology, 91:436–441, 1984.

Dirr, L.Y., et al.: Amaurosis fugax due to pituitary tumor. J. Clinical Neuro-Ophthal., 11:254–258, 1991.

Feinber, A.W.: Recognition and significance of amaurosis fugax. Heart Disease & Stroke, 2:382–385, 1993.

Roy, F.H.: Ocular Syndromes and Systemic Diseases. 2nd Ed. Philadelphia, W.B. Saunders, 1989.

Mader, T.H., et al.: Spontaneous bleeding from a normal-appearing iris: an unusual cause of atypical amaurosis fugax. Annals of Emergency Medicine, 19:1066–1068, 1990.

Snebold, N.G., et al.: Transient visual loss in ornithine transcarbamoylase deficiency. Am. J. Ophthalmol., 104:407–412, 1987.

Xiong, L., et al.: Amaurosis fugax caused by a dural arteriovenous fistula from the ophthalmic artery. Amer. J. Neuroradiology, 14:191–192, 1993.

Sudden Painless Loss of Visual Acuity—One Eye

1. Acute keratoconus
2. Complication of retrobulbar block
3. Injury to the optic nerve
4. Meningeal carcinomatosis
5. Occlusion of central retinal artery (see p. 512)
*6. Retinal detachment
7. Vitreous or retinal hemorrhage

Appen, R.E., et al.: Meningeal carcinomatosis with blindness. Am. J. Ophthalmol., 86:661–665, 1978.

Brookshire, G.L., et al.: Life-threatening Complication of Retrobulbar Block. Ophthalmology, 93:1476–1478, 1986.

Kearne, J.R.: Sudden blindness after ventriculography: Bilateral retinal vascular occlusion superimposed on papilledema. Am. J. Ophthalmol., 78:275–278, 1974.

Post-traumatic Loss of Vision

*1. Acute (angle closure) glaucoma precipitated by emotional trauma of recent accident or from intumescent lens capsular trauma or other blunt trauma
2. Avulsion of optic nerve by lateral orbital wall trauma or contrecoup blow to head
3. Central retinal artery (see p. 512) or vein occlusion (see p. 525) (from markedly increased orbital pressure or embolus)
4. Cortical blindness from hematoma, ischemia or anoxia (patient may be unaware of blindness)
5. Hyphema, vitreous hemorrhage (see p. 474)
6. Hysteria
7. Indirect trauma to optic nerves and/or chiasm
8. Intracranial interruption of visual pathways (hemorrhage, foreign body)
*9. Lid swelling, blood or foreign material covering cornea, corneal damage
10. Malingering
*11. Retinal detachment

* = most important

12. Traumatic cataract, luxation of the lens (see p. 453)

13. Traumatic retinal edema and hemorrhages of retina from direct or contre-coup blows

Deutsch, T.A., and Feller, D.B.: Paton and Goldberg's Management of Ocular Injuries. Philadelphia, W.B. Saunders, 1985.

Decreased Visual Acuity

1. Achromatopsia

2. Amblyopia ex anopsia—disuse

    A. Anisometropia—difference in refractive error between the eyes

    B. Monocular occlusion

    C. Strabismus—esotropia, exotropia, or hypertropia

    D. Unilateral atropinization

3. Anomalous elevation of optic disc with hyperplastic glial tissue and anomalous retinal vessels

4. Apparently normal eye with central fixation with poorer visual acuity in one than other eye—anisometropia

5. Apparently normal eye with normal fixation with disparity between near and distance vision—amblyopia, hysteria, malingering, retrobulbar neuritis, presbyopia, and micronystagmus

6. Apparently normal eye with normal fixation with poor distance and near vision-astigmatism, amblyopia, hyperopia in older persons

7. Drugs including:

acebutolol	aluminum nicotinate
aceclidine	amantadine
acetaminophen	ambenonium
acetanilid	ambutonium
acetazolamide	aminosalicylate(?)
acetohexamide	aminosalicylic acid(?)
acetophenazine	amiodarone
acetyldigitoxin	amithiozone
acid bismuth sodium tartrate(?)	amitriptyline
acyclovir	amobarbital
adiphenine	amodiaquine
adrenal cortex injection	amoxapine
albuterol	amphetamine
alcohol	amphotericin B
aldosterone	amyl nitrite
alkavervir	anisindione
allobarbital	anisotropine
allopurinol	antazoline
alprazolam	antimony lithium thiomalate
alseroxylon	antimony potassium tartrate

antimony sodium tartrate

antimony sodium thioglycollate

antipyrine

aprobarbital

aspirin

atenolol

atropine

azatadine

bacitracin

baclofen

barbital

BCG vaccine

belladonna

bendroflumethiazide

benoxinate

benzathine penicillin G

benzphetamine

benzthiazide

benztropine

betamethasone

betaxolol

biperiden

bismuth oxychloride

bismuth sodium tartrate(?)

bismuth sodium thioglycollate(?)

bismuth sodium triglycollamate(?)

bismuth subcarbonate(?)

bismuth subsalicylate(?)

bromide

bromisovalum

brompheniramine

broxyquinoline

bupivacaine

busulfan

butabarbital

butacaine

butalbital

butallylonal

butaperazine

capreomycin

captopril

carbachol

carbamazepine

carbinoxamine

carbon dioxide

carbromal

carisoprodol

carmustine

carphenazine

cefaclor(?)

cefadroxil(?)

cefamandole(?)

cefazolin(?)

cefonicid(?)

cefoperazone(?)

ceforanide(?)

cefotaxime(?)

cefotetan(?)

cefoxitin(?)

cefsulodin(?)

ceftazidime(?)

ceftizoxime(?)

ceftriaxone(?)

cefuroxime(?)

cephalexin(?)

cephaloglycin(?)

cephaloridine(?)

cephalothin(?)

cephapirin(?)

cephradine(?)

chloral hydrate

chlorambucil

chloramphenicol

chlorcyclizine

chlordiazepoxide

chloroform

chloroprocaine

chloroquine

chlorothiazide

chlorpheniramine

chlorphenoxamine

chlorphentermine

chloroprocaine

chlorpromazine

chlorpropamide

chlorprothixene

chlortetracycline

chlorthalidone

cimetidine

cisplatin

clemastine

clidinium

clofazimine

clofibrate

clomiphene

clomipramine

clonazepam

clonidine

clorazepate

cobalt

cocaine

codeine

colchicine

colloidal silver

cortisone

cryptenamine

cyclizine

cyclobarbital

cyclopentobarbital

cyclopentolate

cyclophosphamide

cycloserine

cyclosporine

cyclothiazide

cycrimine

cyproheptadine

cytarabine

dacarbazine

danazol

dantrolene

dapsone

deferoxamine

demecarium

demeclocycline

deserpidine

desipramine

deslanoside

desoxycorticosterone

dexamethasone

dexbrompheniramine

dexchlorpheniramine

dextroamphetamine

dextrothyroxine

diatrizoate meglumine and sodium

diazepam

diazoxide

dibucaine

dichlorphenamide

dicumarol

dicyclomine

diethazine

diethylpropion

digitalis

digitoxin

digoxin

diltiazem

dimethindene

diphemanil

diphenadione

diphenhydramine

diphenylpyraline

diphtheria and tetanus toxoids adsorbed

diphtheria and tetanus toxoids and pertussis (adsorbed)

diphtheria toxoid (adsorbed)

dipivefrin

disopyramide

disulfiram

doxepin

doxycycline

doxylamine

dronabinol

droperidol

dyclonine

echothiophate

edrophonium

emetine

enalapril

ephedrine

epinephrine

ergonovine

ergot

ergotamine
erythrityl tetranitrate
ethacrynic acid
ethambutol
ethchlorvynol
ether
ethionamide
ethopropazine
ethosuximide
ethoxzolamide
etidocaine
etretinate
fenfluramine
fenoprofen
flecainide
floxuridine
fludrocortisone
fluorometholone
fluorouracil
fluphenazine
fluprednisolone
flurazepam
flurbiprofen
furosemide
gentamicin
gitalin
glutethimide
glyburide
glycerin
glycopyrrolate
griseofulvin
guanethidine
halazepam
haloperidol
hashish
heparin
heptabarbital
hexachlorophene
hexamethonium
hexethal
hexobarbital
hexocyclium
homatropine

hydrabamine penicillin V
hydralazine
hydrochlorothiazide
hydrocortisone
hydroflumethiazide
hydromorphone
hydroxyamphetamine
hydroxychloroquine
ibuprofen
imipramine
indapamide
indomethacin
influenza virus vaccine
insulin
interferon
iodide and iodine solutions and compounds
iodochlorhydroxyquin
iodoquinol
iophendylate
iothalamate meglumine and sodium othalamic acid
iron dextran
isocarboxazid
isoflurophate
isoniazid
isopropamide
isosorbide
isosorbide dinitrate
isotretinoin
kanamycin
ketamine
ketoprofen
labetalol
lanatoside C
levallorphan
levobunolol
levodopa
levothyroxine
lidocaine
liothyronine
liotrix
lithium carbonate
lomustine

lorazepam

lysergide

mannitol

mannitol hexanitrate

maprotiline

marihuana

measles and rubella virus vaccine (live)

measles, mumps and rubella virus vaccine (live)

measles virus vaccine (live)

mecamylamine

mechlorethamine

meclizine

medrysone

mefenamic acid

melphalan

mepenzolate

meperidine

mephenesin

mephobarbital

mepivacaine

meprednisone

meprobamate

mescaline

mesoridazine

methacycline

methadone

methamphetamine

methantheline

methaqualone

metharbital

methazolamide

methdilazine

methitural

methixene

methocarbamol

methohexital

methotrexate

methotrimeprazine

methscopolamine

methsuximide

methyclothiazide

methyl alcohol

methylatropine nitrate

methyldopa

methylene blue

methylergonovine

methylphenidate

methylprednisolone

methyprylon

methysergide

metoclopramide

metolazone

metoprolol

metrizamide

metronidazole

mexiletine

mianserin

midazolam

minocycline

minoxidil

mitomycin

mitotane

morphine

moxalactam(?)

mumps virus vaccine (live)

nadolol

nalidixic acid

nalorphine

naloxone

naltrexone

naphazoline

naproxen

neostigmine

niacin

niacinamide

nialamide

nicotinyl alcohol

nifedipine

nitrazepam

nitrofurantoin

nitroglycerin

nitrous oxide

nortriptyline

nystatin

opium

oral contraceptives
orphenadrine
ouabain
oxazepam
oxprenolol
oxygen
oxymorphone
oxyphenbutazone
oxyphencyclimine
oxyphenonium
oxytetracycline
paraldehyde
paramethasone
pemoline
pentaerythritol tetranitrate
pentazocine
pentobarbital pentolinium
perazine
perhexiline
pericyazine
perphenazine
phenacaine
phenacetin
phencyclidine
phendimetrazine
phenelzine
phenindione
pheniramine
phenmetrazine
phenobarbital
phensuximide
phentermine
phenylbutazone
phenylephrine
phenylpropanolamine
phenytoin
physostigmine
pilocarpine
pimozide
pindolol
pipenzolate
piperacetazine
piperazine

piperidolate
piperocaine
piroxicam
poldine
poliovirus vaccine
polymyxin B
polythiazide
potassium penicillin G
potassium penicillin V
potassium phenethicillin
practolol
pralidoxime
prazepam
prazosin
prednisolone
prednisone
prilocaine
primidone
probarbital
procaine
procaine penicillin G
prochlorperazine
procyclidine
promazine
promethazine
propantheline
proparacaine
propiomazine
propoxycaine
propoxyphene
propanolol
protoveratrines A and B
protriptyline
psilocybin
pyridostigmine
pyrilamine
quinacrine
quinethazone
quinidine
quinine
rabies immune globulin
rabies vaccine
radioactive iodides

ranitidine
rauwolfia serpentina
rescinnamine
reserpine
rifampin
rubella and mumps virus vaccine (live)
rubella virus vaccine (live)
scopolamine
secobarbital
semustine
silver nitrate
silver protein
smallpox vaccine
sodium antimonylgluconate
sodium salicylate
spironolactone
stibocaptate
stibogluconate
stibophen
streptomycin
streptozocin
sulfacetamide
sulfachlorpyridazine
sulfacytine
sulfadiazine
sulfadimethoxine
sulfamerazine
sulfameter
sulfamethazine
sulfamethizole
sulfamethoxazole
sulfamethoxypyridazine
sulfanilamide
sulfaphenazole
sulfapyridine
sulfasalazine
sulfathiazole
sulfisoxazole
sulindac
sulthiame
syrosingopine
talbutal
tamoxifen

temazepam
tetracaine
tetracycline
tetraethylammonium
tetrahydrocannabinol
tetrahydrozoline
thiabendazole
thiamylal
thiethylperazine
thiopental
thiopropazate
thioproperazine
thioridazine
thiothixene
thyroglobulin
thyroid
timolol
tobramycin
tocainide
tolazamide
tolbutamide
tranylcypromine
trazodone
triamcinolone
triazolam
trichlormethiazide
trichloroethylene
tridihexethyl
triethylenemelamine
trifluoperazine
trifluperidol
triflupromazine
trihexyphenidyl
trimeprazine
trimethaphan
trimethidinium
trimipramine
tripelennamine
triprolidine
trolnitrate
tropicamide
tryparsamide
uracil mustard

urea

urethan

verapamil

veratrum viride alkaloids

vinbarbital

vinblastine

warfarin

8. Hysteria

9. Irregular astigmatism—distortions in the anterior corneal surface (scarring, ectasia, edema, ulcer, postinflammatory processes)

10. Macular pathology (including edema, hemorrhage or scar tissue)

11. Malingering

*12. Myopia

13. Myotonic dystrophy—exertional vision loss

14. Nystagmus

15. Opacities of cornea, lens, or vitreous precluding good vision

16. Optic neuritis—retrobulbar and papillitis, including toxic causes such as those due to tobacco, alcohol, and quinine (see p. 641)

17. Sphenoid sinus mucocele

18. Transient refractive errors

    *A. Hyperopia

    B. Myopia—diabetes

Cohen, D.B., and Glasgow, B.J.: Bilateral Optic Nerve Cryptococcosis in Sudden Blindness in Patients with Acquired Immune Deficiency Syndrome. Ophthalmology, 100:1689–1694, 1993.

Fraunfelder, F.T.: Drug-Induced Ocular Side Effects and Drug Interactions. 4th Ed. Philadelphia, Williams & Wilkins, 1996.

Pau, H.: Differential Diagnosis of Eye Diseases. 2nd Ed. New York, Thieme Med. Pub., 1988.

Von Noorden, G.K.: Amblyopia Caused by Unilateral Atropinization. Ophthalmology, 88:131, 1981.

Walsh, F.B., and Hoyt, W.F.: Clinical Neuro-ophthalmology. Vol. 1. 4th Ed. Baltimore, Williams & Wilkins, 1985.

Bilateral Blurring of Vision

1. Drug-induced (see paresis of accommodation p. 467)

2. Intracranial hypertension and advanced papilledema (see p. 653)

*3. Migraine—attacks last 15 to 20 minutes

4. Narcolepsy

5. Refractive error (myopia, hyperopia, presbyopia)

6. Retinal "black-out" experienced by pilots

7. Severe systemic hypertension

8. Systemic hypotension

9. Vertebrobasilar insufficiency

Norman, M.E., and Dyer, J.A.: Ophthalmic manifestations of narcolepsy. Am. J. Ophthalmol., 103:81–86, 1987.

Wylie, E.J., and Ehrenfeld, W.K.: Extracranial Occlusive Cerebrovascular Disease: Diagnosis and Management. Philadelphia, W.B. Saunders, 1970.

* = most important

Cortical Blindness

	Trauma (Subdural Hematoma)	Space-occupying Lesions (Occipital Tumors)	Inflammatory Lesions as Meningitis	Vascular Lesion (Subarachnoid Hemorrhage)	Drugs (Alcohol [Methanol])	Degenerative Condition (Renal Failure)
History						
1. Accidental ingestion					U	
2. Diplopia	S	S	S		U	
3. Formed hallucinations		S		R		
4. Head injury	U			S		
5. Photophobia			U	U		
6. Photopsia			U			
7. Systemic bacterial infection			U			
8. Systemic hypertension				S		U
9. Unformed hallucination		U				
10. Usually in elderly persons		U				
Physical Findings						
1. Blepharoptosis				S		
2. Cataract						S
3. Choroidal ischemic infarcts						S
4. Conjunctivitis			U			
5. Cotton-wool spots						U
6. Exophthalmos				S		
7. Failing visual acuity		U			U	
8. Fixed dilated pupil	U			S		
9. Glaucoma						S
10. Keratitis			U			
11. Lid edema						U
12. Macular edema			S			
13. Miosis			S			
14. Nonrhegmatogenous retinal detachment						S
15. Nystagmus			S		U	
16. Oculomotor paralysis				S		
17. Optic nerve atrophy			U		U	
18. Optic neuritis			S			
19. Panophthalmitis			S			
20. Papilledema	U	U	S	U	U	U
21. Paralysis of sixth cranial nerve	S		S			
22. Paresis of seventh cranial nerve			S			
23. Retinal edema						U
24. Retinal hemorrhage	S			U		U
25. Subhyaloid hemorrhage						
26. Unilateral central retinal vein occlusion					U	S
27. Uveitis			U			

Cortical Blindness *Continued*

	Trauma (Subdural Hematoma)	Space-occupying Lesions (Occipital Tumors)	Inflammatory Lesions as Meningitis	Vascular Lesion (Subarachnoid Hemorrhage)	Drugs (Alcohol [Methanol])	Degenerative Condition (Renal Failure)
Laboratory Data						
1. Cerebral angiography	U	U	S	U		
2. Cerebrospinal fluid abnormal			U	U		
3. Computed tomographic scan of head	U	U		U		
4. Electroencephalogram	R					
5. Pneumoencephalogram	S					
6. Proteinuria/hematuria						U
7. Red blood cell count, white blood cell count, hemoglobin, hematocrit			U		U	
8. Serum blood-urea nitrogen, creatinine potassium, phosphate, sulfate increased						U
9. Serum sodium, calcium CO_2, decreased						U
10. Skull roentgenogram	S	S	S			
11. Subdural tap—children	U					

R = rarely; S = sometimes; and U = usually.

Cortical Blindness (Cerebral Blindness) (Complete Loss of All Visual Sensation, Including All Appreciation of Light and Dark—Loss of Reflex Lid Closure to Bright Illumination and to Threatening Gestures; Retention of Pupil Constriction to Light and Accommodation; Normal Ophthalmoscopic Examination; Normal Motility; May Be Associated with Hemiplegia, Sensory Disorders, Aphasia and Disorientation)

1. Degenerative conditions
    A. Alper progressive gray matter
    B. Cerebral dysgenesis associated with dementia
    C. Creutzfeldt-Jakob disease (corticostrialtospinal degeneration)
    D. Cytomegalic inclusion disease (rare)
    E. Galactosemia
    F. Hodgkin disease
    G. Infantile neuroaxonal dystrophy
    H. Krabbe syndrome
    I. Phenylpyruvic oligophrenia
    J. Pompe disease (generalized glycogenesis)
    K. Porencephaly
    L. Renal failure
    M. Schilder disease (encephalitis periaxialis diffusa)
    N. Scholz subacute cerebral sclerosis
    O. Spongy degeneration of the brain
    P. Subacute sclerosing panencephalitis
    Q. Tay-Sachs disease (familial amaurotic idiocy)
    R. Toxoplasmosis (rare)

2. Drugs including:

alcohol	ketamine(?)	sulfamerazine
bendroflumethiazide(?)	lead poisoning	sulfameter
benzthiazide(?)	meglumine	sulfamethazine
carbon dioxide	methadone	sulfamethizole
carbon monoxide	methyclothiazide(?)	sulfamethoxazole
chloroform(?)	methylergonovine(?)	sulfamethoxypyridazine
chlorothiazide	metolazone(?)	sulfanilamide
corticotropin	metrizamide	sulfaphenazole
chlorthalidone	nifedipine	sulfapyridine
cisplatin	nitroglycerin	sulfasalazine
cyclosporin	nitrous oxide(?)	sulfathiazole
cyclothiazide(?)	polythiazide(?)	sulfisoxazole
ether(?),	quinethazone	tansy poisoning
FK506	sulfacetamide	thiopental(?)
hexamethonium chloride	sulfachlorpyridazine	trichlormethiazide(?)
hydrochlorothiazide(?)	sulfacytine	vinblastine
hydroflumethiazide(?)	sulfadiazine	vincristine
indapamide(?)	sulfadimethoxine	

*3. Inflammatory lesions

    A. Bacterial endocarditis

    B. Encephalitis (including that due to measles and pertussis) and subacute sclerosing panencephalitis

    C. Influenza

    D. Meningococcal meningitis

    E. Mumps

    F. Pneumococcal meningitis

    G. Syphilitic meningitis

4. Space-taking lesions, such as tumors, gummas, abscesses, and cysts

*5. Trauma

    A. Birth trauma including heart dysfunction, postictal, and vertebral artery injury

    B. Chiropractic manipulation of the neck and odontotic subluxation

    C. Posthypoxic syndrome

    D. Subdural hematoma with cerebral edema

    E. Occipital region

    F. Ventriculography and ventriculoatrial shunt operation

*6. Vascular lesions

    A. Air embolism

    B. Angioma of occipital region

    C. Angiospastic lesions, including: hypertension, nephritis, eclampsia, uremia, and chronic lead poisoning (saturnism)

    D. Anoxia from chronic respiratory insufficiency

    E. Anoxia from high altitude

    F. Basilar artery thrombosis

    G. Bilateral posterior cerebral artery occlusion

    H. Blood loss syndrome (acute cerebral hypotension)

    I. Blood transfusion reaction

    J. Cardiac arrest

    K. Cerebral hemorrhage

    L. Electroshock

    M. Following burns and sunstroke

    N. Following cardiac, cerebral or vertebral angiography

    O. Hemorrhage in spastic paralysis

    P. Herniation of hippocampal gyrus associated with subdural hematoma

    Q. Hydrocephalus and microcephaly

    R. Malaria

    S. Obstruction of the local venous sinus, such as from septic thrombosis of superior longitudinal sinus

    T. Periarteritis nodosa

* = most important

   U. Subarachnoid hemorrhage
   V. "Subclavian steal syndrome" with reversal of blood flow through the verte-
      bral artery
   W. Thrombotic thrombocytopenic purpura

Fraunfelder, F.T.: Drug-Induced Ocular Side Effects and Drug Interactions. 4th Ed. Philadelphia,
   Williams & Wilkins, 1996.

Lawerence-Friedl, D., and Bauer, K.M.: Bilateral cortical blindness: an unusual presentation of bacterial endocarditis. Annals of Emergency Medicine, 21:1502–1504, 1992.

Rama, B.N., et al.: Cortical blindness after cardiac catheterization: effect of rechallenge with dye.
   Catheterization & Cardiovascular Diagnosis, 28:149–151, 1993.

Roy, F.H.: Ocular Syndromes and Systemic Diseases. 2nd Ed. Philadelphia, W.B. Saunders, 1989.

Shutter, L.S., et al.: Cortical blindness and white matter lesions in a patient receiving FK after liver
   transplantation. Neurology, 43:2417–2418, 1993.

Walsh, F.B., and Hoyt, W.F.: Clinical Neuro-ophthalmology. 4th Ed. Baltimore, Williams & Wilkins,
   1985.

Wong, V.C.: Cortical blindness in children: a study of etiology and prognosis. Pediatric Neurology,
   7:178–185, 1991.

Blindness in Childhood

   1. Cornea
      A. Hereditary dystrophies
      B. Inflammations such as varicella, rubeola, vaccinia, and gonorrhea, ophthalmia
         neonatorum, and pemphigus
      C. Trauma (abrasion or laceration)
   2. Cortical blindness (see p. 704)
   3. Globe
      A. Anophthalmos (see p. 263)
      B. Buphthalmos (see p. 256)
      C. Congenital, primary infantile, or secondary glaucoma (see p. 351)
      D. Hydrophthalmos
      E. Microphthalmos (see p. 253)
   4. Lens
      A. Aphakia
      B. Congenital cataracts (see syndromes associated with cataracts, p. 459)
   5. Optic nerve
      A. Aplasia
      B. Asphyxia at birth
      C. Associated with widespread disease such as mental deficiency, cerebral palsy,
         or epilepsy
      D. Atrophy (hereditary or secondary) (see p. 625)
      E. Cavernous sinus thrombosis (Foix syndrome)
      F. Cerebral hemorrhage (associated with major brain damage from accidental
         trauma, abuse or birth trauma)

G. Crouzon syndrome (craniofacial dysostosis)

H. Hydrocephalus

I. Inflammatory damage—encephalomyelitis, encephalitis, tuberculous

J. Osteopetrosis (Albers-Schönberg syndrome)

K. Subdural hematoma

L. Trauma-fracture at the orbital canal

M. Tumors

6. Psychic blindness

A. Agnosia

B. Alexia

7. Retina

A. Achromatopsia

B. Albinism

C. Coat disease (retinal telangiectasia)

D. Early chorioretinal heredodegenerations, including Stargardt disease and pigmentary retinopathy (see pseudoretinitis pigmentosa, p. 551)

E. Embryopathies, including rubella, toxoplasmosis, and syphilis

F. High myopia

G. Infantile macular degeneration

H. Pseudoretinitis pigmentosa (see p. 551)

I. Reese retinal dysplasia

J. Retinal detachment

K. Retinoblastoma

L. Retinoschisis

M. Retinopathy of prematurity

N. Tapetoretinal degeneration

8. Syndromes associated with amaurosis or blindness

A. Davidoff single ventricle

B. Laurence-Moon-Bardet-Biedl syndrome (retinitis-pigmentosa-polydactyly-adiposogenital syndrome)

C. Malformative syndrome with cryptophthalmos

D. Marfan syndrome (arachnodactyly dystrophia mesodermalis congenita)

E. Metachromatic leukodystrophy (arylsulfatase A deficiency syndrome)

F. Niemann-Pick syndrome (essential lipoid histiocytosis)

G. Sandoff disease

H. Schilder disease (encephalitis periaxialis diffusa)

9. Uveal tract

A. Chorioretinitis

B. Congenital coloboma

C. Iridocyclitis

10. Vitreous

    A. Persistence of primary vitreous

    B. Pseudoglioma

Brownstein, S., et al.: Sandhoff's disease (Gmgangliosidosis type 2). Arch. Ophthalmol., 98:1089, 1980.

Fraser, G.R., and Friedmann, A.I.: The Causes of Blindness in Childhood. Baltimore, Johns Hopkins Press, 1968.

Nickel, B.L., and Hoyt, C.S.: Leber's congenital amaurosis. Arch. Ophthalmol., 100:1089, 1982.

Pau, H.: Differential Diagnosis of Eye Diseases. 2nd Ed. New York, Thieme Med. Pub., 1988.

Binocular Diplopia (Double Vision Using Both Eyes)

1. Intractable postoperative diplopia

    A. Anomalous retinal correspondence with or without amblyopia (common), which is called paradoxical diplopia

    B. Cyclotropia due to oblique muscle operation

    C. Following surgical treatment of retinal detachment because of symblepharon or limitation of extraocular movement

    D. "Horror fusionis" (rare)—congenital or developmental deficiency of fusion, i.e., absence of sensory correspondence between two eyes (not the same as abnormal retinal correspondence, because visual directions are normal in these cases)

    E. Large surgical overcorrection

2. Other

    A. Aniseikonia

    B. Heterophoria—due to lesions such as orbital tumor and cellulitis

    C. Narcolepsy

    D. Physiologic diplopia

    E. Psychogenic causes

3. Paralysis of one or more extraocular muscles

    A. Fourth-nerve palsy (rare) (see p. 183)

   *B. Sixth-nerve palsy—has no localizing value (see p. 186)

    C. Third-nerve palsy—with isolated muscle paralysis one must suspect a nuclear lesion (hemorrhage, syphilis, multiple sclerosis) or myasthenia gravis (see p. 176)

Norman, M.E., and Dyer, J.A.: Ophthalmic manifestations of narcolepsy. Am. J. Ophthalmol., 103:81–86, 1987.

Norton, E.W.D.: Complications of retinal detachment surgery. Symposium on Retina and Retinal Surgery. Transactions of New Orleans Academy Ophthalmology. St. Louis, C.V. Mosby, 1969.

Binocular Triplopia (Uniocular Diplopia)

1. Abnormal retinal correspondence with single image given two associations of direction, so that the abnormal retinal point is brought into consciousness at the same time as the macula image

2. Central uniocular diplopia (rare)—systemic or neurologic causes include: cerebral aneurysm, abscess or gross degenerative lesions, encephalitis lethargica, postencephalitis, multiple sclerosis, basal meningitis, cerebellar tumor, and vertebrobasilar insufficiency

*3. Malingering, hysteria, or psychogenic causes

4. Optical causes external to the eye
   A. Double or single prism placed in center of pupil before one eye
   *B. Improper correction of a high astigmatism
   *C. Looking through the edge of a bifocal or margin of lens

5. Optical causes in the eye
   A. Air bubbles or transparent foreign bodies in aqueous or vitreous
   B. Complete or partial contraction of the eyelids, in which the eyelids impinge on the cornea (de Schweintz)
   C. Dislocation of the lens or misalignment of corneal and lenticular optical axis
   D. Double pupil
   E. High myopia, probably because of irregular astigmatism
   F. Irregular astigmatism such as pressure on the globe
   G. Irregular spasm of the ciliary muscle
   H. Keratoconus (see p. 328)
   I. Lens abnormalities such as fluid clefts or incipient cataract
   J. Looking through edge of intraocular lens
   *K. Map-dot-fingerprint dystrophy
   L. Megalocornea (see p. 295)
   M. Migration of filtering bleb into the cornea
   N. Multifocal intraocular lens
   O. Postiridectomy
   *P. Refractive surgery
   Q. Retinal detachment
   R. Spherophakia (see p. 448)

Brems, R.N., et al.: Posterior chamber intraocular lenses in a series of autopsy eyes. J. Cataract Refract. Surg., 12:367–375, 1986.

Coffeen, P., and Guyton, D.L.: Monocular diplopia accompanying ordinary refractive errors. Am. J. Ophthalmol., 105:451–459, 1988.

Ellingson, F.T.: Explanation of 3M diffractive intraocular lenses. J. Cataract Refract. Surg., 16:697–702, 1990.

Girard, L.J.: Monocular diplopia accompanying ordinary refractive errors. Am. J. Ophthalmol., 106:369, 1988.

Rubin, M.L.: The woman who saw too much. Surv. Ophthalmol., 16:382–383, 1972.

Wyzinski, P., and O'Dell, L.: Subjective and objective findings after radial keratotomy. Ophthalmology, 96:1608–1611, 1989.

Diplopia following Head Trauma

1. Avulsion, contusion, or transection of extraocular muscles
2. Avulsion of the pulley of the superior oblique

* = most important

3. Decompensation of a pre-existing ocular phoria, becoming a tropia

4. Edema or detachment of the macula (monocular diplopia)

*5. Hematoma in the orbit and/or the ocular muscles

*6. Orbital fracture (particularly blow-out fracture of the floor, causing restricted function of inferior rectus and inferior oblique muscles)

7. Subluxation of the lens (monocular diplopia)

8. Third, fourth, and/or sixth cranial nerve palsies (orbital or intracranial) (see p. 176, 181, or 184)

9. "Whiplash" injury and the diplopias of obscure origin

Deutsch, T.A., and Feller, D.B.: Paton's and Goldberg's Management of Ocular Injuries. Philadelphia, W.B. Saunders, 1985.

Eccentric Vision (Vision Is Best When the Individual Is Not Looking Directly at Object of Regard)

1. Central scotoma

2. Craniopharyngioma

3. Eccentric fixation with amblyopia

4. Ectopic macula such as macula displaced by retinal scarring or fibrous strands, often a result of retinopathy of prematurity

5. Glaucoma—late with only eccentric field remaining

6. Homonymous hemianopia with macular involvement (see p. 680)

*7. Macular scar such as with age related macular degeneration.

Beyer-Machule, C., and Noorden, G.K., von: Atlas of Ophthalmic Surg. Vol. 1: Lids, Orbits, Extraocular Muscles. New York, Thieme Med. Pub., 1984.

Huber, A.: Eye Signs and Symptoms in Brain Tumors. 3rd Ed. St. Louis, C.V. Mosby, 1976.

Decreased Dark Adaptation (Nyctalopia; Night Blindness)

1. Choroideremia

2. Congenital night blindness

*3. May be due to drugs, including:

alcohol	etretinate	methysergide
amodiaquine	hashish	oxygen
carbon dioxide	hydroxychloroquine	pilocarpine
chloroquine	indomethacin(?)	psilocybin
colloidal silver	isotretinoin	silver nitrate
deferoxamine	lysergide	silver protein
dronabinol	marihuana	tetrahydrocannabinol
ergonovine	mescaline	vinblastine
ergotamine	methylergonovine	vincristine

4. Progressive cone rod dystrophy

5. Refsum syndrome (heredopathia atactica polyneuritiformis syndrome)

6. Retinitis pigmentosa (see p. 551)

Fraunfelder, F.T.: Drug-Induced Ocular Side Effects and Drug Interactions. 4th Ed. Philadelphia, Williams & Wilkins, 1996.

Tasman, W., and Jaeger, E., eds: Duane's Clinical Ophthalmology. Philadelphia, J.B. Lippincott, 1990.

Astigmatism—Refractive Power of Eye Varies Along Different Meridians; Steepest Meridian Is Vertical in "with the Rule" (Corrected with Plus Cylinder at Ninety Degrees) and Horizontal in "against the Rule"

  1. Adnexal masses

  2. Anterior segment surgery for cornea, lens or glaucoma

 *3. Chalazion

 *4. Contact lens wear

 *5. Corneal scars

 *6. Following refractive surgery

  7. Keratoconus (see p. 328)

  8. May be dominant inheritance with incomplete penetrance

  9. Nuclear cataract with coloboma of lens, iris, and choroid

10. Oversized, rigid, anterior chamber, intraocular lens implant

11. Physiologic—about 0.5 diopters of "with the rule"

12. Retinal detachment procedures

13. Tilted intraocular lens

Abdel-Hakim, A.S.: Corneal astigmatism induced by oversized rigid anterior chamber implants. Am. Intra. Implant. Soc. J., 11:474–482, 1985.

Binder, P.S.: Optical problems following refractive surgery. Ophthalmology, 93:739–745, 1986.

Bogan, S., et al.: Astigmatism associated with adnexal masses in infancy. Arch. Ophthalmol., 105:1368–1370, 1987.

Deg, J.K., et al.: Delayed corneal wound healing following radial keratotomy. Ophthalmology, 92:734–740, 1985.

Bouzas, A.G.: Anterior Polar Congenital Cataract and Corneal Astigmatism. J. Pediatr. Ophthalmol. Strabismus, 29:210–212, 1993.

Fraunfelder, F.T., and Roy, F.H.: Current Ocular Therapy. 4th Ed. Philadelphia, W.B. Saunders, 1995.

Lakshminarayananm, V., et al.: Refractive changes induced by intraocular lens tilt and longitudinal displacement. Arch. Ophthalmol., 104:90–92, 1986.

Vaughn, L.W., and Schepens, C.L.: Progressive lenticular astigmatism associated with nuclear sclerosis and coloboma of the iris, lens, and choroid. Ann. Ophthalmol., 13:25, 1981.

Visual Allesthesia—Displacement of Image to Opposite Half of Visual Field

  1. Parieto-occipital lobe disease

     A. Neoplasm

     B. Vascular insufficiency

     C. Trauma

     D. Seizure activity

  2. Occipital lobe disease

     A. Neoplasm

* = most important

    B. Vascular insufficiency

    C. Trauma

    D. Seizure activity

Bowen, S.F.: Visual disorientation in allesthesia and palinopsia. J.A.M.A., 239:56, 1978.

Jacobs, L.: Visual allesthesia. Neurology, 30:1059, 1980.

Gaze-evoked Amaurosis (Transient Monocular Loss of Vision Occurring in a Particular Direction of Eccentric Gaze)

   *1. Bone fragment adjacent to optic nerve following orbital fracture

   *2. Central retinal artery occlusion

    3. Optic nerve sheath meningiomas

    4. Orbital cavernous hemangiomas

    5. Orbital osteoma

Hampton, G.R., and Krohel, G.B.: Gaze-evoked blindness. Ann. Ophthalmol., 15:73–76, 1983.

Orcutt, J.C., et al.: Gaze-evoked amaurosis. Ophthalmology, 94:213–218, 1987.

Knapp, M.E., et al.: Gaze-induced amaurosis from central artery compression. Ophthalmology, 99:238–240, 1992.

Visual Acuity Loss after Glaucoma Surgery

    1. Cystoid macular edema

   *2. Hypotony maculopathy

    3. IOP spike

   *4. Lens opacification

    5. Postoperative capsule opacity

    6. Retinal detachment

    7. Suprachoroidal hemorrhage

    8. Unknown

    9. Vitreous hemorrhage

   10. Wipe-out (loss of central fixation)

Costa, V.P., et al.: Loss of Visual Acuity after Trabeculectomy. Ophthalmology, 100:599–612, 1993.

Cristiansson, J.: Ocular Hypotony after fistulizing Glaucoma Surgery. Acta Ophthalmol., 45:837–45, 1967.

Watson, R.G., et al.: The Complications of Trabeculectomy (a year follow-up). Eye, 4: 425–438, 1990.

Sudden Painful Loss of Vision

    1. Acute-angle closure glaucoma

    2. Fracture of the lesser wing of the sphenoid bone

    3. Keratoconus

    4. Optic neuritis

    5. Temporal arteritis

    6. Uveitis

Friedberg, M.A., and Rapuano, C.J.: Office and Emergency Room Diagnosis and Treatment of Eye Disease. J.B. Lippincott Co., Philadelphia, 1990.

Sudden Painless Loss of Vision—Both Eyes

1. Brain injury
2. Brain stem arteriovenous malformations
3. Meningeal carcinomatosis
4. Quinine poisoning
5. Wood alcohol poisoning (methyl)

Friedberg, M.A., and Rapuano, C.J.: Office and Emergency Room Diagnosis and Treatment of Eye Disease. J.B. Lippincott Co., Philadelphia, 1990.

Gradual Painless Loss of Vision

1. Age-related macular degeneration
2. Cataract
3. Chronic corneal disease
4. Diabetic retinopathy
5. Glaucoma, open angle
6. Optic neuropathy/atrophy
7. Refractive error
8. Retinal disease, chronic

Friedberg, M.A., and Rapuano, C.J.: Office and Emergency Room Diagnosis and Treatment of Eye Disease. J.B. Lippincott Co., Philadelphia, 1990.

* = most important

Visual Complaint

KRISTIN TARBET, M.D.

Contents

Photopsia (Scintillations, Sparks or Flashes of Light before the Eyes)

1. Associated with arteriovenous aneurysm
2. Auditory-visual synesthetic phenomena-optic nerve lesion; usually demyelinative
3. Brain concussion
4. Clomiphene citrate (Clomid)
5. Focal lesions of occipital region

6. Glaucoma

7. Idiopathic thrombocytosis

8. Impending retinal detachment

*9. Migraine and epilepsy

10. Moore lightning streak—traction of a partially liquefied vitreous on the retina

11. Oculodigital phenomenon (entopic phenomenon)

12. Paraneoplastic retinopathy

13. Phosphene of quick eye motion (Flick phosphene)

14. Retinal microembolization

15. Retinitis

16. Vertebral basilar insufficiency

Morse, P.H., et al.: Light flashes as a clue to retinal disease. Arch. Ophthalmol., 91:179–180, 1974.

Pau, H.: Differential Diagnosis of Eye Diseases. 2nd ed. New York, Thieme Med. Pub., 1988.

Roy, F.H.: Ocular Autostimulation. Am. J. Ophthalmol., 63:1776, 1967.

Walsh, F.B., and Hoyt, W.F.: Clinical Neuro-ophthalmology. 4th ed. Baltimore, Williams & Wilkins, 1985.

Hallucinations (Formed Images)

1. Blind persons (central or peripheral visual field loss)

2. Bilateral eye covering—such as may be required after an eye operation, especially in elderly patients

3. Ocular lesions as retinal hemorrhage, glaucoma, optic atrophy of tertiary syphilis and choroidal neovascularization.

4. Psychoses

5. Central nervous system lesions

   A. Alzheimer disease

   B. Diffuse irritative lesion of parietotemporal area including: uncinate seizures of the temporal lobe, stimulation of superior colliculus, and optic radiation

   C. Encephalitis

   D. Hippocampus lesions

   E. Hypophyseal duct tumors

   F. Measles

   G. Medulloblastoma

   H. Myxedema

   I. Narcolepsy

   J. Occipital lobe seizures—moving lights and colors, visual and complex hallucinations with formed images

   K. Papilledema (see p. 651)

   L. Peduncular hallucinations with midbrain lesions from vascular, encephalitic, and mass lesions

   M. Pellagra

* = most important

N. Pituitary and optic chiasmal lesion

O. Vertebrobasilar insufficiency/basilar artery migraine

6. Chronic mountain sickness (Monge syndrome)

7. Malignant melanoma

8. Poisonings such as mushroom, psilocin, cannabis, hashish, hemp, camphor, mescaline from peyote, myristica (nutmeg), gasoline, mullet (Hawaiian fish), and ololiuqui (morning glory seeds)

9. Drugs including:

acebutolol

acetaminophen

acetanilid

acetophenazine

acid bismuth sodium tartrate

acyclovir

adrenal cortex injection

albuterol

alcohol

aldosterone

allobarbital

alprazolam

amantadine

amitriptyline

amobarbital

amodiaquine

amoxapine

amphetamine

amyl nitrite

antazoline

aprobarbital

aspirin

atenolol

atropine

azatadine

baclofen

barbital

belladonna

bendroflumethiazide

benzathine penicillin G

benzphetamine

benztropine

betamethasone

betaxolol

biperiden

bismuth oxychloride

bismuth sodium tartrate

bismuth sodium thioglycollate

bismuth sodium triglycollamate

bismuth subcarbonate

bismuth subsalicylate

bromide

brompheniramine

butabarbital

butalbital

butallylonal

butaperazine

butethal

calcitriol

capreomycin

captopril

carbamazepine

carbinoxamine

carbon dioxide

carphenazine

cefaclor

cefadroxil

cefamandole

cefazolin

cefonicid

cefoperazone

ceforanide

cefotaxime

cefotetan

cefoxitin

cefsulodin

ceftazidime

ceftizoxime

ceftriaxone

cefuroxime

cephalexin

cephaloglycin

cephaloridine

cephalothin

cephapirin

cephradine

chloral hydrate

chlorambucil

chlordiazepoxide

chloroquine

chlorpheniramine

chlorphenoxamine

chlorpromazine

chlortetracycline

chlorthalidone

cholecalciferol

cimetidine

clemastine

clomipramine

clonazepam

clonidine

clorazepate

cocaine

codeine

cortisone

cyclizine

cyclobarbital

cyclopentobarbital

cyclopentolate

cycloserine

cyclosporine

cyclothiazide

cycrimine

cyproheptadine

dantrolene

dapsone

demeclocycline

desipramine

desoxycorticosterone

dexamethasone

dexbrompheniramine

dexchlorpheniramine

dextroamphetamine

dextrothyroxine

diazepam

diethazine

diethylpropion

digitalis

digoxin

diltiazem

dimethindene

diphenhydramine

diphenylhydantoin

diphenylpyraline

disopyridamide

disulfiram

ditran

divalproex sodium

doxepin

doxycycline

dronabinol

droperidol

enalapril

ephedrine

ergocalciferol

ethchlorvynol

ethionamide

ethopropazinc

ethosuximide

fenfluramine

flecainide

fludrocortisone

fluphenazine

fluprednisolone

flurazepam

furosemide

gentamicin

glutethimide

glycerin

griseofulvin

halazepam

haloperidol

hashish

heptabarbital

hexethal

hexobarbital

homatropine

hydrabamine penicillin V

penicillin

hydrochlorothiazide

hydrocortisone

hydroflumethiazide

hydroxychloroquine

hydroxyurea

ibuprofen

imipramine

indapamide

indomethacin

interferon

iodide and iodine solutions and compounds

isoniazid

isosorbide

ketamine

ketoprofen

labetalol

levallorphan

levobunolol

levodopa

levothyroxine

lidocaine

liothyronine

liotrix

lithium carbonate

lorazepam

lysergide

mannitol

maprotiline

marihuana

meclizine

meperidine

mephentermine

mephobarbital

meprednisone

mescaline

mesoridazine

methacycline

methamphetamine

methaqualone

metharbital

methdilazine

methitural

methohexital

methotrimeprazine

methscopolamine

methsuximide

methyclothiazide

methyldopa

methylpentynol

methylphenidate

methylprednisolone

methyprylon

methysergide

metolazone

metoprolol

metrizamide

metronidazole

mexiletine

mianserin

midazolam

minocycline

morphine(?)

moxalactam

nadolol

nalidixic acid

nalorphine

naloxone

naltrexone

neostigmine

nialamide

nifedipine

nitrazepam

nitrofurantoin(?)

nitroglycerin(?)

nortriptyline

opium(?)

orphenadrine

oxazepam

oxprenolol

oxyphenbutazone

oxytetracycline

paraldehyde

paramethasone

pargyline

pemoline

penicillin

pentazocine

pentobarbital

pentylenetetrazol

perazine

perhexiline(?)

pericyazine

perphenazine

phenacetin

phencyclidine

phendimetrazine

phenelzine

pheniramine

phenobarbital

phensuximide

phentermine

phenoxymethyl

phenylbutazone

phenylephrine

phenylpropanolamine

phenytoin

pimozide

pindolol

piperacetazine

piperazine

piroxicam

polythiazide

potassium penicillin G

potassium penicillin V

phenoxymethyl penicillin

practolol

prazepam

prazosin

prednisolone

prednisone

primidone

probarbital

procaine penicillin G

prochlorperazine

procyclidine

promazine

promethazine

propiomazine

propoxyphene

propranolol

protriptyline

psilocybin

pyrilamine

quinacrine

quinethazone

quinidine

quinine

radioactive iodides

ranitidine

scopolamine

secobarbital

sodium salicylate

sulfacetamide

sulfachlorpyridazine

sulfacytine

sulfadiazine

sulfadimethoxine

sulfamerazine

sulfameter

sulfamethazine

sulfamethizole

sulfamethoxazole

sulfamethoxypyridazine

sulfanilamide

sulfaphenazole

sulfapyridine

sulfasalazine

sulfisoxazole

sulfathiazole

sulindac(?)

talbutal

temazepam

tetanus immune globulin

tetanus toxoid

tetracycline

tetrahydrocannabinol

thiabendazole

thiamylal

thiethylperazine

thiopental	triflupromazine
thiopropazate	trihexyphenidyl
thioproperazine	trimeprazine
thioridazine	trimipramine
thyroglobulin	tripelennamine
thyroid	triprolidine
timolol	tropicamide
tobramycin	urea
tocainide	valproate sodium
trazodone	valproic acid
triamcinolone	verapamil
triazolam	vidarabine
trichlormethiazide	vinbarbital
trichloroethylene	vinblastine
trifluoperazine	vincristine
trifluperidol	vitamin D

10. Exercise-induced with occipital lobe tumor

11. Patients in seclusion

Fisher, C.M.: Visual hallucinations, atropine toxicity. Am. J. Ophthalmol., 112:368, 1991.

Fraunfelder, F.T.: Drug-Induced Ocular Side Effects and Drug Interactions. 4th Ed. Philadelphia, Williams & Wilkins, 1996.

Gittinger, J.W., et al.: Sugarplum fairies. Visual hallucinations. Surv. Ophthalmol., 27:42, 1982.

Glaser, J.S.: Neuro-Ophthalmology. 2nd ed. Philadelphia, J.B. Lippincott Co., 1989.

Lerner, A.J., et al.: Concomitants of visual hallucinations in Alzheimer's disease. Neurology, 44:523–527, 1994.

Lessell, S., and Kylstra, J.: Exercise-induced visual hallucination: a symptom of occipital lobe tumors. J. Clin. Neuro-ophthalmol., 8:81–84, 1988.

Loewenstein, J.I.: Visual hallucinations in patients with choroidal neovascularization. J.A.M.A., 272:243, 1994.

Norman, M.E., and Dyer, J.A.: Ophthalmic manifestations of narcolepsy. Am. J. Ophthalmol., 103:81–86, 1987.

"Spots" before Eyes (Dots or Filaments that Move with Movement of Eye)

*1. Vitreous opacities—muscae volitantes; associated with preretinal hemorrhage, myopia, posterior vitreous detachment or intraocular inflammations

2. Scotomatous defects

    A. Retinal lesions

    B. Myopia

3. Corneal foreign-body reflection/corneal opacity

4. Carbon tetrachloride poisoning

5. Migraine

Grant, W.M.: Toxicology of the Eye. 2nd ed. Springfield, Ill., Charles C Thomas, 1974.

Vaughan, D., et al.: General Ophthalmology. 14th ed. Norwalk, Conn., Appleton & Lange, 1995.

Colored Halos around Lights (Blue and Violet Are Next to the Stimulating Light and Red Outermost)

1. Glaucoma
    A. Acute-angle closure with stretching of corneal lamellae
    B. Open-angle glaucoma—halo noted on awakening (intraocular pressure is highest in the morning)
2. Mucus on the cornea
3. Corneal scar/corneal edema
4. Krukenberg spindle
5. Lens opacities
6. Vitreous opacities (see p. 480)
7. Any haze of ocular media
8. Drugs probably affecting corneal epithelium including:

acetophenazine	digitalis	methotrimeprazine	promethazine
acetyldigitoxin	digitoxin	methylprednisolone	propiomazine
amiodarone	digoxin	nitroglycerin	quinacrine
amodiaquine	ethopropazine	nitronaphthalene	thiethylperazine
amyl nitrite	ethylene diamine	oral contraceptives	thiopropazate
butaperazine	fluorometholone	ouabain	thioproperazine
carphenazine	fluphenazine	paramethadione	thioridazine
chloroquine	gitalin	perazine	trifluoperazine
chlorine dioxide	hydrocortisone	pericyazine	triflupromazine
chlorpromazine	hydroxychloroquine	perphenazine	trimeprazine
cortisone	lanatoside C	piperacetazine	trimethadione
deslanoside	medrysone	prednisolone	sterile water
dexamethasone	mesoridazine	prochlorperazine	
diethazine	methdilazine	promazine	

9. Physiologic halos—most common when lens acts as diffracting gradient
10. Too intense exposure to light as in snow blindness
11. Asymmetric placement of the intraocular lens in relation to the pupillary aperture

Brems, R.N., et al.: Posterior chamber intraocular lenses in a series of autopsy eyes. J. Cataract Refract. Surg., 12:367–375, 1986.

Fraunfelder, F.T.: Drug-Induced Ocular Side Effects and Drug Interactions. 4th Ed. Philadelphia, Williams & Wilkins. 1996.

Grant, W.M.: Toxicology of the Eye. 2nd Ed. Springfield, Ill., Charles C Thomas, 1974.

Kolker, A.E., and Hetherington, J.: Becker-Shaffer's Diagnosis and Therapy of the Glaucomas. 5th ed. St. Louis, C.V. Mosby, 1983.

Moses, R.A.: Adler's Physiology of the Eye: Clinical Application. 7th ed. St. Louis, C.V. Mosby, 1980.

Light Streaks

1. Cataracts
2. Contact lenses

* = most important

3. Excessive tear meniscus

4. Intraocular lens scratches

5. Lashes

*6. Migraine

7. Posterior capsules—lens fibers and debris-filled corrugations

8. Rapid eye movements (especially in a dark environment)

9. Reflection off edge of intraocular lens

10. Reflection off manipulation holes of intraocular lens

*11. Retinal break/tear or detachment

12. Spectacles

13. Windshields, windows

Holladay, J.T., et al.: Diagnosis and treatment of mysterious light streaks seen by patients following extracapsular cataract extraction. Am. Intra. Implant. Soc. J., 11:21–23, 1985.

Holladay, J.T., et al.: The optimal size of a posterior capsulotomy. Am. Intra. Implant. Soc. J., 11:18–20, 1985.

Photophobia (Painful Intolerance of the Eyes to Light)

1. Aniridia

*2. Ocular, including: conjunctivitis, keratitis, iritis, iridocyclitis, uveitis, and corneal, lenticular, and vitreous opacities, Angelucci syndrome (critical allergic conjunctivitis), acute hemorrhagic conjunctiva, and cone dysfunction syndrome

3. Albinism

4. Total color blindness (achromatopsia)

5. Patients with corneal lesions having diseases characterized by photosensitization (xeroderma pigmentosa, hydroa vacciniforme, and smallpox)

6. Systemic diseases, including botulism, cystinosis, erythropoietic porphyria, hypoparathyroidism, rabies, psittacosis, and schistosomiasis

7. Toxic causes, including mercury poisoning

8. Drugs including:

acetohexamide	belladonna	clidinium
acetophenazine	bendroflumethiazide	clomiphene
adiphenine	benzthiazide	deferoxamine
allobarbital	bromide	demeclocycline
ambutonium	brompheniramine	desipramine
amiodarone	butaperazine	dextrothyroxine
amitriptyline	captopril(?)	diazepam(?)
amobarbital	carbon dioxide	dicyclomine
amodiaquine	carphenazine	diethazine
anisotropine	chloroquine	digitalis
atropine	chlorpromazine	digitoxin
auranofin	chlorpropamide	dimethyl sulfoxide
aurothioglucose	chlortetracycline	diphemanil
aurothioglycanide	cimetidine	dipivefrin

disopyramide
doxepin
doxycycline
edrophonium
enalapril
ethambutol
ethionamide
ethopropazine
ethosuximide
ethotoin
fluphenazine
furosemide(?)
glyburide
glycopyrrolate
gold Au 198
gold sodium thiomalate
gold sodium thiosulfate
hexethal
hexobarbital
hexocyclium
homatropine
hydroxychloroquine
ibuprofen
imipramine
indomethacin
isoniazid
isocarboxazid
isopropamide
levarterenol
levothyroxine
liothyronine
liotrix
mepenzolate
mephenytoin
mesoridazine
methacycline

methantheline
methdilazine
methixene
methotrimeprazine
methoxsalen
methsuximide
methyl alcohol
methylatropine nitrate
methyldopa
metoclopramide
metrizamide
metronidazole
minocycline
nalidixic acid
nialamide
norepinephrine
nortriptyline
oral contraceptives
oxyphenbutazone
oxyphencyclimine
oxyphenonium
oxytetracycline
paramethadione
perazine
pericyazine
perphenazine
phenelzine
phensuximide
phenylbutazone
pipenzolate
piperacetazine
piperidolate
poldine
practolol
procarbazine
prochlorperazine

promazine
promethazine
propantheline
propiomazine
protriptyline
quinacrine
quinidine
quinine
rabies immune globulin
rabies vaccine
streptomycin
tetanus immune globulin
tetanus toxoid
tetracycline
thiethylperazine
thiopropazate
thioproperazine
thioridazine
thyroglobulin thyroid
tolazamide
tolbutamide
tranylcypromine
trichlorethylene
tridihexethyl
trifluoperazine
triflupromazine
trimeprazine
trimethadione
trioxsalen
tripelennamine
vancomycin
vinbarbital
vinblastine
vincristine

9. Normal ocular findings with photophobia

    A. Trigeminal neuralgia (Charlin syndrome)

    B. Migraine

    C. Neurasthenia

    D. Meningitis

    E. Subarachnoid hemorrhage

    F. Acromegaly

* = most important

    G. Associated with hypophyseal tumor, and craniopharyngioma

    H. During and following retrobulbar neuritis

    I. Acrodynia (Feer syndrome)

    J. Following severe head injury

    K. Hypoparathyroidism

    L. Lesions of gasserian ganglion

    M. Tumors of ophthalmic branch of the trigeminal nerve, such as neuroma, middle fossa tumor, and posterior fossa tumor, such as meningioma or acoustic neuroma

    N. Increased intracranial pressure, including subdural hematomas

10. Acrodermatitis chronica atrophicans

11. Avitaminosis B (pellagra)

12. Chediak-Higashi syndrome (anomalous leukocytic inclusions with constitutional stigmata)

13. Danbolt-Closs syndrome (acrodermatitis enteropathica)

14. Elschnig syndrome (meibomian conjunctivitis)

15. Feer syndrome (acrodynia)

16. Folling syndrome (phenylketonuria)

17. Following refractive surgery

18. Gradenigo syndrome (temporal syndrome)

19. Hanhart syndrome (pseudoherpetic keratitis)

20. Hartnup syndrome (niacin deficiency)

21. Hysteria

22. Infantile globoid cell leukodystrophy (Krabbe disease)

23. Keratodermia palmaris et plantaris

24. Photosensitivity and sunburn

25. Reiter syndrome (polyarthritis enterica)

Binder, P.S.: Optical problems following refractive surgery. Ophthalmology, 98:739–745, 1986.

Fraunfelder, F.T.: Drug-Induced Ocular Side Effects and Drug Interactions. 4th ed. Philadelphia, Williams & Wilkins, 1996.

Pau, H.: Differential Diagnosis of Eye Diseases. 2nd ed. New York, Thieme Med. Pub., 1988.

Roy, F.H.: Ocular Syndromes and Systemic Diseases. 2nd ed. Philadelphia, W.B. Saunders, 1989.

Walsh, F.B., and Hoyt, W.F.: Clinical Neuro-ophthalmology. 4th ed. Baltimore, Williams & Wilkins, 1985.

Asthenopia (Uncomfortable Ocular Sensation or Eye Ache)

1. Dazzling from bright light

2. Episcleritis or scleritis

3. Glaucoma

4. Iritis or iridocyclitis

5. Neurasthenia or hysteria

6. Passive congestion

7. Phoria or tropia

8. Retrobulbar neuritis

9. Sinus disease

10. Spasm from muscles held too long in a restricted position

11. Subclinical open angle glaucoma

12. Uncorrected refractive errors, especially hyperopia or astigmatism

13. Unknown

14. Use of miotics

15. Weak accommodation

Otto, J.: Asthenopia and wide-angle glaucoma. Glaucoma, 8:75–77, 1986.

Pau, H.: Differential Diagnosis of Eye Diseases. 2nd ed. New York, Thieme Med. Pub., 1988.

Dazzling or Glare Discomfort

1. Altered pupillary response

2. Asymmetric placement of the intraocular lens in relation to the pupillary aperture

3. Corneal scars or foreign bodies

4. Drugs, such as chloroquine, acetazolamide, or trimethadione (Tridione)

5. Emotional disorders

6. Following refractive surgery

7. Idiopathic

8. Lenticular changes

Brems, R.N., et al.: Posterior chamber intraocular lenses in a series of autopsy eyes. J. Cataract Refract. Surg., 12:367–375, 1986.

Deg, J.K., et al.: Delayed corneal wound healing following radial keratotomy. Ophthalmology, 92:734–740, 1985.

Vaughan, D., et al.: General Ophthalmology. 12th Ed. Norwalk, Conn., Appleton & Lange, 1989.

Chromatopsia (Colored Vision, Objects Are Abnormally Colored)

1. Blue color (cyanopsia)

    A. Drugs, including:

acetyldigitoxin	deslanoside	hydroxyampheta-mine	nalidixic acid
alcohol	digitalis		oral contraceptives
amodiaquine	digitoxin	hydroxychloroquine	ouabain
amphetamine	digoxin	lanatoside C	quinacrine
chloroquine	gitalin	methylene blue	

    B. Pseudophakia

    C. Optic atrophy of tertiary syphilis

2. Red color (erythropsia)

    A. Drugs, including:

acetyldigitoxin	belladonna	digitalis
atropine	deslanoside	digitoxin

digoxin
ergonovine
ergotamine
gitalin
homatropine
lanatoside C
methylergonovine
methysergide
ouabain
quinine

sulfacetamide
sulfachlorpyridazine
sulfadiazine
sulfacytine
sulfadimethoxine
sulfamerazine
sulfameter
sulfamethazine
sulfamethizole
sulfamethoxazole

sulfamethoxypyridazine
sulfanilamide
sulfaphenazole
sulfapyridine
sulfasalazine
sulfathiazole
sulfisoxazole
sulthiame

    B. Hysteria

    C. Optic atrophy of tertiary syphilis

    D. Vitreous or retinal hemorrhage (see pp. or 527)

    E. Pseudophakia and aphakia

    F. Snow blindness or blindness following electric shock

    G. After working with green monochrome video display terminals

    H. Welding arc maculopathy

3. Yellow color (Xanthopsia)

    A. Drugs, including:

acetaminophen
acetanilid
acetophenazine
acetyldigitoxin
allobarbital
alseroxylon
amobarbital amodiaquine
amyl nitrite
aprobarbital
aspirin
barbital
bendroflumethiazide
benzthiazide
butabarbital
butalbital
butallylonal
butaperazine
butethal
carbachol(?)
carbon dioxide
carphenazine
chloramphenicol
chloroquine

chlorothiazide
chlorpromazine
chlortetracycline
chlorthalidone
cimetidine(?)
colloidal silver
cyclobarbital
cyclopentobarbital
cyclothiazide
deserpidine
deslanoside
diethazine
digitalis
digitoxin
digoxin
ethopropazine
fluorescein
fluphenazine
gitalin
hashish
heptabarbital
hexethal
hexobarbital

hydrochlorothiazide
hydroflumethiazide
hydroxychloroquine
lanatoside C
marijuana
mephobarbital
mesoridazine
methaqualone
metharbital methazolamide
methdilazine
methitural
methohexital
methotrimeprazine
methyclothiazide
metolazone
mild silver protein
nalidixic acid
nitrofurantoin(?)
ouabain
pentobarbital
pentylenetetrazol
perazine
pericyazine

perphenazine

phenacetin

phenobarbital

piperacetazine

polythiazide

primidone

probarbital

prochlorperazine

promazine

promethazine

propiomazine

quinacrine

quinethazone

rauwolfia serpentina

rescinnamine

reserpine

secobarbital

silver nitrate

silver protein

sodium salicylate

streptomycin

sulfacetamide

sulfachlorpyridazine

sulfacytine

sulfadiazine

sulfadimethoxine

sulfamerazine

sulfameter

sulfamethazine

sulfamethizole

sulfamethoxazole

sulfamethoxypyridazine

sulfanilamide

sulfaphenazole

sulfapyridine

sulfasalazine

sulfathiazole

sulfisoxazole

syrosingopine

talbutal

tetrahydrocannabinol

THC

thiabendazole

thiamylal

thiethylperazine

thiopental

thiopropazate

thioproperazine

thioridazine

trichlormethiazide

trifluoperazine

triflupromazine

trimeprazine

vinbarbital

vitamin A

   B. Lenticular change

   C. Aphakia

   D. Poisons, including: aconite, dichloro-diphenyl trichloroethane, carbon disulfide, chromic acid, methyl salicylate, aspidium (Felix mas,) santontomin, picric acid

   E. Jaundice

   F. Hysteria

4. Green color (Chloropsia)

   A. Drugs, including:

acetyldigitoxin

allobarbital

amobarbital

amodiaquine

aprobarbital

barbital

butabarbital

butalbital

butallylonal

butethal

chloroquine

cyclobarbital

cyclopentobarbital

deslanoside

digitalis

digitoxin

digoxin

epinephrine

gitalin

griseofulvin

heptabarbital

hexethal

hexobarbital

hydroxychloroquine

iodide and iodine solutions and compounds

lanatoside C

mephobarbital

metharbital

methitural
methohexital
nalidixic acid
ouabain
pentobarbital
phenobarbital
primidone
probarbital

quinacrine
quinine
radioactive iodides
secobarbital
talbutal
thiamylal
thiopental
vinbarbital

   B. Poisons such as santonin

5. Violet color (ianthinopsia)

   A. Drugs, including:

dronabinol
hashish

marijuana
nalidixic acid

quinacrine
tetrahydrocannabinol

   B. Pseudophakia and aphakia

   C. Intracameral air

6. Brown color

   A. Drugs including:

acetophenazine
butaperazine
carphenazine
chlorpromazine
diethazine
ethopropazine
fluphenazine
mesoridazine
methdilazine

methotrimeprazine
perazine
pericyazine
perphenazine
piperacetazine
prochlorperazine
promazine
promethazine
propiomazine

thiethylperazine
thiopropazate
thioproperazine
thioridazine
trifluoperazine
triflupromazine
trimeprazine

   B. Lenticular change

7. White color

   A. Drugs including:

capreomycin
diphenylhydantoin

paramethadione trimethadione

   B. Pseudophakia and aphakia

Fraunfelder, F.T.: Drug-Induced Ocular Side Effects and Drug Interactions. 4th Ed. Philadelphia, Williams & Wilkins, 1996.

Keane, J.R., and Talalla, A.: Post-traumatic intracavernous aneurysms. Arch. Ophthalmol., 87:701–705, 1972.

Uniat, L., et al.: Welding arc maculopathy. Am. J. Ophthalmol., 102:394–395, 1986.

Walraven, J.: Prolonged complementary chromatopsia in users of video display terminals. Am. J. Ophthalmol., 100:350–351, 1985.

Walsh, F.B., and Hoyt, W.F.: Clinical Neuro-ophthalmology. Vol. 1. 4th Ed. Baltimore, Williams & Wilkins, 1985.

Heightened Color Perception

1. Heightened color perception is due to drugs, including:

dronabinol	lysergide	oxygen
ethionamide	marijuana	psilocybin
hashish	mescaline	tetrahydrocannabinol

Fraunfelder, F.T.: Drug-Induced Ocular Side Effects and Drug Interactions. 4th Ed. Philadelphia, Williams & Wilkins, 1996.

Nyctalopia (Night Blindness)

1. Anemia
2. Carbon monoxide poisoning
3. Congenital high myopia
4. Diffuse opacities of media including corneal edema, keratitis and nuclear cataract
5. Following refractive surgery
6. Glaucoma—especially open-angle and angle-closure glaucoma
7. Paraneoplastic retinopathy
8. Psychologic causes—malingering or psychoses
9. Optic atrophy
10. Refsum syndrome (phytanic acid oxidase deficiency)
11. Tapetoretinal degenerations

    A. Choroideremia

    B. Congenital night blindness

        (1) Dominant form

        (2) Recessive form

        (3) Recessive, sex-linked

    C. Detachment of retina including malignant melanoma

    D. Drugs, including:

acetophenazine	hydroxychloroquine	piperacetazine	thioproperazine
amodiaquine	indomethacin	prochlorperazine	thioridazine
butaperazine	mesoridazine	promazine	trifluoperazine
carphenazine	methdilazine	promethazine	triflupromazine
chloroquine	methotrimeprazine	propiomazine	trimeprazine
chlorpromazine	paramethadione	quinidine	trimethadione
diethazine	perazine	quinine	
ethopropazine	pericyazine	thiethylperazine	
fluphenazine	perphenazine	thiopropazate	

    E Drusen (familial)—minimal

    F. Fleck retina—nonprogressive, congenital, rare

    G. Fundus flavimaculatus—minimal

    H. General choroidal sclerosis

    I. Gyrate atrophy

    J. Retinitis pigmentosa

    K. Retinitis punctata albescens

    L. Miner nystagmus

    M. Oguchi disease—may be abnormal

12. Visual field defects

13. Vitamin A deficiency

    A. Dietary deficiencies, including malnutrition and cystic fibrosis

    B. Digestive tract disturbance

        (1) Colitis and enteritis

        (2) Crohn' disease

        (3) Jejunoileal bypass surgery

        (4) In pancreas—such as chronic pancreatitis

        (5) In stomach—achlorhydria, chronic gastritis or diarrhea, peptic ulcer

    C. Liver disease such as chronic cirrhosis

    D. Malaria

    E. Pregnancy

    F. Pulmonary tuberculosis

    G. Skin disorders such as pityriasis rubra pilaris

    H. Thyroid gland disorders such as hyperthyroidism

14. Vitreous opacities including hemorrhage

15. Vitreotapetoretinal degeneration—sex-linked recessive and autosomal recessive

Berson, E.L., and Lessell, S.: Paraneoplastic night blindness with malignant melanoma. Am. J. Ophthalmol., 106:307–311, 1988.

Brown, G.C., et al.: Reversible night blindness associated with intestinal bypass surgery. Am. J. Ophthalmol., 89:776–779, 1980.

Deg, J.K., et al.: Delayed corneal wound healing following radial keratotomy. Ophthalmology, 92:734–740, 1985.

Fraunfelder, F.T.: Drug-Induced Ocular Side Effects and Drug Interactions. 4th Ed. Philadelphia, Williams & Wilkins, 1996.

Gans, M., and Taylor, C.: Reversal of progressive nyctalopia in a patient with Crohn' disease. Canadian J. Ophthal., 25:156–158, 1990.

Merin, S., et al.: Syndrome of congenital high myopia with nyctalopia. Am. J. Ophthalmol., 70:541–547, 1970.

Pau, H.: Differential Diagnosis of Eye Diseases. 2nd Ed. New York, Thieme Med. Pub., 1988.

Hemeralopia (Day Blindness—Inability to See as Distinctly in a Bright Light as in a Dim One)

1. Adie pupil

2. Albinism

3. Aniridia

4. Central opacities of the lens—nuclear or perinuclear cataracts

5. Central scotoma

6. Congenital—autosomal recessive trait usually associated with amblyopia and color deficiency

7. Hereditary retinoschisis

8. Intraocular iron

9. Partial occlusion of the central retinal artery (see p. 512)

10. Refsum syndrome (phytanic acid oxidase deficiency)

11. Total color blindness

Gehrs, K., and Tiedeman, J.: Hemeralopia in an older adult. Survey Ophthal., 37:185–189, 1992.

MacVicar, J.E., and Wilbrandt, H.R.: Hereditary retinoschisis and early hemeralopia. Arch. Ophthalmol., 83:629–636, 1970.

Pau, H.: Differential Diagnosis of Eye Diseases. 2nd Ed. New York, Thieme Med. Pub., 1988.

Oscillopsia (Illusionary Movement of Environment; May Be Unilateral or Bilateral; Usually Because of Acquired Nystagmus)

1. Drugs, including:

2. Fixation and voluntary nystagmus

alcohol	butethal	hexobarbital	probarbital
allobarbital	carbamazepine	mephobarbital	secobarbital
amobarbital	cyclobarbital	metharbital	talbutal
aprobarbital	cyclopentobarbital	methitural	thiamylal
barbital	diphenylhydantoin	methohexital	thiopental
butabarbital	gentamicin	pentobarbital	vinbarbital
butalbital	heptabarbital	phenobarbital	
butallylonal	hexethal	primidone	

3. Defective vestibulo-ocular reflex/vestibular pathway lesion occurs during movement of the head or body

    A. Sectioning of vestibular (VIII) nerve for vertigo

    B. Streptomycin toxicity

    C. Spontaneous loss

4. Head trauma/seizures

5. Intermittent exotropia

6. Involvement of medial longitudinal fasciculus affecting ipsilateral medial rectus in internuclear ophthalmoplegia—monocular oscillopsia

7. Myokymia of the eyelid

8. Opsoclonus and ocular flutter

9. Vertebral artery dissection

Chrousos, G.A., et al.: Two cases of downbeat nystagmus and oscillopsia associated with carbamazepine. Am. J. Ophthalmol., 103:221–224, 1987.

Demer, J.L.: Evaluation of vestibular and visual oculomotor function. Otolary. Head Neck Surg., 112:16–35, 1995.

Fraunfelder, F.T.: Drug-Induced Ocular Side Effects and Drug Interactions. 4th Ed. Philadelphia, Williams & Wilkins, 1996.

Gendeh, B.S., et al: Gentamicin ototoxicity in continuous ambulatory peritoneal dialysis. J. Laryngol. Otol., 107:681–685, 1993.

Glaser, J.S.: Neuro-Ophthalmology. 2nd Ed. Philadelphia, J.B. Lippincott Co., 1989.

Hicks, P.A., et al.: Ophthalmic manifestation of vertebral artery dissection. Patients seen at Mayo clinic from 1976–1992. Ophthal., 101:1786–1792, 1994.

Reinecke, R.D.: Translated myokymia of the lower eyelid causing uniocular vertical pseudonystagmus. Am. J. Ophthalmol., 75:150–151, 1973.

Color Blindness

1. Inherited—stable defect, affecting both eyes

    A. Bassen-Kornzweig syndrome (abetalipoproteinemia)

    B. Congenital dyslexia syndrome (developmental dyslexia syndrome)

    C. Down syndrome (mongolism)

    D. Duane retraction syndrome (Stilling syndrome)

    E. Duchenne muscular dystrophy

    F. Glucose-6-phosphate dehydrogenase deficiency (glycogen storage disease type I)

    G. Guillain-Barré syndrome (acute infectious neuritis)

    H. Hemophilia

    I. "Intrinsic" defect

        (1) Dichromat—two colors mixed to see white

            a. Deuteranope—green deficiency

            b. Protanope—red deficiency

            c. Tritanope—blue deficiency

        (2) Monochromat—one color mixed to see white

            a. Cone deficient

            b. Rod deficient

        (3) Trichromat—three colors mixed to see white

            a. Deuteranomaly—green anomaly

            b. Protanomaly—red anomaly

            c. Tritanomaly—blue anomaly

    J. Kallman syndrome (hypogonadotrophic hypogonadism-anosmia syndrome)

    K. Klinefelter syndrome (XXY) (gynecomastia-aspermatogenesis syndrome)

    L. Turner syndrome (XO) (gonadal dysgenesis)

2. Acquired—defect can increase or decrease; may affect only one eye; impairment of other visual function; often characterized by chromatopsia; hue discrimination primarily affected; yellow-blue defects more common in retinal disease; red-green defects in optic nerve disease

    A. Advanced hypertensive retinopathy

    B. Albinism

    C. Amblyopia

    D. Blue-yellow defect with retinal disorders from drugs, including:

acetophenazine	amodiaquine	benztropine(?)	butaperazine
amiodarone(?)	azathioprine	biperiden(?)	carbamazepine

carphenazine	diethazine	mitotane	quinacrine(?)
cephaloridine(?)	diethylcarbamazine	naproxen(?)	quinine
chloramphenicol	ethambutol	penicillamine	sulindac(?)
chloroquine	ethopropazine	perazine	tamoxifen
chlorphenoxamine(?)	fluphenazine	pericyazine	thiethylperazine
chlorpromazine	hydroxychloroquine	perphenazine	thiopropazate
chlorprothixene	indomethacin(?)	piperacetazine	thioproperazine
cisplatin	ketoprofen(?)	prazosin(?)	thioridazine
clofazimine	mesoridazine	prochlorperazine	thiothixene
clonidine(?)	methdilazine	procyclidine(?)	trifluoperazine
cobalt(?)	methotrexate	promazine	triflupromazine
cycrimine(?)	methotrimeprazine	promethazine	trihexyphenidyl(?)
deferoxamine	minoxidil(?)	propiomazine	trimeprazine

E. Chorioretinitis

F. Color anomia—inability to name colors; may be associated with homonymous hemianopia due to infarct of posterior parietal and corpus callosum

G. Diabetic retinitis

H. Dominantly inherited juvenile optic atrophy

I. Drugs and chemical substances causing optic neuropathy with red-green defect, including:

acetophenazine	butallylonal
alcohol	butaperazine
allobarbital	butethal
alseroxylon(?)	calcitriol
aminosalicylate(?)	carbromal
aminosalicylic acid(?)	carphenazine
amobarbital	chloramphenicol
amodiaquine	chloroprocaine(?)
antimony lithium thiomalate	chloroquine
antimony potassium tartrate	chlorpromazine
antimony sodium tartrate	cholecalciferol
antimony sodium thioglycollate	clindamycin
antipyrine	cobalt(?)
aprobarbital	cortisone
aspirin	cyclobarbital
barbital	cyclopentobarbital
betamethasone	cycloserine(?)
bromide(?)	dapsone
bromisovalum	deferoxamine
broxyquinoline	deserpidine(?)
bupivacaine(?)	dexamethasone
butabarbital	dextrothyroxine(?)
butalbital	diethazine

ergocalciferol
ergonovine(?)
ergot(?)
ergotamine(?)
ethambutol
ethopropazine
etidocaine(?)
ferrocholinate(?)
ferrous fumarate(?)
ferrous gluconate(?)
ferrous succinate(?)
ferrous sulfate(?)
fluorometholone
fluphenazine
gentamycin
heptabarbital
hexachlorophene
hexamethonium
hexethal
hexobarbital
hydrocortisone
hydroxychloroquine
iodide and iodine solutions and compounds
iodochlorhydroxyquin
iodoquinol
iron dextran(?)
iron sorbitex(?)
isoniazid
levothyroxine(?)
lidocaine(?)
liothyronine(?)
liotrix(?)
medrysone
mephobarbital
mepivacaine(?)
mesoridazine
metharbital
methdilazine
methitural
methohexital
methotrexate(?)
methotrimeprazine
methyl alcohol

methylene blue
methylergonovine
methysergide(?)
nitroglycerin(?)
oxyphenbutazone
pentobarbital
perazine
pericyazine
perphenazine
phenobarbital
phenylbutazone
piperacetazine
polysaccharide-iron complex(?)
prednisolone
prilocaine(?)
primidone
probarbital
procaine(?)
prochlorperazine
promazine
promethazine
propiomazine
propoxycaine(?)
propoxyphene
quinine
radioactive iodides
rauwolfia serpentina(?)
rescinnamine(?)
reserpine(?)
secobarbital
sodium antimonylgluconate
sodium salicylate
stibocaptate
stibogluconate
stibophen
streptomycin
sulfacetamide(?)
sulfachlorpyridazine(?)
sulfacytine(?)
sulfadiazine(?)
sulfadimethoxine(?)
sulfamerazine(?)
sulfameter(?)

sulfamethazine
sulfamethizole(?)
sulfamethoxazole(?)
sulfamethoxypyridazine(?)
sulfanilamide(?)
sulfaphenazole(?)
sulfapyridine(?)
sulfasalazine(?)
sulfathiazole(?)
sulfisoxazole(?)
suramin
syrosingopine(?)
talbutal
thiamylal
thiethylperazine
thiopental

thiopropazate
thioproperazine
thioridazine
thyroglobulin(?)
thyroid(?)
tobramycin
trichloroethylene
trifluoperazine
triflupromazine
trimeprazine
tryparsamide
vinbarbital
vinblastine
vincristine
vitamin A
vitamin D

    J. Friedreich ataxia

    K. Glaucoma, including narrow and open angle

    L. Hepatic cirrhosis

    M. Hysteria

    N. Macular lesions, including juvenile degeneration, senile degeneration dystrophy, and edema

    O. Night blindness

    P. Occlusion of retinal vessels

    Q. Oguchi disease

    R. Open angle glaucoma

    S. Ophthalmologist who use argon blue-green lasers or operating microscopes

    T. Optic atrophy

    U. Optic pathways, including brain tumor

    V. Papillitis

    W. Peripheral chorioretinal degeneration

    X. Retinal detachment

    Y. Retinitis pigmentosa

    Z. Retrobulbar optic neuritis

  AA. Snow blindness

Arden, G.B., et al.: A Survey of Color Discrimination in German Ophthalmologists. Ophthalmology, 98:567–575, 1991.

Fraunfelder, F.T.: Drug-Induced Ocular Side Effects and Drug Interactions. 4th Ed. Philadelphia, Williams & Wilkins, 1996.

Pau, H.: Differential Diagnosis of Eye Diseases. 2nd Ed. New York, Thieme Med. Pub., 1988.

Rothstein, T.B., et al.: Dyschromatopsia with hepatic cirrhosis relation to serum Band folic acid. Am. J. Ophthalmol., 75:889–895, 1973.

Roy, F.H.: Ocular Syndromes and Systemic Diseases. 2nd Ed. Philadelphia, W.B. Saunders, 1989.

Sample, P.A., et al.: Isolating the color vision loss in primary open angle glaucoma. Am. J. Ophthalmol., 106:686–691, 1988.

Walsh, F.B., and Hoyt, W.F.: Clinical Neuro-ophthalmology. Vol. 1. 4th Ed. Baltimore, Williams & Wilkins, 1985.

Palinopsia (Persistence or Recurrence of Visual Images after Exciting Stimulus Object Has Been Removed; Patient Has a Hemianopic Field Defect)

1. Acute migraine

2. Encephalitis

3. Epilepsy

4. Intoxications, such as mescal delirium, LSD, trazodone-induced and clomiphene citrate.

5. Kartagener's syndrome

6. Temporal-parietal-occipital lesion

    A. Degenerative

    B. Neoplastic

    C. Traumatic

    D. Vascular

7. Schizophrenia

Hughes, M.S., and Lessell, S.: Trazodone-induced palinopsia. Arch Ophthal., 108:399–400, 1990.

Kawasaki, A., and Purvin, V.: Persistent palinopsia following ingestion of LSD. Arch. Ophthal., 114:47–50, 1996.

Lunardi, P., et al.: Palinopsia: unusual presenting symptom of a cerebral abscess in a man with Kartagener's syndrome. Clinical Neurology & Neurosurgery, 93:337–339, 1991.

Marneros, A. and Korner, J.: Chronic palinopsia in schizophrenia. Psychopathology, 26:236–239, 1993.

Purvin, V.A.: Visual disturbance secondary to clomiphene citrate. Arch. Ophthal., 113:482–484, 1995.

Vertical Reading (Patient Reads from above Downward)

1. Astigmatism—high error of refraction

2. Homonymous hemianopia (see p. 680)

3. Voluntary as oriental script written vertical

O'Brien, C.S.: Ophthalmology, Notes for Students. Iowa City, Athens Press, 1930.

Visual Agnosia—Failure to Recognize Objects by Sight for Animate and Inanimate Objects but Does Not Interfere with Recognition of Language Symbols

1. Drugs including:

benzathine penicillin G	potassium penicillin V
hydrabamine phenoxymethyl penicillin	potassium phenethicillin
phenoxymethyl penicillin	potassium phenoxymethyl penicillin
potassium penicillin G	procaine penicillin G

2. Kluver-Bucy Syndrome (temporal lobectomy behavior syndrome)

3. Lesion of Brodmann area 18

Fraunfelder, F.T.: Drug-Induced Ocular Side Effects and Drug Interactions. 4th Philadelphia, Williams & Wilkins, 1996.

Hooshmand, H., et al.: Kluver-Bucy Syndrome. J.A.M.A., 229:13, 1974.

Scheie, H.G.: Textbook of Ophthalmology. 10th Ed. Philadelphia, W.B. Saunders, 1986.

Ocular Lateropulsion—Eyes Feel Like They Are Drawn toward One Side, but This Problem Can Be Overcome with Conscious Effect; Full Range of Extraocular Muscle Movements

1. Lateral medullary disease including infarction of lateral medullary plate, acoustic neurinoma, posterior fossa meningioma or multiple sclerosis

2. Peripheral vestibular disease

Meyer, K.T., et al.: Ocular lateropulsion. Arch. Ophthalmol., 98:1614–1616, 1980.

Pain In and About Eye

1. Ocular
   A. Angle closure glaucoma
   B. Chronic ocular hypoxia, carotid occlusive disease
   C. Dry eye and tear deficiency syndrome
   D. Local lid, conjunctival, and anterior segment disease
   E. Ocular inflammation

2. Ophthalmic division
   A. Herpes zoster
   B. Migraine, cluster headache
   C. Painful ophthalmoplegia syndrome
   D. Raeder paratrigeminal neuralgia
   E. Referred (dural) pain, including occipital infarction
   F. Sinusitis
   G. Tic douloureux (infrequent in V-1)

3. Mandibular division
   A. Dental disease
   B. Tic douloureux

4. Maxillary division
   A. Dental disease
   B. Nasopharyngeal carcinoma
   C. Sinusitis
   D. Temporomandibular syndrome
   E. Tic douloureux

5. Miscellaneous
   A. Atypical facial neuralgias
   B. Cranial arteritis

C. Pain with medullary lesions

D. Trigeminal tumors

Glaser, J.S.: Neuro-Ophthalmology. 2nd Ed. Philadelphia, J.B. Lippincott Co., 1989.

Hill, L.M., and Hasting, G.: Carotidynia: a pain syndrome. J. Family Practice, 39:71–75, 1994.

Headache

1. Vascular headache of migraine type

    A. Acephalgic migraine (migraine equivalent)—migraine aura without headache

    B. Classic migraine—migraine with aura

    C. Common migraine—migraine without aura

    D. Complicated migraine—hemiplegic migraine and ophthalmoplegia migraine

    E. Cluster headache

    F. Lower-half headache

2. Muscle contraction headache

3. Combined (skeletal vascular)

4. Headache of nasal vasomotor reaction

5. Headache of delusional, conversion or hypochondriacal states

6. Nonmigrainous vascular headaches

    A. Primary or metastatic tumors of meninges, vessels, or brain

    B. Hematomas (epidural, subdural, or parenchymal)

    C. Abscesses (epidural, subdural, or parenchymal)

    D. Post-lumbar puncture headache (leakage, headache)

    E. Pseudomotor cerebri and various causes of brain swelling

7. Headache due to overt cranial inflammation

    A. Intracranial disorders

        (1) Mass

        (2) Meningitis

        (3) Subarachnoid hemorrhage

    B. Extracranial disorders (temporal arteritis)

8. Headache because of diseases of ocular structures

9. Headache because of diseases of aural structures

10. Headache because of diseases of the nasal and sinus structures

11. Headache because of diseases of dental structures

12. Headache because of diseases of other cranial and neck structures

13. Cranial neuritides

14. Cranial neuralgias

        (1) Glossopharyngeal neuralegia

        (2) Trigeminal neuralgia

15. Analgesic/ergotamine rebound headache

Friedman, A.P., et al.: Classification of headache. Neurology, 12:173, 1962.

Glaser, J.S.: Neuro-Ophthalmology. 2nd Ed. Philadelphia., J.B. Lippincott Co., 1989.

Head Position

EDWARD G. BUCKLEY, M.D.

Contents

Head Turn (Face Turn)

1. Head turned toward right (gaze left)
   A. Left Brown's syndrome
   B. Left inferior oblique muscle palsy
   C. Left medial rectus muscle palsy
   D. Left superior oblique muscle palsy
   E. Right Duane's syndrome
   F. Right jerk nystagmus
   G. Right inferior rectus muscle palsy
   H. Right lateral rectus muscle palsy
   I. Right superior rectus muscle palsy
   J. Right supranuclear gaze paresis
2. Head turned toward left (gaze right)
   A. Left Duane's syndrome
   B. Left jerk nystagmus
   C. Left inferior rectus muscle palsy
   D. Left lateral rectus muscle palsy
   E. Left superior rectus muscle palsy
   F. Left supranuclear gaze paresis
   G. Right Brown's syndrome

      H. Right inferior rectus muscle palsy

      I. Right medial rectus muscle palsy

      J. Right superior oblique muscle palsy

3. Head turned toward either left or right

      A. Congenital jerk nystagmus—head turned away from field with least amplitude of nystagmus (i.e., left jerk nystagmus improves in right gaze; left head turn)

      B. Esotropia—head turned in direction of convergent eye (cross fixation)

      C. Hearing defect

      D. One blind eye—head turn away affected side (good eye fixates in adduction)

      E. Photophobia (see p. 722)

      F. Progressive intracranial arterial occlusion syndrome (Taveras syndrome)

      G. Strabismus fixus (general fibrosis syndrome)

      H. Under corrected myope

Hiatt, R.L., and Cope-Troupe, C.: Abnormal head positions due to ocular problems. Ann. Ophthalmol., 10:881–892, 1978.

Kushner, B.J.: Ocular causes of abnormal head postures. Ophthalmology, 86:2115–2125, 1979.

Walsh, F.B., and Hoyt, W.F.: Clinical Neuro-ophthalmology, 4th Ed. Baltimore, Williams & Wilkins, 1985.

Head Tilt (Head Tilted toward Either Shoulder or around an Anteroposterior Axis)

1. Head tilted toward right

      A. Left superior oblique muscle palsy

      B. Left superior rectus muscle palsy

      C. Right inferior oblique muscle palsy

      D. Right inferior rectus muscle palsy

2. Head tilted toward left

      A. Left inferior oblique muscle palsy

      B. Left inferior rectus muscle palsy

      C. Right superior oblique muscle palsy

      D. Right superior rectus muscle palsy

3. Head tilted toward either right or left

      A. Astigmatism

      B. Blow-out fracture

      C. Incorrectly aligned cylinder axis

      D. Monocular torticollis—patching of eyes does not eliminate problem; roentgenogram may help

        (1) Congenital malformation of fracture of cervical spine or vertebral processes

        (2) Fracture of clavicle

        (3) Functional habit and hysteria

        (4) Pain from infection

          a. Adenitis

          b. Arthritis

        c. Mastoiditis

        d. Synovitis

     (5) Paralysis of absent muscles on opposite side of head tilt

     (6) Sandifer syndrome (hiatus hernia-torticollis syndrome)

     (7) Spasm of sternocleidomastoid or contracture of sternocleidomastoid muscle on side of head tilt

     (8) Vestibular defect

        a. Acoustic neuroma

        b. Labyrinthitis

        c. Otitis media

  E. Nystagmus—turned away from field with least amplitude of nystagmus

  F. Superior oblique tendon sheath syndrome (Brown syndrome)

Hiatt, R.L., and Cope-Troupe, C.: Abnormal head positions due to ocular problems. Ann. Ophthalmol., 10:881–892, 1978.

Kattah, J.C., and Dagi, T.F.: Compensatory head tilt in upbeating nystagmus. J. Clinical Neuro-Ophthal., 10: 27–31, 1990.

Nemet, P., et al.: Pitfall of acquired ocular torticollis. J. Pediatr. Ophthalmol., 17:310, 1980.

Rubin, S.E., et al: Ocular Torticolis. Survey Ophthal., 30:366, 1986.

Chin Elevation

1. Adaptive symptom of contact lens wearer

2. A esotropia with fusion in downward gaze

3. Blow-out fracture of orbit

4. Brown syndrome (superior oblique tendon sheath syndrome)

5. Double elevator palsy

6. General fibrosis syndrome (strabismus fixus)

7. Incomplete bilateral ptosis

8. Inferior oblique muscle palsy

9. Parinaud's syndrome (dorsal midbrain syndrome)

10. Superior rectus muscle palsy

11. Supranuclear lesion (upgaze palsy)

12. Thyroidectomy

13. "V" pattern exotropia with fusion in downward gaze

Beyer-Machule, C., and Noorden, G.K., von: Atlas of Ophthalmic Surgery: Vol. 1: Lids, Orbits, Extraocular Muscles. New York, Thieme Med. Pub., 1984.

Hiatt, R.L., and Cope-Troupe, C.: Abnormal head positions due to ocular problems. Ann. Ophthalmol., 10:881–892, 1978.

Nutt, A.B.: Abnormal Head Posture. Br. Orthop. J., 20:18–28, 1963.

Chin Depression

1. "A" pattern exotropia with fusion in upward gaze (A pattern)

2. Inferior rectus muscle palsy

3. Photophobia

4. Progressive supranuclear palsy

5. Superior oblique muscle palsy (bilateral)

6. Supranuclear lesion (down gaze palsy)

7. Uncorrected myope of low degree

8. "V" pattern esotropia with fusion in upward gaze

Beyer-Machule, C., and Noorden, G.K., von: Atlas of Ophthalmic Surgery: Vol. 1: Lids, Orbits, Extraocular Muscles. New York, Thieme Med. Pub., 1984.

Hiatt, R.L., and Cope-Troupe, C.: Abnormal head positions due to ocular problems. Ann. Ophthalmol., 10:881–892, 1978.

Kushner, B.J.: Ocular causes of abnormal head postures. Ophthalmology, 86:2115–2125, 1979.

Head Nodding

1. Benign or familial tremor

2. Bobble head (doll syndrome)—to-and-fro bobbing of the head and trunk, at 2- to 3-second intervals because of cyst of third ventricle

3. Congenital nystagmus

4. Extrapyramidal dysfunction, such as paralysis agitans (Parkinson syndrome)

5. Habit spasm

6. Spasms nutans

Gottlob, I., et al.: Head nodding is compensatory in spasmus nutans. Ophthal., 99:1024–1031, 1992.

Rubin, S.E., and Slavin, M.L.: Head nodding associated with intermittent esotropia. J. Pediatric Ophthal. & Strabismus, 27:250–251, 1990.

Head Tremor

1. Cerebellar system afflictions (benign essential senile tremor)—most common

2. Extrapyramidal disorder

3. Hereditary postural tremor (familial tremor) 4. Postural tremor

Hughes, A.J., et al.: Paroxysmal dystonic head tumor. Movement Disorders, 6:85–86, 1991.

Klawans, H.L.: Rhythmic head tremor. J.A.M.A., 248:1510, 1982.

Head Thrust

1. oculomotor apraxia-defect or horizontal voluntary movements)

2. Ataxia-telangiectasia syndrome

3. Isolated

4. Male predominance

5. Oral-facial-digital syndrome type II

Isenberg, S.J.: The Eye in Infancy. Chicago, Year Book Medical Publishers, 1989.

Index

Page numbers in italics indicate diagnostic tables and charts.